Principles and Labs
for Fitness and Wellness

EIGHTH EDITION

www.wadsworth.com

wadsworth.com is the World Wide Web site for
Wadsworth and is your direct source to dozens
of online resources.

At *wadsworth.com* you can find out about
supplements, demonstration software, and student
resources. You can also send email to many of our
authors and preview new publications and exciting
new technologies.

wadsworth.com
Changing the way the world learns®

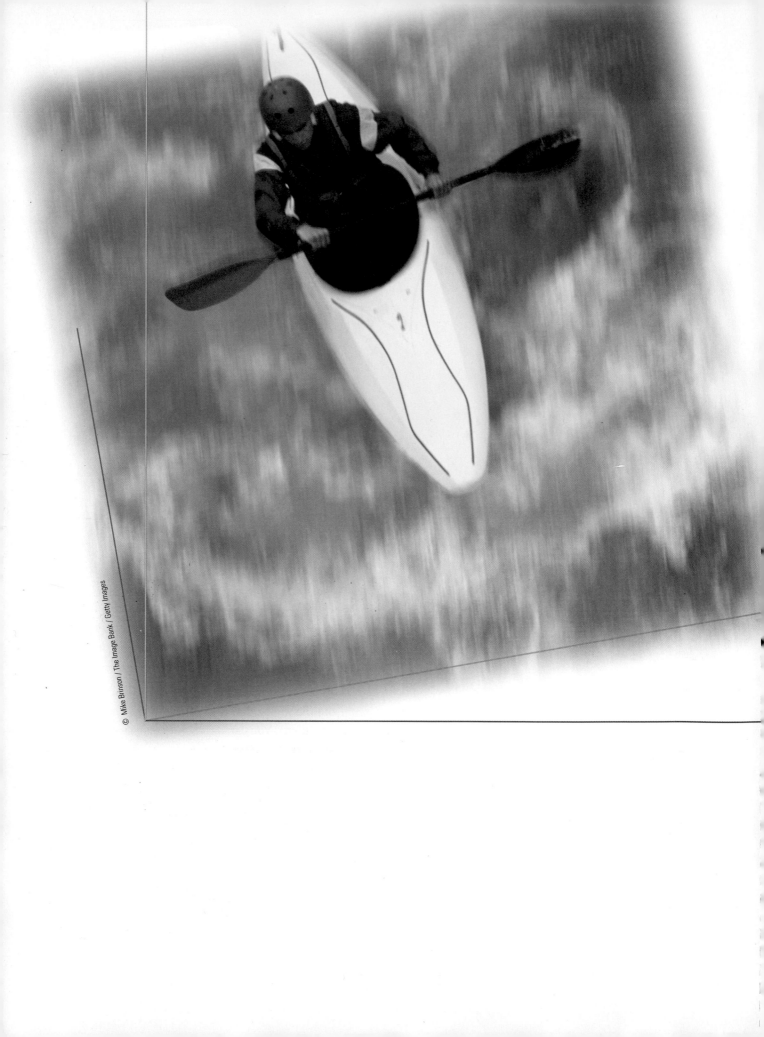

Principles and Labs for Fitness and Wellness

EIGHTH EDITION

Werner W.K. Hoeger Boise State University

Sharon A. Hoeger Fitness & Wellness, Inc.

THOMSON
WADSWORTH

Australia • Canada • Mexico • Singapore • Spain
United Kingdom • United States

THOMSON
WADSWORTH

PRINCIPLES AND LABS FOR FITNESS AND WELLNESS
Eighth Edition
Werner W.K. Hoeger and Sharon A. Hoeger

■ **EXECUTIVE EDITOR:** *Nedah Rose* ■ **ASSISTANT EDITOR:** *Seth Dobrin* ■ **EDITORIAL ASSISTANT:** *Colin Blake*
■ **TECHNOLOGY PROJECT MANAGER:** *Travis Metz* ■ **MARKETING MANAGER:** *Jennifer Somerville* ■ **MARKETING ASSISTANT:** *Michele Colella*
■ **MARKETING COMMUNICATIONS MANAGER:** *Shemika Britt* ■ **PROJECT MANAGER, EDITORIAL PRODUCTION:** *Sandra Craig*
■ **ART DIRECTOR:** *Lee Friedman* ■ **PRINT BUYER:** *Judy Inouye* ■ **PERMISSIONS EDITOR:** *Stephanie Lee*
■ **PRODUCTION AND COMPOSITION:** *Ash Street Typecrafters, Inc.* ■ **TEXT AND COVER DESIGNER:** *Norman Baugher*
■ **PHOTO RESEARCHER:** *Myrna Engler* ■ **COPY EDITOR:** *Carolyn Acheson* ■ **COVER IMAGE:** *Chris Cheadle/Getty Images*
■ **PRINTER:** *Quebecor World / Dubuque*

For more information about our products, contact us at:
Thomson Learning Academic Resource Center
1-800-423-0563
For permission to use material from this text or product, submit a request online at:
http://www.thomsonrights.com
Any additional questions about permissions can be submitted by email to thomsonrights@thomson.com

Library of Congress Control Number: 2004117257

Student Edition: ISBN 0-495-11357-3
Instructor's Edition: ISBN 0-534-60499-4

Thomson Higher Education
10 Davis Drive
Belmont, CA 94002-3098
USA

Asia (including India)
Thomson Learning
5 Shenton Way
#01-01 UIC Building
Singapore 068808

Australia/New Zealand
Thomson Learning Australia
102 Dodds Street
Southbank, Victoria 3006
Australia

Canada
Thomson Nelson
1120 Birchmount Road
Toronto, Ontario M1K 5G4
Canada

UK/Europe/Middle East/Africa
Thomson Learning
High Holborn House
50–51 Bedford Row
London WC1R 4LR
United Kingdom

Latin America
Thomson Learning
Seneca, 53
Colonia Polanco
11560 Mexico
D.F. Mexico

Spain (including Portugal)
Thomson Paraninfo
Calle Magallanes, 25
28015 Madrid, Spain

brief contents

contents

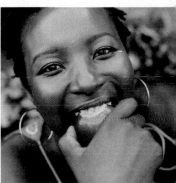

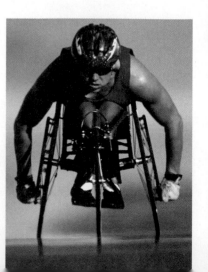

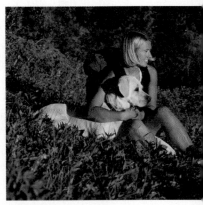

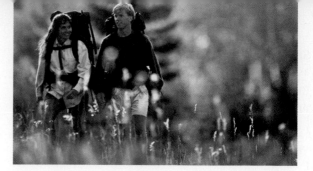

The current North American way of life does not provide the human body with sufficient physical activity to maintain adequate health and improve quality of life. Many present lifestyle patterns are such a serious threat to our health that they actually increase the deterioration rate of the human body and often lead to premature morbidity and mortality.

People who lead an active and healthy lifestyle live longer and enjoy a better quality of life. Most people, however, do not reap the benefit because they are either led astray by a multi-billion dollar "quick fix," fad industry or simply do not know how to develop their own program.

The U.S. Surgeon General has determined that lack of physical activity is detrimental to good health. As a result, the importance of sound fitness programs has assumed an entirely new dimension. The office of the Surgeon General identified physical fitness as a top health priority by stating that: "The nation's top health goals as we begin the new millennium are: exercise, increased consumption of fruits and vegetables, smoking cessation, and the practice of safe sex." All four of these fundamental healthy lifestyle factors are thoroughly addressed in this book.

Principles and Labs for Fitness and Wellness contains 15 chapters and 36 laboratories (labs) that serve as a guide to implement a complete lifetime fitness and wellness program. The book contents point out the need to go beyond the basic components of fitness to achieve total well-being. In addition to a thorough discussion on physical fitness, including all health- and skill-related components, extensive and up-to-date information is provided on behavior modification, nutrition, weight management, stress management, cardiovascular and cancer risk reduction, exercise and aging, prevention of sexually transmitted diseases, and substance abuse control (including tobacco, alcohol, and other psychoactive drugs). Furthermore, the information has been written to provide you with the necessary tools and guidelines for lifetime exercise and a wellness way of life.

As you work through the various chapters and laboratories in the book, you will be able to develop and regularly update your own lifetime program to improve fitness components and personal wellness.

The emphasis throughout the book is on teaching you how to take control of your own personal health and lifestyle habits so that you can make a constant and deliberate effort to stay healthy and achieve the highest potential for well-being.

New and Enhanced Features of the Eighth Edition

The chapters in this edition of *Principles and Labs for Fitness and Wellness* have been revised and updated to include new information reported in literature and at professional health, physical education, and sports medicine meetings. The most significant changes in this new edition are as follows:

■ Chapter 1 was reorganized and updated so that contents flow better. An update on all statistics related to the leading causes of death and the underlying causes of death in the United States, along with new information on chronic lower respiratory diseases, and blood pressure ratings recently released by the National Heart, Lung, and Blood Institute are also included.

■ A section on writing SMART goals has been added to Chapter 2, including a new lab for students to develop two SMART goals and write specific objectives to reach their goals.

■ The contents of Chapter 3, Nutrition for Wellness, have been revised to include the 2005 Dietary Guidelines for Americans, current information on antioxidant nutrients, healthy foods choices, genetically modified crops, and the vegetarian food guide pyramid.

■ The importance of waist circumference to help identify individuals with high abdominal visceral fat and increased risk for disease has been expanded in the body composition chapter. Additional information on overweight and obesity trends in the U.S. during the last four decades is also included.

■ In Chapter 5, Principles of Weight Management, changes include additional information on the health consequences of being overweight or obese; the controversial low carbohydrate/high protein diets; the binge-eating disorder, learning to make healthy food choices; the benefits of dietary calcium on weight management; and the relationship between strength training, diet, and muscle mass. Several behavior modification boxes to clarify misconceptions and help students make healthy-lifestyle decisions were also added throughout the chapter.

■ The concepts of responders, nonresponders, and the principle of individuality have been added to Chapter 8 (cardiorespiratory endurance). The importance of increasing daily physical activity as a means to enhance health and quality of life are also emphasized, including behavior modification techniques to pursue this goal.

■ The discussion on the principle of specificity of training has been expanded in Chapter 7, including the specific adaptation to imposed demand (SAID training) principle. Due to previous users' requests, the normative data for the Muscular Strength and Endurance Test has been reintroduced in this chapter. An introduction to the Pilates exercise system has also been added to the chapter.

■ Several revisions were made to Chapter 8 to incorporate recent developments regarding the benefits of adequate flexibility; the relationship between flexibility and injury prevention; the best time to conduct stretching exercises; and a revision of guidelines for the prevention and treatment of back pain, including the importance of spinal stability exercises, localized muscular endurance, and isometric exercises for back care management.

■ Several questions related to the specific exercise considerations have been updated in Chapter 9, including an expanded discussion on the guidelines for exercise and pregnancy. A new lab on fitness programming case studies has been added to the chapter. This lab allows students to evaluate how well they have learned and are able to apply the concepts of exercise prescription.

■ The characteristics of good stress managers have been added to Chapter 10. An update on the benefits of meditation and yoga on health and wellness are also provided.

■ Statistical updates on the incidence and prevalence of cardiovascular disease and cancer are given in Chapters 11 and 12. Additional information is presented on the coronary heart disease risk factor analysis, C-reactive protein, homocysteine, HDL cholesterol, LDL particles, dietary guidelines to decrease blood lipids, guidelines for the diagnosis of the metabolic syndrome, blood pressure guidelines, sodium and potassium recommendation to manage or prevent high blood pressure, exercise recommendations for hypertensive individuals, and cancer prevention guidelines.

■ In Chapters 13 and 14, the incidence and prevalence of substance abuse and sexually transmitted diseases have been brought up to date according to the latest data available from the Centers for Disease Control and Prevention.

■ Chapter 15 includes updates on the sections on complementary and alternative medicine; quackery and fraud; personal trainers; reliable sources of health, fitness, nutrition, and wellness information; and reliable health web sites. The information on writing objectives under Tips for Behavioral Change in the previous edition of the book has been moved to the section on SMART Goals in Chapter 2.

■ New photography and graphs have been added throughout the book.

Ancillaries

■ **INSTRUCTOR'S MANUAL AND TEST BANK.** The Instructor's Manual and Test Bank helps instructors plan and coordinate their lectures by offering detailed outlines of each chapter with specific transparency and PowerPoint® references. A lab list accompanies Instructor's Activities for each chapter. These activities offer instructors ideas for incorporating the material into classroom activities and discussions. A full test bank containing approximately 50 questions per chapter is also provided.

■ **TRANSPARENCIES.** Approximately 100 color transparency acetates of charts, tables, and illustrations from the text can be used to enhance lectures.

■ **PROFILE PLUS® 2006.** This interactive CD-ROM includes chapter objectives, Assess Your Knowledge questions from the book, practice quizzes, digital video clips demonstrating the different assessment exercises used to generate a personalized fitness and wellness program, and more. In addition to fitness and wellness self-assessments, students can analyze their diets and keep an exercises log to determine their own health status. Profile Plus is packaged FREE with every copy of *Principles and Labs for Fitness and Wellness.*

■ **DIET ANALYSIS PLUS 7.0.** This interactive nutrition-learning tool allows students to create personal profiles and determine the nutritional value of their diet. The program calculates nutrition intakes, goal percentages, and actual percentages of nutrients, vitamins, and minerals, customized according to the student's profile. The information is displayed in colorful, easy-to-read graphs, charts, and spreadsheets.

■ **TESTWELL.** This online assessment tool allows students to complete a 100-question wellness inventory related to the dimensions of wellness. Students can evaluate their nutrition, emotional health, spirituality, sexuality, physical health, self-care, safety, environmental health, occupational health, and intellectual health.

■ **EXAMVIEW®.** Computerized testing. Create, deliver, and customize tests and study guides (both print and online) in minutes with this easy-to-use assessment and tutorial system. ExamView offers a Quick Test Wizard that guides you step-by-step through the process of creating tests, while it allows you to see the test you are creating on the screen exactly as it will print or display online.

■ **MULTIMEDIA MANAGER FOR PRINCIPLES AND LABS SERIES.** This teaching tool contains a lecture presentation tool that features more than 100 PowerPoint slides, including a text outline and resources including the Instructor's Manual and Test Bank. All on one convenient CD-ROM!

■ **CNN TODAY: FITNESS AND WELLNESS.** Enhance your lectures with riveting footage from CNN, the world's leading 24-hour global news network. The CNN Today: Fitness and Wellness video allows you to integrate the news gathering and programming power of CNN into the classroom to show students the relevance of course topics to their everyday lives. The clips are organized by topics introduced in the text and are presented in 2–5 minute segments.

■ **FITNESS AND WELLNESS LECTURE LAUNCHER VIDEO.** Organized by text topics and presented in 2–5 minute segments, this video brings riveting course-related news clips into the classroom.

■ **WADSWORTH VIDEO LIBRARY FOR FITNESS, WELLNESS, AND PERSONAL HEALTH.** This comprehensive library of videos includes such topics as weight control and fitness, AIDS, sexual communication, peer pressure, compulsive and addictive behaviors, and the relationship between alcohol and violence. Available to qualified adopters. Please consult your local sales representative for details.

■ **PERSONAL DAILY LOG.** This log contains an exercise pyramid, ethnic food pyramid, time management strategies and goal setting worksheets, cardiorespiratory exercise record forms, strength training forms, and much more.

■ **HEALTH AND FITNESS & WELLNESS INTERNET EXPLORER.** This handy full-color trifold brochure contains dozens of useful health, fitness, and wellness Internet links.

■ **TRIGGER VIDEO SERIES.** Exclusive to Thomson/ Wadsworth! These videos are designed to promote classroom discussion on a variety of important topics related to physical fitness and stress. Each 60-minute video contains five 8–10 minute clips, followed by questions for answer or discussion and material appropriate to the chapters in Hoeger and Hoeger's text. Available to qualified adopters. Please consult your local sales representative for details.

■ **INFOTRAC® COLLEGE EDITION.** This extensive online library gives professors and students access to the latest news and research articles online—updated daily and spanning 20 years. Conveniently accessible from students' own computers or the campus library, Infotrac College Edition opens the door to the full extent of articles from hundreds of scholarly and popular journals and publications.

■ **THE THOMSON/WADSWORTH HEALTH, HUMAN PERFORMANCE, & PHYSICAL EDUCATION RESOURCE CENTER:** http://health.wadsworth.com. When you adopt *Principles and Labs for Fitness and Wellness*, you and your students will have access to a rich array of teaching and learning resources you won't find anywhere else. This outstanding site features both student and instructor resources for the text, including self-quizzes, Web links, suggested online readings, and discussion forums for students—as well as downloadable supplementary resources, PowerPoint® presentations and more for instructors.

■ **THOMSON LEARNING WEBTUTOR™.** Available on WebCT and Blackboard, this content-rich, Web-based teaching and learning tool is rich with study and mastery tools, communication tools, and course content. WebTutor is filled with preloaded content and is ready to use as soon as you and your students log on. At the same time, you can customize the content in any way you choose, from uploading images and other resources, to adding Web links, to creating your own practice materials.

■ **BEHAVIOR CHANGE WORKBOOK.** This workbook includes a brief discussion of the current theories about making positive lifestyle changes, plus exercises to help students make those changes.

brief author biographies

WERNER W.K. HOEGER is the most successful Fitness and Wellness college textbook author. Dr. Hoeger is a Full Professor and Director of the Human Performance Laboratory at Boise State University. He completed his undergraduate and Master's degrees in physical education at the age of 20 and received his Doctorate degree with an emphasis in exercise physiology at the age of 24. Dr. Werner Hoeger is a fellow of the American College of Sports Medicine. In 2002, he was recognized as the Honored Alumnus from the College of Health and Human Performance at Brigham Young University. He is also the recipient of the first (2004) Presidential Award for Research and Scholarship in the College of Education at Boise State University.

Dr. Hoeger uses his knowledge and personal experiences to write engaging, informative books that thoroughly address today's fitness and wellness issues in a format accessible to students. He has written several textbooks for Thomson/Wadsworth, including *Lifetime Physical Fitness and Wellness*, eighth edition; *Fitness and Wellness*, sixth edition, *Principles and Labs for Physical Fitness*, fifth edition; *Wellness: Guidelines for a Healthy Lifestyle*, fourth edition; and *Water Aerobics for Fitness and Wellness*, third edition (with Terry-Ann Spitzer Gibson).

He was the first author to write a college fitness textbook that incorporated the "wellness" concept. In 1986, with the release of the first edition of *Lifetime Physical Fitness and Wellness*, he introduced the principle that to truly improve fitness, health, quality of life, and achieve wellness, a person needed to go beyond the basic health-related components of physical fitness. His work was so well received that almost every fitness author immediately followed his lead in the field.

As an innovator in the field, Dr. Hoeger has developed many fitness and wellness assessment tools; including fitness tests such as the modified sit-and-reach, total body rotation, shoulder rotation, muscular endurance, and muscular strength and endurance, and "soda pop" coordination tests. Proving that he "practices what he preaches," at 48, he was the oldest male competitor in the 2002 Winter Olympics in Salt Lake City, Utah. He raced in the sport of luge along with his 17-year-old son Christopher. This was the first time in Winter Olympics history that father and son competed in the same event.

SHARON A. HOEGER Sharon A. Hoeger is vice-president of Fitness & Wellness, Inc. of Boise, Idaho. Sharon received her degree in computer science from Brigham Young University. She is the author of the software that accompanies all of their fitness and wellness textbooks. Her innovations in this area since the publication of the first edition of *Lifetime Physical Fitness & Wellness* set the standard for fitness and wellness computer software used in this market today.

Sharon is a coauthor in five of the seven fitness and wellness titles. Husband and wife have been jogging and strength training together for over 28 years. They are the proud parents of five children, all of whom are involved in sports and lifetime fitness activities. Their motto: "Families that exercise together, stay together."

Acknowledgments

Many individuals unselfishly contributed to the creation of this eighth edition of *Principles and Labs for Fitness and Wellness*. In particular we would like to express our most sincere gratitude to:

■ Teachers, students, researchers, coaches, and friends who have shared their expertise, time, talents, and energy with us.

■ Colleagues throughout the U.S. and Canada who evaluated this and previous editions of *Principles and Labs for Fitness and Wellness*. Their feedback and input greatly enhanced the preparation of this edition:

Helaine Alessio, Miami University
Helaine Cigal, John Jay College of Criminal Justice
Dale DeVoe, Colorado State University
Kevin Harper, University of Texas
Lance Lamport, St. Petersburg College
Julie A. Lombardi, Millersville University
Pamela Meyers, Kennesaw State University
Vincent E. Mumford, University of Central Florida
Willie J. Warren, Miami Dade Community College—Mitchell Wolfson Campus
Paul A. Smith, McMurry University

■ Joanne Saliger, Patricia Govro, and Elaine McFarlane for their unwavering commitment to the production of the most remarkable books in the field.

■ Carolyn Acheson for exceptional editing.

■ Nedah Rose, Jennifer Somerville, Sandra Craig, and Jean Thompson for their valuable input and patience in the development, production, and marketing of this edition.

■ John Kelly, Lynda Johnson, Ryan Johnson, Jim Moore, Morgan Turner, and Julianne Hoeger; all of whom contributed to the new photography in this eighth edition.

Chapter 1

Physical Fitness and Wellness

Objectives

- Define physical fitness and list health-related and skill-related components.
- Explain the differences between physical fitness and wellness.
- Define wellness and list its dimensions.
- Distinguish between health fitness standards and physical fitness standards.
- Identify the major health problems in the United States.
- Understand the benefits and significance of participating in a lifetime fitness and wellness program.
- Identify risk factors that may interfere with safe participation in exercise.
- Learn to assess resting heart rate and blood pressure.

Profile Plus CD Connections

- Chronicle your daily activities using the exercise log.
- Determine your heart rate and blood pressure.
- Check how well you understand the chapter's concepts.

© Dan Cutrona

Widespread interest in **health** and preventive medicine over the last three decades has led to an increase in the number of people participating in organized fitness and wellness programs. From an initial fitness fad in the early 1970s, physical activity and wellness programs became a trend that now is very much a part of the North American way of life. The growing number of participants is attributed primarily to scientific evidence linking regular physical activity and positive lifestyle habits to better health, longevity, quality of life, and total well-being.

Research findings in the last few years have shown that physical inactivity and a negative lifestyle seriously threaten health and hasten the deterioration rate of the human body. Physically active people live longer than their inactive counterparts, even if activity begins later in life. United States estimates indicate that more than 400,000 deaths yearly are attributed to poor diet and physical inactivity.[1] Similar trends are found in most industrialized nations throughout the world.

The human organism needs movement and activity to grow, develop, and maintain health. Advances in modern technology, however, have almost completely eliminated the necessity for physical exertion in daily life. Physical activity is no longer a natural part of our existence. We live in an automated society, where most of the activities that used to require strenuous exertion can be accomplished by machines with the simple pull of a handle or push of a button. This epidemic of physical inactivity is the second greatest threat to U.S. public health and has been termed **Sedentary Death Syndrome**, or **SeDS**[2] (the number-one threat is tobacco use—the largest cause of preventable deaths).

At the beginning of the 20th century, **life expectancy** for a child born in the United States was only 47 years. The most common health problems in the Western world were infectious diseases, such as tuberculosis, diphtheria, influenza, kidney disease, polio, and other illnesses of infancy. Progress in the medical field largely eliminated these diseases. Then, as more North American people started to enjoy the "good life" (sedentary living and overuse of alcohol, fatty foods, excessive sweets, tobacco, drugs), we saw an increase in deaths resulting from **chronic diseases** such as hypertension, coronary heart disease, atherosclerosis, strokes, diabetes, cancer, emphysema, and cirrhosis of the liver (see Figure 1.1).

As the incidence of chronic diseases climbed, we recognized that prevention is the best medicine. Consequently, a fitness and wellness movement developed gradually in the 1980s. People began to realize that good health is mostly self-controlled and that the leading causes of illness and premature death in North America could be prevented by adhering to positive lifestyle habits. Whereas we all desire to live

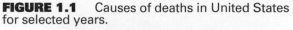

FIGURE 1.1 Causes of deaths in United States for selected years.

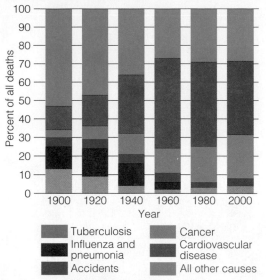

Tuberculosis
Influenza and pneumonia
Accidents
Cancer
Cardiovascular disease
All other causes

Source: National Center for Health Statistics, Division of Vital Statistics.

a long life, wellness programs focus on enhancing the overall quality of life—for as long as we live.

Life Expectancy Versus Healthy Life Expectancy

Presently, the average life expectancy in the United States is about 77.4 years (about 74.7 for men and 79.9 for women). In a break with tradition, for the first time in the year 2000, the World Health Organization (WHO) calculated **healthy life expectancy (HLE)** estimates for 191 nations. HLE is obtained by subtracting the years of ill health from total life expectancy. The United States ranked 24th in this report, with an HLE of 70 years; Japan was first with an HLE of 74.5 years (see Figure 1.2). This was a major surprise, given the Unites States' status as a developed country with one of the best medical care systems in the world. The rating indicates that Americans die earlier and spend more time disabled than people in most other advanced countries. The WHO report points to several factors that may account for this unexpected finding:

1. The extremely poor health of some groups, such as Native Americans, rural African Americans, and the inner-city poor. Their health status is more characteristic of poor developing nations than a rich industrialized country.
2. The HIV epidemic, which causes more deaths and disabilities in the United States than in other developed nations.

FIGURE 1.2 Life expectancy and healthy life expectancy for selected countries.

Country	Healthy life expectancy	Life expectancy
Ireland	69.6	75.8
USA	70.0	76.8
Germany	70.4	76.9
United Kingdom	71.7	77.2
Austria	71.6	77.4
Belgium	71.6	77.9
Greece	72.5	78.0
Netherlands	72.0	78.1
Norway	71.7	78.6
Spain	72.8	78.7
Italy	72.7	78.8
Canada	72.0	79.1
Switzerland	72.5	79.3
France	73.1	79.3
Sweden	73.0	79.5
Japan	74.5	81.0

Years (60, 65, 70, 75, 80)

■ Healthy life expectancy ■ Life expectancy

Source: World Health Organization, http://www.who.int/inf-pr-2000/en/pr2000-life.html. Retrieved June 4, 2000.

FIGURE 1.3 Leading causes of death in United States in 2002.

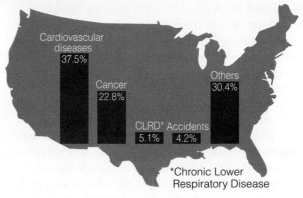

Cardiovascular diseases 37.5%
Cancer 22.8%
Others 30.4%
CLRD* 5.1% Accidents 4.2%

*Chronic Lower Respiratory Disease

Source: U. S. Department of Health and Human Services, Centers for Disease Control and Prevention, National Center for Health Statistics, National Vital Statistics Reports, *Deaths: Final Data for 2002*, 53:5 (October 12, 2004).

3. The high incidence of tobacco use.
4. The high incidence of coronary heart disease.
5. Fairly high levels of violence, notably homicides, compared with other developed countries.

Leading Health Problems in the United States

The leading causes of death in the United States today are largely lifestyle-related (see Figure 1.3). More than 60 percent of all deaths in the United States are caused by cardiovascular disease and cancer.[3] Almost 80 percent of these deaths could be prevented through a healthy lifestyle program. The third and fourth leading causes of death are chronic lower respiratory disease and accidents, respectively.

In the United States, the most prevalent degenerative diseases are those of the cardiovascular system. Of all deaths, 38 percent are attributed to diseases of the heart and blood vessels. According to the American Heart Association, 64.4 million people in the United States were afflicted with diseases of the cardiovascular system in 2004, including 50 million with hypertension (high blood pressure) and 13.2 million with coronary heart disease (many of these people have more than one type of cardiovascular disease). About 1.2 million people have heart attacks each year, and more than 500,000 of them die as a result. The estimated cost of heart and blood vessel disease in 2004 exceeded $368 billion.[4] A complete cardiovascular disease prevention program is outlined in Chapter 11.

The second leading cause of death in the United States is cancer. Even though cancer is not the number-one killer, it is the number-one health fear of the American people. About 23 percent of all deaths in the United States are attributable to cancer. More than 563,700 people died from this disease in 2004, and an estimated 1,368,030 new cases were reported the same year.[5] The major contributor to the increase in incidence of cancer during the last five decades is lung cancer, and 87 percent of lung cancer is caused by tobacco use. Furthermore,

Health A state of complete well-being, and not just the absence of disease or infirmity.

Sedentary Death Syndrome (SeDS) A term used to describe deaths that are attributed to a lack of regular physical activity.

Life expectancy Number of years a person is expected to live based on the person's birth year.

Chronic diseases Illnesses that develop and last a long time.

Healthy Life Expectancy (HLE) Number of years a person is expected to live in good health; this number is obtained by subtracting ill-health years from overall life expectancy.

smoking accounts for more than 30 percent of all deaths from cancer. Another 33 percent of deaths are related to nutrition, physical inactivity, excessive body weight, and other faulty lifestyle habits.

According to the American Cancer Society, the most influential factor in fighting cancer today is prevention through health education programs. Evidence indicates that as much as 80 percent of all human cancer can be prevented through positive lifestyle behaviors. A comprehensive cancer prevention program is presented in Chapter 12.

The third cause of death, **chronic lower respiratory disease (CLRD)**, is a general term that includes chronic obstructive pulmonary disease, emphysema, and chronic bronchitis (all diseases of the respiratory system). Although CLRD is related mostly to tobacco use (see Chapter 13 for discussion on how to stop smoking), lifetime non-smokers can also develop CLRD. Precautions to prevent CLRD include:[6]

1. Consuming a low-fat, low-sodium, nutrient-dense diet (similar to a cardio- and cancer-protective diet).
2. Staying physically active.
3. Not smoking and staying clear of cigarette smoke.
4. Avoiding swimming pools for chlorine-vapor-sensitive individuals.
5. Getting a pneumonia vaccine if over 50 and a current or ex-smoker.

Accidents are the fourth leading cause of death. Even though not all accidents are preventable, many are. Fatal accidents are often related to abusing drugs and not wearing seat belts.

Most people do not perceive accidents as a health problem. Even so, accidents affect the total well-being of millions of Americans each year. Accident prevention and personal safety are part of a health-enhancement program aimed at achieving a better quality of life. Proper nutrition, exercise, stress management, and abstinence from cigarette smoking are of little help if the person is involved in a disabling or fatal accident as a result of distraction, a single reckless decision, or not wearing seat belts properly.

Accidents do not just happen. We cause accidents, and we are victims of accidents. Although some factors in life, such as earthquakes, tornadoes, and airplane crashes, are completely beyond our control, more often than not, personal safety and accident prevention are a matter of common sense. Most accidents stem from poor judgment and confused mental states, which occur when people are upset, are not paying attention to the task at hand, or are abusing alcohol or other drugs.

Alcohol abuse is the number-one cause of all accidents. About 50 percent of accidental deaths and suicides in the United States are alcohol-related. Further, alcohol intoxication is the leading cause of

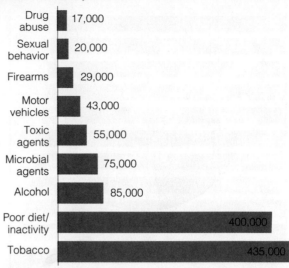

FIGURE 1.4 Underlying causes of death in United States, year 2000.

Cause	Deaths
Drug abuse	17,000
Sexual behavior	20,000
Firearms	29,000
Motor vehicles	43,000
Toxic agents	55,000
Microbial agents	75,000
Alcohol	85,000
Poor diet/inactivity	400,000
Tobacco	435,000

Source: Centers for Disease Control and Prevention, Atlanta, GA, 2003.

fatal automobile accidents. Other commonly abused drugs alter feelings and perceptions, generate mental confusion, and impair judgment and coordination, greatly enhancing the risk for accidental **morbidity** and mortality (see Chapter 13).

The underlying causes of death in the United States (see Figure 1.4) indicate that 8 of the 9 causes are related to lifestyle and lack of common sense. Of the approximate 2.4 million yearly deaths in the U.S., the "big three"—tobacco use, poor diet and inactivity, and alcohol abuse—are responsible for more than 900,000 deaths each year.

Lifestyle as a Health Problem

As the incidence of chronic diseases rose, it became obvious that prevention was—and remains—the best medicine. According to Dr. David Satcher, former U.S. Surgeon General, more than 50 percent of the people who die in this country each year die because of what they do.

According to estimates, more than half of disease is lifestyle-related, a fifth is attributed to the environment, and a tenth is influenced by the health care the individual receives. Only 16 percent is related to genetic factors (see Figure 1.5).[7] Thus, the individual controls as much as 84 percent of his or her vulnerability to disease—and, thus, quality of life. The data also indicate that 83 percent of deaths before age 65 are preventable. In essence, most people in the United States are threatened by the very lives they lead today.

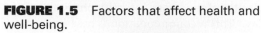

FIGURE 1.5 Factors that affect health and well-being.

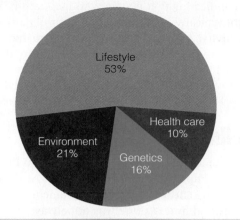

Lifestyle
53%

Health care
10%

Environment
21%

Genetics
16%

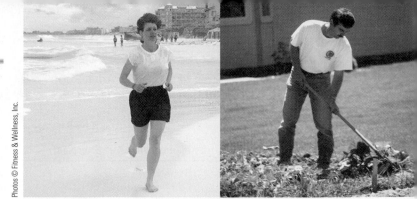

Exercise and an active lifestyle increases health, quality of life, and longevity.

Because of the unhealthy lifestyles that many young adults lead, their bodies may be middle-aged or older! Healthy choices made today influence health for decades. Many physical education programs do not emphasize the skills necessary for youth to maintain a high level of fitness and health throughout life. The intent of this book is to provide those skills and help to prepare you for a lifetime of physical fitness and wellness. A healthy lifestyle is self-controlled, and you can learn how to be responsible for your own health and fitness.

Physical Activity and Exercise Defined

Abundant scientific research over the last three decades has established a distinction between physical activity and exercise. **Physical activity** is bodily movement produced by skeletal muscles. It requires energy expenditure and produces progressive health benefits. Physical activity typically requires only a low to moderate intensity of effort. Examples of physical activity are walking to and from work, taking the stairs instead of elevators and escalators, gardening, doing household chores, dancing, and washing the car by hand. Physical inactivity, on the other hand, implies a level of activity that is lower than that required to maintain good health.

Exercise is a type of physical activity that requires planned, structured, and repetitive bodily movement to improve or maintain one or more components of physical fitness. Examples of exercise are walking, running, cycling, aerobics, swimming, and strength training. Exercise is usually viewed as an activity that requires a high-intensity effort.

Surgeon General's Report on Physical Activity and Health

According to a 1996 landmark report by the U.S. Surgeon General, poor health because of the lack of physical activity is a serious public health problem that we must meet head-on at once.[8] More than 60 percent of adults do not achieve the recommended amount of physical activity (see Table 1.1), and 25 percent are not physically active at all. Further, almost half of all people between 12 and 21 years of age are not vigorously active on a regular basis. The report also stated that physical inactivity is more prevalent in

1. Women than men
2. African Americans and Hispanic Americans than whites
3. Older than younger adults
4. Less affluent than more affluent people
5. Less educated than more educated adults.

Furthermore, the number of people who are not physically active is more than twice the number of people who have hypertension, have high cholesterol, or smoke cigarettes. This report became a nationwide call to action.

The report states that regular **moderate physical activity** can prevent premature death, unnecessary illness, and disability. It could provide

Chronic Lower Respiratory Disease (CLRD) A general term that includes chronic obstructive pulmonary disease, emphysema, and chronic bronchitis (all diseases of the respiratory system).

Morbidity A condition related to, or caused by, illness or disease.

Physical activity Bodily movement produced by skeletal muscles; requires expenditure of energy and produces progressive health benefits.

Exercise A type of physical activity that requires planned, structured, and repetitive bodily movement with the intent of improving or maintaining one or more components of physical fitness.

Moderate physical activity Activity that uses 150 calories of energy per day, or 1,000 calories per week.

TABLE 1.1 Percent of Total U.S. Adult Population That Regularly Participates in Physical Activity

	Moderate Intensity*	High Intensity** (Exercise)
Overall	20%	14%
By Gender		
Men	21	13
Women	19	16
By Ethnicity		
White	21	15
African American	15	9
Hispanic American	20	12

*A minimum of 5 days per week for at least 30 minutes per session.

**A minimum of 3 days per week for a minimum of 20 minutes.

Source: U.S. Department of Health and Human Services, *Physical Activity and Health: A Report of the Surgeon General* (Atlanta: Centers for Disease Control and Prevention, National Center for Chronic Disease Prevention and Health Promotion, 1996).

substantial benefits in health and well-being for the vast majority of people who are not physically active. Individuals who are already moderately active can achieve even greater health benefits by increasing their amount of physical activity.

Among the benefits listed in the report are significantly reduced risks for developing or dying from heart disease, diabetes, colon cancer, and high blood pressure. Regular physical activity also is important for the health of muscles, bones, and joints, and it seems to reduce symptoms of depression and anxiety, improve mood, and enhance one's ability to perform daily tasks throughout life. It also can help control health-care costs and help to maintain a high quality of life into old age.

The 1996 report defined moderate physical activity as using 150 calories of energy per day, or 1,000 calories per week. It recommended that people strive to achieve at least 30 minutes of physical activity per day most days of the week. Examples of moderate physical activity are walking, cycling, playing basketball or volleyball, swimming, water aerobics, dancing fast, pushing a stroller, raking leaves, shoveling snow, washing or waxing a car, washing windows or floors, and even gardening.

Because of the ever-growing epidemic of obesity in the United States, a 2002 guideline by American and Canadian scientists from the Institute of Medicine of the National

CRITICAL THINKING

Do you consciously incorporate physical activity into your daily lifestyle? Can you provide examples? Do you think you get sufficient daily physical activity to maintain good health?

Academy of Sciences increased the recommendation to 60 minutes of moderate-intensity physical activity every day.[9] This recommendation is based on evidence indicating that people who maintain healthy weight typically accumulate one hour of daily physical activity. Although health benefits are derived with 30 minutes per day, it takes an hour of daily activity to prevent weight gain. Further, one hour a day provides additional health benefits, including a lower risk for cardiovascular disease and diabetes.

Wellness

Most people recognize that participating in fitness programs improves their quality of life. At the end of the 20th century, however, we came to realize that physical fitness alone was not always sufficient to lower the risk for disease and ensure better health. For example, individuals who run 3 miles (about 5 km) a day, lift weights regularly, participate in stretching exercises, and watch their body weight might be easily classified as having good or excellent fitness. Offsetting these good habits, however, might be **risk factors**, including high blood pressure, smoking, excessive stress, drinking excessive alcohol, and eating too many fatty foods. These factors place people at risk for cardiovascular disease and other chronic diseases of which they may not be aware.

Even though most people are aware of their unhealthy behaviors, they seem satisfied with life as long as they are free from symptoms of disease or illness. They do not contemplate change until they suffer a major health problem. Present lifestyle habits, however, dictate the health and well-being of tomorrow.

Good health is no longer viewed as simply the absence of illness. The notion of good health has evolved notably in the last few years and continues to change as scientists learn more about lifestyle factors that bring on illness and affect wellness. Furthermore, once the idea took hold that fitness by itself would not always decrease the risk for disease and ensure better health, the **wellness** concept developed. Wellness living requires implementing positive programs to change behavior to improve health and quality of life, prolong life, and achieve total well-being.

The Seven Dimensions of Wellness

Wellness has seven dimensions: physical, emotional, mental, social, environmental, occupational, and spiritual* (see Figure 1.6). These dimensions are interrelated: One frequently affects the others. For example, a person who is emotionally down often has no desire to exercise, study, socialize with

* Adapted from W. W. K. Hoeger, L. W. Turner, and B. Q. Hafen, *Wellness: Guidelines for a Healthy Lifestyle* (Belmont, CA: Wadsworth/Thomson Learning, 2002).

FIGURE 1.6 Dimensions of wellness.

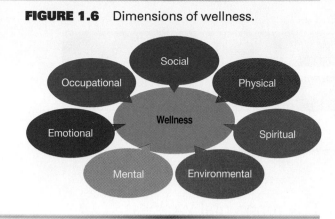

Physical Wellness

Physical wellness is the dimension most commonly associated with being healthy. It entails confidence and optimism about one's ability to protect one's physical health and take care of health problems.

Physically well individuals are active, exercise regularly, eat a well-balanced diet, maintain recommended body weight, get sufficient sleep, practice safe sex, minimize exposure to environmental contaminants, avoid harmful drugs (including tobacco and excessive alcohol), and seek medical care and exams as needed. Physically well people also exhibit good cardiorespiratory endurance, adequate muscular strength and flexibility, proper body composition, and the ability to carry out ordinary and unusual demands of daily life safely and effectively. These concepts are discussed in subsequent chapters.

friends, attend church, and may be more susceptible to illness and disease.

The seven dimensions of wellness show how the concept clearly goes beyond the absence of disease. Wellness incorporates factors such as adequate fitness, proper nutrition, stress management, disease prevention, spirituality, not smoking or abusing drugs, personal safety, regular physical examinations, health education, and environmental support.

For a wellness way of life, not only must individuals be physically fit and manifest no signs of disease, but they must also be free of risk factors for disease (such as hypertension, hyperlipidemia, cigarette smoking, negative stress, faulty nutrition, careless sex). The relationship between adequate fitness and wellness is illustrated in the continuum in Figure 1.7. Even though an individual tested in a fitness center may demonstrate adequate or even excellent fitness, indulgence in unhealthy lifestyle behaviors will still increase the risk for chronic diseases and diminish the person's well-being.

Emotional Wellness

Emotional wellness involves the ability to understand one's own feelings, accept one's limitations, and achieve emotional stability. Furthermore, it implies the ability to express emotions appropriately, adjust to change, cope with stress in a healthy way, and enjoy life despite its occasional disappointments and frustrations.

Emotional wellness brings with it a certain stability, an ability to look both success and failure squarely in the face and to keep moving along a predetermined course. When success is evident, the emotionally well person radiates the expected joy and confidence. When failure seems evident, the emotionally well person responds by making the best of circumstances and moving beyond the failure. Wellness enables one to move ahead with optimism and energy instead of spending time and talent worrying about failure. You learn from it, identify ways to avoid it in the future, and then go on with the business at hand.

And emotional wellness involves happiness—an emotional anchor that gives meaning and joy to life. Happiness is a long-term state of mind that permeates the various facets of life and influences our outlook. Although there is no simple recipe for creating happiness, researchers agree that happy people are usually participants in some category of a supportive family unit where they feel loved themselves. Healthy, happy people enjoy friends, work hard at something fulfilling, get plenty of exercise, and enjoy play and leisure time. They know how to laugh, and they laugh often. They give of themselves freely to others and seem to have found deep meaning in life.

An attitude of true happiness signals freedom from the tension and depression that many people endure. Emotionally well people are obviously subject to the same kinds of depression and unhappiness that occasionally plague us all, but the difference lies in their ability to bounce back. Emotionally well people take minor setbacks in stride and have the ability to enjoy life despite it all. They don't waste energy or time recounting the situation, wondering how they could have changed it, or dwelling on the past.

Risk factors Lifestyle and genetic variables that may lead to disease.

Wellness The constant and deliberate effort to stay healthy and achieve the highest potential for well-being. It encompasses seven dimensions—physical, emotional, mental, social, environmental, occupational, and spiritual—and integrates them all into a quality life.

Physical wellness Good physical fitness and confidence in one's personal ability to take care of health problems.

Emotional wellness The ability to understand one's own feelings, accept limitations, and achieve emotional stability.

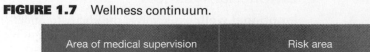

FIGURE 1.7 Wellness continuum.

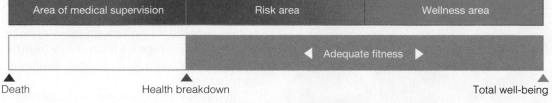

Mental Wellness

Mental wellness, also referred to as intellectual wellness, implies that the mentally well person can apply the things he or she has learned, create opportunities to learn more, and engage the mind in lively interaction with the outside world. When you are mentally well, you are not intimidated by facts and figures with which you are unfamiliar but instead embrace the chance to learn something new. Your confidence and enthusiasm enables you to approach any learning situation with eagerness that leads to success.

Mental wellness brings with it vision and promise. More than anything else, mentally well people are open-minded and accepting of others. Instead of being threatened by people who are different from themselves, they show respect and curiosity without feeling they have to conform. They are faithful to their own ideas and philosophies and allow others the same privilege. Their self-confidence guarantees that they can take their place among others in the world without having to give up part of themselves and without requiring others to do the same.

Social Wellness

Social wellness, with its accompanying positive self-image, endows a person with the ease and confidence to be outgoing, friendly, and affectionate toward others. Social wellness involves not only a concern for oneself but also an interest in humanity and the environment as a whole.

One of the hallmarks of social wellness is the ability to relate to others and to reach out to other people both within the family and outside it. Similar to emotional wellness, it involves being comfortable with one's emotions and thus helps the socially well person understand and accept the emotions of others. One's own balance and sense of self enables extending respect and tolerance to others. Healthy people are honest and loyal. This dimension of wellness leads to the ability to maintain close relationships with other people.

Environmental Wellness

Environmental wellness refers to the effect that our surroundings have on our well-being. Our planet is a delicate **ecosystem**, and its health depends on the continuous recycling of its elements. Unfortunately, the man-made toxicity of the environment has a direct effect on personal wellness.

To enjoy health, we require clean air, pure water, quality food, adequate shelter, satisfactory work conditions, personal safety, and healthy relationships. Health is negatively affected when we live in a polluted, toxic, unkind, and unsafe environment. Unfortunately, a national survey of first-year college students showed that less than 20 percent were concerned about the health of the environment.[10] To enjoy environmental wellness, it is our personal responsibility not only to educate and protect ourselves against environmental hazards but also to protect the environment so that we, our children, and future generations can enjoy a safe and clean environment.

Occupational Wellness

Occupational wellness is not tied to high salary, prestigious position, or extravagant working conditions. Any job can bring occupational wellness if it provides rewards that are important to the individual. Salary might be the most important factor to one person, whereas another might place a much greater value on creativity. People who are occupationally well have their own "ideal" job, which allows them to thrive.

People who are occupationally well face demands on the job, but they also have some say over demands that are placed on them. Any job has routine demands, but occupational wellness means that routine demands are mixed with new, unpredictable challenges that keep a job exciting. Occupationally well people are able to maximize their skills, and they have the opportunity to broaden their existing skills or gain new ones. Their occupation offers opportunities for advancement and recognition for achievement. Occupational wellness encourages collaboration and interaction among co-workers, which fosters a sense of teamwork and support.

Spiritual Wellness

Spiritual wellness provides a unifying power that integrates all dimensions of wellness. Basic characteristics of spiritual people include a sense of meaning and direction in life and a relationship to a higher being. This leads to personal freedom and encompasses prayer, faith, love, closeness to others, peace, joy, and fulfillment, and altruism. Although not everyone claims affiliation with a certain religion or denomination, based on recent national Gallup polls, 95 percent of the U.S. population believes in God or a universal spirit functioning as God.

Several studies have reported positive relationships among spiritual well-being, emotional well-being, and satisfaction with life. People who attend church and regularly participate in religious organizations enjoy better health, have a lower incidence of chronic diseases, handle stress more effectively, and seem to live longer.[11]

Although the ways by which religious affiliation enhances wellness are difficult to determine, possible benefits include the promotion of healthy lifestyle behaviors, social support, assistance in times of crisis and need, and counseling to overcome weaknesses. Spiritual beliefs also seem to help people overcome crises and aid them in developing better coping techniques to deal with future trauma.

PRAYER

Prayer is a signpost of our spirituality, at the core of most spiritual experiences. It is communication with a higher power. Prayers are said for a multiplicity of reasons, including requests for guidance, wisdom, strength, protection, and health, as well as thanksgiving.

Research has shown that for prayers to be effective, a person needs to accept the efficacy of prayer and pray with sincerity, humility, and love. At least 200 studies have been conducted on the effects of prayer on health. About two-thirds of these studies have linked prayer to positive health outcomes, as long as these prayers are offered with love, empathy, and compassion. Some studies have shown faster healing time and fewer complications in patients who didn't even know that they were being prayed for, as compared to patients who were not prayed for.[12]

ALTRUISM

Altruism, a key attribute of spiritual people, seems to enhance health and longevity. Studies indicate that people who perform regular volunteer work live longer. Doing good for others is good for oneself, especially for the immune system. Research has found that health benefits of altruism are so powerful

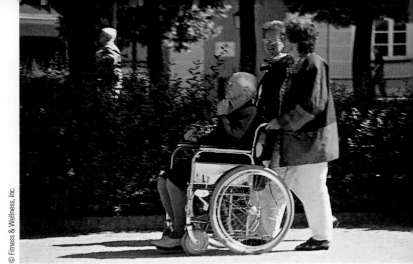

Altruism enhances health and well-being.

that even watching films of altruistic endeavors enhances the formation of an immune-system chemical that helps fight disease.

Wellness requires a balance among all of its seven dimensions. The relationship between spirituality and wellness, therefore, is meaningful in our quest for a better quality of life. As with the other parameters listed above, optimum wellness requires development of the spiritual dimension to its fullest potential.

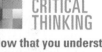

CRITICAL THINKING

Now that you understand the seven dimensions of wellness, rank them in order of importance to you and explain your rationale in doing so.

Wellness, Fitness, and Longevity

During the second half of the 20th century, scientists began to realize the importance of good fitness and improved lifestyle in the fight against chronic

Mental wellness A state in which one's mind is engaged in lively interaction with the surrounding world; also called intellectual wellness.

Social wellness The ability to relate well to others, both within and outside the family unit.

Environmental wellness The capability to live in a clean and safe environment that is not detrimental to health.

Ecosystem A community of organisms interacting with each other in an environment.

Occupational wellness The ability to perform one's job skillfully and effectively under conditions that provide personal and team satisfaction and adequately reward each individual.

Spiritual wellness The sense that life is meaningful, that life has purpose, and that some power brings all humanity together; the ethics, values, and morals that guide one and give meaning and direction to life.

Prayer Sincere and humble communication with a higher power.

Altruism True concern for the welfare of others.

diseases, particularly those of the cardiovascular system. Because of more participation in wellness programs, cardiovascular mortality rates dropped: The decline began in about 1963, and between 1960 and 2000 the incidence of cardiovascular disease dropped by 26 percent. This decrease is credited to higher levels of wellness and better health care in the United States. More than half of the decline is specifically attributed to improved diet and reduction in smoking.

Furthermore, several studies have showed an inverse relationship between physical activity and premature mortality rates. The first major study in this area was conducted among 16,936 Harvard alumni, linking physical activity habits and mortality rates.[13] The results showed that as the amount of weekly physical activity increased, the risk of cardiovascular deaths decreased. The largest decrease in cardiovascular deaths was observed among alumni who used more than 2,000 calories per week through physical activity. Figure 1.8 graphically illustrates the study results.

A landmark study subsequently conducted at the Aerobics Research Institute in Dallas upheld the findings of the Harvard alumni study.[14] Based on data from 13,344 people followed over an average of 8 years, the study revealed a graded and consistent inverse relationship between physical activity levels and mortality, regardless of age and other risk factors. As illustrated in Figure 1.9, the higher the level of physical activity, the longer the lifespan. The death rate during the 8-year study from all causes for the least-fit men was 3.4 times higher than that of the most-fit men. For the least-fit women, the death rate was 4.6 times higher than that of most fit women.

The same study also reported a greatly reduced rate of premature death, even at moderate fitness levels that most adults can achieve easily. Greater protection is attained by combining higher fitness levels with reduction in other risk factors such as hypertension, high serum cholesterol, cigarette smoking, and excessive body fat.

A 5-year follow-up study on fitness and mortality found a substantial (44 percent) reduction in mortality risk when people abandoned a **sedentary** lifestyle and become moderately fit.[15] The lowest death rate was found in people who were fit at the start of the study and remained fit; and the highest death rate was found in men who were unfit at the beginning of the study and remained unfit.

In another major research study, a healthy lifestyle was shown to contribute to some of the lowest mortality rates ever reported in the literature.[16] The investigators in this study looked at three general health habits among the participants: regular physical

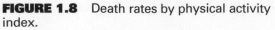

FIGURE 1.8 Death rates by physical activity index.

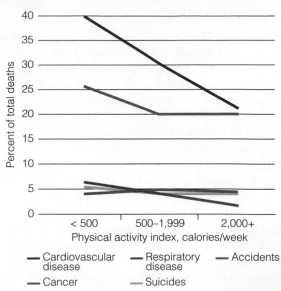

Note: The graph represents cause-specific death rates per 10,000 person-years of observation among 16,936 Harvard alumni, 1962–1978, by physical activity index; adjusted for differences in age, cigarette smoking, and hypertension.

Source: R. S. Paffenbarger, R. T. Hyde, A. L. Wing, and C. H. Steinmetz, "A Natural History of Athleticism and Cardiovascular Health," *Journal of the American Medical Association* 252 (1984): 491–495. Used by permission.

activity, sufficient sleep, and lifetime abstinence from smoking. In addition, study participants abstained from alcohol, drugs, and all forms of tobacco.

Compared with the general white population, this group of more 10,000 people had much lower cancer, cardiovascular, and overall death rates. Men in the study had one-third the death rate from cancer, one-seventh the death rate from cardiovascular disease, and one-fifth the rate of overall mortality. Women had about half the rate of cancer and overall mortality and one-third the death rate from cardiovascular disease. Life expectancies for 25-year-olds who adhered to the three health habits were 85 and 86 years, respectively, compared with 74 and 80 for the average U.S. white man and woman. The additional 6 to 11 "golden years" are precious—and more enjoyable—for those who maintain a lifetime wellness program.

The results of these studies clearly indicate that fitness improves wellness, quality of life, and longevity. **Vigorous activity** is preferable to the extent of one's capabilities because it is most clearly associated with longer life.

FIGURE 1.9 Death rates by physical fitness groups.

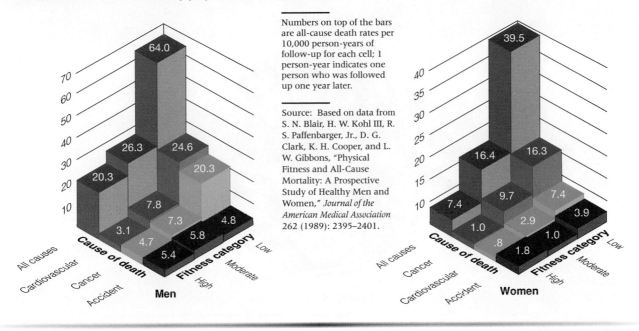

Numbers on top of the bars are all-cause death rates per 10,000 person-years of follow-up for each cell; 1 person-year indicates one person who was followed up one year later.

Source: Based on data from S. N. Blair, H. W. Kohl III, R. S. Paffenbarger, Jr., D. G. Clark, K. H. Cooper, and L. W. Gibbons, "Physical Fitness and All-Cause Mortality: A Prospective Study of Healthy Men and Women," *Journal of the American Medical Association* 262 (1989): 2395–2401.

Types of Physical Fitness

As the fitness concept grew at the end of the last century, it became clear that several specific components contribute to an individual's overall level of fitness. **Physical fitness** can be classified into health-related and motor skill-related fitness.

The four **health-related fitness** components are (see Figure 1.10):

1. cardiorespiratory (aerobic) endurance
2. muscular strength and endurance
3. muscular flexibility
4. body composition.

The **skill-related fitness** components consist of (see Figure 1.11):

1. agility
2. balance
3. coordination
4. power
5. reaction time
6. speed

These skill-related fitness components are related primarily to athletic success and may not be as crucial as the health-related components to better health.

In terms of preventive medicine, the main emphasis of fitness programs should be on the health-related components. Nevertheless, total fitness is achieved by taking part in specific programs to improve both health-related and skill-related components.

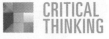

CRITICAL THINKING

What role do the four health-related components of physical fitness play in your life? Can you rank them in order of importance to you and explain the rationale you used?

Sedentary A lifestyle characterized by relative inactivity and a lot of sitting.

Vigorous activity Any exercise that requires a MET level equal to or greater than 6 METs (21 ml/kg/min); 1 MET is the energy expenditure at rest, 3.5 ml/kg/min, whereas METs are defined as multiples of the resting metabolic rate (examples of activities that require a 6-MET level are aerobics, walking uphill at 3.5 mph, cycling at 10 to 12 mph, playing doubles in tennis, and vigorous strength training).

Physical fitness The ability to meet the ordinary as well as the unusual demands of daily life safely and effectively without being overly fatigued and still have energy left for leisure and recreational activities.

Health-related fitness Fitness programs that are prescribed to improve the individual's overall health; components are cardio-respiratory endurance, muscular strength and endurance, muscular flexibility, and body composition.

Skill-related fitness Fitness components important for success in activities and athletic events requiring high skill levels; encompasses agility, balance, coordination, power, reaction time, and speed.

FIGURE 1.10 Health-related components of physical fitness.

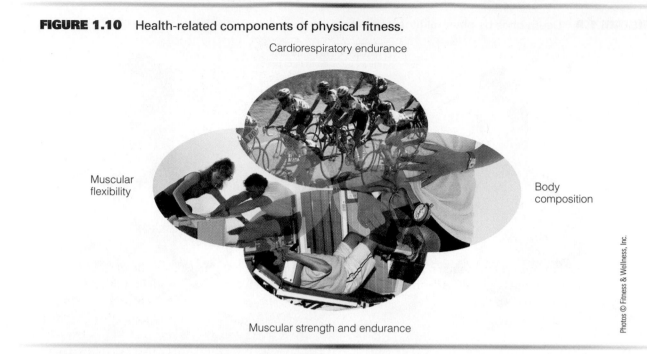

Cardiorespiratory endurance

Muscular flexibility

Body composition

Muscular strength and endurance

FIGURE 1.11 Motor skill-related components of physical fitness.

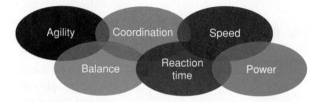

Agility Coordination Speed

Balance Reaction time Power

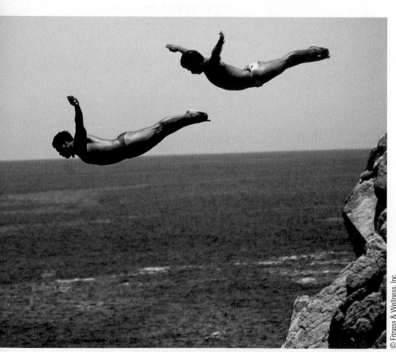

Good health- and skill-related fitness are required to participate in highly skilled activities.

Fitness Standards: Health Versus Physical Fitness

The assessments of fitness components are presented in Chapters 4, 6, 7, 8, and 9. A meaningful debate regarding age- and gender-related fitness standards, however, has resulted in two standards: health fitness (also referred to as criterion-referenced fitness) and physical fitness.

Health Fitness Standards

The **health fitness standards** proposed here are based on data linking minimum fitness values to disease prevention and health. Attaining the health fitness standard requires only moderate physical activity. For example, a 2-mile walk in less than 30 minutes, 5 or 6 times per week, seems to be sufficient to achieve the health-fitness standard for cardiorespiratory endurance.

As illustrated in Figure 1.12, significant health benefits can be reaped with such a program, although improvements in fitness, expressed in terms of oxygen uptake or VO_{2max} (explained on page 13 and in Chapter 6) are not as notable. Nevertheless, health improvements are quite striking, and only slightly greater benefits are obtained with a more intense exercise program. These benefits include reduction in blood lipids, lower blood pressure, weight loss, stress release, decreased risk for diabetes, and lower risk for disease and premature mortality.

FIGURE 1.12 Health and fitness benefits based on type of lifestyle and physical activity program.

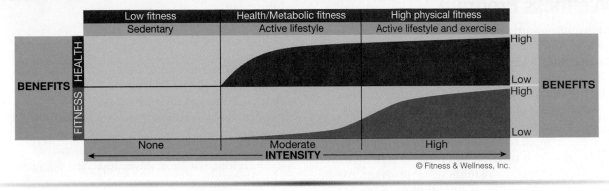

© Fitness & Wellness, Inc.

More specifically, improvements in the **metabolic profile** (measured by insulin sensitivity, glucose tolerance, and improved cholesterol levels) can be notable despite little or no weight loss or improvement in aerobic capacity. **Metabolic fitness** can be attained through an active lifestyle and moderate physical activity.

An assessment of health-related fitness uses **cardiorespiratory endurance**, measured in terms of the maximal amount of oxygen the body is able to utilize per minute of physical activity (maximal oxygen uptake, or VO_{2max}), essentially, a measure of how efficiently the heart, lungs, and muscles can operate during aerobic exercise (see Chapter 6). VO_{2max} is commonly expressed in milliliters (ml) of oxygen (volume of oxygen) per kilogram (kg) of body weight per minute (ml/kg/min). Individual values can range from about 10 ml/kg/min in cardiac patients to more than 80 ml/kg/min in world-class runners, cyclists, and cross-country skiers.

Research data from the study presented in Figure 1.9 reported that achieving VO_{2max} values of 35 and 32.5 ml/kg/min for men and women, respectively, may be sufficient to lower the risk for all-cause mortality significantly. Although greater improvements in fitness yield a slightly lower risk for premature death, the largest drop is seen between the least fit and the moderately fit. Therefore, the 35 and 32.5 ml/kg/min values could be selected as the health fitness standards.

Physical Fitness Standards

Physical fitness standards are set higher than the health fitness standards and require a more intense exercise program. Physically fit people of all ages have the freedom to enjoy most of life's daily and recreational activities to their fullest potential. Current health fitness standards may not be enough to achieve these objectives.

Sound physical fitness gives the individual a measure of independence throughout life that many people in the United States no longer enjoy. Most adults should be able to carry out activities similar to those they conducted in their youth, though not with the same intensity. These standards do not require being a championship athlete, but activities such as changing a tire, chopping wood, climbing several flights of stairs, playing basketball, mountain biking, playing soccer with children or grandchildren, walking several miles around a lake, and hiking through a national park do require more than the current "average fitness" level in the United States.

Your own personal objectives will determine the fitness program you use. If the main objective of your fitness program is to lower the risk of disease, attaining the health fitness standards may be enough to ensure better health. If, however, you want to participate in vigorous fitness activities, achieving a high physical fitness standard is recommended. This book gives both health fitness standards and physical fitness standards for each fitness test so you can personalize your approach.

Health fitness standards The lowest fitness requirements for maintaining good health, decreasing the risk for chronic diseases, and lowering the incidence of muscular-skeletal injuries; also referred to as criterion-referenced standards.

Metabolic profile A measurement to assess risk for diabetes and cardiovascular disease through plasma insulin, glucose, lipid, and lipoprotein levels.

Metabolic fitness Denotes improvements in the metabolic profile through a moderate-intensity exercise program in spite of little or no improvement in physical fitness standards.

Cardiorespiratory endurance The ability of the lungs, heart, and blood vessels to deliver adequate amounts of oxygen to the cells to meet the demands of prolonged physical activity.

Physical fitness standards A fitness level that allows a person to sustain moderate-to-vigorous physical activity without undue fatigue and the ability to closely maintain this level throughout life.

Benefits of a Comprehensive Wellness Program

An inspiring story illustrating what fitness can do for a person's health and well-being is that of George Snell from Sandy, Utah. At age 45, Snell weighed approximately 400 pounds, his blood pressure was 220/180, he was blind because of undiagnosed diabetes, and his blood glucose level was 487.

Snell had determined to do something about his physical and medical condition, so he started a walking/jogging program. After about 8 months of conditioning, Snell had lost almost 200 pounds, his eyesight had returned, his glucose level was down to 67, and he was taken off medication. Just 2 months later—less than 10 months after beginning his personal exercise program—he completed his first marathon, a running course of 26.2 miles!

Health Benefits

Most people exercise because it improves their personal appearance and makes them feel good about themselves. Although many benefits accrue from participating in a regular fitness and wellness program and active people generally live longer, the greatest benefit of all is that physically fit individuals enjoy a better quality of life. These people live life to its fullest, with fewer health problems than inactive individuals (who may also indulge in other negative lifestyle behaviors). Although it would be difficult to compile an all-inclusive list, participating in a fitness and wellness program:

- Improves and strengthens the cardiorespiratory system.
- Maintains better muscle tone, muscular strength, and endurance.
- Improves muscular flexibility.
- Enhances athletic performance.
- Helps to maintain recommended body weight.
- Helps to preserve lean body tissue.
- Increases resting metabolic rate.
- Improves the body's ability to use fat during physical activity.
- Improves posture and physical appearance.
- Improves functioning of the immune system.
- Lowers the risk for chronic diseases and illness (such as cardiovascular diseases and cancer).
- Decreases the mortality rate from chronic diseases.
- Thins the blood so it doesn't clot as readily (thereby decreasing the risk for coronary heart disease and strokes).
- Helps the body to manage cholesterol levels more effectively.
- Prevents or delays the development of high blood pressure and lowers blood pressure in people with hypertension.
- Helps to prevent and control diabetes.
- Helps to achieve peak bone mass in young adults and maintain bone mass later in life, thereby decreasing the risk for osteoporosis.
- Helps people sleep better.
- Helps to prevent chronic back pain.
- Relieves tension and helps in coping with life stresses.
- Raises levels of energy and job productivity.
- Extends longevity and slows down the aging process.
- Promotes psychological well-being; better morale, self-image, and self-esteem.
- Reduces feelings of depression and anxiety.
- Encourages positive lifestyle changes (improving nutrition, quitting smoking, controlling alcohol and drug use).
- Speeds recovery time following physical exertion.
- Speeds recovery following injury or disease.
- Regulates and improves overall body functions.
- Improves physical stamina and counteracts chronic fatigue.
- Helps to maintain independent living, especially in older adults.
- Enhances quality of life; adherents feel better and live a healthier and happier life.

Economic Benefits

Sedentary living can have a strong impression on a nation's economy. As the need for physical exertion in Western countries decreased steadily during the last century, health-care expenditures increased dramatically. Health-care costs in the United States rose from $12 billion in 1950 to $1.7 trillion in 2003 (Figure 1.13), or about 13 percent of the gross national product (GNP). In 1980, health care costs represented 8.8 percent of the GNP, and they are projected to reach about 16 percent by the year 2010.

In terms of yearly health care costs per person, as illustrated in Figure 1.14, the United States spends more per person than any other industrialized nation. In 2003, U.S. health care costs per capita rose to $5,800, and are expected to reach almost $9,000 in 2010. Yet, overall, the U.S. health care system ranks only 37th in the world. One of the reasons for the low overall ranking is the overemphasis on state-of-the art cures instead of prevention programs. The United States is the best place in the world for people to receive treatment once they are sick, but the system does a poor job at keeping people healthy in the first place. The United States also fails to provide good health care for all: More than 44 million residents do not have health insurance.

Research indicates that adhering to the following 12 life-style habits will significantly improve health and extend life.

1. *Participate in a lifetime physical activity program.* Exercise regularly at least 3 times per week and try to accumulate a minimum of 60 minutes of moderate-intensity physical activity each day of your life. The 60 minutes should include 20 to 30 minutes of aerobic exercise at least 3 times per week, along with strengthening and stretching exercises 2 to 3 times per week.

2. *Do not smoke cigarettes.* Cigarette smoking is the largest preventable cause of illness and premature death in the United States. If we include all related deaths, smoking is responsible for more than 440,000 unnecessary deaths each year.

3. *Eat right.* Eat a good breakfast and two additional well-balanced meals every day. Avoid eating too many calories and foods with a lot of sugar, fat, and salt. Increase your daily consumption of fruits, vegetables, and whole-grain products.

4. *Avoid snacking.* Some researchers recommend refraining from frequent between-meal snacks. Every time a person eats, insulin is released to remove sugar from the blood. Such frequent spikes in insulin may contribute to the development of heart disease. Less frequent increases of insulin are more conducive to good health.

5. *Maintain recommended body weight through adequate nutrition and exercise.* This is important in preventing chronic diseases and in developing a higher level of fitness.

6. *Get enough rest.* Sleep 7 to 8 hours each night.

7. *Lower your stress levels.* Reduce your vulnerability to stress and practice stress management techniques as needed.

8. *Be wary of alcohol.* Drink alcohol moderately or not at all. Alcohol abuse leads to mental, emotional, physical, and social problems.

9. *Surround yourself with healthy friendships.* Unhealthy friendships contribute to destructive behaviors and low self-esteem. Associating with people who strive to maintain good fitness and health reinforces a positive outlook in life and encourages positive behaviors. Constructive social interactions enhance well-being. Researchers have also found that mortality rates are much higher among people who are socially isolated. People who aren't socially integrated are more likely to "give up when seriously ill"—which accelerates dying.

10. *Be informed about the environment.* Seek clean air, clean water, and a clean environment. Be aware of pollutants and occupational hazards: asbestos fibers, nickel dust, chromate, uranium dust, and so on. Take precautions when using pesticides and insecticides.

11. *Increase education.* Data indicates that people who are more educated live longer. The theory is that as education increases, so do the number of connections between nerve cells. The increased number of connections in turn help the individual make better survival (healthy lifestyle) choices.

12. *Take personal safety measures.* Although not all accidents are preventable, many are. Taking simple precautionary measures—such as using seat belts and keeping electrical appliances away from water—lessens the risk for avoidable accidents.

Unhealthy behaviors are contributing to the staggering U.S. health care costs. Risk factors for disease such as obesity and smoking carry a heavy price tag. Estimates also indicate that 1 percent of the people account for 30 percent of health care costs.[17] Half of the people use up about 97 percent of health-care dollars. Furthermore, the average health-care cost per person in the United States is almost twice as high as that in most other industrialized nations.

Scientific evidence now links participation in fitness and wellness programs not only to better health but also to lower medical costs and higher job productivity. As a result of the recent staggering rise in medical costs, many organizations are beginning to realize that keeping employees healthy costs less than treating them once they are sick.

A survey by the American Institute for Preventive Medicine found that large corporations are reaping health-cost savings by implementing health promotion programs.[18] Cost savings per dollar spent on health promotion programs ranged from $1.20 at the Adolph Coors Company to $6.00 at the Pontiac Division of General Motors.

Another reason some organizations are offering wellness programs to their employees—overlooked by many because it does not seem to affect the bottom line directly—is simply top management's concern for employees' physical well-being. Whether the program lowers medical costs is not the main issue; more important is that wellness programs help individuals feel better about themselves and improve their quality of life.

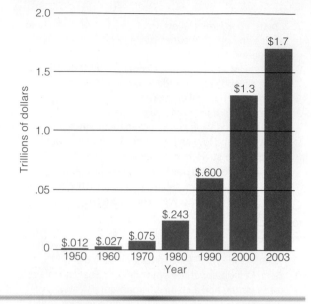

FIGURE 1.13 U.S. health care cost increments since 1950.

FIGURE 1.14 Estimated 1989 and 1997 health-care costs per person for selected countries.

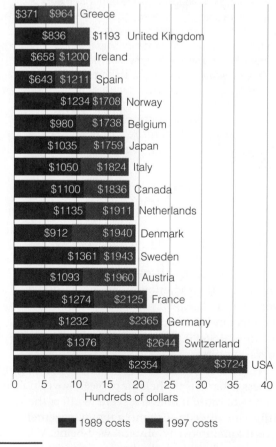

1989 costs   1997 costs

Sources: "Daten Der Woche," Welt am Sonntag 25 (1991): 35. World Health Organization, *The World Health Report 2000—Health Systems: Improving Performance* (2000): Annex Table 8.

The Wellness Challenge of the 21st Century

Because a better and healthier life is something every person should strive for, our biggest challenge as we begin the new century is to teach people how to take control of their personal health habits and adhere to a positive lifestyle. A wealth of information on the benefits of fitness and wellness programs indicates that improving the quality and possible length of our lives is a matter of personal choice.

Even though people in the United States believe a positive lifestyle has a great impact on health and longevity, most do not reap the benefits because they don't know how to implement a safe and effective fitness and wellness program. Others are exercising incorrectly and, therefore, are not reaping the full benefits of their program. How, then, can we meet the health challenges of the 21st century? That is the focus of this book—to provide the tools necessary to enable you to write, implement, and regularly update your personal lifetime fitness and wellness program.

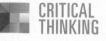

CRITICAL THINKING

What are your feelings about lifestyle habits that enhance health and longevity? How important are they to you? What obstacles keep you from adhering to such habits or incorporating new ones into your life?

National Health Objectives for the Year 2010

Every 10 years, the U.S. Department of Health and Human Services releases a list of objectives for preventing disease and promoting health. Since its initiation in 1980, this 10-year plan has helped to instill a new sense of purpose and focus for public health and preventive medicine. These national health objectives are intended to be realistic goals to improve the health of all Americans. Two unique goals of the 2010 objectives emphasize increased quality and years of healthy life and seek to eliminate health disparities among all groups of people (see Figure 1.15). The objectives address three important points:[19]

1. *Personal responsibility for health behavior*. Individuals need to become ever more health-conscious. Responsible and informed behavior is the key to good health.
2. *Health benefits for all people and all communities*. Lower socioeconomic conditions and poor health often are interrelated. Extending the benefits of good health to all people is crucial to the health of the nation.
3. *Health promotion and disease prevention*. A shift from treatment to preventive techniques will

drastically cut health care costs and help all Americans achieve a better quality of life.

Development of these health objectives typically involves more than 10,000 people representing 300 national organizations, including the Institute of Medicine of the National Academy of Sciences, all state health departments, and the federal Office of Disease Prevention and Health Promotion. A summary of key 2010 objectives is provided in Figure 1.16. Living the fitness and wellness principles provided in this book will enhance the quality of your life and also will allow you to be an active participant in achieving the Healthy People 2010 Objectives.

Wellness Education: Using this Book

Most people go to college to learn how to make a living, but a fitness and wellness course will teach you how to *live*—how to truly live life to its fullest potential. Some people seem to think that success is measured by how much money they make. Making a good living will not help you unless you live a wellness lifestyle that will allow you to enjoy what you earn.

Although everyone would like to enjoy good health and wellness, most people don't know how to reach this objective. Lifestyle is the most important factor affecting personal well-being. Granted, some people live long because of genetic factors, but quality of life during middle age and the "golden

FIGURE 1.15 National Health Objectives 2010: Healthy People in Healthy Communities.

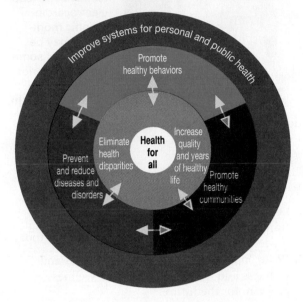

FIGURE 1.16 Selected Health Objectives for the Year 2010.

1. Increase quality and years of healthy life.
2. Eliminate health disparities.
3. Improve the health, fitness, and quality of life of all Americans through the adoption and maintenance of regular, daily physical activity.
4. Promote health and reduce chronic disease risk, disease progression, debilitation, and premature death associated with dietary factors and nutritional status among all people in the United States.
5. Reduce disease, disability, and death related to tobacco use and exposure to secondhand smoke.
6. Increase the quality, availability, and effectiveness of educational and community-based programs designed to prevent disease and improve the health and quality of life of the American people.
7. Promote health for all people through a healthy environment.
8. Reduce the incidence and severity of injuries from unintentional causes, as well as violence and abuse.
9. Promote worker health and safety through prevention.
10. Improve access to comprehensive, high quality health care.
11. Ensure that every pregnancy in the United States is intended.
12. Improve maternal and pregnancy outcomes and reduce rates of disability in infants.
13. Improve the quality of health-related decisions through effective communication.
14. Decrease the incidence of functional limitations due to arthritis, osteoporosis, and chronic back conditions.
15. Decrease cancer incidence, morbidity, and mortality.
16. Promote health and prevent secondary conditions among persons with disabilities.
17. Enhance the cardiovascular health and quality of life of all Americans through prevention and control of risk factors and promotion of healthy lifestyle behaviors.
18. Prevent HIV transmission and associated morbidity and mortality.
19. Improve the mental health of all Americans.
20. Raise the public's awareness of the signs and symptoms of lung disease.
21. Increase awareness of healthy sexual relationships and prevent all forms of sexually transmitted diseases.
22. Reduce the incidence of substance abuse by all people, especially children.

years" is more often related to wise choices initiated during youth and continued throughout life. In a few short years, lack of wellness can lead to a loss of vitality and gusto for life, as well as premature morbidity and mortality.

A Personalized Approach

Because fitness and wellness needs vary significantly from one individual to another, all exercise and wellness prescriptions must be personalized to obtain best results. The Wellness Lifestyle Questionnaire in Lab 1A will provide an initial rating of your current efforts to stay healthy and well. Subsequent chapters of this book and their respective laboratory experiences present the components of a wellness lifestyle and set forth the necessary guidelines that will allow you to develop a personal lifetime program that will improve your fitness and promote your own preventive health care and personal wellness.

The laboratory experiences have been prepared on tear-out sheets so they can be turned in to class instructors. As you study this book and complete the respective worksheets, you will learn to do the following:

- Implement motivational and behavior modification techniques that will help you adhere to a lifetime fitness and wellness program.
- Determine whether medical clearance is needed for your safe participation in exercise.
- Conduct nutritional analyses and follow the recommendations for adequate nutrition.
- Write sound diet and weight-control programs.
- Assess the health-related components of fitness (cardiorespiratory endurance, muscular strength and endurance, muscular flexibility, and body composition).
- Write exercise prescriptions for cardiorespiratory endurance, muscular strength and endurance, and muscular flexibility.
- Assess the skill-related components of fitness (agility, balance, coordination, power, reaction time, and speed).
- Understand the relationship between fitness and aging.
- Determine your levels of tension and stress, lessen your vulnerability to stress, and implement a stress management program, if necessary.
- Determine your potential risk for cardiovascular disease and implement a risk-reduction program.
- Follow a cancer risk-reduction program.
- Implement a smoking cessation program, if applicable.
- Avoid chemical dependency and know where to find assistance, if needed.

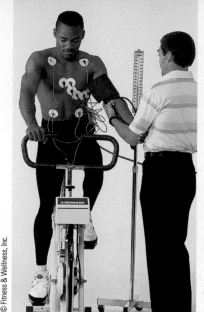

An exercise tolerance test (stress test) with 12-lead electrocardiographic monitoring may be required of some individuals prior to initiating an exercise program.

© Fitness & Wellness, Inc.

- Learn the health consequences of sexually transmitted diseases, including HIV/AIDS, and guidelines for preventing STDs.
- Write objectives to improve your fitness and wellness and learn how to chart a wellness program for the future.
- Differentiate myths and facts of exercise and health-related concepts.

Exercise Safety

Even though testing and participation in exercise are relatively safe for most apparently healthy individuals under age 45, the reaction of the cardiovascular system to higher levels of physical activity cannot be totally predicted.[20] Consequently, a small but real risk exists for exercise-induced abnormalities in people with a history of cardiovascular problems and those who are at higher risk for disease. These include abnormal blood pressure, irregular heart rhythm, fainting, and, in rare instances, a heart attack or cardiac arrest.

Before you start to engage in an exercise program or participate in any exercise testing, you should fill out the questionnaire in Lab 1B. If your answer to any of the questions is yes, you should see a physician before participating in a fitness program. Exercise testing and participation is not wise under some of the conditions listed in Lab 1B and may require a medical evaluation, including a stress electrocardiogram (ECG) test. If you have any questions regarding your current health status, consult your doctor before initiating, continuing, or increasing your level of physical activity.

Resting Heart Rate and Blood Pressure Assessment

In Lab 1C you will learn how to determine your heart rate and blood pressure. Heart rate can be obtained by counting your pulse either on the wrist over the radial artery or over the carotid artery in the neck (see Chapter 6, page 167).

You may count your pulse for 30 seconds and multiply by 2 or take it for a full minute. The heart rate usually is at its lowest point (resting heart rate) late in the evening after you have been sitting quietly for about half an hour watching a relaxing TV show or reading in bed, or early in the morning just before you get out of bed.

Unless you have a pathological condition, a lower resting heart rate indicates a stronger heart. To adapt to cardiorespiratory or aerobic exercise, blood volume increases, the heart enlarges, and the muscle gets stronger. A stronger heart can pump more blood with fewer strokes.

Resting heart rate ratings are given in Table 1.2. Although resting heart rate decreases with training, the extent of **bradycardia** depends not only on the amount of training but also on genetic factors. Although most highly trained athletes have a resting heart rate around 40 beats per minute, occasionally, one of these athletes has a resting heart rate in the 60s or 70s even during peak training months of the season. For most individuals, however, the resting heart rate decreases as the level of cardiorespiratory endurance increases.

Blood pressure is assessed using a **sphygmomanometer** and a stethoscope. Use a cuff of the appropriate size to get accurate readings. Size is determined by the width of the inflatable bladder, which should be about 40 percent of the circumference of the midpoint of the arm.

Blood pressure usually is measured while the person is in the sitting position, with the forearm and the manometer at the same level as the heart. At first, the pressure is recorded from each arm, and after that from the arm with the highest reading.

The cuff should be applied approximately an inch above the antecubital space (natural crease of the elbow), with the center of the bladder directly over the medial (inner) surface of the arm. The stethoscope head should be applied firmly, but with little pressure, over the brachial artery in the antecubital space. The arm should be flexed slightly and placed on a flat surface.

To determine how high the cuff should be inflated, the person recording the blood pressure monitors the subject's radial pulse with one hand, and with the other hand inflates the manometer's bladder to about 30 to 40 mm Hg above the point at which the feeling of the pulse in the wrist disappears.

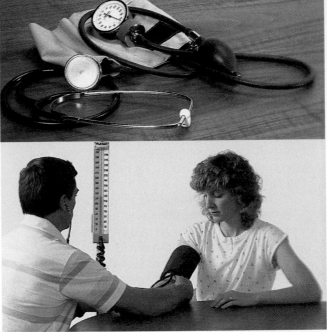

A mercury gravity manometer can be used to measure blood pressure.

TABLE 1.2 Resting Heart Rate Ratings

Heart Rate (beats/minute)	Rating
≤59	Excellent
60–69	Good
70–79	Average
80–89	Fair
≥90	Poor

Next, the pressure is released, followed by a wait of about one minute, and then the bladder is inflated to the predetermined level to take the blood pressure reading. The cuff should not be overinflated, as this may cause blood vessel spasm, resulting in higher blood pressure readings. The pressure should be released at a rate of 2 to 4 mm Hg per second.

As the pressure is released, **systolic blood pressure** is recorded as the point where the sound of the pulse becomes audible. The **diastolic blood**

Bradycardia Slower heart rate than normal.

Sphygmomanometer Inflatable bladder contained within a cuff and a mercury gravity manometer (or aneroid manometer) from which the pressure is read.

Systolic blood pressure Pressure exerted by blood against walls of arteries during forceful contraction (systole) of the heart.

Diastolic blood pressure Pressure exerted by the blood against the walls of the arteries during the relaxation phase (diastole) of the heart.

pressure is the point where the sound disappears. The recordings should be expressed as systolic over diastolic pressure—for example, 124/80.

If you take more than one reading, be sure the bladder is completely deflated between readings and allow at least a full minute should before making the next recording. The person measuring the pressure also should note whether the pressure was recorded from the left or the right arm. Resting blood pressure ratings are given in Table 1.3.

In some cases the pulse sounds become less intense (point of muffling sounds) but still can be heard at a lower pressure (50 or 40 mm Hg) or even all the way down to zero. In this situation the diastolic pressure is recorded at the point of a clear, definite change in the loudness of the sound (also referred to as fourth phase), and at complete disappearance of the sound (fifth phase) (for example, 120/78/60 or 120/82/0).

TABLE 1.3 Blood Pressure Guidelines (expressed in mm Hg)

Rating	Systolic	Diastolic
Normal	≤120	≤80
Prehypertension	120–139	80–89
Hypertension	≥140	≥90

Source: National Heart, Lung and Blood Institute.

To establish the real values for resting blood pressure, have different people take readings at different times of the day. A single reading may not be an accurate value because of the various factors that can affect blood pressure.

Profile Plus

Evaluate how well you understand the concepts presented in this chapter using the "Assess Your Knowledge" and "Practice Quizzes" options on your CD-ROM.

ASSESS YOUR KNOWLEDGE

1. Bodily movement produced by skeletal muscles is called
   a. physical activity.
   b. kinesiology.
   c. exercise.
   d. aerobic exercise.
   e. muscle strength.

2. Most people in the United States
   a. get adequate physical activity on a regular basis.
   b. meet health-related fitness standards.
   c. regularly participate in skill-related activities.
   d. Choices a, b, and c are correct.
   e. do not get sufficient physical activity to maintain good health.

3. The constant and deliberate effort to stay healthy and achieve the highest potential for well-being is defined as
   a. health.
   b. physical fitness.
   c. wellness.
   d. health-related fitness.
   e. metabolic fitness.

4. The ability to understand your own feelings and accept your limitations is known as
   a. mental wellness.
   b. social wellness.
   c. intellectual wellness.
   d. spiritual wellness.
   e. emotional wellness.

5. Research on the effects of fitness on mortality indicates that the largest drop in premature mortality is seen between
   a. the average and excellent fitness groups.
   b. the least fit and moderately fit groups.
   c. the good and high fitness groups.
   d. the moderately fit and good fitness groups.
   e. the drop is similar between all fitness groups.

6. Which of the following is *not* a component of health-related fitness?
   a. cardiorespiratory endurance
   b. body composition
   c. agility
   d. muscular strength and endurance
   e. muscular flexibility

7. Metabolic fitness can be achieved
   a. with an active lifestyle and moderate physical activity.
   b. through a high-intensity speed-training program.
   c. through an increased basal metabolic rate.
   d. with anaerobic training.
   e. through an increase in lean body mass.

8. The leading cause of death in the United States is
   a. cancer.
   b. accidents.
   c. CLRD.
   d. diseases of the cardiovascular system.
   e. drug-related deaths.

9. During the last decade, health care costs in the United States
   a. have decreased.
   b. have stayed about the same.
   c. have continued to increase.
   d. have increased in some years and decreased in others.
   e. are unknown.

10. What is the greatest benefit of being physically fit?
   a. absence of disease
   b. a higher quality of life
   c. improved sports performance
   d. better personal appearance
   e. maintenance of ideal body weight

Correct answers can be found at the back of the book.

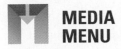

MEDIA MENU

PROFILE PLUS CD CONNECTIONS

■ Chronicle your daily activities using the exercise log.

■ Determine the safety of exercise participation.

■ Check how well you understand the chapter's concepts.

INTERNET CONNECTIONS

■ Healthy People 2010. Healthy People, a national health promotion and disease prevention initiative, lists national goals for improving health of all Americans by the year 2010.

http://www.health.gov/healthypeople

■ The National Association for Health and Fitness (NAHF). This non-profit organization promotes physical fitness, sports, and healthy lifestyles; it fosters and supports governors' and state councils on physical fitness and sports in every state and U.S. territory. NAHF is also the national sponsor of the largest U.S. worksite health and fitness event: "Let's Get Physical" (the national fitness challenge), and "Make Your Move!" (an incentive-based health promotion campaign).

http://www.physicalfitness.org

■ Aerobics and Fitness Association of America: This interactive site features Exercise Gets Personal™ where you can create a customized exercise program that includes activities you select, geared to your current level of fitness activity. Exercises include aerobics, muscular conditioning, and flexibility with descriptions and precautions for each activity.

http://www.aerobics.com

■ Lifescan Health Risk Appraisal. This site was created by Bill Hettler, M.D., of the National Wellness Institute and features questions to help you identify the specific lifestyle factors that can impair your health and longevity.

http://wellness.uwsp.edu/other/lifescan/index.htm

Notes

1. A. H. Mokdad, J. S. Marks, D. F. Stroup, and J. L. Gerberding, "Actual Causes of Death in the United States, 2000," *Journal of the American Medical Association* 291 (2004): 1238–1241.

2. Frank Booth, et al., "Physiologists Claim 'SeDS' Is Second Greatest Threat to U.S. Public Health," *Medical Letter on CDC & FDA*, June 24, 2001.

3. U.S. Department of Health and Human Services, Centers for Disease Control and Prevention, National Center for Health Statistics, *National Vital Statistics Reports: Deaths, Final Data for 2002* 53, no. 5 (October 12, 2004).

4. Heart Disease and Stroke Statistics—2004 Update (Dallas: American Heart Association, 2003).

5. American Cancer Society, 2004 *Cancer Facts and Figures* (New York: ACS, 2004).

6. N. Schachter, "Lung Disease Can Affect All Adults," *Bottom Line/Health* 17 (May 2003): 13–14.

7. T. A. Murphy and D. Murphy, *The Wellness for Life Workbook* (San Diego: Fitness Publications, 1987).

8. U.S. Department of Health and Human Services, *Physical Activity and Health: A Report of the Surgeon General* (Atlanta: Centers for Disease Control and Prevention, National Center for Chronic Disease Prevention and Health Promotion, 1996).

9. National Academy of Sciences, Institute of Medicine, *Dietary Reference Intakes for Energy, Carbohydrates, Fiber, Fat, Protein and Amino Acids (Macronutrients).* (Washington, DC: National Academy Press, 2002).

10. L. Sax, et al., *The American Freshman: National Norms for Fall 2000* (Los Angeles: UCLA, Higher Education Research Institute, 2000).

11. H. G. Koenig, "The Healing Power of Faith," *Bottom Line/Health* 18 (May 2004): 3–4.

12. L. Dossey, "Can Spirituality Improve Your Health?" *Bottom Line/Health* 15 (July 2001): 11–13.

13. R. S. Paffenbarger, Jr., R. T. Hyde, A. L. Wing, and C. H. Steinmetz, "A Natural History of Athleticism and Cardiovascular Health," *Journal of the American Medical Association* 252 (1984): 491–495.

14. S. N. Blair, H. W. Kohl III, R. S. Paffenbarger, Jr., D. G. Clark, K. H. Cooper, and L. W. Gibbons, "Physical Fitness and All-Cause Mortality: A Prospective Study of Healthy Men and Women," *Journal of the American Medical Association* 262 (1989): 2395–2401.

15. S. N. Blair, H. W. Kohl III, C. E. Barlow, R. S. Paffenbarger, Jr., L. W. Gibbons, and C. A. Macera, "Changes in Physical Fitness and All-Cause Mortality: A Prospective Study of Healthy and Unhealthy Men," *Journal of the American Medical Association* 273 (1995): 1193–1198.

16. J. E. Enstrom, "Health Practices and Cancer Mortality Among Active California Mormons," *Journal of the National Cancer Institute* 81 (1989): 1807–1814.

17. "Wellness Facts," *University of California at Berkeley Wellness Letter* (Palm Coast, FL: The Editors, April 1995).

18. Robert C. Chadbourne, "Fit for Hire," *Fitness Management* 12, no. 2 (1996): 28–30.

19. U.S. Department of Health and Human Services, *Healthy People 2010* (Washington DC: U.S. Government Printing Office, November 2000).

20. American College of Sports Medicine, *Guidelines for Exercise Testing and Prescription* (Baltimore: Williams & Wilkins, 2000).

Suggested Readings

American College of Sports Medicine. ACSM Fit Society Page. http://acsm.org/health+fitness/fit_society.htm.

Blair, S. N., et al. "Influences of Cardiorespiratory Fitness and Other Precursors on Cardiovascular Disease and All-cause Mortality in Men and Women." *Journal of the American Medical Association* 276 (1996): 205–210.

Booth, F. W., and B. S. Tseng. "America Needs to Exercise for Health." *Medicine and Science in Sports and Exercise* 27 (1995): 462–465.

Hales, D. *An Invitation to Health*. Belmont, CA: Wadsworth/ Thomson Learning, 2003.

Hoeger, W. W. K., L. W. Turner, and B. Q. Hafen. *Wellness: Guidelines for a Healthy Lifestyle*. Belmont, CA: Wadsworth/ Thomson Learning, 2002.

National Academy of Sciences, Institute of Medicine. *Dietary Reference Intakes for Energy, Carbohydrates, Fiber, Fat, Protein and Amino Acids (Macronutrients)*. Washington, DC: National Academy Press, 2002.

Nieman, D. C. *The Exercise-Health Connection*. Champaign, IL: Human Kinetics, 1998.

Pate, R., et al. "Physical Activity and Public Health: A Recommendation from the Centers for Disease Control and Prevention and the American College of Sports Medicine." *Journal of the American Medical Association* 273 (1995): 402–407.

U.S. Department of Health and Human Services, *Physical Activity and Health: A Report of the Surgeon General*. Atlanta: Centers for Disease Control and Prevention, National Center for Chronic Disease Prevention and Health Promotion, 1996.

U.S. Department of Health and Human Services, Public Health Service, *Healthy People 2010: Conference Edition*. (http://www.health.gov/healthypeople/Document/ tableofcontents.htm).

Lab 1A

WELLNESS LIFESTYLE QUESTIONNAIRE

Name:		Date:		Grade:	
Instructor:		Course:		Section:	

Necessary Lab Equipment
None.

Objective
To analyze current lifestyle habits and help determine changes necessary for future health and wellness.

Instructions
Check the appropriate answer to each question and obtain a final score according to the guidelines provided at the end of the questionnaire.

	Always	Nearly always	Often	Seldom	Never
1. I participate in vigorous aerobic activity for 20 minutes on three or more days per week, and I accumulate at least 30 minutes of moderate intensity physical activity on a minimum of three additional days per week.	5	4	3	2	1
2. I participate in strength training exercises, using a minimum of eight different exercises, two or more days per week.	5	4	3	2	1
3. I perform flexibility exercises a minimum of three days per week.	5	4	3	2	1
4. I maintain recommended body weight (includes avoidance of excessive body fat, excessive thinness, or frequent fluctuations in body weight).	5	4	3	2	1
5. Every day, I eat three regular meals that include a wide variety of foods.	5	4	3	2	1
6. I limit the amount of fat and saturated fat in my diet on most days of the week.	5	4	3	2	1
7. I eat a minimum of five servings of fruits and vegetables and six servings from grain products on a daily basis.	5	4	3	2	1
8. I regularly avoid snacks, especially those that are high in calories and fat and low in nutrients and fiber.	5	4	3	2	1
9. I avoid cigarettes or tobacco in any other form.	5	4	3	2	1
10. I avoid alcoholic beverages. If I drink, I do so in moderation (one daily drink for women and two for men), and I do not combine alcohol with other drugs.	5	4	3	2	1
11. I avoid addictive drugs or needles that have been used by others.	5	4	3	2	1
12. I use prescription drugs and over-the-counter drugs sparingly, only when needed, and I follow all directions for their proper use.	5	4	3	2	1
13. I readily recognize when I am under excessive tension and stress (distress).	5	4	3	2	1
14. I am able to perform effective stress management techniques.	5	4	3	2	1
15. I have close friends and relatives that I can discuss personal problems with and approach for help when needed, and with whom I can express my feelings freely.	5	4	3	2	1
16. I spend most of my daily leisure time in wholesome recreational activities.	5	4	3	2	1
17. I sleep 7 to 8 hours each night.	5	4	3	2	1
18. I floss my teeth every day and brush them at least twice daily.	5	4	3	2	1
19. I avoid overexposure to the sun, and I use sunscreen and appropriate clothing when I am out in the sun for extended periods of time.	5	4	3	2	1
20. I avoid using products that have not been shown by science to be safe and effective (this includes anabolic steroids and unproven nutrient or weight loss supplements).	5	4	3	2	1
21. I stay current with the warning signs for heart attack, stroke, and cancer.	5	4	3	2	1

22. I practice monthly breast/testicle self-exams, get recommended screening tests (blood lipids, blood pressure, Pap tests), and seek a medical evaluation when I am not well or disease symptoms arise.   [5] [4] [3] [2] [1]

23. I have a dental checkup at least once a year, and I get regular medical exams according to age recommendations.   [5] [4] [3] [2] [1]

24. I am not sexually active / I practice safe sex.   [5] [4] [3] [2] [1]

25. I can effectively deal with disappointments and temporary feelings of sadness, loneliness, and depression. If I am unable to deal with these feelings, I seek professional help.   [5] [4] [3] [2] [1]

26. I can work out emotional problems without turning to alcohol or other drugs.   [5] [4] [3] [2] [1]

27. I associate with people who have a positive attitude about life.   [5] [4] [3] [2] [1]

28. I respond to temporary setbacks by making the best of the circumstances and by moving ahead with optimism and energy. I do not spend time and talent worrying about failures.   [5] [4] [3] [2] [1]

29. I wear a seat belt whenever I am in a car, I ask others in my vehicle to do the same, and I make sure that children are in an infant seat or wear a shoulder harness.   [5] [4] [3] [2] [1]

30. I do not drive under the influence of alcohol or other drugs, and I make an effort to keep others from doing the same.   [5] [4] [3] [2] [1]

31. I avoid being alone in public places, especially after dark; I seek escorts when I visit or exercise in unfamiliar places.   [5] [4] [3] [2] [1]

32. I seek to make my living quarters accident-free, and I keep doors and windows locked, especially when home alone.   [5] [4] [3] [2] [1]

33. I try to minimize environmental pollutants, and I support community efforts to minimize pollution.   [5] [4] [3] [2] [1]

34. I keep my living quarters clean and organized.   [5] [4] [3] [2] [1]

35. I study and/or work in a clean environment (including avoidance of second-hand smoke).   [5] [4] [3] [2] [1]

36. I participate in recycling programs for paper, cardboard, glass, plastic, and aluminum.   [5] [4] [3] [2] [1]

How to Score

Enter the score you have circled for each question in the spaces provided below. Next, total the score for each specific wellness lifestyle category and obtain a rating for each category according to the criteria provided below.

Health-Related Fitness	Nutrition	Avoiding Chemical Dependency	Stress Management	Personal Hygiene/Health	Disease Prevention	Emotional Well-being	Personal Safety	Environmental Health & Protection
1.	5.	9.	13.	17.	21.	25.	29.	33.
2.	6.	10.	14.	18.	22.	26.	30.	34.
3.	7.	11.	15.	19.	23.	27.	31.	35.
4.	8.	12.	16.	20.	24.	28.	32.	36.
Total:								
Rating:								

Category Rating

Excellent (E) = ≥17 Your answers show that you are aware of the importance of this category to your health and wellness. You are putting your knowledge to work for you by practicing good habits. As long as you continue to do so, this category should not pose a health risk. You are also setting a good example for family and friends to follow. Because you got a very high test score on this part of the test, you may want to consider other categories where your score indicates room for improvement.

Good (G) = 13–16 Your health practices in this area are good, but there is room for improvement. Look again at the items you answered with a 4 or below and identify changes that you can make to improve your lifestyle. Even small changes can often help you achieve better health.

Needs Improvement (NI) ≤12 Your health risks are showing. You may be taking serious and unnecessary risks with your health. Perhaps you are not aware of the risks and what to do about them. Most likely you need additional information and help in deciding how to successfully make the changes you desire. You can easily get the information that you need to improve, if you wish. The next step is up to you.

Please note that no final overall rating is provided for the entire questionnaire, because it may not be indicative of overall wellness. For example, an excellent rating in most categories will not offset the immediate health risks and life-threatening consequences of using addictive drugs or not wearing a seat belt.

Lab 1B

CLEARANCE FOR EXERCISE PARTICIPATION

Name: _____   Date: _____   Grade: _____

Instructor: _____   Course: _____   Section: _____

Necessary Lab Equipment
None.

Objective
To determine the safety of exercise participation.

Introduction
Although exercise testing and exercise participation are relatively safe for most apparently healthy individuals under the age of 45, the reaction of the cardiovascular system to increased levels of physical activity cannot always be totally predicted. Consequently, there is a small but real risk of certain changes occurring during exercise testing and participation. Some of these changes may be abnormal blood pressure, irregular heart rhythm, fainting, and in rare instances a heart attack or cardiac arrest. Therefore, you must provide honest answers to this questionnaire. Exercise may be contraindicated under some of the conditions listed below; others may simply require special consideration. **If any of the conditions apply, consult your physician before you participate in an exercise program.** Also, promptly report to your instructor any exercise-related abnormalities that you may experience during the course of the semester.

A. Have you ever had or do you now have any of the following conditions?

☐ 1. A myocardial infarction.

☐ 2. Coronary artery disease.

☐ 3. Congestive heart failure.

☐ 4. Elevated blood lipids (cholesterol and triglycerides).

☐ 5. Chest pain at rest or during exertion.

☐ 6. Shortness of breath.

☐ 7. An abnormal resting or stress electrocardiogram.

☐ 8. Uneven, irregular, or skipped heartbeats (including a racing or fluttering heart).

☐ 9. A blood embolism.

☐ 10. Thrombophlebitis.

☐ 11. Rheumatic heart fever.

☐ 12. Elevated blood pressure.

☐ 13. A stroke.

☐ 14. Diabetes.

☐ 15. A family history of coronary heart disease, syncope, or sudden death before age 60.

☐ 16. Any other heart problem that makes exercise unsafe.

B. Do you have any of the following conditions?

☐ 1. Arthritis, rheumatism, or gout.

☐ 2. Chronic low-back pain.

☐ 3. Any other joint, bone, or muscle problems.

☐ 4. Any respiratory problems.

☐ 5. Obesity (more than 30 percent overweight).

☐ 6. Anorexia.

☐ 7. Bulimia.

☐ 8. Mononucleosis.

☐ 9. Any physical disability that could interfere with safe participation in exercise.

C. Do any of the following conditions apply?

☐ 1. Do you smoke cigarettes?

☐ 2. Are you taking any prescription drug?

☐ 3. Are you 45 years or older?

D. Do you have any other concern regarding your ability to safely participate in an exercise program? If so, explain:

_____

_____

Student's Signature: _____   Date: _____

Personal Challenge

In your own words, indicate what the Wellness Lifestyle Questionnaire in Lab 1A tells you about your current state of wellness. Also, identify categories where you can personally make changes in the next few months and indicate what may help you accomplish your goals.

Lab 1A suggests that _____

_____

_____

_____

I can make these changes in the next few months: _____

_____

_____

_____

The following could help me accomplish my goals: _____

_____

_____

_____

_____

Do you feel that it is safe for you to proceed with an exercise program? Explain any concerns or limitations that you may have regarding your safe participation in a comprehensive exercise program that will target cardiorespiratory endurance, muscular strength, muscular flexibility, and weight management.

I believe ☐ it is ☐ is not safe for me to exercise. I have the following concerns or limitations: _____

_____

_____

_____

_____

_____

Lab 1C

RESTING HEART RATE AND BLOOD PRESSURE ASSESSMENT

Name:		Date:		Grade:	
Instructor:		Course:		Section:	

Necessary Lab Equipment
Stopwatches, stethoscopes, and blood pressure sphygmomanometers.

Objective
To determine resting heart rate and blood pressure.

Preparation
The instructions to determine heart rate and blood pressure are given on pages 19–20. Many factors can affect heart rate and blood pressure. Factors such as excitement, nervousness, stress, food, smoking, pain, temperature, and physical exertion all can alter heart rate and blood pressure significantly. Therefore, whenever possible, readings should be taken in a quiet, comfortable room following a few minutes of rest in the recording position. Avoid any form of exercise several hours prior to the assessment. Wear exercise clothing, including a shirt with short or loose-fitting sleeves to allow for placement of the blood pressure cuff around the upper arm.

I. Resting Heart Rate and Blood Pressure

Determine your resting heart rate and blood pressure in the right and left arms while sitting comfortably in a chair.

Resting Heart Rate: [____] bpm   Rating (see Table 1.2, page 19): [____]

Blood Pressure:	Right Arm	Rating (from Table 1.3, page 20)	Left Arm	Rating (from Table 1.3, page 20)
Systolic				
Diastolic				

II. Standing, Walking, Jogging Heart Rate and Blood Pressure

Have one individual measure your heart rate and another individual your blood pressure immediately after standing for one minute, after walking for one minute, and after jogging in place for one minute. For blood pressure assessment use the arm that showed the highest reading in the sitting position (in Part I, above).

Activity	Heart Rate (bpm)	Systolic/Diastolic Blood Pressure (mm Hg)	
Standing			/
Walking			/
Jogging			/

III. Effects of Aerobic Activity on Resting Heart Rate

Using your actual resting heart rate (RHR) from Part I of this lab, compute the total number of times your heart beats each day and each year:

A. Beats per day = _____ (RHR bpm) × 60 (min per hour) × 24 (hours per day) = _____ beats per day

B. Beats per year = _____ (heart rate in beats per day, use item A) × 365 = _____ beats per year

If your RHR dropped 20 bpm through an aerobic exercise program, determine the number of beats that your heart would save each year at that lower RHR:

C. Beats per day = _____ (RHR, use your current RHR) − 20 × 60 × 24 = _____ beats per day

D. Beats per year = _____ (heart rate in beats per day, use item C) × 365 = _____ beats per year

E. Number of beats saved per year (B − D) = _____ − _____ = _____ beats saved per year

Assuming that you will reach the average U.S. life expectancy of 80 years for women or 73 for men, determine the additional number of "heart rate life years" available to you if your RHR was 20 bpm lower:

F. Years of life ahead = _____ (use 80 for women and 73 for men) − _____ (current age) = _____ years

G. Number of beats saved = _____ (use item E) × _____ (use item F) = _____ beats saved

H. Number of heart rate life years based on the lower RHR = _____ (use item G) ÷ _____ (use item D) = _____ years

IV. Mean Blood Pressure Computation

During a normal resting contraction/relaxation cycle of the heart, the heart spends more time in the relaxation (diastolic) phase than in the contraction (systolic) phase. Accordingly, mean blood pressure (MBP) cannot be computed by taking an average of the systolic (SBP) and diastolic (DBP) blood pressures. The following equations are, therefore, used to determine MBP:

MBP = DBP + ⅓ PP   Where PP = pulse pressure or the difference between the systolic and diastolic pressures.

A. Compute your MBP using your own blood pressure results:

PP = _____ (systolic) − _____ (diastolic) = _____ mm Hg

MBP = _____ (DBP) + $\dfrac{\text{(PP)}}{3}$ = _____ mm Hg

B. Determine the MBP for a person with a BP of 130/80 and a second person with a BP of 120/90.

130/80

120/90

Which subject has the lower MBP? _____

V. What I Learned

Draw conclusions based on your observed resting and activity heart rates and blood pressures. Discuss the importance of a lower resting heart rate to your health and comment on the effects of a higher systolic versus diastolic blood pressure on the mean arterial blood pressure.

Behavior Modification

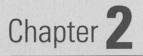

Objectives

- Learn the effects of environment on human behavior.
- Understand obstacles that hinder the ability to change behavior.
- Explain the concepts of motivation and locus of control.
- Identify the stages of change.
- Describe the processes of change.
- Explain techniques that will facilitate the process of change.
- Describe the role of SMART goal setting in the process of change.
- Be able to write specific objectives for behavioral change.

Profile Plus CD Connections

- Prepare for a healthy change in lifestyle.
- Check how well you understand the chapter's concepts.

Research studies during the last three decades have convincingly documented the benefits of physical activity and healthy lifestyles. Although 97 percent of Americans accept that exercise is beneficial to health and see a need to incorporate it into their lives,[1] 70 percent of new and returning exercisers are at risk for early dropout.[2] And, although the scientific evidence continues to mount each day and the data are impressive, most people still do not adhere to a healthy lifestyle program.

Let's look at an all-too-common occurrence on college campuses. Most students understand that they should be exercising and they contemplate enrolling in a fitness course. The motivating factor might be enhanced physical appearance, health benefits, or simply fulfillment of a college requirement. They sign up for the course, participate for a few months, finish the course—and stop exercising! A wide array of excuses are offered: too busy, no one to exercise with, already have the grade, inconvenient open-gym hours, or job conflicts. A few months later they realize once again that exercise is vital and repeat the cycle (see Figure 2.1).

The information in this book will be of little value to you if you are unable to abandon negative habits and adopt and maintain new, healthy behaviors. Before looking at physical fitness and wellness guidelines, you will need to take a critical look at your behaviors and lifestyle—and most likely make some permanent changes to promote your overall health and wellness.

The science of behavioral therapy has established that most of the behaviors we adopt are a product of our environment—the forces of social influences we encounter and the thought processes we go through. This environment includes family, friends, peers, homes, schools, workplaces, television, radio, and movies, as well as our communities, country, and culture in general.

Unfortunately, when it comes to fitness and wellness, we live in a "toxic environment." From a young age, we are transported by parents, relatives, and friends who drive us nearly any place we need to go. We also watch them drive short distances to run errands. We see them take escalators and elevators and ride moving sidewalks at malls and airports. We notice that they use remote controls, pagers, and cell phones. We observe as they stop at fast-food restaurants and pick up super-sized, calorie-dense, high-fat meals. They watch television and surf the Net for hours at a time. Some smoke, some drink heavily, and some have hard-drug addictions. Others engage in risky behaviors by not wearing seat belts, drinking and driving, and having unprotected sex. All of these unhealthy habits can be passed along, unquestioned, to the next generation.

Even modern-day architecture reinforces unhealthy behaviors, and elevators and escalators are

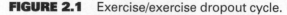

FIGURE 2.1 Exercise/exercise dropout cycle.

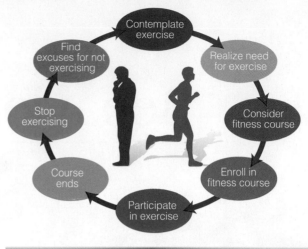

often of the finest workmanship and located in convenient places. Many of our newest, showiest shopping centers and convention centers don't provide accessible stairwells, so people are all but forced to ride escalators. If they want to walk up the escalator, they can't because the people in front of them obstruct the way. Entrances to buildings provide electric sensors and automatic door openers. Without a second thought, people walk through automatic doors instead of taking the time to push a door open.

Walking, jogging, and bicycle trails are too sparse in our cities, further discouraging physical activity. Places for safe exercise are hard to find in many metropolitan areas, motivating many people to remain indoors during leisure hours for fear of endangering their personal safety and well-being.

Food portions in restaurants have substantially increased in size. Patrons consume huge amounts of food, almost as if this were the last meal they will ever have. They drink entire pitchers of soda pop or beer instead of the traditional 8-ounce cup size. Most restaurants are colorful, well-lit, and nicely decorated to enhance comfort and appetite and increase the length of stay to entice more eating.

All of these examples influence our thought process and hinder our ability to be physically active and adopt healthy behaviors. From childhood through young adulthood, we observe, we learn, we emulate, and gradually, without realizing it, we incorporate many of these unhealthy behaviors into our personal lifestyle.

Let's look at weight gain. Most people do not start life with a weight problem. By age 20, a man may weigh 160 pounds. A few years later, the weight starts to climb and may reach 170 pounds. He now adapts and accepts 170 pounds as his weight.

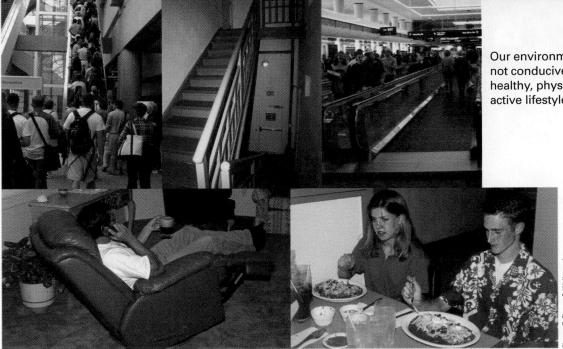

Our environment is not conducive to a healthy, physically active lifestyle.

He may go on a diet but not make the necessary lifestyle changes. Gradually his weight climbs to 180, 190, 200 pounds. Although he may not like it and would like to weigh less, once again he adapts and accepts 200 pounds as his stable weight.

The time comes, usually around middle age, when most people want to make changes in their lives but find this difficult to accomplish, illustrating the adage that "old habits die hard." Acquiring positive behaviors that will lead to better health and well-being is a long-lasting process and requires continual effort. Understanding why so many people are unsuccessful at changing their behaviors and are unable to live a healthy lifestyle may increase your readiness and motivation for change. Next we will examine barriers to change, what motivates people to change, the various stages of change, the process of change, techniques for change, and actions required to make permanent changes in behavior.

Barriers to Change

In spite of the best intentions, people make unhealthy choices daily. The most common reasons are:

1. **Procrastination.** People seem to think that tomorrow, next week, or after the holiday is the best time to start change.

    Tip to initiate change. Ask yourself: Why wait until tomorrow when you can start changing today? Lack of motivation is a key factor in procrastination (motivation is discussed on pages 33–34).

2. **Preconditioned cultural beliefs.** If we accept the principle that we are a product of our environment, our cultural beliefs and our physical surroundings pose significant barriers to change. In Salzburg, Austria, people of both genders and all ages use bicycles as a primary mode of transportation. In the United States, few people other than children ride bicycles.

    Tip to initiate change. Find a like-minded partner. In the pre-Columbian era, people thought the world was flat. Few dared to sail long distances for fear that they would fall off the edge. If your health and fitness are at stake, preconditioned cultural beliefs shouldn't keep you from making changes. Finding people who are willing to "sail" with you will help overcome this barrier.

3. **Gratification.** People prefer instant gratification to long-term benefits. Therefore, they will overeat (instant pleasure) instead of using self-restraint to eat moderately to prevent weight gain (long-term satisfaction). We like tanning (instant gratification) and avoid paying much attention to skin cancer (long-term consequence).

    Tip to initiate change. Think ahead and ask yourself the following questions: How did you feel the last time you engaged in this behavior? How did it affect you? Did you really feel good about yourself or about the results? In retrospect, was it worth it?

4. **Risk complacency.** Consequences of unhealthy behaviors often don't manifest themselves until years later. People tell themselves, "If I get heart disease, I'll deal with it then. For now, let me eat, drink, and be merry."

    Tip to initiate change. Ask yourself these questions: How long do you want to live? How do you want to live the rest of your life and

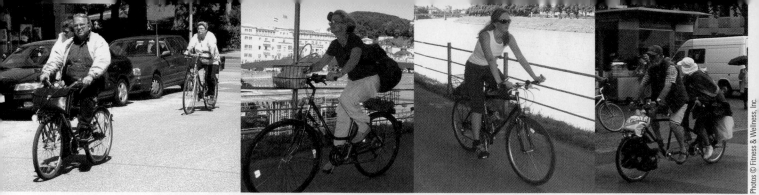

Bicycles are the preferred mode of transportation for local residents in many European cities.

what type of health do you want to have? What do you want to be able to do when you are 60, 70, or 80 years old?

5. **Complexity.** People think the world is too complicated, with too much to think about. If you are living the typical lifestyle, you may feel overwhelmed by everything that seems to be required to lead a healthy lifestyle, for example:

- Getting exercise
- Decreasing saturated fat intake
- Eating high-fiber meals and cutting total calories
- Controlling use of substances
- Managing stress
- Wearing seat belts
- Practicing safe sex
- Getting annual physicals, including blood tests, Pap smears, and so on
- Fostering spiritual, social, and emotional wellness

Tip to initiate change. Take it one step at a time. Work on only one or two behaviors at a time so the task won't seem insurmountable.

6. **Indifference and helplessness.** A defeatist thought process often takes over, and we may believe that the way we live won't really affect our health, that we have no control over our health, or that our destiny is all in our genes (also see discussion of locus of control, pages 33–34).

Tip to initiate change. As much as 84 percent of the leading causes of death in the United States are preventable. Realize that only you can take control over your personal health and lifestyle habits and affect the quality of your life. Implementing many of the behavioral modification strategies and programs outlined in this book will get you started on a wellness way of life.

7. **Rationalization.** Even though people are not practicing healthy behaviors, they often tell themselves that they do get sufficient exercise, that their diet is fine, that they have good solid relationships, or that they really don't smoke/drink/get high enough to affect their health.

Tip to initiate change. Learn to recognize when you're glossing over or minimizing a problem. You'll need to face the fact that you have a problem before you can really commit to change. Your health and your life are at stake. Monitoring lifestyle habits through daily logs and then analyzing the results can help you make necessary changes in self-defeating behaviors.

8. **Illusions of invincibility.** At times people believe that unhealthy behaviors will not harm them. Young adults often have the attitude that "I can smoke now, and in a few years I'll quit before it causes any damage." Unfortunately, nicotine is one of the most addictive drugs known to us, so quitting smoking is not an easy task. Health problems may arise before you quit, and the risk of lung cancer lingers for years after you quit. Another example is drinking and driving. The feeling of "I'm in control" or "I can handle it" while under the influence is a deadly combination.

Others perceive low risk when engaging in negative behaviors with people they like (for example, sex with someone you've recently met and feel attracted to) but perceive themselves at risk just by being in the same classroom with an HIV-infected person.

Tip to initiate change. No one is immune to sickness, disease, and tragedy. The younger you are when you implement a healthy lifestyle, the better are your odds for a long and healthy life. Thus, initiating change right now will help you enjoy the best possible quality of life for as long as you live.

When health and appearance begin to deteriorate—usually around middle age—people seek out health care professionals in search of a "magic pill" to reverse and cure the many ills accumulated during years of abuse and overindulgence. The sooner we implement a healthy lifestyle program,

CRITICAL THINKING

What barriers to exercise do you encounter most frequently? How about barriers that keep you from managing your daily caloric intake?

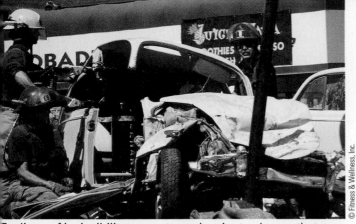

Feelings of invincibility are a strong barrier to change that can bring about life-threatening consequences.

© Fitness & Wellness, Inc.

the greater will be the health benefits and quality of life that lie ahead.

Motivation and Locus of Control

The explanation given for why some people succeed and others do not is often **motivation**. Although motivation comes from within, external factors trigger the inner desire to accomplish a given task. These external factors, then, control behavior.

When studying motivation, understanding **locus of control** is helpful. People who believe they have control over events in their lives are said to have an *internal locus of control*. People with an *external locus of control* believe that what happens to them is a result of chance or the environment and is unrelated to their behavior. People with an internal locus of control generally are healthier and have an easier time initiating and adhering to a wellness program than those who perceive that they have no control and think of themselves as powerless and vulnerable. The latter people also are at greater risk for illness. When illness does strike a person, establishing a sense of control is vital to recovery.

Few people have either a completely external or a completely internal locus of control. They fall somewhere along a continuum. The more external one's locus of control is, the greater is the challenge to change and adhere to exercise and other healthy lifestyle behaviors. Fortunately, people can develop a more internal locus of control. Understanding that most events in life are not determined genetically or environmentally helps people pursue goals and gain control over their lives. Three impediments, however, can keep people from taking action: lack of competence, confidence, and motivation.[3]

1. *Problems of competence.* Lacking the skills to get a given task done leads to reduced competence. If your friends play basketball regularly but you don't know how to play, you might be inclined not to participate. The solution to this problem of competence is to master the skills you need

to participate. Most people are not born with all-inclusive natural abilities, including playing sports.

Another alternative is to select an activity in which you are skilled. It may not be basketball, but it well could be aerobics. Don't be afraid to try new activities. Similarly, if your body weight is a problem, you could learn to cook healthy, low-calorie meals. Try different recipes until you find foods that you like.

2. *Problems of confidence.* Problems with confidence arise when you have the skill but don't believe you can get it done. Fear and feelings of inadequacy often interfere with ability to perform the task. You shouldn't talk yourself out of something until you have given it a fair try. If the skills are there, the sky is the limit. Initially, try to visualize yourself doing the task and getting it done. Repeat this several times, then actually try it. You will surprise yourself.

Sometimes, lack of confidence arises when the task seems insurmountable. In these situations, dividing a goal into smaller, more realistic objectives helps to accomplish the task. You might know how to swim but may need to train for several weeks to swim a continuous mile. Set up your training program so you swim a little farther each day until you are able to swim the entire mile. If you don't meet your objective on a given day, try it again, reevaluate, cut back a little, and, most important, don't give up.

3. *Problems of motivation.* With problems of motivation, both the competence and the confidence are there, but individuals are unwilling to change because the reasons to change are not important to them. For example, people begin contemplating a smoking cessation program only when the reasons for quitting outweigh the reasons for smoking. The primary causes of unwillingness to change are lack of knowledge and lack of goals. Knowledge often determines goals, and goals determine motivation. How badly you want something dictates how hard you'll work at it.

Many people are unaware of the magnitude of the benefits of a wellness program. When it comes to a healthy lifestyle, however, you may not get a second chance. A stroke, a heart attack, or cancer can have irreparable or fatal consequences. Greater understanding of what leads to disease may be all you need to initiate change.

Motivation The desire and will to do something.

Locus of control A concept examining the extent to which a person believes he or she can influence the external environment.

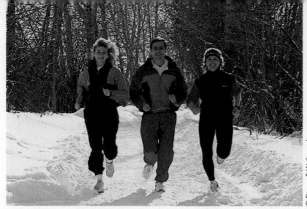

The higher quality of life experienced by people who are physically fit is hard to explain to someone who has never achieved good fitness.

Also, feeling physically fit is difficult to explain unless you have experienced it yourself. Feelings of fitness, self-esteem, confidence, health, and better quality of life cannot be conveyed to someone who is constrained by sedentary living. In a way, wellness is like reaching the top of a mountain. The quiet, the clean air, the lush vegetation, the flowing water in the river, the wildlife, and the majestic valley below are difficult to explain to someone who has spent a lifetime within city limits.

Changing Behavior

Psychotherapy has been used successfully to help change behavior. The great majority of people, however, do not seek professional help. They usually attempt change by themselves with limited or no knowledge of the process itself.

The simplest model of change is the two-stage model of unhealthy behavior and healthy behavior. This model states that either you do it or you don't. Most people who use this model attempt self-change but end up asking themselves why they're unsuccessful: They just can't do it (exercise, perhaps, or quitting smoking). Their intention to change may be good, but to accomplish it, they need knowledge about how to achieve change. The following discussion may help.

The Transtheoretical Model

For most people, changing chronic/unhealthy behaviors to stable/healthy behaviors is a challenging process. Change usually does not happen all at once. It is a gradual process that involves several stages. To aid with the process of self-change, psychologists James Prochaska, John Norcross, and Carlo DiClemente developed the Transtheoretical Model of Stages of Change.[4]

The transtheoretical model identifies five stages in the process of willful change. These stages describe underlying processes that people go through to change most problem behaviors and adopt healthy behaviors, and understanding the five stages will help you use this process. A sixth stage (termination/adoption) has subsequently been added to this model. Most frequently, the model is used to change health-related behaviors such as physical inactivity, smoking, poor nutrition, weight problems, stress, and alcohol abuse.

The six stages of change are precontemplation, contemplation, preparation, action, maintenance, and termination/adoption (see Figure 2.2). After years of study, researchers indicate that applying specific behavioral-change processes during each stage of the model increases the success rate for change (specific processes for each stage are shown in Table 2.1, page 37). Understanding each stage of this model will help you determine where you are in relation to your personal healthy-lifestyle behaviors. It will also help you identify processes to make successful changes.

Precontemplation

People in the **precontemplation stage** are not considering change or do not want to change a given behavior. They typically deny having a problem and have no intention of changing in the immediate future. These people are usually unaware or under-aware of the problem. Other people around them, including family, friends, health care practitioners, and co-workers, however, identify the problem clearly. Precontemplators do not care about the problem behavior and may even avoid information and materials that address the issue. They tend to avoid free screenings and workshops that might help identify and change the problem, even if they receive financial compensation for attendance. These people frequently have an active resistance to change and seem resigned to accepting the unhealthy behavior as their "fate."

Precontemplators are the most difficult people to inspire toward behavioral change. Many think that change isn't even a possibility. At this stage, knowledge is power. Educating them about the problem behavior is critical to help them start contemplating the process of change. The challenge is to find ways to help them realize that they are ultimately responsible for the consequences of their behavior. Typically, they initiate change only when people they respect or job requirements pressure them to do so.

Contemplation

In the **contemplation stage**, people acknowledge that they have a problem and begin to think seriously about overcoming it. Although they are not quite

FIGURE 2.2 Stages of change model.

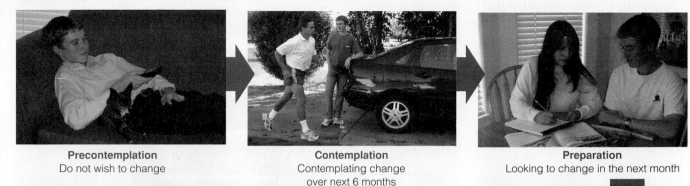

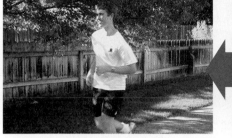

Precontemplation
Do not wish to change

Contemplation
Contemplating change
over next 6 months

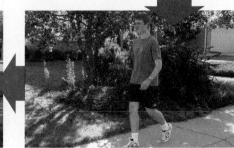

Preparation
Looking to change in the next month

Termination/Adoption
Change has been maintained
for more than 5 years

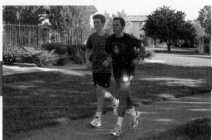

Maintenance
Maintaining change for 5 years

Action
Implementing change for 6 months

ready for change, they are weighing the pros and cons of changing. Even though people may remain in this stage for years, in their minds they are planning to take some action within the next 6 months. Education and peer support remain valuable during this stage.

Preparation

In the **preparation stage**, people are seriously considering change and planning to change a behavior within the next month. They are taking initial steps for change and may even try the new behavior for a short while, such as stopping smoking for a day or exercising a few times during the month. During this stage, people define a general goal for behavioral change (for example, to quit smoking by the last day of the month) and write specific objectives to accomplish this goal (see the section on "Goal Setting" later in this chapter). Continued peer and environmental support are helpful during the preparation stage.

Action

This stage requires the greatest commitment of time and energy on the part of the individual. Here people are actively doing things to change or modify the problem behavior or to adopt a new health behavior. The **action stage** requires that the person follow the specific guidelines set forth for that behavior. For example, a person has actually stopped smoking completely, is exercising aerobically three times per week according to exercise prescription guidelines, or is maintaining a healthy diet. Relapse is common during this stage, and the individual may regress to previous stages. Once people maintain the action stage for 6 consecutive months, they move into the maintenance stage.

Precontemplation stage Stage of change in the transtheoretical model in which people are unwilling to change behavior.

Contemplation stage Stage of change in the transtheoretical model in which people are considering changing behavior within the next 6 months.

Preparation stage Stage of change in the transtheoretical model in which people are getting ready to make a change within the next month.

Action stage Stage of change in the transtheoretical model in which people are actively changing a negative behavior or adopting a new, healthy behavior.

Maintenance

During the **maintenance stage**, the person continues the new behavior for up to 5 years. The maintenance phase requires continued adherence to the specific guidelines that govern the behavior (such as complete smoking cessation, exercising aerobically three times per week, practicing proper stress management techniques). At this time, the person works to reinforce the gains made through the various stages of change and strives to prevent lapses and relapse.

Termination/Adoption

Once a behavior has been maintained for more than 5 years, a person is said to be in the **termination** or **adoption stage** and exits from the cycle of change without fear of relapse. In the case of negative behaviors that are terminated, the stage of change is referred to as *termination*. If a positive behavior has been successfully adopted for over 5 years, this stage is designated as *adoption*. Some researchers have also labeled this stage the "transformed" stage of change because the word literally means "to have changed."[5]

Many experts believe that, once an individual enters the termination/adoption stage, former addictions, problems, or lack of compliance with healthy behaviors no longer present an obstacle in the quest for wellness. The change has now become part of one's lifestyle. This phase is the ultimate goal for all people searching for a healthier lifestyle.

For addictive behaviors such as alcoholism and hard drug use, however, many health care practitioners believe that the individual never enters the termination stage. Chemical dependency is so strong that most former alcoholics and hard-drug users must make a lifetime effort to prevent relapse. Similarly, some behavioral scientists suggest that the adoption stage might not be applicable to health behaviors such as exercise and weight control, because the likelihood of relapse is always high.[6]

Use the guidelines provided in Lab 2A to determine where you stand in respect to behaviors you want to change or new ones you wish to adopt. As you follow the guidelines, you will realize that you might be at different stages for different behaviors. For instance, you might be in the preparation stage for aerobic exercise and smoking cessation, in the action stage for strength training, but only in the contemplation stage for a healthy diet. Realizing where you are with respect to different behaviors will help you design a better action plan for a healthy lifestyle.

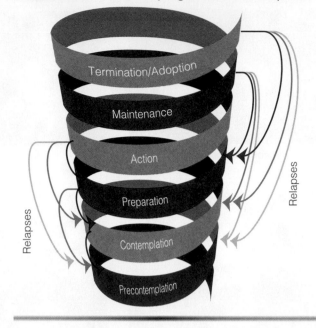

FIGURE 2.3 Model of progression and relapse.

Relapse

After the precontemplation stage, **relapse** may occur at any level of the model. Even individuals in the maintenance and termination/adoption stages may regress to any of the first three stages of the model (see Figure 2.3). Relapse, however, does not mean failure. Failure comes only to those who give up and don't use prior experiences as a building block for future success. The chances of moving back up to a higher stage of the model are far better for someone who has previously made it into one of those stages.

The Process of Change

Using the same plan for every individual who wishes to change a behavior will not work. With exercise, for instance, we provide different prescriptions to people of varying fitness levels (see Chapter 6). The same prescription would not provide optimal results for a person who has been inactive for 20 years, compared to one who already walks regularly three times each week. This principle also holds true for people who are attempting to change behaviors.

Timing is also important in the process of willful change. People respond more effectively to selected **processes of change** according to the stage of change they have reached at any given time.[7] Thus, applying appropriate processes at each stage of change enhances the likelihood of changing behavior permanently. The following description of 14 of the

TABLE 2.1   Applicable Processes of Change During Each Stage of Change

Precontemplation	Contemplation	Preparation	Action	Maintenance	Termination/Adoption
Consciousness-raising	Consciousness-raising	Consciousness-raising			
Social liberation	Social liberation	Social liberation	Social liberation		
	Self-analysis	Self-analysis			
	Emotional arousal	Emotional arousal			
	Positive outlook	Positive outlook	Positive outlook		
		Commitment	Commitment	Commitment	Commitment
		Behavior analysis	Behavior analysis		
		Goal setting	Goal setting	Goal setting	
		Self-reevaluation	Self-reevaluation	Self-reevaluation	
			Countering	Countering	
			Monitoring	Monitoring	Monitoring
			Environment control	Environment control	Environment control
			Helping relationships	Helping relationships	Helping relationships
			Rewards	Rewards	Rewards

Source: Adapted from J. O. Prochaska, J. C. Norcross, and C. C. DiClemente, *Changing for Good*, (New York: William Morrow, 1994); and W. W. K. Hoeger and S. A. Hoeger, *Fitness & Wellness* (Belmont, CA: Wadsworth/Thomson Learning, 2002).

most common processes of change will help you develop a personal plan for change. The respective stages of change where each process works best are summarized in Table 2.1.

Consciousness-Raising

The first step in a **behavior modification** program is consciousness-raising. This process involves obtaining information about the problem so you can make a better decision about the problem behavior. For example, the problem could be physical inactivity. Learning about the benefits of exercise or the difference in benefits between physical activity and exercise (see Chapter 1) can help you decide the type of fitness program (health or high fitness) that you want to pursue. It is also possible that you don't even know that a certain behavior is a problem, such as unawareness of saturated and total fat content in many fast-food items. Consciousness-raising may continue from the precontemplation stage through the preparation stage.

Social Liberation

Social liberation stresses external alternatives that make you aware of problem behaviors and contemplate change. Examples of social liberation include pedestrian-only traffic areas, non-smoking areas, health-oriented cafeterias and restaurants, advocacy

groups, civic organizations, policy interventions, and self-help groups. Social liberation often provides opportunities to get involved, stir up emotions, and enhance self-esteem—helping you gain confidence in your ability to change.

Self-Analysis

The next process in modifying behavior is a decisive desire to do so, called self-analysis. If you have no interest in changing a behavior, you won't do it. You will remain a precontemplator or a contemplator. A person who has no intention of quitting smoking will not quit, regardless of what anyone may say or how strong the evidence in favor of quitting may be. In your self-analysis, you may want to prepare a list of reasons for continuing or discontinuing the

Maintenance stage   Stage of change in the transtheoretical model in which people maintain behavioral change for up to 5 years.

Termination/adoption stage   Stage of change in the transtheoretical model in which people have eliminated an undesirable behavior or maintained a positive behavior for more than 5 years.

Relapse (v.)   To slip or fall back into unhealthy behavior(s); or (n.) failure to maintain healthy behaviors.

Processes of change   Actions that help you achieve change in behavior.

Behavior modification   The process of permanently changing negative behaviors to positive behaviors that will lead to better health and well-being.

behavior. When the reasons for changing outweigh the reasons for not changing, you are ready for the next stage—either the contemplation stage or the preparation stage.

Emotional Arousal

In emotional arousal, a person experiences and expresses feelings about the problem and its solutions. Also referred to as "dramatic release," this process often involves deep emotional experiences. Watching a loved one die from lung cancer caused by cigarette smoking may be all that is needed to make a person quit smoking. As other examples, emotional arousal might be prompted by a dramatization of the consequences of drug use and abuse, a film about a person undergoing open-heart surgery, or a book illustrating damage to body systems as a result of unhealthy behaviors.

Positive Outlook

Having a positive outlook means taking an optimistic approach from the beginning and believing in yourself. Following the guidelines in this chapter will help you design a plan so you can work toward change and remain enthused about your progress. Also, you may become motivated by looking at the outcome—how much healthier you will be, how much better you will look, or how far you will be able to jog.

Commitment

Upon making a decision to change, you accept the responsibility to change and believe in your ability to do so. During the commitment process, you engage in preparation and may draw up a specific plan of action. Write down your goals and, preferably, share them with others. In essence, you are signing a behavioral contract for change. You will be more likely to adhere to your program if others know you are committed to change.

Behavior Analysis

Now you determine the frequency, circumstances, and consequences of the behavior to be altered or implemented, called behavior analysis. If the desired outcome is to consume less saturated fat, you first must find out what foods in your diet are high in saturated fat, when you eat them, and when you don't eat them—all part of the preparation stage. Knowing when you don't eat them points to circumstances under which you exert control of your diet and will help as you set goals.

Goals

Goals motivate change in behavior. The stronger the goal or desire, the more motivated you'll be either to change unwanted behaviors or to implement new, healthy behaviors. The discussion on goal setting (pages 41–43) will help you write goals and prepare an action plan to achieve those goals. This will aid with behavior modification.

Self-Reevaluation

During the process of self-evaluation, individuals analyze their feelings about a problem behavior. The pros and cons or advantages and disadvantages of a certain behavior can be reevaluated at this time. For example, you may decide that strength training will help you tone up and boost your metabolism, but implementing this change will require you to stop watching an hour of TV three times per week. If you presently have a weight problem and are unable to lift certain objects around the house, you may feel good about weight loss and enhanced physical capacity as a result of a strength-training program. You might also visualize what it would be like if you were successful at changing.

Countering

The process whereby you substitute healthy behaviors for a problem behavior, known as countering, is critical in changing behaviors as part of the action and maintenance stages. You need to replace unhealthy behaviors with new, healthy ones. You can use

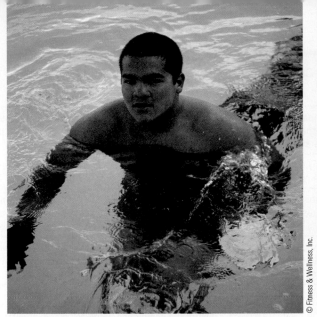

Countering: Substituting healthy behaviors for problem behaviors facilitates change.

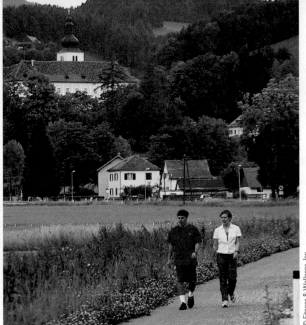

Rewarding oneself when a goal is achieved, such as scheduling a weekend getaway, is a powerful tool during the process of change.

exercise to combat sedentary living, smoking, stress, or overeating. You may also use exercise, diet, yard-work, volunteer work, or reading to prevent over-eating and achieve recommended body weight.

Monitoring

During the action and maintenance stages, continuous behavior monitoring increases awareness of the desired outcome. Sometimes this process of monitoring is sufficient in itself to cause change. For example, keeping track of daily food intake reveals sources of excessive fat in the diet. This can help you gradually cut down or completely eliminate high-fat foods. If the goal is to increase daily intake of fruit and vegetables, keeping track of the number of servings consumed each day raises awareness and may help increase intake.

Environment Control

In environment control, the person restructures the physical surroundings to avoid problem behaviors and decrease temptations. If you don't buy alcohol, you can't drink any. If you shop on a full stomach, you can reduce impulse-buying of junk food.

Similarly, you can create an environment in which exceptions become the norm, and then the norm can flourish. Instead of bringing home cookies for snacks, bring fruit. Place notes to yourself on the refrigerator and pantry to avoid unnecessary snacking. Place baby carrots or sugarless gum where you used to place cigarettes. Post notes around the house to remind you of your exercise time. Leave exercise shoes and clothing by the entry way so they are visible as you walk into your home. Put an electric

timer on the TV so it will shut off automatically at 7:00 P.M. All of these tactics will be helpful throughout the action, maintenance, and termination/adoption stages.

Helping Relationships

Surrounding yourself with people who will work toward a common goal with you or those who care about you and will encourage you along the way—helping relationships—will be helpful during the action, maintenance, and termination/adoption stages.

Attempting to quit smoking, for instance, is easier when a person is around others who are trying to quit as well. The person could also get help from friends who have quit smoking already. Losing weight is difficult if meal planning and cooking are shared with roommates who enjoy foods that are high in fat and sugar. This situation can be even worse if a roommate also has a weight problem and does not desire to lose weight.

Peer support is a strong incentive for behavioral change. During this process, the individual should avoid people who will not be supportive. Friends who have no desire to quit smoking or to lose weight, or whatever behavior a person is trying to change, may tempt one to smoke or overeat and encourage relapse into unwanted behaviors.

People who have achieved the same goal already may not be supportive either. For instance, someone may say, "I can do 6 consecutive miles." Your response should be, "I'm proud that I can jog 3 consecutive miles."

TABLE 2.2 Sample Techniques for Use With Processes of Change

Process	Techniques
Consciousness-Raising	Become aware that there is a problem, read educational materials about the problem behavior or about people who have overcome this same problem, find out about the benefits of changing the behavior, watch an instructional program on television, visit a therapist, talk and listen to others, ask questions, take a class.
Social Liberation	Seek out advocacy groups (Overeaters Anonymous, Alcoholics Anonymous), join a health club, buy a bike, join a neighborhood walking group, work in nonsmoking areas.
Self-Analysis	Become aware that there is a problem, question yourself on the problem behavior, express your feelings about it, analyze your values, list advantages and disadvantages of continuing (smoking) or not implementing a behavior (exercise), take a fitness test, do a nutrient analysis.
Emotional Arousal	Practice mental imagery of yourself going through the process of change, visualize yourself overcoming the problem behavior, do some role-playing in overcoming the behavior or practicing a new one, watch dramatizations (a movie) of the consequences or benefits of your actions, visit an auto salvage yard or a drug rehabilitation center.
Positive Outlook	Believe in yourself, know that you are capable, know that you are special, draw from previous personal successes.
Commitment	Just do it, set New Year's resolutions, sign a behavioral contract, set start and completion dates, tell others about your goals, work on your action plan.
Behavior Analysis	Prepare logs of circumstances that trigger or prevent a given behavior and look for patterns that prompt the behavior or cause you to relapse.
Goal Setting	Write goals and objectives; design a specific action plan.
Self-Reevaluation	Determine accomplishments and evaluate progress, rewrite goals and objectives, list pros and cons, weigh sacrifices (can't eat out with others) versus benefits (weight loss), visualize continued change, think before you act, learn from mistakes, and prepare new action plans accordingly.
Countering	Seek out alternatives: Stay busy, walk (don't drive), read a book (instead of snacking), attend alcohol-free socials, carry your own groceries, mow your yard, dance (don't eat), go to a movie (instead of smoking), practice stress management.
Monitoring	Use exercise logs (days exercised, sets and resistance used in strength training), keep journals, conduct nutrient analyses, count grams of fat, count number of consecutive days without smoking, list days and type of relaxation technique(s) used.
Environment Control	Rearrange your home (no TVs, ashtrays, large-sized cups), get rid of unhealthy items (cigarettes, junk food, alcohol), then avoid unhealthy places (bars, happy hour), avoid relationships that encourage problem behaviors, use reminders to control problem behaviors (post notes indicating "don't snack after dinner" or "lift weights at 8:00 PM"). Frequent healthy environments (a clean park, a health club, restaurants with low-fat/low-calorie/nutrient-dense menus, friends with goals similar to yours).
Helping Relationships	Associate with people who have and want to overcome the same problem, form or join self-help groups, join community programs specifically designed to deal with your problem (eating disorders, substance abuse control, smoking cessation).
Rewards	Go to a movie, buy a new outfit or shoes, buy a new bike, go on a weekend get-away, reassess your fitness level, use positive self-talk ("good job," "that felt good," "I did it," "I knew I'd make it," "I'm good at this").

Rewards

People tend to repeat behaviors that are rewarded and disregard those that are not rewarded or are punished. Rewarding oneself or being rewarded by others is a powerful tool during the process of change in all stages. If you have successfully cut down your caloric intake during the week, reward yourself by going to a show or buying a new pair of shoes. Do not reinforce yourself with destructive behaviors such as eating a high-fat/calorie-dense dinner. If you fail to change a desired behavior (or to implement a new one), you may want to put off buying those new shoes you had planned for that week. When a positive behavior becomes habitual, give yourself an even better reward. Treat yourself to a weekend away from home or buy a new bicycle.

Techniques of Change

Not to be confused with the processes of change, you can apply any number of **techniques of change** within each process to help you through that specific process (see Table 2.2). For example, following dinner, people with a weight problem often can't resist continuous snacking during the rest of the evening until it is time to retire for the night. In the process of countering, for example, you can use various techniques to avoid unnecessary snacking. Examples include going for a walk, flossing

FIGURE 2.4   Stage of change identification and behavior modification outline.

Please indicate which response most accurately describes your current [_____] behavior (in the blank space identify the behavior: smoking, physical activity, stress, nutrition, weight control). Next, select the statement below (select only one) that best represents your current behavior pattern. To select the most appropriate statement, fill in the blank for one of the first three statements if your current behavior is a problem behavior. (For example, you may say, "I currently smoke and I do *not* intend to change in the foreseeable future," or "I currently *do not exercise* but I am contemplating changing in the next 6 months.") If you have already started to make changes, fill in the blank in one of the last three statements. (In this case, you may say: "I currently *eat a low-fat diet* but I have only done so within the last 6 months," or "I currently *practice adequate stress management techniques* and I have done so for over 6 months.") As you can see, you may use this form to identify your stage of change for any type of health-related behavior.

1.   I currently [_____], and I do not intend to change in the foreseeable future.

2.   I currently [_____], but I am contemplating changing in the next 6 months.

3.   I currently [_____] regularly, but I intend to change in the next month.

4.   I currently [_____], but I have done so only within the last 6 months.

5.   I currently [_____], and I have done so for more than 6 months.

6.   I currently [_____], and I have done so for more than 5 years.

---

and brushing your teeth right after dinner, going for a drive, playing the piano, going to a show, or going to bed earlier.

As you develop a behavior modification plan, you need to identify specific techniques that may work for you within each process of change. A list of techniques for each process is provided in Table 2.2. This is only a sample list; dozens of other techniques may be used as well. For example, Behavior Modification and Adherence to a Weight Management Program is found on page 144, Getting Started and Adhering to a Lifetime Exercise Program is presented on page 180, stress management techniques are provided in Chapter 10, and tips to help stop smoking on pages 409–410. Some of the techniques can also be used with more than one process, visualization, for example, is helpful in emotional arousal and self-reevaluation.

Now that you are familiar with the stages of change in the process of behavior modification, use Figure 2.4 and Lab 2A to identify two problem behaviors in your life. In this lab you will be asked to determine your stage of change for two behaviors according to six standard

CRITICAL THINKING

Your friend John is a 20-year-old student who is not physically active. Exercise has never been a part of his life, and it has not been a priority in his family. He has decided to start a jogging and strength-training course in 2 weeks. Can you identify his current stage of change and list processes and techniques of change that will help him maintain a regular exercise behavior?

TABLE 2.3   Stage of Change Classification

Selected Statement (see Figure 2.4 and Lab 2A)	Classification
1	Precontemplation
2	Contemplation
3	Preparation
4	Action
5	Maintenance
6	Termination/Adoption

statements. Based on your selection, determine the stage of change classification according to the ratings provided in Table 2.3. Next, develop a behavior modification plan according to the processes and techniques for change that you have learned in this chapter. (Similar exercises to identify stages of change for other fitness and wellness behaviors are provided in labs for subsequent chapters.)

Goal Setting

To initiate change, **goals** are essential, as goals motivate behavioral change. Whatever you set out to accomplish, setting goals will provide the road map

Techniques of change   Methods or procedures used during each process of change.

Goals   The ultimate aims toward which effort is directed.

to help make your dreams a reality. Setting goals, however, is not as simple as it looks. Setting goals is more than just deciding what you want to do. A vague statement such as, "I will lose weight," is not sufficient to help you achieve this goal.

SMART Goals

Only a well-conceived action plan will help you attain goals. Determining what you want to accomplish is the starting point, but to reach your goal you need to write **SMART** goals. The SMART acronym is used in reference to goals that are *S*pecific, *M*easurable, *A*cceptable, *R*ealistic, and *T*ime-specific. In Lab 2B you will have an opportunity to set SMART goals for two behaviors that you wish to change or adopt.

1. *Specific.* When writing goals, state exactly and in a positive manner what you would like to accomplish. For example, if you are overweight at 150 pounds and at 27 percent body fat, to simply state "I will lose weight," is not a specific goal. Instead, re-write your goal to state "I will reduce my body fat to 20 percent body fat (137 pounds) in 12 weeks."

    Be sure to write down your goals. An unwritten goal is simply a wish. A written goal, in essence, becomes a contract with yourself. Show this goal to a friend or an instructor and have him or her witness the contract you made with yourself by signing alongside your signature.

    Once you have identified and written down a specific goal, write the specific **objectives** that will help you reach that goal. These objectives are the necessary steps required to reach your goal. For example, a goal might be to achieve recommended body weight. Several specific objectives could be to

    (a) lose an average of 1 pound (or 1 fat percentage point) per week
    (b) monitor body weight before breakfast every morning
    (c) assess body composition every 2 weeks
    (d) limit fat intake to less than 25 percent of total daily caloric intake
    (e) eliminate all pastries from the diet during this time, and
    (f) walk/jog in the proper target zone for 60 minutes, six times per week.
2. *Measurable.* Whenever possible, goals and objectives should be measurable. For example, "I will lose weight" is not measurable, but "to reduce body fat to 20 percent" is measurable. Also note that all of the sample specific objectives (a) through (f) in Item 1 above are measurable.

For instance, you can figure out easily whether you are losing a pound or a percentage point per week; you can conduct a nutrient analysis to assess your average fat intake; or you can monitor your weekly exercise sessions to make sure you are meeting this specific objective.

3. *Acceptable.* Goals that you set for yourself are more motivational than goals that someone else sets for you. These goals will motivate and challenge you and should be consistent with other goals that you have. As you set an acceptable goal, ask yourself: Do I have the time, commitment, and necessary skills to accomplish this goal? If not, you need to restate your goal so that it is acceptable to you.

    In instances where successful completion of a goal involves others, such as an athletic team or an organization, an acceptable goal must be compatible with those of the other people involved. If a team's practice schedule is set Monday through Friday from 4:00 to 6:00 P.M., it is unacceptable for you to train only three times per week or at a different time of the day.

    Acceptable goals are also embraced with positive thoughts. Visualize and believe in your success. As difficult as some tasks may seem, where there's a will, there's a way. A plan of action, prepared according to the guidelines in this chapter, will help you achieve your goals.

4. *Realistic.* Goals should be within reach. If you currently weigh 190 pounds and your target weight (at 20 percent body fat) is 137 pounds, setting a goal to lose 53 pounds in a month would be unsound, if not impossible. Such a goal does not allow for the implementation of adequate behavior modification techniques or ensure weight maintenance at the target weight. Unattainable goals only set you up for failure, discouragement, and loss of interest.

    On the other hand, do not write goals that are too easy to achieve and do not challenge you. If a goal is too easy, you may lose interest and stop working toward it.

    You can write both short-term and long-term goals. If the long-term goal is to attain recommended body weight and you are 53 pounds overweight, you might set a short-term goal of losing 10 pounds and write specific objectives to accomplish this goal. Then the immediate task will not seem as overwhelming and will be easier.

    At times, problems arise even with realistic goals. Try to anticipate potential difficulties as much as possible, and plan for ways to deal with them. If your goal is to jog for 30 minutes on six consecutive days, what are the alternatives if the weather turns bad? Possible solutions are to jog in the rain, find an indoor track, jog at a different time of day when the weather is better, or participate in a different aerobic activity such as stationary cycling, swimming, or step aerobics.

Monitoring your progress as you move toward a goal also reinforces behavior. Keeping an exercise log or doing a body composition assessment periodically enables you to determine your progress at any given time.

5. *Time-specific.* A goal always should have a specific date set for completion. The above example to reach 20 percent body fat in 12 weeks is time-specific. The chosen date should be realistic but not too distant in the future. Allow yourself enough time to achieve the goal, but not too much time, as this could affect your performance. With a deadline, a task is much easier to work toward.

Goal Evaluation

In addition to the SMART guidelines provided above, you should conduct periodic evaluations of your goals. Reevaluations are vital for success. You may find that after you have fully committed and put all your effort into a goal, that goal may be unreachable. If so, reassess the goal.

Recognize that you will face obstacles, and you will not always meet your goals. Use your setbacks and learn from them. Rewrite your goal and create a plan that will help you get around self-defeating behaviors in the future. Once you achieve a goal, set a new one to improve upon or maintain what you have achieved. Goals keep you motivated.

SMART An acronym used in reference to *S*pecific, *M*easurable, *A*ttainable, *R*ealistic, and *T*ime-specific goals.

Objectives Steps required to reach a goal.

ofile
us

ing the
ssess Your
owledge"
d "Practice
izzes" op-
ns on your
)-ROM,
aluate how
ell you
derstand
e concepts
esented in
s chapter.

 ## ASSESS YOUR KNOWLEDGE

1. Most of the behaviors that people adopt in life are
   a. a product of their environment.
   b. learned early in childhood.
   c. learned from parents.
   d. genetically determined.
   e. the result of peer pressure.

2. Instant gratification is
   a. a barrier to change.
   b. a factor that motivates change.
   c. one of the six stages of change.
   d. the end result of successful change.
   e. a technique in the process of change.

3. The desire and will to do something is referred to as
   a. invincibility.
   b. confidence.
   c. competence.
   d. external locus of control.
   e. motivation.

4. People who believe they have control over events in their lives
   a. tend to rationalize their negative actions.
   b. exhibit problems of competence.
   c. often feel helpless over illness and disease.
   d. have an internal locus of control.
   e. often engage in risky lifestyle behaviors.

5. A person who is unwilling to change a negative behavior because the reasons for change are not important enough is said to have problems of
   a. competence.
   b. conduct.
   c. motivation.
   d. confidence.
   e. risk complacency.

6. Which of the following is a stage of change in the Transtheoretical Model?
   a. recognition
   b. motivation
   c. relapse
   d. preparation
   e. goal setting

7. A precontemplator is a person who
   a. has no desire to change a behavior.
   b. is looking to make a change in the next 6 months.
   c. is preparing for change in the next 30 days.
   d. willingly adopts healthy behaviors.
   e. is talking to a therapist to overcome a problem behavior.

8. An individual who is trying to stop smoking and has not smoked for 3 months is in the
   a. maintenance stage.
   b. action stage.
   c. termination stage.
   d. adoption stage.
   e. evaluation stage.

9. The process of change where an individual obtains information to make a better decision about a problem behavior is known as
   a. behavior analysis.
   b. self-reevaluation.
   c. commitment.
   d. positive outlook.
   e. consciousness-raising.

10. A goal is effective when it is
   a. specific.
   b. measurable.
   c. time-specific.
   d. realistic.
   e. all of the above.

Correct answers can be found at the back of the book.

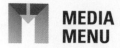

MEDIA MENU

PROFILE PLUS CD CONNECTIONS
■ Prepare for a healthy change in lifestyle.
■ Check how well you understand the chapter's concepts.

INTERNET CONNECTIONS
■ Transtheoretical Model as described by its originators, James O. Prochaska, Ph.D., and Carlo C. DiClemente, Ph.D. This site, from the University of South Florida Community and Family Health, describes the historical development of the transtheoretical model and features several useful print references.

http://www.med.usf.edu/~kmbrown/Stages_of_Change_Overview htm

■ Transtheoretical Model—Cancer Prevention Research Center. This site describes the transtheoretical model, including descriptions of effective interventions to promote health behavior change, focusing on the individual's decision-making strategies.

http://www.uri.edu/research/cprc/TTM/detailedoverview.htm

■ Behavior Change Theories. This very comprehensive site, by the Department of Health Promotion at California Polytechnic University at Pomona, describes all of the theories of behavioral change, including Learning Theories, Transtheoretical Model, Health Belief Model, Relapse Prevention Model, Reasoned Action and Planned Behavior, Social Learning/Social Cognitive Theory, and Social Support.

http://www.csupomona.edu/~jvgrizzell/best_practices/bctheory.html

■ How to Fit Exercise into Your Daily Routine. Sponsored by the Centers for Disease Control and Prevention, this site describes how you can incorporate simple exercises into your daily schedule—whether you're at home, at work, or spending time away with the family. Make time to exercise!

http://www.cdc.gov/nccdphp/dnpa/phys_act.htm

Notes

1. U.S. Department of Health and Human Services, *Physical Activity and Health: A Report of the Surgeon General* (Atlanta: Centers for Disease Control and Prevention, National Center for Chronic Disease Prevention and Health Promotion, 1996).

2. J. Annesi, "Using Emotions to Empower Members for Long-Term Exercise Success," *Fitness Management* 17 (2001): 54–58.

3. G. S. Howard, D. W. Nance, and P. Myers, *Adaptive Counseling and Therapy* (San Francisco: Jossey–Bass, 1987).

4. J. O. Prochaska, J. C. Norcross, and C. C. DiClemente, *Changing for Good* (New York: William Morrow, 1994).

5. B. J. Cardinal, "Extended Stage Model of Physical Activity Behavior," *Journal of Human Movement Studies* 37 (1999): 37–54.

6. See note 5.

7. See note 4. Also in B. H. Marcus, et al., "Evaluation of Motivationally Tailored vs. Standard Self-help Physical Activity Interventions at the Workplace," *American Journal of Health Promotion* 12 (1998): 246–253.

Suggested Readings

Bouchard, C., et al. *Physical Activity, Fitness, and Health.* Champaign, IL: Human Kinetics, 1994.

Blair, S. N., et al. *Active Living Every Day.* Champaign, IL: Human Kinetics, 2001.

Brehm, B. *Successful Fitness Motivation Strategies.* Champaign, IL: Human Kinetics, 2004.

Dishman, R. *Advances in Exercise Adherence.* Champaign, IL: Human Kinetics, 1994.

Marcus, B., and L. Forsyth. *Motivating People To Be Physically Active.* Champaign, IL: Human Kinetics, 2003.

Prochaska, J. O., J. C. Norcross, and C. C. DiClemente. *Changing for Good.* New York: William Morrow, 1994.

Samuelson, M. "Stages of Change: From Theory to Practice." *The Art of Health Promotion* 2 (1998): 1–7.

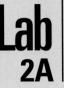

Lab 2A

BEHAVIOR MODIFICATION:
STAGES, PROCESSES, AND TECHNIQUES FOR CHANGE

Name: _____ Date: _____ Grade: _____

Instructor: _____ Course: _____ Section: _____

Necessary Lab Equipment
None required.

Lab Preparation
Chapter 2 must be read prior to this lab.

Objective
To help you identify the stage of change for two problem behaviors and the processes and techniques for change.

I. Stages of Change Instructions

Please indicate which response most accurately describes your current _____ behavior (in the blank space identify the behavior: smoking, physical activity, stress, nutrition, weight control). Next, select the statement below (select only one) that best represents your current behavior pattern. To select the most appropriate statement, fill in the blank for one of the first three statements if your current behavior is a problem behavior. For example, you may say:

"I currently <u>smoke</u>, and I do not intend to change in the foreseeable future" or

"I currently <u>do not exercise</u>, but I am contemplating changing in the next 6 months."

If you have already started to make changes, fill in the blank in one of the last three statements. In this case you may say:

"I currently <u>eat a low-fat diet</u>, but I have only done so within the last 6 months" or

"I currently <u>practice adequate stress management techniques</u>, and I have done so for over 6 months."

You may use this form to identify your stage of change for any health-related behavior. After identifying two problem behaviors, look up your stage of change for each one using Table 2.3 (on page 41).

Behavior #1. Fill in only one blank.

☐ 1. I currently _____, and do not intend to change in the foreseeable future.

☐ 2. I currently _____, but I am contemplating changing in the next 6 months.

☐ 3. I currently _____ regularly, but I intend to change in the next month.

☐ 4. I currently _____, but I have only done so within the last 6 months.

☐ 5. I currently _____, and I have done so for over 6 months.

☐ 6. I currently _____, and I have done so for over 5 years.

Stage of change: _____ (see Table 2.3 on page 41).

Behavior #2. Fill in only one blank.

1. I currently _____, and do not intend to change in the foreseeable future.

2. I currently _____, but I am contemplating changing in the next 6 months.

3. I currently _____ regularly, but I intend to change in the next month.

4. I currently _____, but I have only done so within the last 6 months.

5. I currently _____, and I have done so for over 6 months.

6. I currently _____, and I have done so for over 5 years.

Stage of change: _____ (see Table 2.3 on page 41).

II. Processes of Change

According to your stage of change for the two behaviors identified above, list the processes of change that apply to each behavior (see Table 2.1 on page 37).

Behavior #1: _____

_____

Behavior #2: _____

_____

III. Techniques for Change

List a minimum of three techniques that you will use with each process of change (see Table 2.2 on page 40).

Behavior #1: 1. _____

2. _____

3. _____

Behavior #2: 1. _____

2. _____

3. _____

Today's date: _____   Completion Date: _____   Signature: _____

Lab 2B

SETTING SMART GOALS

Name: _____ **Date:** _____ **Grade:** _____

Instructor: _____ **Course:** _____ **Section:** _____

Objective

To learn to write SMART goals.

Instructions

In lab 2A you identified two behaviors that you wish to change. Using SMART goal guidelines, write goals and objectives that will provide a road map for behavioral change. In the spaces provided in this lab, indicate how your stated goals meet each one of the SMART goal guidelines.

I. SMART Goals

Goal 1:

_____

_____

Indicate what makes your goal specific.

_____

_____

How is your goal measurable?

_____

_____

Why is this an acceptable goal?

_____

_____

State why you consider this goal realistic.

_____

_____

How is this goal time-specific?

_____

_____

Goal 2:

_____

_____

Indicate what makes your goal specific.

_____

How is your goal measurable?

_____

Why is this an acceptable goal?

_____

State why you consider this goal realistic.

_____

How is this goal time-specific?

_____

_____

II. Specific Objectives

Write a minimum of five specific objectives that will help you reach your two SMART goals.

Goal 1:

Objectives:

1.

2.

3.

4.

5.

Goal 2:

Objectives:

1.

2.

3.

4.

5.

Nutrition for Wellness

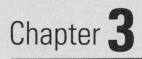

Objectives

■ Define nutrition and describe its relationship to health and well-being.

■ Learn to use the USDA MyPyramid guidelines for healthier eating.

■ Describe the functions of the nutrients—carbohydrates, fiber, fats, proteins, vitamins, minerals, and water—in the human body.

■ Define the various energy production mechanisms of the human body.

■ Be able to conduct a comprehensive nutrient analysis and implement changes to meet the Dietary Reference Intakes (DRIs).

■ Identify myths and fallacies regarding nutrition.

■ Become aware of guidelines for nutrient supplementation.

■ Describe the national Dietary Guidelines for Americans.

Profile Plus CD Connections

■ Analyze your diet and plan for a healthy change.

■ Check how well you understand the chapter's concepts.

Scientific evidence has long linked good **nutrition** to overall health and well-being. Proper nutrition means that a person's diet supplies all the essential nutrients needed to carry out normal tissue growth, repair, and maintenance. The diet should also provide enough **substrates** to produce the energy necessary for work, physical activity, and relaxation. These **nutrients** should be obtained from a wide variety of sources. Figure 3.1 shows MyPyramid nutrition guidelines and recommended daily food amounts according to various caloric requirements. To lower the risk for chronic disease, an effective wellness program must incorporate healthy eating guidelines. These guidelines will be discussed throughout this chapter and in later chapters of this book.

Too much or too little of any nutrient can precipitate serious health problems. The typical U.S. diet is too high in calories, sugar, fat, saturated fat, and sodium, and not high enough in fiber—factors that undermine good health. Food availability is not the problem. The problem is overconsumption.

According to the first report on nutrition and health issued by the U.S. Surgeon General in 1988, diseases of dietary excess and imbalance are among the leading causes of death in the United States. Similar trends are observed in developed countries throughout the world. In the report, based on more than 2,000 scientific studies, the Surgeon General said that dietary changes can bring better health to all Americans. Other surveys reveal that, on a given day, nearly half of the people in the United States eat no fruit and almost a fourth eat no vegetables.

Diet and nutrition often play a crucial role in the development and progression of chronic diseases. A diet high in saturated fat and cholesterol increases the risk for atherosclerosis and coronary heart disease. In sodium-sensitive individuals, high salt intake has been linked to high blood pressure. Some researchers believe that 30 to 50 percent of all cancers are diet-related. Obesity, diabetes, and osteoporosis also have been associated with faulty nutrition.

To lower the risk for chronic disease, an effective wellness program must incorporate the dietary recommendations for Americans, as follows:

■ Let the current nutrition recommendations guide your food choices.
■ Eat a variety of foods daily, especially whole grains, fruits, and vegetables. Many of these foods are high in nutrients, starch, and fiber.
■ Avoid too much fat, saturated fat, trans fatty acids, and cholesterol.
■ Avoid too much sugar and sodium.
■ Maintain adequate calcium intake.
■ Keep food safe to eat—which means that the food poses little risk of food-borne illness.

■ Maintain recommended body weight.
■ Drink alcoholic beverages in moderation, if at all.

These guidelines will be discussed throughout this chapter and in later chapters of this book.

Nutrients

The essential nutrients the human body requires are carbohydrates, fat, protein, vitamins, minerals, and water. The first three are called *fuel nutrients* because they are the only substances the body uses to supply the energy (commonly measured in calories) needed for work and normal body functions. The three others—vitamins, minerals, and water—are regulatory nutrients. They have no caloric value, but still are necessary for a person to function normally and maintain good health. Many nutritionists add to this list a seventh nutrient: fiber. This nutrient has received a great deal of attention recently. Recommended amounts seem to provide protection against several diseases, including cardiovascular disease and some cancers.

Carbohydrates, fats, proteins, and water are termed *macronutrients* because we need them in proportionately large amounts daily. Vitamins and minerals are required in only small amounts—grams, milligrams, and micrograms instead of, say, ounces—and nutritionists refer to them as *micronutrients*.

Depending on the amount of nutrients and calories they contain, foods can be classified by their **nutrient density**. Foods that contain few or a moderate number of calories but are packed with nutrients are said to have high nutrient density. Foods that have a lot of calories but few nutrients are of low nutrient density and are commonly called "junk food."

A **calorie** is the unit of measure indicating the energy value of food to the person who consumes it. It is also used to express the amount of energy a person expends in physical activity. Technically, a kilocalorie (kcal), or large calorie, is the amount of heat necessary to raise the temperature of 1 kilogram of water 1 degree Centigrade. For simplicity, people

Nutrition Science that studies the relationship of foods to optimal health and performance.

Substrates Substances acted upon by an enzyme (examples: carbohydrates, fats).

Nutrients Substances found in food that provide energy, regulate metabolism, and help with growth and repair of body tissues.

Nutrient density A measure of the amount of nutrients and calories in various foods.

Calorie The amount of heat necessary to raise the temperature of 1 gram of water 1 degree Centigrade; used to measure the energy value of food and cost (energy expenditure) of physical activity.

FIGURE 3.1 MyPyramid: Steps to a Healthier You.

The colors of the pyramid illustrate variety: each color represents one of the five food groups, plus one for oils. Different band widths suggest the proportional contribution of each food group to a healthy diet.

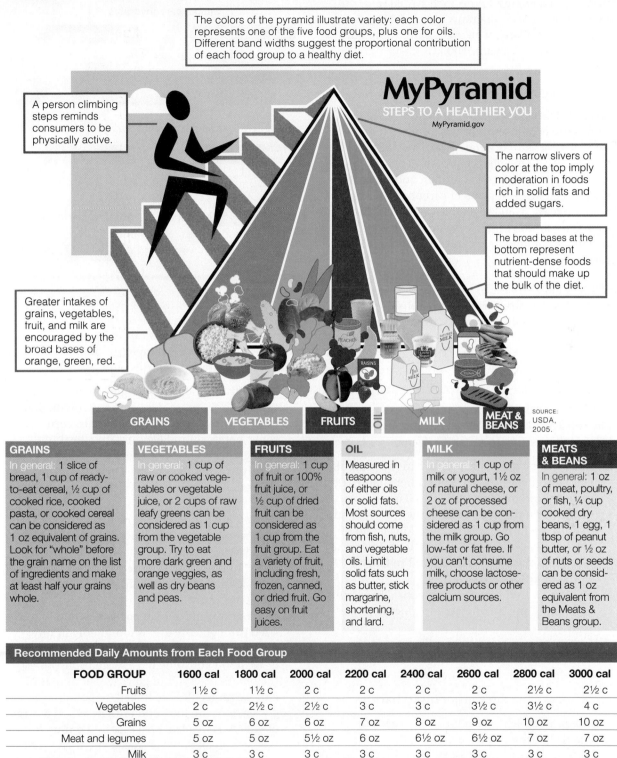

A person climbing steps reminds consumers to be physically active.

The narrow slivers of color at the top imply moderation in foods rich in solid fats and added sugars.

The broad bases at the bottom represent nutrient-dense foods that should make up the bulk of the diet.

Greater intakes of grains, vegetables, fruit, and milk are encouraged by the broad bases of orange, green, red.

MyPyramid
STEPS TO A HEALTHIER YOU
MyPyramid.gov

GRAINS | VEGETABLES | FRUITS | OIL | MILK | MEAT & BEANS

SOURCE: USDA, 2005.

GRAINS
In general: 1 slice of bread, 1 cup of ready-to-eat cereal, ½ cup of cooked rice, cooked pasta, or cooked cereal can be considered as 1 oz equivalent of grains. Look for "whole" before the grain name on the list of ingredients and make at least half your grains whole.

VEGETABLES
In general: 1 cup of raw or cooked vegetables or vegetable juice, or 2 cups of raw leafy greens can be considered as 1 cup from the vegetable group. Try to eat more dark green and orange veggies, as well as dry beans and peas.

FRUITS
In general: 1 cup of fruit or 100% fruit juice, or ½ cup of dried fruit can be considered as 1 cup from the fruit group. Eat a variety of fruit, including fresh, frozen, canned, or dried fruit. Go easy on fruit juices.

OIL
Measured in teaspoons of either oils or solid fats. Most sources should come from fish, nuts, and vegetable oils. Limit solid fats such as butter, stick margarine, shortening, and lard.

MILK
In general: 1 cup of milk or yogurt, 1½ oz of natural cheese, or 2 oz of processed cheese can be considered as 1 cup from the milk group. Go low-fat or fat free. If you can't consume milk, choose lactose-free products or other calcium sources.

MEATS & BEANS
In general: 1 oz of meat, poultry, or fish, ¼ cup cooked dry beans, 1 egg, 1 tbsp of peanut butter, or ½ oz of nuts or seeds can be considered as 1 oz equivalent from the Meats & Beans group.

Recommended Daily Amounts from Each Food Group

FOOD GROUP	1600 cal	1800 cal	2000 cal	2200 cal	2400 cal	2600 cal	2800 cal	3000 cal
Fruits	1½ c	1½ c	2 c	2 c	2 c	2 c	2½ c	2½ c
Vegetables	2 c	2½ c	2½ c	3 c	3 c	3½ c	3½ c	4 c
Grains	5 oz	6 oz	6 oz	7 oz	8 oz	9 oz	10 oz	10 oz
Meat and legumes	5 oz	5 oz	5½ oz	6 oz	6½ oz	6½ oz	7 oz	7 oz
Milk	3 c	3 c	3 c	3 c	3 c	3 c	3 c	3 c
Oils	5 tsp	5 tsp	6 tsp	6 tsp	7 tsp	8 tsp	8 tsp	10 tsp
Discretionary calorie allowance	132 cal	195 cal	267 cal	290 cal	362 cal	410 cal	426 cal	512 cal

*Discretionary calorie allowance: At each calorie level, people who consistently choose calorie-dense foods may be able to meet their nutrient needs without consuming their full allotment of calories. The difference between the calories needed to supply nutrients and those needed for energy is known as the *discretionary calorie allowance*.

Source: http://mypyramid.gov/   Additional information on MyPyramid can be obtained at this site, including an online individualized MyPyramid eating plan based on your age, gender, and activity level.

call it a calorie rather than a kcal. For example, if the caloric value of a food is 100 calories (that is, 100 kcal), the energy in this food would raise the temperature of 100 kilograms of water 1 degree Centigrade. Similarly, walking 1 mile would burn about 100 calories (again, 100 kcal).

Carbohydrates

Carbohydrates constitute the major source of calories the body uses to provide energy for work, maintain cells, and generate heat. They also help regulate fat and metabolize protein. Each gram of carbohydrates provides the human body with 4 calories. The major sources of carbohydrates are breads, cereals, fruits, vegetables, and milk and other dairy products. Carbohydrates are classified into simple carbohydrates and complex carbohydrates (Figure 3.2).

SIMPLE CARBOHYDRATES

Often called "sugars," **simple carbohydrates** have little nutritive value. Examples are candy, soda, and cakes. Simple carbohydrates are divided into monosaccharides and disaccharides. These carbohydrates—whose names end with "-ose"—often take the place of more nutritive foods in the diet.

Monosaccharides The simplest sugars are **monosaccharides**. The three most common monosaccharides are glucose, fructose, and galactose.

1. *Glucose* is a natural sugar found in food and also is produced in the body from other simple and complex carbohydrates. It is used as a source of energy, or it may be stored in the muscles and liver in the form of glycogen (a long chain of glucose molecules hooked together). Excess glucose in the blood is converted to fat and stored in **adipose tissue**.
2. *Fructose*, or fruit sugar, occurs naturally in fruits and honey and is converted to glucose in the body.
3. *Galactose* is produced from milk sugar in the mammary glands of lactating animals and is converted to glucose in the body.

Disaccharides The three major **disaccharides** are:

1. *Sucrose* or table sugar (glucose + fructose).
2. *Lactose* (glucose + galactose).
3. *Maltose* (glucose + glucose).

These disaccharides are broken down in the body, and the resulting simple sugars (monosaccharides) are used as indicated above.

COMPLEX CARBOHYDRATES

Complex carbohydrates are also called *polysaccharides*. Anywhere from about ten to thousands of

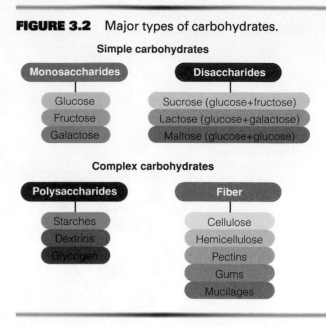

FIGURE 3.2 Major types of carbohydrates.

Simple carbohydrates

Monosaccharides	Disaccharides
Glucose	Sucrose (glucose+fructose)
Fructose	Lactose (glucose+galactose)
Galactose	Maltose (glucose+glucose)

Complex carbohydrates

Polysaccharides	Fiber
Starches	Cellulose
Dextrins	Hemicellulose
Glycogen	Pectins
	Gums
	Mucilages

monosaccharide molecules can unite to form a single polysaccharide. Examples of complex carbohydrates are starches, dextrins, and glycogen.

1. *Starch*, the storage form of glucose in plants, is needed to promote their earliest growth. Starch is commonly found in grains, seeds, corn, nuts, roots, potatoes, and legumes. In a healthful diet, grains, the richest source of starch, should supply most of the energy. Once eaten, starch is converted to glucose for the body's own energy use.
2. *Dextrins* are formed from the breakdown of large starch molecules exposed to dry heat, such as in baking bread or producing cold cereals. These complex carbohydrates of plant origin provide many valuable nutrients and can be an excellent source of fiber.
3. **Glycogen** is the animal polysaccharide synthesized from glucose and is found only in tiny amounts in meats. In essence, we manufacture it; we don't consume it. Glycogen constitutes the body's reservoir of glucose. Thousands of glucose molecules are linked, to be stored as glycogen in the liver and muscle. When a surge of energy is needed, enzymes in the muscle and the liver break down glycogen and thereby make glucose readily available for energy transformation. (This process is discussed under "Nutrition for Athletes," starting on page 79.)

FIBER

Fiber is a form of complex carbohydrate. A high-fiber diet gives a person a feeling of fullness without adding too many calories to the diet. **Dietary fiber** is present mainly in plant leaves, skins, roots, and seeds. Processing and refining foods removes almost all of their natural fiber. In our diet, the main sources of fiber are whole-grain cereals and breads, fruits, vegetables, and legumes.

Fiber is important in the diet because it decreases the risk for cardiovascular disease and cancer. Increased fiber intake also may lower the risk for coronary heart disease, because saturated fats often take the place of fiber in the diet, increasing the absorption and formation of cholesterol. Other health disorders that have been tied to low intake of fiber are constipation, diverticulitis, hemorrhoids, gallbladder disease, and obesity.

The recommended fiber intake for adults 50 years and younger is 25 grams per day for women and 38 grams for men. As a result of decreased food consumption in people over 50 years of age, 21 and 30 grams of fiber per day, respectively, are recommended.[1] Most people in the United States eat only 15 grams of fiber per day, putting them at increased risk for disease.

A person can increase fiber intake by eating more fruits, vegetables, legumes, whole grains, and whole-grain cereals. Research provides evidence that increasing fiber intake to 30 grams per day leads to a significant reduction in heart attacks, cancer of the colon, breast cancer, diabetes, and diverticulitis. Table 3.1 provides the fiber content of selected foods. A practical guideline to obtain your fiber intake is to eat at least five daily servings of

TABLE 3.1 Dietary Fiber Content of Selected Foods

Food (gm)	Serving Size	Dietary Fiber
Almonds, shelled	¼ cup	3.9
Apple	1 medium	3.7
Banana	1 small	1.2
Beans (red kidney)	½ cup	8.2
Blackberries	½ cup	4.9
Beets, red, canned (cooked)	½ cup	1.4
Brazil nuts	1 oz	2.5
Broccoli (cooked)	½ cup	3.3
Brown rice (cooked)	½ cup	1.7
Carrots (cooked)	½ cup	3.3
Cauliflower (cooked)	½ cup	5.0
Cereal		
All Bran	1 oz	8.5
Cheerios	1 oz	1.1
Cornflakes	1 oz	0.5
Fruit and Fibre	1 oz	4.0
Fruit Wheats	1 oz	2.0
Just Right	1 oz	2.0
Wheaties	1 oz	2.0
Corn (cooked)	½ cup	2.2
Eggplant (cooked)	½ cup	3.0
Lettuce (chopped)	½ cup	0.5
Orange	1 medium	4.3
Parsnips (cooked)	½ cup	2.1
Pear	1 medium	4.5
Peas (cooked)	½ cup	4.4
Popcorn (plain)	1 cup	1.2
Potato (baked)	1 medium	4.9
Strawberries	½ cup	1.6
Summer squash (cooked)	½ cup	1.6
Watermelon	1 cup	0.1

Carbohydrates A classification of dietary nutrient containing carbon, hydrogen, and oxygen; the major source of energy for the human body.

Simple carbohydrates Formed by simple or double sugar units with little nutritive value; divided into monosaccharides and disaccharides.

Monosaccharides The simplest carbohydrates (sugars), formed by five- or six-carbon skeletons. The three most common monosaccharides are glucose, fructose, and galactose.

Adipose tissue Fat cells in the body.

Disaccharides Simple carbohydrates formed by two monosaccharide units linked together, one of which is glucose. The major disaccharides are sucrose, lactose, and maltose.

Complex carbohydrates Carbohydrates formed by three or more simple sugar molecules linked together; also referred to as polysaccharides.

Glycogen Form in which glucose is stored in the body.

Dietary fiber A complex carbohydrate in plant foods that is not digested but is essential to the digestion process.

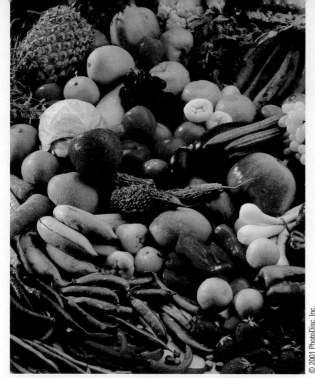

High-fiber foods are essential in a healthy diet.

fruits and vegetables and three servings of whole-grain foods (whole-grain bread, cereal, and rice).

Fiber is typically classified according to solubility in water. *Soluble fiber* dissolves in water and forms a gel-like substance that encloses food particles. This property allows soluble fiber to bind and excrete fats from the body. This type of fiber has been shown to lower blood cholesterol and blood sugar levels. Soluble fiber is found primarily in oats, fruits, barley, legumes, and psyllium (an ancient Indian grain added to some breakfast cereals).

Insoluble fiber is not easily dissolved in water, and the body cannot digest it. This type of fiber is important because it binds water, causing a softer and bulkier stool that increases **peristalsis**, the involuntary muscle contractions of intestinal walls that force the stool through the intestines and enable quicker excretion of food residues. Speeding the passage of food residues through the intestines seems to lower the risk for colon cancer, mainly because it reduces the amount of time that cancer-causing agents are in contact with the intestinal wall. Insoluble fiber is also thought to bind with carcinogens (cancer-producing substances), and more water in the stool may dilute the cancer-causing agents, lessening their potency. Sources of insoluble fiber include wheat, cereals, vegetables, and skins of fruits.

The most common types of fiber are:

1. *Cellulose*, water-soluble fiber found in plant cell walls.
2. *Hemicellulose*, water-soluble fiber found in cereal fibers.
3. *Pectins*, water-insoluble fiber found in vegetables and fruits.
4. *Gums and mucilages*, water-insoluble fiber also found in small amounts in foods of plant origin.

Surprisingly, excessive fiber intake can be detrimental to health. It can produce loss of calcium, phosphorus, and iron, not to mention gastrointestinal discomfort. If your fiber intake is below the recommended amount, increase your intake gradually over several weeks to avoid gastrointestinal disturbances. While increasing fiber intake, be sure to drink more water to avoid constipation and even dehydration.

Fats

The human body uses **fats** as a source of energy. Fat is the most concentrated energy source. Each gram of fat supplies 9 calories to the body (in contrast to 4 for carbohydrates). Fats are a part of the human cell structure. Deposits of fat cells are used as stored energy and as an insulator to preserve body heat. They absorb shock, supply essential fatty acids, and carry the fat-soluble vitamins A, D, E, and K. Fats can be classified into three main groups: simple, compound, and derived (see Figure 3.3). The most familiar sources of fat are whole milk and other dairy products, meats, and meat alternatives such as eggs and nuts.

SIMPLE FATS

A simple fat consists of a glyceride molecule linked to one, two, or three units of fatty acids. Depending on the number of fatty acids attached, simple fats are divided into *monoglycerides* (one fatty acid), *diglycerides* (two fatty acids), and *triglycerides* (three fatty acids). More than 90 percent of the weight of fat in foods and more than 95 percent of the stored fat in the human body are in the form of triglycerides.

The length of the carbon atom chain and the amount of hydrogen saturation (that is, the number of hydrogen molecules attached to the carbon chain) in fatty acids varies. Based on the extent of saturation, fatty acids are said to be saturated or unsaturated. Unsaturated fatty acids are classified further into monounsaturated and polyunsaturated. Saturated fatty acids are mainly of animal origin; unsaturated fats are found mostly in plant products.

Saturated Fats   In saturated fatty acids (often called "saturated fats"), the carbon atoms are fully saturated with hydrogen atoms; only single bonds link the carbon atoms on the chain (see Figure 3.4). Foods high in saturated fatty acids are meats, animal fat, lard, whole milk, cream, butter, cheese, ice cream, hydrogenated oils (hydrogenation makes oils saturated), coconut oil, and palm oils. Saturated fats

FIGURE 3.3 Major types of fats (lipids).

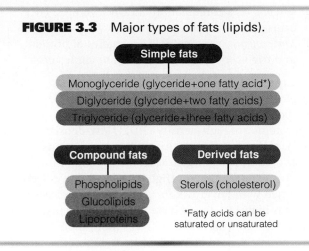

Simple fats
- Monoglyceride (glyceride+one fatty acid*)
- Diglyceride (glyceride+two fatty acids)
- Triglyceride (glyceride+three fatty acids)

Compound fats
- Phospholipids
- Glucolipids
- Lipoproteins

Derived fats
- Sterols (cholesterol)

*Fatty acids can be saturated or unsaturated

FIGURE 3.4 Chemical structure of saturated and unsaturated fats.

Saturated Fatty Acid

Monounsaturated Fatty Acid

Double Bond

Polyunsaturated Fatty Acid

Double Bonds

*Glyceride component

typically do not melt at room temperature. Coconut and palm oils are exceptions. In general, saturated fats raise the blood cholesterol level.

Unsaturated Fats   In unsaturated fatty acids (often called "unsaturated fats"), double bonds form between unsaturated carbons. In monounsaturated fatty acids (MUFA), only one double bond is found along the chain. Examples of monounsaturated fatty acids are olive, canola, rapeseed, peanut, and sesame oils. Polyunsaturated fatty acids (PUFA) contain two or more double bonds between unsaturated carbon atoms along the chain. Corn, cottonseed, safflower, walnut, sunflower, and soybean oils are high in polyunsaturated fatty acids. Unsaturated fats usually are liquid at room temperature. Shorter fatty acid chains also tend to be liquid at room temperature.

Polyunsaturated and monounsaturated fats tend to lower blood cholesterol. When unsaturated fats replace saturated fats in the diet, the former tend to stimulate the liver to clear cholesterol from the blood.

Other Fatty Acids   Hydrogen is often added to monounsaturated and polyunsaturated fats to increase shelf life and to solidify them so they are more spreadable. During this process, called "partial hydrogenation," the position of hydrogen atoms may be changed along the carbon chain, transforming the fat into a **trans fatty acid**.

Margarine and spreads, crackers, cookies, dairy products, meats, and fast foods often contain trans fatty acids. Trans fatty acids are not essential and provide no known health benefit. In fact, health-conscious people minimize their intake of these types of fats, because diets high in trans fatty acids elevate cholesterol. Paying attention to food labels is important, because the words "partially hydrogenated" and "trans fatty acids" indicate that the product carries a health risk just as high as that of

saturated fat. Starting in 2006, the Food and Drug Administration requires that food labels list trans fatty acids so consumers can make healthier choices.

A type of polyunsaturated fatty acids that has gained attention in recent years are the **omega-3 fatty acids** (specifically alpha-linolenic acid), which are heart-healthy. Fish—especially fresh or frozen mackerel, herring, tuna, salmon, and lake trout—and flaxseed contain omega-3 fatty acids. Canned fish is not recommended for this purpose, because the canning process destroys most of the omega-3 oil. These fatty acids are also found, but to a lesser extent, in milk, canola oil, walnuts, soybeans, and wheat germ.

One of the simplest ways to increase omega-3 fatty acids is to consume flaxseed, which is also high in fiber and plant chemicals known as *lignans*. The

Peristalsis   Involuntary muscle contractions of intestinal walls that facilitate excretion of wastes.

Fats   A classification of nutrients containing carbon, hydrogen, some oxygen, and sometimes other chemical elements.

Trans fatty acid   Solidified fat formed by adding hydrogen to monounsaturated and polyunsaturated fats to increase shelf life.

Omega-3 fatty acids   Polyunsaturated fatty acids found primarily in cold-water seafood, flaxseed, and flaxseed oil; thought to lower blood cholesterol and triglycerides.

oil in flaxseed is high in alpha-linolenic acid and has been shown to reduce abnormal heart rhythms and prevent blood clots.[2]

Studies are being conducted to investigate the potential cancer-fighting ability of lignans. In one report, the addition of a daily ounce (3 to 4 tablespoons) of ground flaxseeds to the diet seemed to lead to a decrease in the onset of tumors, preventing their formation, and even led to a shrinkage of tumors.[3]

Amounts of flaxseed in the diet higher than recommended, however, is not recommended. High doses actually may be detrimental to health. Pregnant and lactating women, especially, should not consume large amounts of flaxseed.

Because flaxseeds have a hard outer shell, they should be ground to obtain the nutrients; whole seeds will pass through the body undigested. Flavor and nutrients are best preserved by grinding the seeds just before use. Pre-ground seeds should be kept sealed and refrigerated. Ground flaxseeds can be mixed with salad dressings, salads, wheat flour, pancakes, muffins, cereals, rice, cottage cheese, and yogurt. Flaxseed oil also may be used, but the oil must be kept refrigerated because it spoils quickly. The oil cannot be used for cooking either, because it scorches easily. A drawback of flaxseed oils is that they have little or no fiber and lignans.

Other essential unsaturated fatty acids are the **omega-6** group, in particular linoleic acid. Our diets are typically high in omega-6-rich oils, found in corn, sunflower, and most oils in processed foods. We usually consume 10 to 20 times more omega-6 than omega-3. Excessive omega-6 fatty acids amplify inflammatory processes that can damage organs in the body.

In 2002, for the first time, the National Academy of Sciences set recommended intakes for alpha-linolenic acid and linoleic acid. For alpha-linolenic acid, the recommendations are 1.6 and 1.1 grams per day for men and women, respectively. The standard for linoleic acid has been set at 17 grams per day for men and 12 grams for women.

Some data suggest that the amount of fish oil obtained by eating one or two servings of fish weekly lessens the risk for coronary heart disease. However, people who have diabetes or a history of hemorrhaging or strokes, who are on aspirin or blood-thinning therapy, and who are presurgical patients should not consume fish oil except under a physician's instruction.

COMPOUND FATS

Compound fats are a combination of simple fats and other chemicals. Examples are:

1. *Phospholipids:* similar to triglycerides, except that choline (or another compound) and phosphoric acid take the place of one of the fatty acid units.

2. *Glucolipids:* a combination of carbohydrates, fatty acids, and nitrogen.
3. *Lipoproteins:* water-soluble aggregates of protein and triglycerides, phospholipids, or cholesterol.

Lipoproteins (a combination of lipids and proteins) are especially important because they transport fats in the blood. The major forms of lipoproteins are high-density (HDL), low-density (LDL), and very-low-density (VLDL) lipoproteins. Lipoproteins play a large role in developing or in preventing heart disease. High HDL levels have been associated with lower risk for coronary heart disease, whereas high LDL levels have been linked to increased risk for this disease. HDL is more than 50 percent protein and contains little cholesterol; LDL is approximately 25 percent protein and nearly 50 percent cholesterol. VLDL contains about 50 percent triglycerides, only about 10 percent protein, and 20 percent cholesterol.

DERIVED FATS

Derived fats combine simple and compound fats. **Sterols** are an example. Although sterols contain no fatty acids, they are considered lipids because they do not dissolve in water. The most often mentioned sterol is cholesterol, which is found in many foods or can be manufactured in the body—primarily from saturated fats.

Proteins

Proteins are the main substances the body uses to build and repair tissues such as muscles, blood, internal organs, skin, hair, nails, and bones. They form a part of hormone, antibody, and **enzyme** molecules. Enzymes play a key role in all of the body's processes. Because all enzymes are formed by proteins, this nutrient is necessary for normal functioning. Proteins also help maintain the normal balance of body fluids.

Proteins can be used as a source of energy, too, but only if sufficient carbohydrates are not available. Each gram of protein yields 4 calories of energy (the same as carbohydrates). The main sources of protein are meats and alternatives, and milk and other dairy products. Excess proteins may be converted to glucose or fat, or even excreted in the urine.

The human body uses 20 **amino acids** to form different types of protein. Amino acids contain nitrogen, carbon, hydrogen, and oxygen. Of the 20 amino acids, 9 are called "essential amino acids" because the body cannot produce them. The other 11, termed "nonessential amino acids," can be manufactured in the body if food proteins in the diet provide enough nitrogen (see Table 3.2). For the body to function normally, all amino acids shown in the table must be present in the diet.

TABLE 3.2 Amino Acids

Essential Amino Acids*	Nonessential Amino Acids
Histidine	Alanine
Isoleucine	Arginine
Leucine	Asparagine
Lysine	Aspartic acid
Methionine	Cysteine
Phenylalanine	Glutamic acid
Threonine	Glutamine
Tryptophan	Glycine
Valine	Proline
	Serine
	Tyrosine

*Must be provided in the diet, because the body cannot manufacture them.

Proteins that contain all the essential amino acids, known as "complete" or "higher-quality" protein, are usually of animal origin. If one or more of the essential amino acids is missing, the proteins are termed "incomplete" or "lower-quality" protein. Individuals have to take in enough protein to ensure nitrogen for adequate production of amino acids and also to get enough high-quality protein to obtain the essential amino acids.

Protein deficiency is not a problem in the typical U.S. diet. Two glasses of skim milk combined with about 4 ounces of poultry or fish meet the daily protein requirement. Too much animal protein, on the other hand, can cause serious health problems. Some people eat twice as much protein as they need. Protein foods from animal sources are often high in fat, saturated fat, and cholesterol, which can lead to cardiovascular disease and cancer. Too much animal protein also decreases blood enzymes that prevent precancerous cells from developing into tumors.

As mentioned earlier, a well-balanced diet contains a variety of foods from all five basic food groups, including wise selection of foods from animal sources (see also "Balancing the Diet," pages 60–61). Based on current nutrition data, meat (poultry and fish included) should be replaced by grains, legumes, vegetables, and fruits as main courses. Meats should be used more for flavoring than for volume. Daily consumption of beef, poultry, or fish should be limited to 3 ounces (about the size of a deck of cards) to 6 ounces.

Vitamins

Vitamins are necessary for normal bodily metabolism, growth, and development. Vitamins are classified into two types based on their solubility: fat-soluble (A, D, E, and K) and water-soluble (B complex and C). The body does not manufacture most vitamins, so they can be obtained only through a well-balanced diet. To decrease loss of vitamins during cooking, natural foods should be microwaved or steamed rather than boiled in water that is thrown out later.

A few exceptions, such as vitamins A, D, and K, are formed in the body. Vitamin A is produced from beta-carotene, found mainly in yellow foods such as carrots, pumpkin, and sweet potatoes. Vitamin D is created when ultraviolet light from the sun transforms 7-dehydrocholesterol, a compound in human skin. Vitamin K is created in the body by intestinal bacteria. The major functions of vitamins are outlined in Table 3.3.

Vitamins C, E, and beta-carotene also function as antioxidants, which are thought to play a key role in preventing chronic diseases. The specific function of these antioxidant nutrients and of the mineral selenium (also an antioxidant) are discussed under "Antioxidants" (page 73) and "Folate," (page 76).

Minerals

Approximately 25 **minerals** have important roles in body functioning. Minerals are inorganic substances contained in all cells, especially those in hard parts of the body (bones, nails, teeth). Minerals are crucial to maintaining water balance and the acid–base balance. They are essential components of respiratory pigments, enzymes, and enzyme systems, and they regulate muscular and nervous tissue impulses, blood clotting, and normal heart rhythm.

The four minerals mentioned most often are calcium, iron, sodium, and selenium. Calcium

Omega-6 fatty acids Polyunsaturated fatty acids found primarily in corn and sunflower oils and most oils in processed foods.

Lipoproteins Lipids covered by proteins, they transport fats in the blood; types are LDL, HDL, and VLDL.

Sterols Derived fats, of which cholesterol is the best-known example.

Proteins A classification of nutrients consisting of complex organic compounds containing nitrogen and formed by combinations of amino acids; the main substances used in the body to build and repair tissues.

Enzymes Catalysts that facilitate chemical reactions in the body.

Amino acids Chemical compounds that contain nitrogen, carbon, hydrogen, and oxygen; the basic building blocks the body uses to build different types of protein.

Vitamins Organic nutrients essential for normal metabolism, growth, and development of the body.

Minerals Inorganic nutrients essential for normal body functions; found in the body and in food.

TABLE 3.3 Major Functions of Vitamins

Nutrient	Good Sources	Major Functions	Deficiency Symptoms
Vitamin A	Milk, cheese, eggs, liver, yellow and dark green fruits and vegetables	Required for healthy bones, teeth, skin, gums, and hair; maintenance of inner mucous membranes, thus increasing resistance to infection; adequate vision in dim light.	Night blindness; decreased growth; decreased resistance to infection; rough, dry skin
Vitamin D	Fortified milk, cod liver oil, salmon, tuna, egg yolk	Necessary for bones and teeth; needed for calcium and phosphorus absorption.	Rickets (bone softening), fractures, muscle spasms
Vitamin E	Vegetable oils, yellow and green leafy vegetables, margarine, wheat germ, whole grain breads and cereals	Related to oxidation and normal muscle and red blood cell chemistry.	Leg cramps, red blood cell breakdown
Vitamin K	Green leafy vegetables, cauliflower, cabbage, eggs, peas, potatoes	Essential for normal blood clotting.	Hemorrhaging
Vitamin B$_1$ (Thiamin)	Whole grain or enriched bread, lean meats and poultry, fish, liver, pork, poultry, organ meats, legumes, nuts, dried yeast	Assists in proper use of carbohydrates, normal functioning of nervous system, maintenance of good appetite.	Loss of appetite, nausea, confusion, cardiac abnormalities, muscle spasms
Vitamin B$_2$ (Riboflavin)	Eggs, milk, leafy green vegetables, whole grains, lean meats, dried beans and peas	Contributes to energy release from carbohydrates, fats, and proteins; needed for normal growth and development, good vision, and healthy skin.	Cracking of the corners of the mouth, inflammation of the skin, impaired vision
Vitamin B$_6$ (Pyridoxine)	Vegetables, meats, whole grain cereals, soybeans, peanuts, potatoes	Necessary for protein and fatty acids metabolism and for normal red blood cell formation.	Depression, irritability, muscle spasms, nausea
Vitamin B$_{12}$	Meat, poultry, fish, liver, organ meats, eggs, shellfish, milk, cheese	Required for normal growth, red blood cell formation, nervous system and digestive tract functioning.	Impaired balance, weakness, drop in red blood cell count
Niacin	Liver and organ meats, meat, fish, poultry, whole grains, enriched breads, nuts, green leafy vegetables, and dried beans and peas	Contributes to energy release from carbohydrates, fats, and proteins; normal growth and development; and formation of hormones and nerve-regulating substances.	Confusion, depression, weakness, weight loss
Biotin	Liver, kidney, eggs, yeast, legumes, milk, nuts, dark green vegetables	Essential for carbohydrate metabolism and fatty acid synthesis.	Inflamed skin, muscle pain, depression, weight loss
Folic Acid	Leafy green vegetables, organ meats, whole grains and cereals, dried beans	Needed for cell growth and reproduction and for red blood cell formation.	Decreased resistance to infection
Pantothenic Acid	All natural foods, especially liver, kidney, eggs, nuts, yeast, milk, dried peas and beans, green leafy vegetables	Related to carbohydrate and fat metabolism.	Depression, low blood sugar, leg cramps, nausea, headaches
Vitamin C (Ascorbic acid)	Fruits, vegetables	Helps protect against infection; required for formation of collagenous tissue, normal blood vessels, teeth, and bones.	Slow-healing wounds, loose teeth, hemorrhaging, rough scaly skin, irritability

deficiency may result in osteoporosis, and low iron intake can induce iron-deficiency anemia (both are discussed under "Special Nutrient Needs of Women," pages 82–85). High sodium intake may contribute to high blood pressure. Selenium seems to be important in preventing certain types of cancer. Specific functions of some of the most important minerals are given in Table 3.4

Water

The most important nutrient is **water**, as it is involved in almost every vital body process: in digesting and absorbing food, in energy production, in the circulatory process, in body heat regulation, in removing waste products, in building and rebuilding cells, and in transporting other nutrients. Approximately 60 percent of total body weight is water (see Figure 3.5).

Water is contained in almost all foods, but primarily in liquid foods, fruits, and vegetables. Although for decades the recommendation was to consume at least 8 cups of water per day, a panel of scientists of the Institute of Medicine of the National Academy of Sciences indicated in 2004 that people are getting enough water from the liquids (milk,

TABLE 3.4 Major Functions of Minerals

Nutrient	Good Sources	Major Functions	Deficiency Symptoms
Calcium	Milk, yogurt, cheese, green leafy vegetables, dried beans, sardines, salmon	Required for strong teeth and bone formation; maintenance of good muscle tone, heartbeat, and nerve function.	Bone pain and fractures, periodontal disease, muscle cramps
Copper	Seafood, meats, beans, nuts, whole grains	Helps with iron absorption and hemoglobin formation; required to synthesize the enzyme cytochrome oxidase.	Anemia (although deficiency is rare in humans)
Iron	Organ meats, lean meats, seafoods, eggs, dried peas and beans, nuts, whole and enriched grains, green leafy vegetables	Major component of hemoglobin; aids in energy utilization.	Nutritional anemia, overall weakness
Phosphorus	Meats, fish, milk, eggs, dried beans and peas, whole grains, processed foods	Required for bone and teeth formation and for energy release regulation.	Bone pain and fracture, weight loss, weakness
Zinc	Milk, meat, seafood, whole grains, nuts, eggs, dried beans	Essential component of hormones, insulin, and enzymes; used in normal growth and development.	Loss of appetite, slow-healing wounds, skin problems
Magnesium	Green leafy vegetables, whole grains, nuts, soybeans, seafood, legumes	Needed for bone growth and maintenance, carbohydrate and protein utilization, nerve function, temperature regulation.	Irregular heartbeat, weakness, muscle spasms, sleeplessness
Sodium	Table salt, processed foods, meat	Needed for body fluid regulation, transmission of nerve impulses, heart action.	Rarely seen
Potassium	Legumes, whole grains, bananas, orange juice, dried fruits, potatoes	Required for heart action, bone formation and maintenance, regulation of energy release, acid-base regulation.	Irregular heartbeat, nausea, weakness
Selenium	Seafood, meat, whole grains	Component of enzymes; functions in close association with vitamin E.	Muscle pain, possible heart muscle deterioration, possible hair and nail loss

FIGURE 3.5 Approximate proportions of nutrients in the human body.

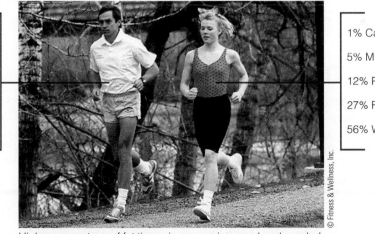

1% Carbohydrates
6% Minerals
16% Protein
17% Fat
61% Water

1% Carbohydrates
5% Minerals
12% Protein
27% Fat
56% Water

© Fitness & Wellness, Inc.

Higher percentage of fat tissue in women is normal and needed for reproduction.

juices, sodas, coffee) and the moisture content of solid foods. Most Americans and Canadians remain well-hydrated simply by using thirst as their guide. Caffeine-containing drinks are also acceptable as a water source because data indicate that people who

Water The most important classification of essential body nutrients, involved in almost every vital body process.

TABLE 3.5 The American Diet: Current and Recommended Carbohydrate, Fat, and Protein Intake Expressed as a Percentage of Total Calories

	Current %	Recommended %*
Carbohydrates:	50%	45–65%
Simple	26%	Less than 25%
Complex	24%	20–40%
Fat:	34%	20–35%**
Monounsaturated:	11%	Up to 20%
Polyunsaturated:	10%	Up to 10%
Saturated:	13%	Less than 7%
Protein:	16%	10–35%

* 2002 recommended guidelines by the National Academy of Sciences.

** Less than 30% recommended by most health organizations. A higher amount may be indicated for people with metabolic syndrome.

regularly consume such beverages do not have a greater 24-hour urine output than those who don't.

An exception of not waiting for the thirst signal to replenish water loss is when an individual exercises in the heat or does so for an extended time (see Chapter 9, page 279). Water lost under these conditions must be replenished regularly. If you wait for the thirst signal, you may have lost too much water already. At 2 percent of body weight lost, a person is dehydrated. At 5 percent, one may become dizzy and disoriented, have trouble with cognitive skills and heart function, and even lose consciousness.

Balancing the Diet

One of the fundamental ways to enjoy good health and live life to its fullest is through a well-balanced diet. Several guidelines have been published to help you accomplish this. As illustrated in Table 3.5, the 2002 recommended guidelines by the National Academy of Sciences (NAS) state that daily caloric intake should be distributed so that 45 to 65 percent of the total calories come from carbohydrates (mostly complex carbohydrates and less than 25 percent from sugar), 20 to 35 percent from fat, and 10 to 35 percent from protein.[4] These new ranges offer greater flexibility in planning diets according to individual health and physical activity needs.

In addition to the macronutrients, the diet must include all of the essential vitamins, minerals, and water. The source of fat calories is also critical. The National Cholesterol Education Program recommends that, of total calories, saturated fat constitutes less than 7 percent, polyunsaturated up to 10 percent, and monounsaturated fat up to 20 percent.

BEHAVIOR MODIFICATION PLANNING

CALORIC AND FAT CONTENT OF SELECTED FAST FOOD ITEMS

	Calories	Total Fat (grams)	Saturated Fat (grams)	Percent Fat Calories
Burgers				
McDonald's Big Mac	590	34	11	52
McDonald's Big N' Tasty with Cheese	590	37	12	56
McDonald's Quarter Pounder with Cheese	530	30	13	51
Burger King Whopper	760	46	15	54
Burger King Bacon Double Cheeseburger	580	34	18	53
Burger King BK Smokehouse Cheddar Griller	720	48	19	60
Burger King Whopper with Cheese	850	53	22	56
Burger King Double Whopper	1,060	69	27	59
Burger King Double Whopper with Cheese	1,150	76	33	59
Sandwiches				
Arby's Regular Roast Beef	350	16	6	41
Arby's Super Roast Beef	470	23	7	44
Arby's Roast Chicken Club	520	28	7	48
Arby's Market Fresh Roast Beef & Swiss	810	42	13	47
McDonald's Crispy Chicken	430	21	8	43
McDonald's Filet-O-Fish	470	26	5	50
McDonald's Chicken McGrill	400	17	3	38
Wendy's Chicken Club	470	19	4	36
Wendy's Breast Fillet	430	16	3	34
Wendy's Grilled Chicken	300	7	2	21
Burger King Specialty Chicken	560	28	6	45
Subway Veggie Delight*	226	3	1	12
Subway Turkey Breast	281	5	2	16
Subway Sweet Onion Chicken Teriyaki	374	5	2	12
Subway Steak & Cheese	390	14	5	32
Subway Cold Cut Trio	440	21	7	43
Subway Tuna	450	22	6	44
Mexican				
Taco Bell Crunchy Taco	170	10	4	53
Taco Bell Taco Supreme	220	14	6	57
Taco Bell Soft Chicken Taco	190	7	3	33
Taco Bell Tostada	250	12	5	43
Taco Bell Bean Burrito	370	12	4	29
Taco Bell Fiesta Steak Burrito	370	12	4	29
Taco Bell Grilled Steak Soft Taco	290	17	4	53
Taco Bell Double Decker Taco	340	14	5	37
French Fries				
Wendy's, biggie (5½ oz.)	440	19	7	39
McDonald's, large (6 oz.)	540	26	9	43
Burger King, large (5½ oz)	500	25	13	45
Shakes				
Wendy's Frosty, medium (16 oz.)	440	11	7	23
McDonald's McFlurry, small (12 oz.)	610	22	14	32
Burger King, Old Fashioned Ice Cream Shake, medium (22 oz)	760	41	29	49
Hash Browns				
McDonald's Hash Browns (2 oz.)	130	8	4	55
Burger King, Hash Browns, small (2½ oz.)	230	15	9	59

* 6-inch sandwich with no mayo

Source: Adapted from *Restaurant Confidential* by Michael F. Jacobson and Jayne Hurley (Workman, 2002), by permission of Center for Science in the Public Interest.

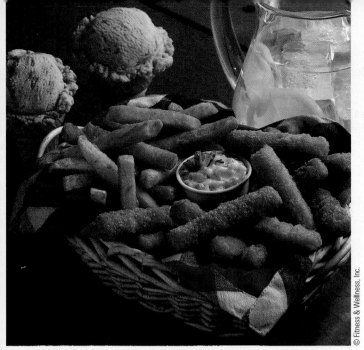

The typical American diet is too high in fat intake.

Rating a particular diet accurately is difficult without a complete nutrient analysis. You have an opportunity to perform this analysis in Lab 3A.

The 2002 NAS guidelines are in sharp contrast to those of major national health organizations, which recommend 50 to 60 percent of total calories from carbohydrates, less than 30 percent from fat, and about 15 percent from protein. These percentages are within the ranges recommended by the NAS. The most drastic difference appears in the NAS allowed range of fat intake, up to 35 percent of total calories. This higher percentage was included to accommodate individuals with metabolic syndrome (see Chapter 11, page 346) who have an abnormal insulin response to carbohydrates and may need additional fat in the diet.

The NAS recommendations will be effective only if people consistently replace saturated and trans fatty acids with unsaturated fatty acids. The latter will require dramatic changes in the typical "unhealthy" American diet, which is generally high in red meats, whole dairy products, and fast foods—all of which are high in saturated and/or trans fatty acids.

Diets in most developed countries have changed significantly since the turn of the 20th century. Today, people eat more calories and fat, fewer carbohydrates, and about the same amount of protein. People also weigh more than they did in 1900, an indication that they are eating more calories and are not as physically active as their ancestors were.

Diets also were much healthier at the turn of the 20th century. In the United States, at the beginning of the 20th century, carbohydrates accounted for 57 percent of the total daily caloric intake, 67 percent

of which were complex carbohydrates. Today, carbohydrate intake has decreased to 50 percent and complex carbohydrates account for only 24 percent of this intake. The proportion of fat has risen from 32 percent to 34 percent, but a higher proportion is in the form of saturated and trans fatty acids.

Nutrition Standards

Nutritionists use a variety of nutrient standards. The most widely known nutrient standard is the RDA, or Recommended Dietary Allowances. This, however, is not the only standard. Among others are the Dietary Reference Intakes and the Daily Values on food labels. Each standard has a different purpose and utilization in dietary planning and assessment.

Dietary Reference Intakes

To help people meet dietary guidelines, the National Academy of Sciences developed a set of dietary nutrient intakes for healthy people in the United States and Canada, the **Dietary Reference Intakes (DRIs)**. The DRIs are based on a review of the most current research on nutrient needs of healthy people. The DRI reports are written by the Food and Nutrition Board of the Institute of Medicine in cooperation with scientists from Canada.

The general term DRIs includes four types of reference values for planning and assessing diets and for establishing adequate amounts and maximum safe nutrient intakes in the diet: Estimated Average Requirement (EAR), Recommended Dietary Allowance (RDA), Adequate Intakes (AI), and Tolerable Upper Intake Levels (UL) . The type of reference value used for a given nutrient and a specific age/gender group is determined according to available scientific information and the intended use of the dietary standard.

EAR

The **Estimated Average Requirement (EAR)** is the amount of a nutrient that is estimated to meet the nutrient requirement of half the healthy people in specific age and gender groups. At this nutrient intake level, 50 percent of the people do not have

Dietary Reference Intakes (DRIs) A general term that describes four types of nutrient standards that establish adequate amounts and maximum safe nutrient intakes in the diet. These standards are Estimated Average Requirements (EAR), Recommended Dietary Allowances (RDA), Adequate Intakes (AI), and Tolerable Upper Intake Levels (UL).

Estimated Average Requirements (EAR) The amount of a nutrient that meets the dietary needs in half the people.

TABLE 3.6 Dietary Reference Intakes (DRIs): Recommended Dietary Allowances (RDA) and Adequate Intakes (AI) for Selected Nutrients

	Recommended Dietary Allowances (RDA)													**Adequate Intakes (AI)**					
	Thiamin (mg)	Riboflavin (mg)	Niacin (mg NE)	Vitamin B_6 (mg)	Folate (mcg DFE)	Vitamin B_{12} (mcg)	Phosphorus (mg)	Magnesium (mg)	Vitamin A (mcg)	Vitamin C (mg)	Vitamin E (mg)	Selenium (mcg)	Iron (mcg)	Calcium (mg)	Vitamin D (mcg)	Fluoride (mg)	Pantothenic acid (mg)	Biotin (mg)	Choline (mg)
Males																			
14–18	1.2	1.3	16	1.3	400	2.4	1,250	410	900	75	15	55	11	1,300	5	3	5.0	25	550
19–30	1.2	1.3	16	1.3	400	2.4	700	400	900	90	15	55	8	1,000	5	4	5.0	30	550
31–50	1.2	1.3	16	1.3	400	2.4	700	420	900	90	15	55	8	1,000	5	4	5.0	30	550
51–70	1.2	1.3	16	1.7	400	2.4	700	420	900	90	15	55	8	1,200	10	4	5.0	30	550
>70	1.2	1.3	16	1.7	400	2.4	700	420	900	90	15	55	8	1,200	15	4	5.0	30	550
Females																			
14–18	1.0	1.0	14	1.2	400	2.4	1,250	360	700	65	15	55	15	1,300	5	3	5.0	25	400
19–30	1.1	1.1	14	1.3	400	2.4	700	310	700	75	15	55	18	1,000	5	3	5.0	30	425
31–50	1.1	1.1	14	1.3	400	2.4	700	320	700	75	15	55	18	1,000	5	3	5.0	30	425
51–70	1.1	1.1	14	1.5	400	2.4	700	320	700	75	15	55	8	1,200	10	3	5.0	30	425
>70	1.1	1.1	14	1.5	400	2.4	700	320	700	75	15	55	8	1,200	15	3	5.0	30	425
Pregnant	1.4	1.4	18	1.9	600	2.6	*	+40	750	85	15	60	27	*	*	3	6.0	30	450
Lactating	1.5	1.6	17	2.0	500	2.8	*	*	1,300	120	19	70	10	*	*	3	7.0	35	550

* Values for these nutrients do not change with pregnancy or lactation. Use the value listed for women of comparable age.

Source: Adapted with permission from *Recommended Dietary Allowances*, 10th Edition, and the *Dietary Reference Intakes* series. Copyright © 1989 and 2002, respectively, by the National Academy of Sciences. Courtesy of the National Academies Press, Washington, DC.

their nutritional requirements met. If, for example, we look at 300 healthy women at age 26, the EAR would meet the nutritional requirement for only half of these women.

RDA

The **Recommended Dietary Allowance (RDA)** is the daily amount of a nutrient considered adequate to meet the known nutrient needs of nearly all healthy people in the United States. Because the committee must decide what level of intake to recommend for everybody, the RDA is set well above the EAR and covers about 98 percent of the population. Stated another way, the RDA recommendation for any nutrient is well above almost everyone's actual requirement. The RDA could be considered a goal for adequate intake. The process for determining the RDA depends on being able to set an EAR, because RDAs are statistically determined from the EAR values. If an EAR cannot be set, no RDA can be established.

AI

When data are insufficient or inadequate to set an EAR, an **Adequate Intakes (AI)** value is determined instead of the RDA. The AI value is derived from approximations of observed nutrient intakes by a group or groups of healthy people. The AI value for children and adults is expected to meet or exceed the nutritional requirements of a corresponding healthy population.

Nutrients for which daily DRIs have been set are presented in Table 3.6.

TABLE 3.7 Tolerable Upper Intake Levels (UL) of Selected Nutrients for Adults (19–70 years)

Nutrient	UL per Day
Calcium	2.5 gr
Phosphorus	4.0 gr*
Magnesium	350 mg
Vitamin D	50 mcg
Fluoride	10 mg
Niacin	35 mg
Iron	45 mg
Vitamin B₆	100 mg
Folate	1,000 mcg
Choline	3.5 gr
Vitamin A	3,000 mcg
Vitamin C	2,000 mg
Vitamin E	1,000 mg
Selenium	400 mcg

* 3.5 gr per day for pregnant women.

UL

The **Upper Intake Level (UL)** establishes the highest level of nutrient intake that seems to be safe for most healthy people, beyond which exists an increased risk of adverse effects. As intakes increase above the UL, so does the risk of adverse effects. In general terms, the optimum nutrient range for healthy eating is between the RDA and the UL. The established ULs are presented in Table 3.7.

Daily Values

The **Daily Values (DVs)** are reference values for nutrients and food components for use on food labels. The DVs include fat, saturated fat, and carbohydrates (as a percent of total calories); cholesterol, sodium, and potassium (in milligrams); and fiber and protein (in grams). The DVs for total fat, saturated fat, and carbohydrate are expressed as percentages for a 2,000-calorie diet and may therefore require adjustments depending on an individual's daily **Estimated Energy Requirement (EER)** in calories. For example, on a 2,000-calorie diet (EER), recommended carbohydrate intake is about 300 grams (about 60 percent of EER), and fat is 65 grams (about 30 percent of EER) (see Figure 3.6). The vitamin, mineral, and protein DVs were adapted from the RDAs. The DVs are also not as specific for age and gender groups as are the DRIs. Both the DRIs and the DVs apply only to healthy adults. They are not intended for people who are ill and may require additional nutrients.

Figure 3.6 shows the food label with U.S. Recommended Daily Values.

Nutrient Analysis

The first step in evaluating your diet is to conduct a nutrient analysis. This can be quite educational, because most people do not realize how harmful and non-nutritious many common foods are. The analysis covers calories, carbohydrates, fats, cholesterol, and sodium, as well as eight crucial nutrients: protein, calcium, iron, vitamin A, thiamin, riboflavin, niacin, and vitamin C. If the diet has enough of these eight nutrients, the foods consumed in natural form to provide these nutrients typically contain all the other nutrients the human body needs.

Profile Plus
You are what you eat. Analyze your current diet and plan for a healthy change using the activity on your CD-ROM.

To do your own nutrient analysis, keep a 3-day record of everything you eat using the form in Lab 3A (make additional copies of this form as needed). At the end of each day, look up the nutrient content for those foods in the list of Nutritive Values of Selected Foods (located in Appendix A). Record this information on the form in Figure 3A.1. If you do not find a food in Appendix A, the information may be on the food container itself.

When you have recorded the nutritive values for each day, add up each column and write the totals at the bottom of the chart. After the third day, fill in your totals on Figure 3A.2 and compute an average for the 3 days. To rate your diet, compare your figures with those in the Recommended Dietary Allowances (RDA) (Table 3.6). The results will give a good indication of areas of strength and deficiency in your current diet.

Recommended Dietary Allowances (RDA) The daily amount of a nutrient (statistically determined from the EARs) considered adequate to meet the known nutrient needs of almost 98 percent of all healthy people in the United States.

Adequate Intakes (AI) The recommended amount of a nutrient intake when sufficient evidence is not available to calculate the EAR and subsequent RDA.

Upper Intake Level (UL) The highest level of nutrient intake that appears safe for most healthy people, beyond which exists an increased risk of adverse effects.

Daily Values (DVs) Reference values for nutrients and food components used in food labels.

Estimated Energy Requirement (EER) The average dietary energy (caloric) intake that is predicted to maintain energy balance in a healthy adult of defined age, gender, weight, height, and level of physical activity, consistent with good health.

FIGURE 3.6 Food label with U.S. Recommended Daily Values.

1 Better by Design
How to recognize the new food labels

The new food labels feature a revamped nutrition panel titled "Nutrition Facts," with nutrient listings that reflect current health concerns. Now you'll be able to find information on fat, fiber, and other food components fundamental to lowering your risk of cancer and other chronic diseases. Listings for nutrients like thiamin and riboflavin will no longer be required, because Americans generally eat enough of them these days.

2 Size Up the Situation
All serving sizes are created equal

Now you can compare similar products and know that their serving sizes are basically identical. So when you realize how much fat is packed into that carton of double-dutch-chocolate-caramel-chew ice cream you're eyeing, you might opt for low-fat frozen yogurt instead. Serving sizes will also be standardized, so manufacturers can't make nutrition claims for unrealistically small portions. That means a chocolate cake, for example, must be divided into 8 servings sized to satisfy the average person—not 16 servings sized to satisfy the average munchkin.

3 Look Before You Leap
Use the Daily Values

You will find the Daily Values on the bottom half of the "Nutrition Facts" panel. Some represent maximum levels of nutrients that should be consumed each day for a healthful diet (as with fat) while others refer to minimum levels that can be exceeded (as with carbohydrates). They are based on both a 2,000 and 2,500 calorie diet. Your own needs may be more or less, but these figures give you a point from which to compare. For example, the sample label indicates that someone with a 2,000 calorie diet should eat no more than 65 grams of fat per day. This is based on a diet getting 30 percent of calories as fat. If you normally eat less calories, or want to eat less than 30 percent of calories as fat, your daily fat consumption will be lower.

4 Rate It Right
Scan the % Daily Values

The % Daily Values make judging the nutritional quality of a food a snap. For instance, you can look at the % Daily Value column and find that a food has 25 percent of the Daily Value for fiber. This means the product will give you a substantial portion of the recommended amount of fiber for the day. You can also use this column to compare nutrients in similar products. The % Daily Values are based on a 2,000 calorie diet.

5 Trust Adjectives
Descriptors have legal definitions

Terms like "low," "high," and "free" have long been used on food labels. What these words actually mean, however, could vary. Thanks to the new labeling laws, such descriptions must now meet legal definitions. For example, you may be shopping for foods high in vitamin A, which has been linked to lower risk of certain cancers. Under the new label laws, a food described as "high" in a particular nutrient must contain 20 percent or more of the Daily Value for that nutrient. So if the bottle of juice you're thinking of buying says "high in vitamin A,'" you can now feel confident that it really is a good source of the vitamin.

6 Read Health Claims with Confidence
The nutrient link to disease prevention

You can also expect to see food packages with health claims linking certain nutrients to reduced risk of cancer and other diseases. The federal government has approved three health claims dealing with cancer prevention: a low-fat diet may reduce your risk for cancer; high fiber foods may reduce your risk for cancer; and fruits and vegetables may reduce your risk for cancer. A food may not make such a health claim for one nutrient if it contains other nutrients that undermine its health benefits. A high fiber, but high fat, jelly doughnut cannot carry a health claim!

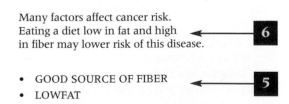

Nutrition Facts

Serving Size ½ cup (91g)
Servings Per Container 5

Amount Per Serving

Calories 58	Calories from Fat 0

	% Daily Value*
Total Fat 0g	**0%**
Saturated Fat 0g	**0%**
Cholesterol 0mg	**0%**
Sodium 45mg	**2%**
Total Carbohydrate 12g	**4%**
Dietary Fiber 3g	**12%**
Sugars 3g	
Protein 3g	

Vitamin A	92%	•	Vitamin C	16%
Calcium	2%	•	Iron	5%

* Percent Daily Values are based on a 2,000 calorie diet. Your daily values may be higher or lower depending on your calorie needs:

	Calories	2,000	2,500
Total Fat	Less than	65g	80g
Sat Fat	Less than	20g	25g
Cholesterol	Less than	300mg	300mg
Sodium	Less than	2,400mg	2,400mg
Total Carbohydrate		300g	375g
Fiber		25g	30g

Calories per gram:
Fat 9 • Carbohydrates 4 • Protein 4

Many factors affect cancer risk. Eating a diet low in fat and high in fiber may lower risk of this disease.

- GOOD SOURCE OF FIBER
- LOWFAT

Reprinted with permission from the American Institute for Cancer Research.

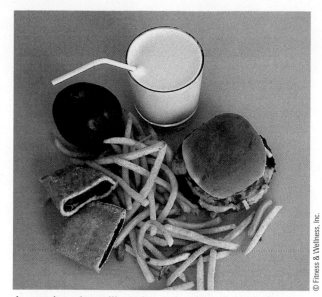

An apple a day will not keep the doctor away if most meals are high in fat content.

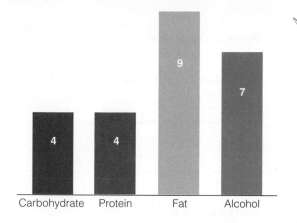

FIGURE 3.7 Caloric value of food (fuel nutrients).

© Fitness & Wellness, Inc.

If you are using the software available with this book to conduct a nutrient analysis, type in the food name and the number of servings based on the standard amounts given in the list of selected foods in Appendix A (see form provided in Figure 3A.3 of Lab 3A or follow the instructions given in the ProfilePlus software program on your CD-ROM).

Some of the most revealing information learned in a nutrient analysis is the source of fat intake in the diet. The average daily fat consumption in the U. S. diet is about 34 percent of the total caloric intake, much of it from saturated and trans fatty acids, which increases the risk for chronic diseases such as cardiovascular disease, cancer, diabetes, and obesity. Although fat provides a smaller percentage of our total daily caloric intake as compared to two decades ago (37 percent), the decrease in the percentage is simply because Americans now eat more calories than 20 years ago (335 additional daily calories for women and 170 for men).

As illustrated in Figure 3.7, 1 gram of carbohydrates or of protein supplies the body with 4 calories, and fat provides 9 calories per gram consumed (alcohol yields 7 calories per gram). Therefore, looking at only the total grams consumed for each type of food can be misleading.

For example, a person who eats 160 grams of carbohydrates, 100 grams of fat, and 70 grams of protein has a total intake of 330 grams of food. This indicates that 30 percent of the total grams of food

is in the form of fat (100 grams of fat ÷ 330 grams of total food = .30; .30 × 100 = 30 percent)—and, in reality, almost half of that diet is in the form of fat calories.

In the sample diet, 640 calories are derived from carbohydrates (160 grams × 4 calories per gram), 280 calories from protein (70 grams × 4 calories per gram), and 900 calories from fat (100 grams × 9 calories per gram), for a total of 1,820 calories. If 900 calories are derived from fat, almost half of the total caloric intake is in the form of fat (900 ÷ 1,820 × 100 = 49.5 percent).

Each gram of fat provides 9 calories—more than twice the calories of a gram of carbohydrates or protein. When figuring out the percent fat calories of individual foods, you may find Figure 3.8 a useful guideline. Multiply the Total Fat grams by 9 and divide by the total calories in that particular food (per serving). Then multiply that number by 100 to get the percentage. For example, the food label in Figure 3.8 lists a total of 120 calories and 5 grams of fat, and the equation below it shows the fat content to be 38 percent of total calories. This simple guideline can help you decrease the fat in your diet.

The fat content of selected foods, given in grams and as a percent of total calories, is presented in Figure 3.9. The percentage of fat is further subdivided into saturated, monounsaturated, polyunsaturated, and other fatty acids.

Beware of products labeled "97 percent fatfree." These products use weight, and not percent of total calories, as a measure of fat. Many of these foods still are in the range of 30 percent fat calories.

FIGURE 3.8 Computation for fat content in food.

Nutrition Facts

Serving Size 1 cup (240 ml)
Servings Per Container 4

Amount Per Serving

Calories 120   Calories from Fat 45

	% Daily Value*
Total Fat 5g	**8%**
Saturated Fat 3g	**15%**
Cholesterol 20mg	**7%**
Sodium 120mg	**5%**
Total Carbohydrate 12g	**4%**
Dietary Fiber 0g	**0%**
Sugars 12g	
Protein 8g	

Vitamin A	10%	• Vitamin C	4%
Calcium	30%	• Iron	0%

*Percent Daily Values are based on a 2,000 calorie diet. Your daily values may be higher or lower depending on your calorie needs:

		Calories	2,000	2,500
Total Fat	Less than		65g	80g
Sat Fat	Less than		20g	25g
Cholesterol	Less than		300mg	300mg
Sodium	Less than		2,400mg	2,400mg
Total Carbohydrate			300g	375g
Fiber			25g	30g

Calories per gram:
Fat 9   •   Carbohydrate 4   •   Protein 4

Percent fat calories = (grams of fat × 9) ÷ calories per serving × 100

5 grams of fat × 9 calories per grams of fat = 45 calories from fat

45 calories from fat ÷ 120 calories per serving × 100 = 38% fat

Achieving a Balanced Diet

Anyone who has completed a nutrient analysis and has given careful attention to Tables 3.3 (vitamins) and 3.4 (minerals) will probably realize that a well-balanced diet entails eating a variety of nutrient-dense foods and monitoring total daily caloric intake. The MyPyramid healthy eating guide in Figure 3.1 (page 51) contains five major food groups and oils. The food groups are grains, vegetables, fruits, milk, and meats and beans.

Whole grains, vegetables, fruits, and milk provide the nutritional base for a healthy diet. When increasing the intake of these food groups, it is important to decrease the intake of low-nutrient-dense foods to effectively balance caloric intake with energy needs.

Whole grains are a major source of fiber as well as other nutrients. Whole grains contain the entire grain kernel (the bran, germ, and endosperm). Examples include whole-wheat flour, whole corn-meal, oatmeal, cracked wheat (bulgur), and brown rice. Refined grains have been milled, a process that removes the bran and germ. The process also removes fiber, iron, and many B vitamins. Refined grains include white flour, white bread, white rice, and degermed cornmeal. Refined grains are often *enriched* to add back B vitamins and iron. Fiber, however, is not added back.

In addition to providing nutrients crucial to health, fruits and vegetables are the sole source of **phytochemicals** ("phyto" comes from the Greek word for plant). These compounds, recently discovered by scientists, show promising results in the fight against cancer and heart disease. More than 4,000 phytochemicals have been identified. The main function of phytochemicals in plants is to protect them from sunlight.

In humans, phytochemicals seem to have a powerful ability to block the formation of cancerous tumors. Their actions are so diverse that, at almost every stage of cancer, phytochemicals have the ability to block, disrupt, slow down, or even reverse the process. In terms of heart disease, they may reduce inflammation, inhibit blood clots, or prevent the oxidation of LDL cholesterol.

The consistent message is to eat a diet with ample fruits and vegetables. The recommended five to nine servings of fruits and vegetables daily has absolutely no substitute. Science has not yet found a way to allow people to eat a poor diet, pop a few pills, and derive the same benefits.

Milk, poultry, fish, and meats are to be consumed in moderation. Milk and milk products should be low-fat. The recommendation is to consume 3 ounces of poultry, fish, or meat and not to exceed 6 ounces daily. All visible fat and skin should be trimmed off meats and poultry before cooking. Fruits are recommended for dessert.

These are all strategies to help you enjoy a healthy diet, prevent disease, and improve your overall quality of life.

Pro-vitamin A compound that can be converted into a vitamin.

Phytochemicals Chemical compounds thought to prevent and fight cancer; found in large quantities in fruits and vegetables.

FIGURE 3.9 Fat content of selected foods.

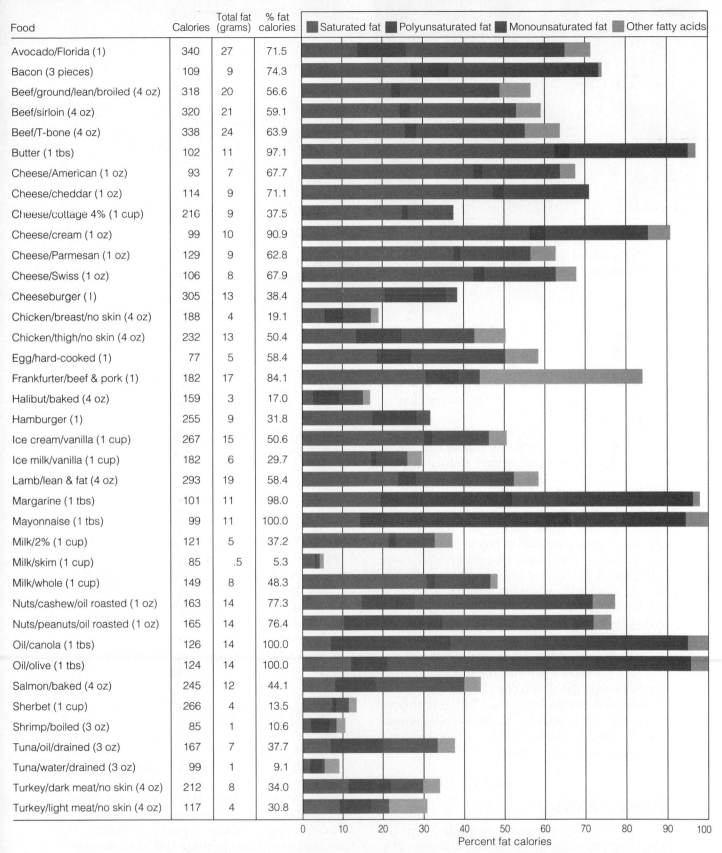

Food	Calories	Total fat (grams)	% fat calories
Avocado/Florida (1)	340	27	71.5
Bacon (3 pieces)	109	9	74.3
Beef/ground/lean/broiled (4 oz)	318	20	56.6
Beef/sirloin (4 oz)	320	21	59.1
Beef/T-bone (4 oz)	338	24	63.9
Butter (1 tbs)	102	11	97.1
Cheese/American (1 oz)	93	7	67.7
Cheese/cheddar (1 oz)	114	9	71.1
Cheese/cottage 4% (1 cup)	216	9	37.5
Cheese/cream (1 oz)	99	10	90.9
Cheese/Parmesan (1 oz)	129	9	62.8
Cheese/Swiss (1 oz)	106	8	67.9
Cheeseburger (1)	305	13	38.4
Chicken/breast/no skin (4 oz)	188	4	19.1
Chicken/thigh/no skin (4 oz)	232	13	50.4
Egg/hard-cooked (1)	77	5	58.4
Frankfurter/beef & pork (1)	182	17	84.1
Halibut/baked (4 oz)	159	3	17.0
Hamburger (1)	255	9	31.8
Ice cream/vanilla (1 cup)	267	15	50.6
Ice milk/vanilla (1 cup)	182	6	29.7
Lamb/lean & fat (4 oz)	293	19	58.4
Margarine (1 tbs)	101	11	98.0
Mayonnaise (1 tbs)	99	11	100.0
Milk/2% (1 cup)	121	5	37.2
Milk/skim (1 cup)	85	.5	5.3
Milk/whole (1 cup)	149	8	48.3
Nuts/cashew/oil roasted (1 oz)	163	14	77.3
Nuts/peanuts/oil roasted (1 oz)	165	14	76.4
Oil/canola (1 tbs)	126	14	100.0
Oil/olive (1 tbs)	124	14	100.0
Salmon/baked (4 oz)	245	12	44.1
Sherbet (1 cup)	266	4	13.5
Shrimp/boiled (3 oz)	85	1	10.6
Tuna/oil/drained (3 oz)	167	7	37.7
Tuna/water/drained (3 oz)	99	1	9.1
Turkey/dark meat/no skin (4 oz)	212	8	34.0
Turkey/light meat/no skin (4 oz)	117	4	30.8

Legend: ■ Saturated fat ■ Polyunsaturated fat ■ Monounsaturated fat ■ Other fatty acids

X-axis: Percent fat calories (0 10 20 30 40 50 60 70 80 90 100)

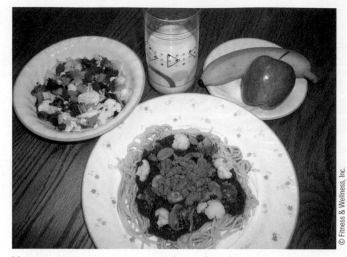

You can restructure your meals so that rice, pasta, beans, breads, and vegetables constitute the major portion of your meal; meats are added primarily for flavoring; fruits are used for desserts; and low- or nonfat milk products are used.

© Fitness & Wellness, Inc.

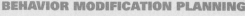
As an aid to balancing your diet, the form in Lab 3B enables you to record your daily food intake. (This record is much easier to keep than the complete dietary analysis in Lab 3A). Make one copy for each day you wish to record.

To start the activity, go to http://mypyramid.gov/ and establish your personal MyPyramid Plan based on your age, sex, and activity level. Record this information on the form provided in Lab 3B. Next, whenever you have something to eat, record the food and the amount eaten according to the MyPyramid standard amounts (oz, c, or tsp—see Figure 3.1). Do this immediately after each meal so you will be able to keep track of your actual food intake more easily. At the end of the day, evaluate your diet by checking whether you ate the minimum required amounts for each food group. If you meet the minimum required servings at the end of each day and your caloric intake is in balance with the recommended amount, you are taking good "Steps to a Healthier You."

Once you have completed the nutrient analysis and the healthy diet plan (Labs 3A and 3B), you may conduct a self-evaluation of your current nutritional habits. Also in Lab 3B, you can assess your current stage of change regarding healthy nutrition and list strategies to help you improve your diet.

Vegetarianism

More than 12 million people in the United States follow vegetarian diets. **Vegetarians** rely primarily on foods from the bread, cereal, rice, pasta, and fruit and vegetable groups and avoid most foods from animal sources in the dairy and protein groups. The five basic types of vegetarians are as follows:

1. **Vegans** eat no animal products at all.
2. **Ovovegetarians** allow eggs in the diet.
3. **Lactovegetarians** allow foods from the milk group.
4. **Ovolactovegetarians** include egg and milk products in the diet.
5. **Semivegetarians** do not eat red meat, but do include fish and poultry in addition to milk products and eggs in their diet.

Vegetarian diets can be healthful and consistent with the Dietary Guidelines for Americans and can meet the DRIs for nutrients. However, vegetarians who do not select their food combinations properly can develop nutritional deficiencies of protein, vitamins, minerals, and even calories. Even greater attention should be paid when planning vegetarian diets for infants and children. Unless carefully planned, a strict plant-based diet will prevent proper growth and development.

Nutrient Concerns

Protein deficiency can be a concern in some vegetarian diets. Vegans in particular must be careful to eat foods that provide a balanced distribution of essential amino acids, such as grain products and legumes. Strict vegans also need a supplement of vitamin B_{12}. This vitamin is not found in plant foods; its only source is animal foods. Deficiency of this vitamin can lead to anemia and nerve damage.

The key to a healthful vegetarian diet is to eat foods that possess complementary proteins. Most plant-based products lack one or more essential amino acids in adequate amounts. For example, both grains and legumes are good protein sources, but neither provides all the essential amino acids. Grains and cereals are low in the amino acid lysine, and legumes lack methionine. Foods from these two groups—such as combinations of tortillas and beans, rice and beans, rice and soybeans, or wheat bread and peanuts—complement each other and provide all required protein nutrients. These complementary proteins may be consumed over the course of one day, but it is best if they are consumed during the same meal.

Other nutrients likely to be deficient in vegetarian diets—and ways to overcome them—are as follows:

- Vitamin D can be obtained from moderate exposure to the sun or by taking a supplement.
- Riboflavin can be found in green leafy vegetables, whole grains, and legumes.
- Calcium can be obtained from fortified soybean milk or fortified orange juice, calcium-rich tofu, and selected cereals. A calcium supplement is also an option.
- Iron can be found in whole grains, dried fruits and nuts, and legumes. To enhance iron absorption, a good source of vitamin C should be consumed with these foods (calcium and iron are the most difficult nutrients to consume in sufficient amounts in a strict vegan diet).
- Zinc can be obtained from whole grains, wheat germ, beans, nuts, and seeds.

MyPyramid can also be used as a guide for vegetarians. The key is food variety. Most vegetarians today consume dairy products and eggs. Meat can be replaced with legumes, nuts, seeds, eggs, and meat substitutes (tofu, tempeh, soy milk, and commercial meat replacers such as veggie burgers and soy hot dogs). Additional MyPyramid healthy eating tips for vegetarians and how to get enough of the previously mentioned nutrients, go to http://my pyramid.gov/. Those who are interested in vegetarian diets are encouraged to consult additional resources, because special vegetarian diet planning cannot be covered adequately in a few paragraphs.

Nuts

Consumption of nuts, commonly used in vegetarian diets, has received considerable attention in recent years. A few years ago, most people regarded nuts as especially high in fat and calories. Although they are 70 to 90 percent fat, most of it is unsaturated fat. And research indicates that people who eat nuts several times a week have a lower incidence of heart disease. Eating 2 to 3 ounces (about one-half cup) of almonds, walnuts, or macadamia

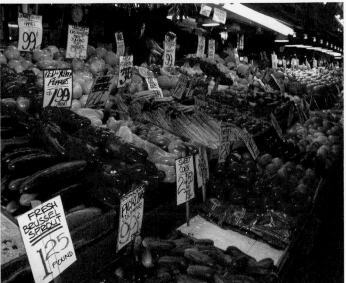

Most fruits and vegetables contain large amounts of cancer-preventing phytochemicals.

nuts a day may decrease high blood cholesterol by about 10 percent. Nuts can even enhance the cholesterol-lowering effects of the **Mediterranean diet** (discussed in the next section).

Heart-health benefits are attributed not only to the unsaturated fats, but to other nutrients found in nuts, such as vitamin E and folic acid. And nuts are also packed with additional B vitamins, calcium, copper, potassium, magnesium, fiber, and phytochemicals. Many of these nutrients are cancer- and cardio-protective, help lower homocysteine levels, and act as antioxidants, discussed in "Antioxidants" (page 73) and "Folate" (page 76).

Nuts do have a drawback: They are high in calories. A handful of nuts provides as many calories as a piece of cake, so nuts should be avoided as a snack. Excessive weight gain is a risk factor for

Vegetarians Individuals whose diet is of vegetable or plant origin.

Vegans Vegetarians who eat no animal products at all.

Ovovegetarians Vegetarians who allow eggs in their diet.

Lactovegetarians Vegetarians who eat foods from the milk group.

Ovolactovegetarians Vegetarians who include eggs and milk products in their diet.

Semivegetarians Vegetarians who include milk products, eggs, and fish and poultry in the diet.

Mediterranean diet Typical diet of people around the Mediterranean region that focuses on olive oil, red wine, grains, legumes, vegetables, and fruits, with limited amounts of meat, fish, milk, and cheese.

FIGURE 3.10 Vegetarian Food Guide Pyramid.[a]

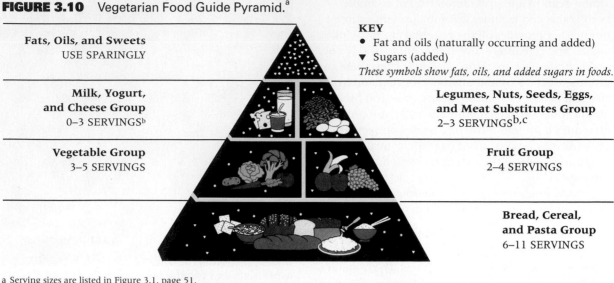

KEY
- ● Fat and oils (naturally occurring and added)
- ▼ Sugars (added)

These symbols show fats, oils, and added sugars in foods.

Fats, Oils, and Sweets
USE SPARINGLY

Milk, Yogurt, and Cheese Group
0–3 SERVINGS[b]

Legumes, Nuts, Seeds, Eggs, and Meat Substitutes Group
2–3 SERVINGS[b,c]

Vegetable Group
3–5 SERVINGS

Fruit Group
2–4 SERVINGS

Bread, Cereal, and Pasta Group
6–11 SERVINGS

a Serving sizes are listed in Figure 3.1, page 51.
b Vegans and other vegetarians who include no eggs, milk, or milk products must obtain calcium, vitamin D, and vitamin B$_{12}$ from other sources. See text for details.
c Meat substitutes include soybean products, such as tofu, tempeh, and soy milk, and commercial meat replacers.

Source: Adapted from the USDA Food Guide Pyramid and Food Guide Pyramid for Vegetarian Meal Planning in Position of the American Dietetic Association: Vegetarian diets, *Journal of the American Dietetic Association* 97 (1997): 1317–1321.

cardiovascular disease. Nuts are recommended for use in place of high-protein foods such as meats, bacon, eggs, or as part of a meal in fruit or vegetable salads, homemade bread, pancakes, casseroles, yogurt, and oatmeal. Peanut butter is also healthier than cheese or some cold cuts in sandwiches.

Soy Products

The increased popularity of soy foods, including use in vegetarian diets, is attributed primarily to Asian research that points to less heart disease, lower cholesterol levels, and fewer hormone-related cancers in people who regularly consume soy foods. The benefits of soy lie in its high protein content and plant chemicals, known as *isoflavones*, that act as antioxidants and may protect against estrogen-related cancers (breast, ovarian, and endometrial). The compound *genistein*, one of many phytochemicals in soy, helps to reduce the risk for breast cancer, and soy consumption also has been linked to a lower risk for prostate cancer.

In addition, soy proteins can lower blood cholesterol to a greater extent than would be expected just from its low-fat and high-fiber content. The evidence of heart-protecting benefits from soy foods is so strong that the FDA now allows the following claim on food labels: "25 grams of soy proteins a day, as part of a diet low in saturated fat and cholesterol, may reduce the risk of heart disease." One to two cups of soy milk, 1/2 cup of tofu, 1½ tablespoons of soy protein isolate, or 1/4 cup of soy flour provide about 10 grams of soy protein.

Mediterranean Diet

Much attention has been given recently to the Mediterranean diet, because people in that region have notably lower rates of diet-linked diseases and a longer life expectancy. The diet focuses on olive oil, grains (whole, not refined), legumes, vegetables, fruits, and, in moderation, fish, red wine, nuts, and dairy products. Although it is a semivegetarian diet, up to 40 percent of the total daily caloric intake may come from fat—mostly monounsaturated fat from olive oil. Moderate intake of red wine is included with meals. The dietary plan also encourages regular physical activity (see Figure 3.11).

More than a "diet," the Mediterranean diet is a dietary pattern that has existed for centuries. According to the largest and most comprehensive research on this dietary pattern, the health benefits and decreased mortality are not linked to any specific component of the diet (such as olive oil or red wine) but are achieved through the interaction of

FIGURE 3.11 The Traditional Healthy Mediterranean Diet Pyramid.

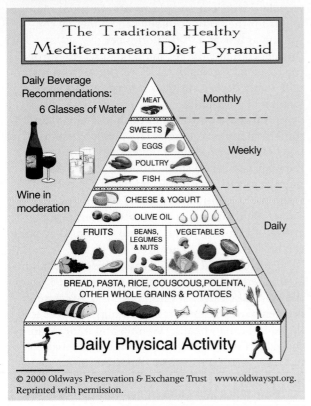

The Traditional Healthy Mediterranean Diet Pyramid

Daily Beverage Recommendations:
6 Glasses of Water

Wine in moderation

MEAT — Monthly

SWEETS
EGGS
POULTRY — Weekly
FISH

CHEESE & YOGURT
OLIVE OIL

FRUITS | BEANS, LEGUMES & NUTS | VEGETABLES — Daily

BREAD, PASTA, RICE, COUSCOUS, POLENTA, OTHER WHOLE GRAINS & POTATOES

Daily Physical Activity

© 2000 Oldways Preservation & Exchange Trust   www.oldwayspt.org. Reprinted with permission.

all the components of the pattern.[5] Those who adhere most closely to the dietary pattern had a lower incidence of heart disease (33 percent) and deaths from cancer (24 percent). While most people in the United States focus on the olive oil component of the diet, olive oil is used mainly as a means to increase consumption of vegetables because sauteed vegetables in oil taste better than steamed vegetables.

Ethnic Diets

As people migrate, they take their dietary practices with them. Many ethnic diets are healthier than the typical American diet, because they emphasize consumption of complex carbohydrates and limit fat intake. The predominant minority ethnic groups in America are African American, Hispanic American, and Asian American. Unfortunately, the generally healthier ethnic diets quickly become Americanized when these minority people enter the United States. Often, they cut back on vegetables and add meats and salt to their diet in conformity with the American consumer.

Ethnic dishes, nonetheless, can be prepared at home. They are easy to make and much healthier when using the typical (original) variety of vegetables, corn, rice, spices, and condiments. Ethnic health recommendations also encourage daily physical activity and suggest no more than two alcoholic drinks per day.

The African American diet (soul food) is based on the regional cuisine of the American South. Soul food includes yams, black-eyed peas, okra, and peanuts. The latter have been combined with American foods such as corn products and pork. Today, most people think of soul food as meat, fried chicken, sweet potatoes, and chitterling.

Hispanic dishes arrived with the conquistadores and evolved through combinations with other ethnic diets and local foods available in Latin America. For example, the Cuban cuisine combined Spanish, Chinese, and native foods; Puerto Rican cuisine developed from Spanish, African, and native products; Mexican diets evolved from Spanish and native food. Prominent in all of these diets were corn, beans, squash, chili peppers, avocados, papayas, and fish. Rice and citrus foods were added later by the colonists. Today, the Hispanic diet incorporates a wide variety of foods, including red meat, but the staple still includes rice, corn, and beans.

Asian-American diets are characteristically rich in vegetables and use minimal meat and fat. The Okinawan diet in Japan, where some of the healthiest and oldest people in the world live, is high in fresh (versus pickled) vegetables, high in fiber, and low in fat and salt. The Chinese cuisine includes more than 200 vegetables, and fat-free sauces and seasoning are used to enhance flavor. The Chinese diet varies somewhat within regions of China. The lowest in fat is that of southern China, with most meals containing fish, seafood, and stir-fried vegetables. Chinese food in American restaurants contains a much higher percentage of fat and protein than the traditional Chinese cuisine.

Table 3.8 provides a list of healthier foods to choose from when dining at selected ethnic restaurants.

All healthy diets have similar characteristics: They are high in fruits, vegetables, and grains, and low in fat and saturated fat. Healthy diets also use low-fat or fat-free dairy products, and they emphasize portion control—essential in a healthy diet plan.

Many people now think that if a food item is labeled "low-fat" or "fat-free," they can consume it in large quantities. "Low-fat" or "fat-free" does not imply "calorie-free." Many people who consume low-fat diets eat more (and thus increase their caloric intake), which in the long term leads to obesity and its associated health problems.

TABLE 3.8 Ethnic Eating Guide

	Choose Often	Choose Less Often

Chinese	Beef with broccoli
	Chinese greens
	Steamed rice, brown
	  or white
	Steamed beef with
	  pea pods
	Stir-fry dishes
	Teriyaki beef or chicken
	Wonton soup
		Crispy duck
		Egg rolls
		Fried rice
		Kung pao chicken (fried)
		Peking duck
		Pork spareribs

Japanese	Chiri nabe (fish stew) Grilled scallops Sushi, sashimi (raw fish) Teriyaki Yakitori (grilled chicken)	Tempura (fried chicken, shrimp, or vegetables) Tonkatsu (fried pork)

Italian	Cioppino (seafood stew)
	Minestrone
	  (vegetarian soup)
	Pasta with marinara sauce
	Pasta primavera
	  (pasta with vegetables)
	Steamed clams
		Antipasto
		Cannelloni, ravioli
		Fettuccini alfredo
		Garlic bread
		White clam sauce

Mexican	Beans and rice Black bean/vegetable soup Burritos, bean Chili Enchiladas, bean Fajitas Gazpacho Taco salad Tamales Tortillas, steamed	Chili rellenos Chimichangas Enchiladas, beef or cheese Flautas Guacamole Nachos Quesadillas Tostadas Sour cream (as topping)
Middle Eastern	Tandoori chicken Curry (yogurt-based) Rice pilaf Lentil soup Shish kebab	Falafel
French	Poached salmon Spinach salad Consommé Salad niçoise	Beef Wellington Escargot French onion soup Sauces in general

Soul Food	Baked chicken
	Baked fish
	Roasted pork
	  (not smothered
	  or "etouffe")
	Sauteed okra
	Baked sweet potato
		Fried chicken
		Fried fish
		Smothered pork
		  tenderloin
		Okra in gumbo
		Sweet potato casserole
		  or pie

Greek	Gyros Pita Lentil soup	Baklava Moussaka

Source: Adapted from P. A. Floyd, S. E. Mimms, and C. Yelding-Howard. *Personal Health: Perspectives & Lifestyles* (Belmont, CA: Wadsworth/Thomson Learning, 1998).

Nutrient Supplementation

Approximately half of all adults in the United States take daily nutrient **supplements**. Nutrient requirements for the body normally can be met by consuming as few as 1,200 calories per day, as long as the diet contains the recommended servings from the five food groups in the Food Guide Pyramid. Still, many people consider it necessary to take vitamin supplements.

It's true that our bodies cannot retain water-soluble vitamins as long as fat-soluble vitamins. The body excretes excessive intakes readily, although the body can retain small amounts for weeks or months in various organs and tissues. Fat-soluble vitamins, by contrast, are stored in fatty tissue. Therefore, daily intake of these vitamins is not as crucial. Too much vitamin A and vitamin D actually can be detrimental to health.

People should not take **megadoses** of vitamins and minerals. For some nutrients, a dose of 5 times the RDA taken over several months may create problems. For other nutrients, it may not pose a threat to human health. Vitamin and mineral doses should not exceed the ULs. For nutrients that do not have an established UL, a person should take a dose no higher than 3 times the RDA.

Iron deficiency (determined through blood testing) is more common in women than men. Iron supplementation is frequently recommended for women who have heavy menstrual flow. Some pregnant and lactating women also may require supplements. The average pregnant woman who eats an adequate amount of a variety of foods should take a low dose of iron supplement daily. Women who are pregnant with more than one baby may need additional supplements. Folate supplements also are encouraged prior to and during pregnancy to prevent certain birth defects (see following discussions of antioxidants and folates). In the above instances, supplements should be taken under a physician's supervision.

Other people who may benefit from supplementation are those with nutrient deficiencies (including low calcium intake), alcoholics and street-drug users who do not have a balanced diet, smokers, vegans (strict vegetarians), individuals on extremely low-calorie diets (fewer than 1,200 calories per day), older adults who don't eat balanced meals regularly, newborn infants (who usually are given a single dose of vitamin K to prevent abnormal bleeding), and people with disease-related disorders or who are taking medications that interfere with proper nutrient absorption.

Although some supplements are encouraged (see discussion that follows), most supplements do not seem to provide additional benefits for healthy

TABLE 3.9 Antioxidant Nutrients, Sources, and Functions

Nutrient	Good Sources	Antioxidant Effect
Vitamin C	Citrus fruit, kiwi fruit, cantaloupe, strawberries, broccoli, green or red peppers, cauliflower, cabbage	Appears to deactivate oxygen free radicals.
Vitamin E	Vegetable oils, yellow and green leafy vegetables, margarine, wheat germ, oatmeal, almonds, whole-grain breads, cereals	Protects lipids from oxidation.
Beta-carotene	Carrots, squash, pumpkin, sweet potatoes, broccoli, green leafy vegetables	Soaks up oxygen free radicals.
Selenium	Seafood, Brazil nuts, meat, whole grains	Helps prevent damage to cell structures.

people who eat a balanced diet. They do not help people run faster, jump higher, relieve stress, improve sexual prowess, cure a common cold, or boost energy levels.

Antioxidants

Much research is being done to study the effectiveness of **antioxidants** in thwarting several chronic diseases. Although foods probably contain more than 4,000 antioxidants, the four more studied antioxidants are vitamins C, E, and beta-carotene (a precursor to vitamin A), and the mineral selenium (see Table 3.9).

Oxygen is used during metabolism to change carbohydrates and fats into energy. During this process, oxygen is transformed into stable forms of water and carbon dioxide. A small amount of oxygen, however, ends up in an unstable form, referred to as **oxygen free radicals**.

A free radical molecule has a normal proton nucleus with a single unpaired electron. Having only one electron makes the free radical extremely reactive, and it looks constantly to pair its electron with one from another molecule. When a free radical steals a second electron from another molecule, that other molecule in turn becomes a free radical. This chain reaction goes on until two free radicals meet to form a stable molecule.

Free radicals attack and damage proteins and lipids, in particular cell membranes and DNA. This damage is thought to contribute to the development of conditions such as cardiovascular disease, cancer, emphysema, cataracts, Parkinson's disease, and premature aging. Solar radiation, cigarette smoke, air pollution, radiation, some drugs, injury, infection, chemicals (such as pesticides), and other environmental factors also seem to encourage the formation of free radicals. Antioxidants are thought to offer protection by absorbing free radicals before they can cause damage and also by interrupting the sequence of reactions once damage has begun, thwarting certain chronic diseases (see Figure 3.12).

The body's own defense systems typically neutralize free radicals so they don't cause any damage. When free radicals are produced faster than the body can neutralize them, however, they can damage the cells.

Antioxidants are found abundantly in food, especially in fruits and vegetables. Unfortunately, most Americans do not eat the minimum five daily servings of fruits and vegetables (five to nine is the recommendation in the Food Guide Pyramid). The benefits of antioxidants are obtained primarily from food sources themselves, and controversy surrounds the benefits of antioxidants taken in supplement form.

Some researchers believe that taking antioxidant supplements further prevents free-radical damage. In 2001, the editorial board of the *University of California at Berkeley Wellness Letter* updated its daily antioxidant nutrient intake recommendations to include[6]

- 250 to 500 mg of vitamin C
- 200 to 400 **IU (international units)** of vitamin E (look for natural vitamin E, because the body does not use synthetic forms well).

Supplements Tablets, pills, capsules, liquids, or powders that contain vitamins, minerals, amino acids, herbs, or fiber that are taken to increase the intake of these nutrients.

Megadoses For most vitamins, 10 times the RDA or more; for vitamins A and D, 5 and 2 times the RDA, respectively.

Antioxidants Compounds such as vitamins C and E, beta-carotene, and selenium that prevent oxygen from combining with other substances in the body to form harmful compounds.

Oxygen free radicals Substances formed during metabolism that attack and damage proteins and lipids, in particular the cell membrane and DNA, leading to diseases such as heart disease, cancer, and emphysema.

International unit (IU) Measure of nutrients in foods.

FIGURE 3.12 Antioxidant protection: blocking and absorbing oxygen free radicals to prevent chronic disease.

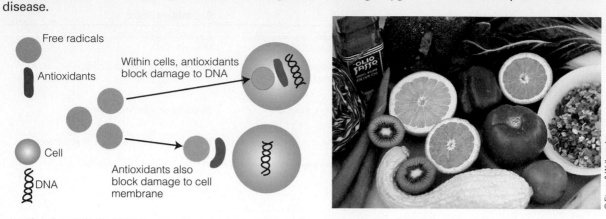

Vitamin C

Based on the above recommendations, people who consume five or more daily servings of fresh fruits and vegetables can get their daily vitamin C requirements through the diet alone. Studies have shown that vitamin C offers benefits against heart disease, cancer, cataracts, and several other health disorders.

Vitamin C is water-soluble, and the body eliminates it in about 12 hours. For best results, consume vitamin C-rich foods twice a day or divide your vitamin C supplement in half and take it twice a day. High intake of a vitamin C supplement (above 500 mg per day) is no longer recommended. More than 500 daily mg is unnecessary, given that research at the National Institutes of Health showed that the body absorbs very little vitamin C beyond the first 200 mg per serving or dose.

Selenium may interfere with the body's absorption of vitamin C, so the two should be taken separately. Wait about an hour following vitamin C intake before taking selenium.

Vitamin E

Vitamin E belongs to a group of eight compounds (four tocopherols and four tocotrienols) of which alpha-tocopherol is the most active form. The antioxidant recommendation for vitamin E is much higher than the RDA (15 mg or 22 IU). To obtain the daily recommended guideline for vitamin E through diet alone, however, is practically impossible. Vitamin E is found primarily in oil-rich seeds and vegetable oils. As shown in Table 3.10, vitamin E is not easily found in large quantities in foods typically consumed in the diet.

Among the benefits of Vitamin E, it may help prevent atherosclerosis in healthy people and diabetics, it seems to lower the risk of stroke, and it improves immune function. Some evidence has suggested that supplemental intake of vitamin E reduces the risk of heart disease, but it may not offer additional protection to people who already have the disease. Healthy people who take vitamin E may have fewer heart problems, and the vitamin seems to slow the progression of plaque (atherosclerosis) in the arteries. Other research, however, has questioned the health benefits of vitamin E supplementation. Thus, controversy exists regarding the benefits of supplementation and additional research is necessary before final recommendations can be made concerning vitamin E supplementation.

Vitamin E supplements from natural sources contain d-alpha tocopherol, which is better absorbed by the body than dl-alpha tocopherol, a synthetic form composed of a variety of E compounds. Because vitamin E is fat-soluble, it should be taken with a meal that has some fat in it. Vitamin E also enhances the effects of selenium, so these should be taken together for best results. Antioxidant nutrients often work in conjunction with other nutrients in food that may further enhance their beneficial actions.

Beta-carotene

Beta-carotene supplementation was encouraged in the early 1990s. It is better, however, to obtain the daily recommended dose of beta-carotene (20,000 IU) from food sources rather than supplements. Clinical trials have found that beta-carotene supplements offered no protection against heart disease and cancer or provided any other health benefits.

TABLE 3.10 Antioxidant Content of Selected Foods

Beta-Carotene	IU
Apricot (1 medium)	675
Broccoli (½ cup, frozen)	1,740
Broccoli (½ cup, raw)	680
Cantaloupe (1 cup)	5,160
Carrot (1 medium, raw)	20,255
Green peas (½ cup, frozen)	535
Mango (1 medium)	8,060
Mustard greens (½ cup, frozen)	3,350
Papaya (1 medium)	6,120
Spinach (½ cup, frozen)	7,395
Sweet potato (1 medium, baked)	24,875
Tomato (1 medium)	1,395
Turnip greens (½ cup, boiled)	3,960

Vitamin C	mg
Acerola (1 cup, raw)	1,640
Acerola juice (8 oz)	3,864
Cantaloupe (½ melon, medium)	90
Cranberry juice (8 oz)	90
Grapefruit (½, medium, white)	52
Grapefruit juice (8 oz)	92
Guava (1 medium)	165
Kiwi (1 medium)	75
Lemon juice (8 oz)	110
Orange (1 medium)	66
Orange juice (8 oz)	120
Papaya (1 medium)	85
Pepper (½ cup, red, chopped, raw)	95
Strawberries (1 cup, raw)	88

Vitamin E	IU	mg*
Almond oil (1 tbsp)		5.3
Almonds (1 oz)	10.1	
Canola oil (1 tbsp)		9.0
Cottonseed oil (1 tbsp)		5.2
Hazelnuts (1 oz)	4.4	
Kale (1 cup)	15.0	
Margarine (1 tbsp)		2.0
Peanuts (1 oz)	3.0	
Shrimp (3 oz, boiled)	3.1	
Sunflower seeds (1 oz, dry)	14.2	
Sunflower seed oil (1 tbsp)		6.9
Sweet potato (1 medium, baked)	7.2	
Wheat germ oil (1 tbsp)		20.0

Selenium	mcg
Brazil nuts (1)	100
Bread, whole wheat enriched (1 slice)	15
Beef (3 oz)	33
Cereals (3½ oz)	20
Chicken breast, roasted, no skin (3 oz)	24
Cod, baked (3 oz)	57
Egg, hard boiled (1 large)	15
Fruits (3½ oz)	1
Noodles, enriched, boiled (1 cup)	50
Oatmeal, cooked (1 cup)	23
Red snapper (3 oz)	150
Rice, long grain, cooked (1 cup)	20
Salmon, baked (3 oz)	35
Spaghetti w/meat sauce (1 cup)	36
Tuna, canned, water, drained (3 oz)	68
Turkey breast, roasted, no skin (3 oz)	28
Walnuts, black, chopped (¼ cup)	5
Vegetables (3½ oz)	1

* Vitamin E values for oils are commonly expressed in milligrams (mg). One mg is almost equal to 1 IU (international unit).

Therefore, it is recommended that you "skip the pill and eat the carrot." One medium raw carrot contains about 20,000 IU of beta-carotene.

Selenium

Adequate intake of the mineral selenium is encouraged. Studies indicate that individuals who take 200 micrograms (mcg) of selenium daily decreased their risk of prostate cancer by 63 percent, colorectal cancer by 58 percent, and lung cancer by 46 percent.[7] Data also point to decreased risk of breast, liver, and digestive tract cancers. According to Dr. Edward Giovannucci of the Harvard Medical School, the evidence for the benefits of selenium in reducing prostate cancer risk is so strong that public health officials should recommend that people increase their selenium intake.

One Brazil nut (unshelled) that you crack yourself provides about 100 mcg of selenium. Shelled nuts found in supermarkets average only about 20 mcg each. Based on the current body of research, a dose of 100 to 200 mcg per day seems to provide the necessary amount of antioxidant for this nutrient. There is no reason to take more than 200 mcg daily. In fact, the UL for selenium has been set at 400 mcg. Too much selenium can damage cells rather than protect them. If you choose to take supplements, take an organic form of selenium from yeast and not selenium selenite. The selenium content of various foods is provided in Table 3.10.

Although much interest has been generated by the previously mentioned supplements, multivitamins are still the preferred supplement of the American people. A multivitamin complex that provides 100 percent of the DV for most nutrients can help fill in certain dietary deficiencies.[8] Some evidence suggests that regular intake decreases the risk for heart disease and stroke.

Multivitamins, however, are not magic pills. They can help, but they don't provide a license to eat carelessly. Multivitamins don't provide energy, fiber, phytochemicals, or the recommended daily dose of vitamin C (250 to 500 mg) and vitamin E (200 to 400 IU).

Folate

Although it is not an antioxidant, 400 mcg of **folate** (a B vitamin) is recommended for all premenopausal women. Folate helps prevent certain birth defects and seems to offer protection against colon and cervical cancers. Women who might become pregnant should plan on taking a folate supplement, because studies have shown that folate intake (400 mcg per day) during early pregnancy can prevent serious birth defects.

Increasing evidence also indicates that taking 400 mcg of folate along with vitamins B_6 and B_{12} prevents heart attacks by reducing homocysteine levels in the blood (see Chapter 11). High concentrations of homocysteine accelerate the process of plaque formation (atherosclerosis) in the arteries. Five servings of fruits and vegetables per day usually meet the needs for these nutrients. Currently, almost 9 of 10 adults in the United States do not obtain the recommended 400 mcg of folate per day. Because of the critical role of folate in preventing heart disease, some experts recommend a daily vitamin B complex that includes 400 mcg of folate.

Side Effects

Toxic effects from antioxidant supplements are rare when they are taken in the recommended amounts. The daily UL for adults 19 to 70 years of age for vitamin C has been set at 2,000 mg, for vitamin E at 1,000 mg, and for selenium at 400 mcg. If any of the following side effects arise, you should stop supplementation and check with your physician:

- Vitamin E: gastrointestinal disturbances, increase in blood lipids (determined through blood tests)
- Vitamin C: nausea, diarrhea, abdominal cramps, kidney stones, liver problems
- Selenium: nausea, vomiting, diarrhea, irritability, fatigue, flu-like symptoms, lesions of the skin and nervous tissue, loss of hair and nails, respiratory failure, liver damage.

Substantial supplementation of vitamin E is not recommended for individuals on **anticoagulant** therapy. Vitamin E is an anticoagulant in itself. Therefore, if you are on such therapy, check with your physician. Pregnant women need a physician's approval prior to beta-carotene supplementation. Vitamin E also may be unsafe if taken with alcohol or by people who drink more than 4 ounces of pure alcohol per day (the equivalent of 8 beers).

Benefits of Foods

Even though you may consider taking some supplements, fruits and vegetables are the richest sources of antioxidants and phytochemicals. Researchers at the U.S. Department of Agriculture compared the antioxidant effects of vitamins C and E with those of various common fruits and vegetables. The results indicated that three-fourths cup of cooked kale (which contains only 11 IU of vitamin E and 76 mg of vitamin C) neutralized as many free radicals as approximately 800 IU of vitamin E or 600 mg of vitamin C. Other excellent sources of antioxidants found by these researchers include blueberries, strawberries, spinach, Brussels sprouts, plums, broccoli, beets, oranges, and grapes. A list of top antioxidant foods is presented in Figure 3.13.

Many people who regularly eat foods high in fat content or too many sweets think they need supplementation to balance their diet. This is another fallacy about nutrition. The problem here is not necessarily a lack of vitamins and minerals, but a diet too high in calories, fat, and sodium. Vitamin, mineral, and fiber supplements do not supply all of the nutrients and other beneficial substances present in food and needed for good health. Supplements will provide added health benefits, but by no means will they replace a well-balanced diet.

Wholesome foods contain vitamins, minerals, carbohydrates, fiber, proteins, fats, phytochemicals, and other substances not yet discovered. Researchers do not know if the protective effects are caused by the antioxidants alone, or in combination with other nutrients (such as phytochemicals), or by some other nutrients in food that have not been investigated yet. Many nutrients work in **synergy**, enhancing chemical processes in the body.

Supplementation will not offset poor eating habits. Pills are no substitute for common sense.

If you think your diet is not balanced, you first need to conduct a nutrient analysis (see Lab 3A) to determine which nutrients you lack in sufficient amounts. Eat more of them, as well as

CRITICAL THINKING

Do you take supplements? If so, for what purposes are you taking them—and do you think you could restructure your diet so you could do without them?

FIGURE 3.13 Top antioxidant foods.

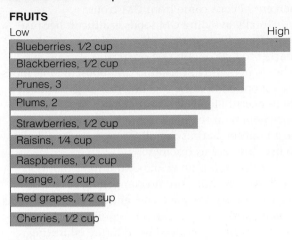

FRUITS

Low — High

- Blueberries, 1/2 cup
- Blackberries, 1/2 cup
- Prunes, 3
- Plums, 2
- Strawberries, 1/2 cup
- Raisins, 1/4 cup
- Raspberries, 1/2 cup
- Orange, 1/2 cup
- Red grapes, 1/2 cup
- Cherries, 1/2 cup

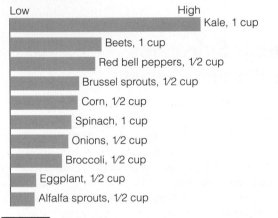

VEGETABLES

Low — High

- Kale, 1 cup
- Beets, 1 cup
- Red bell peppers, 1/2 cup
- Brussel sprouts, 1/2 cup
- Corn, 1/2 cup
- Spinach, 1 cup
- Onions, 1/2 cup
- Broccoli, 1/2 cup
- Eggplant, 1/2 cup
- Alfalfa sprouts, 1/2 cup

Source: Adapted from USDA, Agricultural Research Service, *Food & Nutrition Research Briefs*, April 1999 (downloaded from www.ars.usda.gov/is/np/fnrb).

A tomato, for example, is a functional food because it contains the phytochemical lycopene, thought to reduce the risk for prostate cancer. Other examples of functional foods are kale, broccoli, blueberries, red grapes, and green tea.

The term *functional food*, however, has been used primarily as a marketing tool by the food industry to attract consumers. Unlike **fortified foods**, which have been modified to help prevent nutrient deficiencies, the food industry is creating functional foods by adding ingredients aimed at treating or preventing symptoms or disease. In functional foods, the added ingredient(s) is often not typically found in the particular food item in its natural form but is added to allow manufacturers to make appealing health claims.

In most cases, only one extra ingredient is added (a vitamin, mineral, phytochemical, or herb). An example is calcium added to orange juice to make the claim that this brand offers protection against osteoporosis. Food manufacturers now offer cholesterol-lowering margarines (enhanced with plant stanol), cancer-protective (lycopene-fortified) ketchup, memory-boosting (ginkgo-added) candy, calcium-fortified chips, and corn chips containing kava-kava (to enhance relaxation).

The use of some functional foods, however, may undermine good nutrition. Margarines still may contain saturated fats or partially hydrogenated oils. Regular ketchup consumption on top of large orders of fries adds many calories and fat to the diet. Sweets are also high in calories and sugar. Chips are high in calories, salt, and fat. In all of these cases, the consumer would be better off taking the specific ingredient in a supplement form rather than consuming the functional food with its extra calories, sugar, salt, and/or fat.

Functional foods can provide added benefits, however, if used in conjunction with a healthful diet. You may use nutrient-dense functional foods foods that are high in antioxidants and phytochemicals. Following a nutrient assessment, a **registered dietician** can help you decide what supplement(s) might be necessary. If you take supplements in pill form, look for products that meet the USP (U.S. Pharmacopoeia) disintegration standards on the bottle. The USP symbol suggests that the supplement should completely dissolve in 45 minutes or less. Supplements that do not dissolve, of course, cannot get into the bloodstream.

Functional Foods

Functional foods are any food or food ingredient that offers specific health benefits beyond those supplied by the traditional nutrients it contains. Many functional foods come in their natural form.

Folate One of the B vitamins.

Anticoagulant Any substance that inhibits blood clotting.

Synergy A reaction in which the result is greater than the sum of its two parts.

Registered dietician (RD) A person with a college degree in dietetics who meets all certification and continuing education requirements of the American Dietetic Association or Dietitians of Canada.

Functional foods Foods or food ingredients containing physiologically active substances that provide specific health benefits beyond those supplied by basic nutrition.

Fortified foods Foods that have added nutrients that either were not present or were present in insignificant amounts with the intent of preventing nutrient deficiencies.

in your overall wellness plan as an adjunct to health-promoting strategies and treatments.

Genetically Modified Crops

A genetically modified organism (GMO) is one whose DNA (or basic genetic material) is manipulated to obtain certain results. This is done by inserting genes with desirable traits from one plant, animal, or microorganism into another one to either introduce new traits or enhance existing ones.

Crops are genetically modified to make them better resist disease and extreme environmental conditions (such as heat and frost), require less fertilizers and pesticides, last longer, and improve their nutrient content and taste. Such crops could help save billions of dollars by producing more crops and helping to feed the hungry in developing countries around the world.

Concerns over the safety of **genetically modified foods** (GM foods) have created heated public debates in Europe and, to a lesser extent, in the United States. The concern is that genetic modifications create "transgenic" organisms that have not previously existed and that have potentially unpredictable effects on the environment and on humans. Also, there is some concern that GM foods may cause illness or allergies in humans and that cross-pollination may destroy other plants or create "superweeds" with herbicide-resistant genes.

Genetically modified crops were first introduced in the United States in 1996. This technology is moving forward so rapidly that the USDA has already approved more than 50 GM crops. In 2003, about 40 percent of the U.S. cropland produced GM foods. Now, more than 80 percent of our soybeans, 73 percent of cotton, 50 percent of canola, and 40 percent of corn come from GM crops.

Totally avoiding GM foods is difficult because more than 60 percent of processed foods on the market today contain GM organisms. For people who do not wish to consume GM foods, organic foods are an option because organic trade organizations do not certify foods with genetic modifications. Produce bought at the local farmers' market also may be an option, because small farmers are less likely to use this new technology.

At this point, no evidence indicates that GM foods are harmful—but no compelling evidence guarantees that they are safe, either. Many questions remain, and much research is required in this field. As a consumer, you need to continue educating yourself as more evidence becomes available in the next few years.

Energy Substrates for Physical Activity

The two main fuels that supply energy for physical activity are glucose (sugar) and fat (fatty acids). The body uses amino acids, derived from proteins, as an energy substrate when glucose is low, such as during fasting, prolonged aerobic exercise, or a low-carbohydrate diet.

Glucose is derived from foods high in carbohydrates such as breads, cereals, grains, pasta, beans, fruits, vegetables, and sweets in general. Glucose is stored as glycogen in muscles and the liver. Fatty acids (discussed on pages 54–56) are the product of the breakdown of fats. Unlike glucose, an almost unlimited supply of fatty acids, stored as fat in the body, can be used during exercise.

Energy (ATP) Production

The energy derived from food is not used directly by the cells. It is first transformed into **adenosine triphosphate (ATP)**. The subsequent breakdown of this compound provides the energy used by all energy-requiring processes of the body (also see Figure 3.14). ATP must be recycled continually to sustain life and work. ATP can be resynthesized in three ways:

1. *ATP and ATP-CP system.* The body stores small amounts of ATP and creatine phosphate (CP). These stores are used during all-out activities such as sprinting, long jumping, and weight lifting. The amount of stored ATP provides energy for just 1 or 2 seconds. During brief all-out efforts, ATP is resynthesized from CP, another

FIGURE 3.14 Contributions of the energy formation mechanisms during various forms of physical activity.

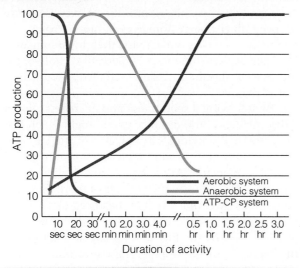

high-energy phosphate compound. This is the ATP-CP, or phosphagen, system.

Depending on the amount of physical training, the concentration of CP stored in cells is sufficient to allow maximum exertion for up to 10 seconds. Once the CP stores are depleted, the person is forced to slow down or rest to allow ATP to form through anaerobic and aerobic pathways.

2. *Anaerobic or* **lactic acid** *system.* During maximal-intensity exercise that is sustained between 10 and 180 seconds, ATP is replenished from the breakdown of glucose through a series of chemical reactions that do not require oxygen (hence "anaerobic"). In the process, though, lactic acid is produced. As lactic acid accumulates, it leads to muscular fatigue.

Because of the accumulation of lactic acid with high-intensity exercise, the formation of ATP during anaerobic activities is limited to about 3 minutes. A recovery period is then necessary to allow for the removal of lactic acid. Formation of ATP through the anaerobic system requires glucose (carbohydrates).

3. *Aerobic system.* The production of energy during slow-sustained exercise is derived primarily through aerobic metabolism. Glucose (carbohydrates), fatty acids (fat), and oxygen (hence "aerobic") are required to form ATP using this process and, under steady-state exercise conditions, lactic acid accumulation is minimal.

Because oxygen is required, a person's capacity to utilize oxygen is crucial for successful athletic performance in aerobic events. The higher one's maximal oxygen uptake (VO_{2max}), the greater one's capacity to generate ATP through the aerobic system—and the better the athletic performance in long distance events.

From the previous discussion, it becomes evident that, for optimal performance, both recreational and highly competitive athletes make the required nutrients a part of their diet.

Nutrition for Athletes

During resting conditions, fat supplies about two-thirds of the energy to sustain the body's vital processes. During exercise, the body uses both glucose (glycogen) and fat in combination to supply the energy demands. The proportion of fat to glucose changes with the intensity of exercise. When a person is exercising below 60 percent of his or her maximal work capacity (VO_{2max}), fat is used as the primary energy substrate. As the intensity of exercise increases, so does the percentage of glucose utilization—up to 100 percent during maximal work that can be sustained for only 2 to 3 minutes.

In general, athletes do not require special supplementation or any other special type of diet. Unless the diet is deficient in basic nutrients, no special secret, or magic diet will help people perform better or develop faster as a result of what they eat. As long as the diet is balanced—that is, based on a large variety of nutrients from all basic food groups—athletes do not require additional supplements. Even in strength training and body building, protein in excess of 20 percent of total daily caloric intake is not necessary. The recommended daily protein intake ranges from 0.8 grams per kilogram of body weight for sedentary people to 1.5 grams per kilogram for extremely active individuals (see Table 3.11).

The main difference between a sensible diet for a sedentary person and a sensible diet for a highly active individual is the total number of calories required daily and the amount of carbohydrate intake needed during prolonged physical activity. People in training consume more calories because of their

Genetically modified foods (GM foods) Foods whose basic genetic material (DNA) is manipulated by inserting genes with desirable traits from one plant, animal, or microorganism into another one either to introduce new traits or to enhance existing ones.

Adenosine triphosphate (ATP) A high-energy chemical compound that the body uses for immediate energy.

Lactic acid End product of anaerobic glycolysis (metabolism).

TABLE 3.11 Recommended Daily Protein Intake

Activity level	Intake in grams per kg (2.2 lb) of body weight
Sedentary	0.8
Lightly active	0.9
Moderately active	1.1
Very active	1.3
Extremely active	1.5

greater energy expenditure—which is required as a result of intense physical training.

Carbohydrate Loading

On a regular diet, the body is able to store between 1,500 and 2,000 calories in the form of glycogen. About 75 percent of this glycogen is stored in muscle tissue. This amount, however, can be increased greatly through **carbohydrate loading**.

A regular diet should be altered during several days of heavy aerobic training or when a person is going to participate in a long-distance event of more than 90 minutes (for example, marathon, triathlon, or road cycling). For events shorter than 90 minutes, carbohydrate loading does not seem to enhance performance.

During prolonged exercise, glycogen is broken down into glucose, which then is readily available to the muscles for energy production. In comparison to fat, glucose frequently is referred to as the "high-octane fuel," because it provides about 6 percent more energy per unit of oxygen consumed.

Heavy training over several consecutive days leads to depletion of glycogen faster than it can be replaced through the diet. Glycogen depletion with heavy training is common in athletes. Signs of depletion include chronic fatigue, difficulty in maintaining accustomed exercise intensity, and lower performance.

On consecutive days of exhaustive physical training (this means several hours daily), a carbohydrate-rich diet—70 percent of total daily caloric intake or 8 grams of carbohydrate per kilogram (2.2 pounds) of body weight—is recommended. This diet often restores glycogen levels in 24 hours. Along with the high-carbohydrate diet, a day of rest often is needed to allow the muscles to recover from glycogen depletion following days of intense training. For people who exercise less than an hour a day, a 60 percent carbohydrate diet or 6 grams of carbohydrate per

kilogram of body weight is enough to replenish glycogen stores.

Following an exhaustive workout, eating a combination of carbohydrates and protein (such as a tuna sandwich) within 30 minutes of exercise seems to speed up glycogen storage even more. Protein intake increases insulin activity, thereby enhancing glycogen replenishment. A 70 percent carbohydrate intake then should be maintained throughout the rest of the day.

By following a special diet and exercise regimen 5 days before a long-distance event, highly (aerobically) trained individuals are capable of storing two to three times the amount of glycogen found in the average person. Athletic performance may be enhanced for long-distance events of more than 90 minutes by eating a regular balanced diet (50 to 60 percent carbohydrates) along with intensive physical training the fifth and fourth days before the event, followed by a diet high in carbohydrates (about 70 percent) and a gradual decrease in training intensity over the last three days before the event.

The amount of glycogen stored as a result of a carbohydrate-rich diet does not seem to be affected by the proportion of complex and simple carbohydrates. Intake of simple carbohydrates (sugars) can be raised while on a 70 percent carbohydrate diet, as long as they don't exceed 25 percent of the total calories. Complex carbohydrates provide more nutrients and fiber, making them a better choice for a healthier diet.

On the day of the long-distance event, carbohydrates are still the recommended choice of substrate. As a general rule, athletes should consume 1 gram of carbohydrate for each kilogram (2.2 pounds) of body weight 1 hour prior to exercise (that is, if you weigh 160 pounds, you should consume 160 ÷ 2.2 = 72 grams). If the pre-event meal is eaten earlier, the amount of carbohydrate can be increased to 2, 3, or 4 grams per kilogram of weight 2, 3, or 4 hours, respectively, before exercise.

During the long-distance event, researchers recommend that 30 to 60 grams of carbohydrates (120 to 240 calories) be consumed every hour. This is best accomplished by drinking 8 ounces of a 6- to 8 percent–carbohydrate sports drink every 15 minutes (check labels to ensure proper carbohydrate concentration). This also lessens the chance of dehydration during exercise, which hinders performance and endangers health. The percentage of the carbohydrate drink is determined by dividing the amount of carbohydrate (in grams) by the amount of fluid (in ml) and then multiplying by 100. For example, 18 grams of carbohydrate in 240 ml (8 oz) of fluid yields a drink that is 7.5 percent (18 ÷ 240 × 100) carbohydrate.

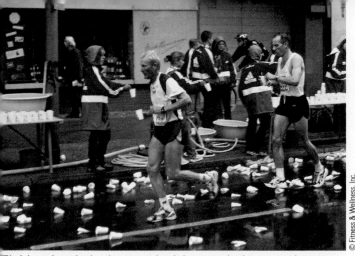

Fluid and carbohydrate replenishment during exercise are essential when participating in long-distance aerobic endurance events, such as a marathon or a triathlon.

© Fitness & Wellness, Inc.

Creatine Supplementation

Creatine is an organic compound obtained in the diet primarily from meat and fish. In the human body, creatine combines with inorganic phosphate and forms the high-energy compound **creatine phosphate (CP).** CP is then used to resynthesize ATP during short bursts of all-out physical activity. Individuals on a normal mixed diet consume an average of 1 gram of creatine per day. Each day, 1 additional gram is synthesized from various amino acids. One pound of meat or fish provides approximately 2 grams of creatine.

Creatine supplementation has become popular in recent years among individuals who want to increase muscle mass and improve athletic performance. Creatine monohydrate—a white, tasteless powder that is mixed with fluids prior to ingestion—is the form most popular among people who use the supplement. Supplementation can result in an approximate 20 percent increase in the amount of creatine that is stored in muscles. Most of this creatine binds to phosphate to form CP, and 30 to 40 percent remains as free creatine in the muscle. Increased creatine storage is believed to enable individuals to train more intensely—thus building more muscle mass and enhancing performance in all-out activities of very short duration (less than 30 seconds).

Creatine supplementation has two phases: the *loading phase* and the *maintenance phase.* During the loading phase, the person consumes between 20 and 25 grams (1 teaspoonful is about 5 grams) of creatine per day for 5 to 6 days, divided into 4 or 5 dosages of 5 grams each throughout the day (this amount represents the equivalent of consuming 10 or more pounds of meat per day). Research also suggests that the amount of creatine stored in muscle

is enhanced by taking creatine in combination with a high-carbohydrate food. Once the loading phase is complete, taking 2 grams per day seems to be sufficient to maintain the increased muscle stores.

To date, no serious side effects have been documented in people who take up to 25 grams of creatine per day for 5 days. Stomach distress and cramping has been reported only in rare instances. The 2 grams taken per day during the maintenance phase is just slightly above the average intake in our daily diet. Long-term effects of creatine supplementation on health, however, have not been established.

A frequently documented result following 5 to 6 days of creatine loading is an increase of 2 to 3 pounds in body weight. This increase appears to be related to increased water retention necessary to maintain the additional creatine stored in muscles. Some data, however, suggest that the increase in stored water and CP stimulates protein synthesis, leading to an increase in lean body mass.

The benefits of elevated creatine stores may be limited to high-intensity/short-duration activities such as sprinting, strength training (weight lifting), and sprint cycling. Supplementation is most beneficial during exercise training itself, rather than as an aid to enhance athletic performance a few days before competition.

Enhanced creatine stores do not benefit athletes competing in aerobic endurance events, because CP is not used in energy production for long-distance events. In fact, the additional weight can be detrimental in long-distance running and swimming events, because the athlete must expend more energy to carry the extra weight during competition.

Amino Acid Supplements

A myth regarding athletic performance is that protein (amino acid) supplements will increase muscle mass. The claims and safety of these products have not been proven scientifically. The RDA for protein is .8 grams per kilogram of body weight per day. That is, if you weigh 154 pounds (70 kilograms, 154 ÷ 2.2), you should consume 56 grams (70 × .8) of protein.

Carbohydrate loading Increasing intake of carbohydrates during heavy aerobic training or prior to aerobic endurance events that last longer than 90 minutes.

Creatine An organic compound derived from meat, fish, and amino acids that combines with inorganic phosphate to form creatine phosphate.

Creatine phosphate (CP) A high-energy compound that the cells use to resynthesize ATP during all-out activities of very short duration.

Most athletes, including weight lifters and body builders, increase their caloric intake automatically during intense training. As caloric intake increases, so does the intake of protein, often approaching 2 or more grams per kilogram of body weight. This amount is more than enough to build and repair muscle tissue. Typically, athletes in strength training consume between 3 and 4 grams per kilogram of body weight. In response, supplement manufacturers have created expensive "free-amino acid supplements."

People who buy costly free-amino acid supplements are led to believe that these contribute to the development of muscle mass. The human body, however, cannot distinguish between amino acids obtained from food or through supplements. Excess protein either is used for energy or is turned into fat. With amino acid supplements, each capsule provides up to 500 milligrams of amino acids and no additional nutrients. In contrast, 3 ounces of meat or fish provide more than 20,000 milligrams of amino acids, along with other essential nutrients such as iron, niacin, and thiamin. The benefits of natural foods to health and budget are clear.

Proponents of free-amino acid supplements further claim that only a small amount of amino acids in food is absorbed and that free-amino acids are absorbed more readily than are protein foods. Neither claim is correct. The human body absorbs and utilizes between 85 and 99 percent of all protein from food intake. The body handles whole, natural proteins better than single amino acids that have been predigested in the laboratory setting.

Amino acid supplementation can even be dangerous: An excess of a single amino acid or a group of chemically similar amino acids often prevents the absorption of other amino acids. Needed amino acids then pass through the body unabsorbed, potentially causing critical imbalances and toxicities. Long-term risks associated with amino acid supplementation have not been determined.

The advertised rate of absorption provides no additional benefit, because building muscle takes hours, not minutes. Muscle overload through heavy training, not supplementation, builds muscle. Expensive protein supplements benefit only those who sell them.

Special Nutrient Needs of Women

Three considerations specific to women are bone health, hormone replacement therapy beginning at menopause, and iron supplementation to offset the iron lost through menstruation.

Bone Health and Osteoporosis

Osteoporosis, literally meaning "porous bones," is a condition in which bones lack the minerals required to keep them strong. In osteoporosis, bones —primarily of the hip, wrist, and spine—become so weak and brittle that they fracture readily. The process begins slowly in the third and fourth decades of life. Women are especially susceptible after menopause because of the accompanying loss of **estrogen**, which increases the rate at which bone mass is broken down.

Approximately 22 million U. S. women have osteoporosis, and 16 million don't know that they have this disease. About 30 percent of post-menopausal women have osteoporosis, but only about 2 percent are actually diagnosed and treated for this condition.[9]

Osteoporosis is the leading cause of serious morbidity and functional loss in the elderly population. One of every two women and one in eight men over age 50 will have an osteoporotic-related fracture at some point in their lives. The chances of a post-menopausal woman developing osteoporosis is much greater than her chances of developing breast cancer or suffering a heart attack or stroke.

According to Stanford University researchers, an estimated 3.6 million Americans in 2003 had been diagnosed with osteoporosis. Up to 20 percent of people who have a hip fracture die within a year because of complications related to the fracture. As alarming as these figures are, they do not convey the pain and loss of quality of life in people who suffer the crippling effects of osteoporotic fractures.

Although osteoporosis is viewed primarily as a women's disease, more than 30 percent of all men will be affected by age 75. About 100,000 of the yearly 300,000 hip fractures in the United States occur in men.

Despite the strong genetic component, osteoporosis is preventable. Maximizing bone density at a young age and subsequently decreasing the rate of bone loss later in life are critical factors in preventing osteoporosis.

Normal hormone levels prior to menopause and adequate calcium intake and physical activity throughout life cannot be overemphasized. These factors are all crucial to preventing osteoporosis. The absence of any one of these three factors leads to bone loss for which the other two factors never completely compensate. Smoking, excessive use of alcohol, and corticosteroid drugs also accelerate the rate of bone loss in women and men alike. Osteoporosis is also more common in whites, Asians, and people with small frames. Figure 3.15 depicts these variables.

Bone health begins at a young age. Some experts have called osteoporosis a "pediatric disease."

FIGURE 3.15 Threats to bone health (osteoporosis).

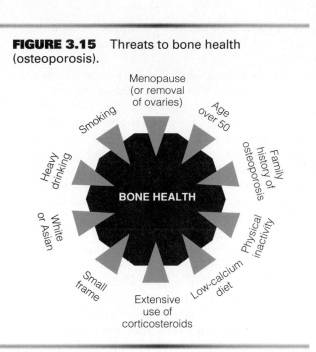

Menopause (or removal of ovaries)

Age over 50

Smoking

Family history of osteoporosis

Heavy drinking

BONE HEALTH

Physical inactivity

White or Asian

Low-calcium diet

Small frame

Extensive use of corticosteroids

TABLE 3.12 Recommended Daily Calcium Intake

Age	Amount (mg)
1–8	800
9–24	1,300
25–50	1,000
Women over 50	1,500
Men 51–65	1,200
Men over 65	1,500

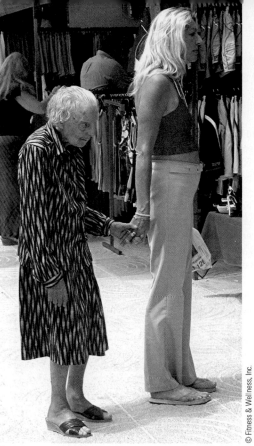

Osteoporosis is a leading cause of morbidity and functional loss in older adults.

Bone density can be promoted early in life by making sure the diet has sufficient calcium and participating in weight-bearing activities. Adequate calcium intake in both women and men is also associated with a reduced risk for colon cancer.[10] The RDA for calcium is between 1,000 and 1,300 mg per day, but leading researchers in this area recommend higher intakes (see Table 3.12). Although the recommended daily intakes can be met easily through diet alone, some experts recommend calcium supplements even for children before puberty.

To obtain your daily calcium requirement, get as much calcium as possible from calcium-rich foods, including calcium-fortified foods. If you don't get enough (most people don't), take calcium supplements.

Supplemental calcium can be obtained in the form of calcium citrate and calcium carbonate. Calcium citrate seems to be equally well absorbed with or without food, whereas calcium carbonate is not well absorbed without food. Thus, if your

supplement contains calcium carbonate, always take the supplement with meals. Do not take more than 500 mg at a time, because larger amounts are not well absorbed. And don't forget vitamin D, which is vital for calcium absorption.

Avoid taking calcium supplements with an iron-rich meal or in conjunction with an iron-containing multivitamin. Unfortunately, calcium interferes with iron absorption, thus it is best to separate the intake of these two minerals. The benefit of taking your calcium supplement without food (calcium citrate) is that, in a young menstruating woman who needs iron, calcium won't interfere with the absorption of iron.

Table 3.13 provides a list of selected foods and their calcium content. Along with having an adequate calcium intake, taking 400 to 800 IU of vitamin D daily is recommended for optimal calcium absorption. People over age 50 may require 800

Osteoporosis Softening, deterioration, or loss of bone mineral density that leads to disability, bone fractures, and even death from medical complications.

Estrogen Female sex hormone essential for bone formation and conservation of bone density.

TABLE 3.13 Low-Fat Calcium-Rich Foods

Food	Amount	Calcium (mg)	Calories
Beans, red kidney, cooked	1 cup	70	218
Beet, greens, cooked	½ cup	82	19
Bok choy (Chinese cabbage)	1 cup	158	20
Broccoli, cooked, drained	1 cup	72	44
Burrito, bean (no cheese)	1	57	225
Cottage cheese, 2% low-fat	½ cup	78	103
Ice milk (vanilla)	½ cup	102	100
Instant breakfast, nonfat milk	1 cup	407	216
Kale, cooked, drained	1 cup	94	36
Milk, nonfat, powdered	1 tbs	52	15
Milk, skim	1 cup	296	88
Oatmeal, instant, fortified, plain	½ cup	109	70
Okra, cooked, drained	½ cup	74	23
Orange juice, fortified	1 cup	300	110
Soy milk, fortified, fat free	1 cup	400	110
Spinach, raw	1 cup	56	12
Turnip greens, cooked	1 cup	197	29
Tofu (some types)	½ cup	138	76
Yogurt, fruit	1 cup	372	250
Yogurt, low-fat, plain	1 cup	448	155

to 1,000 IU. About 40 percent of these adults are deficient in vitamin D.[11]

Excessive protein intake also may affect the body's absorption of calcium. The more protein that is eaten, the higher is the calcium content in the urine (that is, the more calcium excreted). This might be the reason why countries with a high protein intake, including the United States, also have the highest rates of osteoporosis. Aim to achieve the RDA for protein, nonetheless, because people who consume too little protein (less than 35 grams per day) lose more bone mass than those who eat too much (more than 100 grams per day). The RDA for protein is about 50 grams per day for women and 63 for men.

Soft drinks, coffee, and alcoholic beverages can also contribute to a loss in bone density if consumed in large quantities. They may not cause the damage directly but, rather, because they take the place of dairy products in the diet.

Exercise plays a key role in preventing osteoporosis by decreasing the rate of bone loss following the onset of menopause. Active people are able to maintain bone density much more effectively than their inactive counterparts. A combination of weight-bearing exercises, such as walking or jogging and weight training, is especially helpful.

The benefits of exercise go beyond maintaining bone density. Exercise strengthens muscles, ligaments, and tendons—all of which provide support to the bones (skeleton). Exercise also improves balance and coordination, which can help prevent falls and injuries.

Current studies indicate that people who are active have denser bone mineral than inactive people do. Similar to other benefits of participating in exercise, there is no such thing as "bone in the bank." To have good bone health, people need to participate in a regular lifetime exercise program.

Prevailing research also tells us that estrogen is the most important factor in preventing bone loss. Lumbar bone density in women who have always had regular menstrual cycles exceeds that of women with a history of **oligomenorrhea** and **amenorrhea** interspersed with regular cycles. Furthermore, the lumbar density of these two groups of women is higher than that of women who have never had regular menstrual cycles.

For instance, athletes with amenorrhea (who have lower estrogen levels) have lower bone mineral density than even nonathletes with normal estrogen levels. Studies have shown that amenorrheic athletes at age 25 have the bones of women older than 50. Over the last few years, it has become clear that sedentary women with normal estrogen levels have better bone mineral density than active amenorrheic athletes. Many experts believe the best predictor of bone mineral content is the history of menstrual regularity.

As a baseline, women age 65 and older should have a bone density test to establish the risk for osteoporosis. Younger women who are at risk for osteoporosis should discuss a bone density test with their physician at menopause. The test also can be used to monitor changes in bone mass over time and to predict the risk of future fractures. The bone density test is a painless scan requiring only a small amount of radiation to determine bone mass of the spine, hip, wrist, heel, or fingers. The amount of radiation is so low that technicians administering the test can sit right next to the person receiving it. The procedure often takes less than 10 minutes.

Following menopause, every woman should consider some type of therapy to prevent bone loss. The various therapy modalities available should be discussed with a physician.

Hormone Replacement Therapy

For decades, hormone-replacement therapy (HRT) was the most common treatment modality to prevent bone loss following menopause. A large study (16,000 healthy women, ages 50 to 79) was recently terminated 3 years early because the results showed that taking estrogen and progestin, a common form of HRT, actually increased the risk for disease.[12] The study was the first major long-term (8-year) clinical trial investigating the association between HRT and age-related diseases that included cardiovascular disease, cancer, and osteoporosis. Although the risk for hip fractures and colorectal cancer decreased, the risk for developing breast cancer, blood clots, strokes, and heart attacks increased.

HRT may still be the most effective treatment for the relief of acute (short-term) symptoms of menopause, such as hot flashes, mood swings, sleep difficulties, and vaginal dryness. Researchers and physicians, however, must now determine how long women can remain on HRT, how to best taper off treatment to provide maximal physical and emotional relief, and how to protect women from osteoporosis and other age-related diseases. Women who believed that HRT would help them strengthen bones and ward off age-related diseases must now seek other treatments.

New alternative treatments to prevent bone loss are being developed. Miacalcin, a synthetic form of the hormone calcitonin, is FDA-approved for women who suffer from osteoporosis and are at least 5-year post-menopausal. Calcitonin is a thyroid hormone that helps maintain the body's delicate balance of calcium by taking calcium from the blood and depositing it in the bones. Though it is effective in preventing bone loss, it does not help much in re-building bone. The drug seems to have no side effects. It is available in injectable and nasal spray forms.

Two promising nonhormonal drugs, alendronate (Fosamax) and risedronate (Actonel), not only prevent bone loss but actually help increase bone mass. Alendronate is recommended for women who already have osteoporosis. Alendronate is used pri-marily for bone health and does not provide benefits to the cardiovascular system. Although the research is limited, this drug seems to be safe and effective.

Selective estrogen receptor modulators (SERMs) are also used to prevent bone loss. These com-pounds have a positive effect on blood lipids and pose no risk to breast and uterine tissue. SERMs, however, do not help increase bone density. One SERM currently used to prevent osteoporosis is raloxifene (Evista).

Adequate Iron Intake

Iron is a key element of **hemoglobin** in blood. The RDA of iron for adult women is between 15 and 18 mg per day (8 to 11 mg for men). Inadequate iron intake is often seen in children, teenagers, women of childbearing age, and endurance athletes. If iron absorption does not compensate for losses or dietary intake is low, iron deficiency develops. As many as 50 percent of American women suffer from iron deficiency. Over time, excessive depletion of iron stores in the body leads to iron-deficiency anemia, a condition in which the concentration of hemoglobin in the red blood cells is lower than it should be.

Physically active individuals, in particular women, have a greater-than-average need for iron. Heavy training creates a demand for iron that is higher than the recommended intake because small amounts of iron are lost through sweat, urine, and stools. Mechanical trauma, caused by the pounding of the feet on the pavement during extensive jog-ging, may also lead to destruction of iron-containing red blood cells.

A large percentage of female endurance athletes are reported to have iron deficiency. The blood **ferritin** levels of women who participate in intense physical training should be checked frequently.

The rates of iron absorption and iron loss vary from person to person. In most cases, though, people can get enough iron by eating more iron-rich foods such as beans, peas, green leafy vegetables, enriched grain products, egg yolk, fish, and lean meats. Al-though organ meats, such as liver, are especially good sources, they also are high in cholesterol. A list of foods high in iron is given in Table 3.14.

Dietary Guidelines for Americans

The Dietary Guidelines for Americans provide science-based advice to promote health and to reduce risk for major chronic diseases through diet and physical activity. The Secretaries of the Department of Health and Human Services (HHS) and the Department of Agriculture (USDA) issue a report at least every five years that contain nutri-tional and dietary information and guidelines for the general public. Every five years, an expert Dietary Guidelines Advisory Committee is appointed to make recommendations concerning revision of Dietary Guidelines for Americans. The recommen-dations are to be targeted to the general public age 2 years and older and based on the preponderance of scientific and medical knowledge that is current at the time of publication of the committee's report. The main focus of these guidelines is health promo-tion and disease risk reduction.

The topics that the committee addressed in depth included meeting recommended nutrient

Oligomenorrhea Irregular menstrual cycles.

Amenorrhea Cessation of regular menstrual flow.

Hemoglobin Protein–iron compound in red blood cells that transports oxygen in the blood.

Ferritin Iron stored in the body.

TABLE 3.14 Iron-Rich Foods

Food	Amount	Iron (mg)	Calories	Cholesterol	% Calories From Fat
Beans, red kidney, cooked	1 cup	3.2	218	0	4
Beef, ground lean (21% fat)	3 oz	2.1	237	86	57
Beef, sirloin, lean only	3 oz	2.9	171	76	36
Beef, liver, fried	3 oz	5.3	184	409	33
Beet, greens, cooked	½ cup	1.4	19	0	—
Broccoli, cooked, drained	1 cup	1.3	44	0	—
Burrito, bean (no cheese)	1	2.3	225	2	28
Egg, hard-cooked	1	.7	77	212	58
Farina (Cream of Wheat), cooked	½ cup	5.2	65	0	—
Instant breakfast, nonfat milk	1 cup	4.8	216	9	4
Peas, frozen, cooked, drained	½ cup	1.3	62	0	—
Shrimp, boiled	3 oz	2.7	87	172	10
Spinach, raw	1 cup	1.5	12	0	—
Vegetables, mixed, cooked	1 cup	1.5	108	0	—

intakes; physical activity; energy balance; relationships of fats, carbohydrates, selected food groups, and alcohol with health; and consumer aspects of food safety. The committee was especially interested in finding strong scientific support for dietary and physical activity measures that could reduce the Nation's major diet-related health problems: overweight and obesity, hypertension, abnormal blood lipids, diabetes, coronary heart disease (CHD), certain types of cancer, and osteoporosis.

The committee's extensive review of the evidence and deliberations led to the development of a set of nine key messages. These messages should be useful to nutrition-related program providers, healthcare providers, and educators, as well as to those charged with the responsibility to produce the publication *Dietary Guidelines for Americans, 2005 (6th) Edition*. The committee's findings support the development of dietary guidelines that convey the following nine major messages (additional information on these guidelines are posted at www.health.gov/dietaryguidelines):

■ *Consume a variety of foods within and among the basic food groups while staying within energy needs.*

The recommendations for nutrient intakes consider the prevention of chronic disease as well as basic nutrient needs. Meeting those recommendations provides a firm foundation for health and for reducing chronic disease risk. For most nutrients, intakes by Americans appear adequate. However, efforts are warranted to promote increased dietary intakes of vitamin E, calcium, magnesium, potassium, and fiber by children and adults and to promote increased dietary intakes of

vitamins A and C by adults. Meeting the recommended nutrient intakes while staying within energy needs is a basic premise of dietary guidance.

■ *Control calorie intake to manage body weight.*

Calorie intake and physical activity go hand in hand in controlling a person's weight. To stem the obesity epidemic, most Americans need to reduce the amount of calories they consume. When it comes to weight control, calories do count. Limiting portion sizes and monitoring weight regularly to adjust food intake as necessary is recommended.

■ *Be physically active every day.*

Making moderate physical activity a part of an adult's daily routine for at least 30 minutes per day promotes fitness and reduces the risk of chronic health conditions. Moderate physical activity for an hour each day can increase energy expenditure by about 150 to 200 calories, depending on body size. According to the committee, many adults need to participate in up to 60 minutes of moderate to vigorous physical activity on most days to prevent unhealthy weight gain; while adults who have previously lost weight may need 60 and up to 90 minutes of moderate physical activity daily to help avoid regain of weight. Compared with moderate physical activity, vigorous physical activity provides greater benefits for physical fitness and burns more calories per unit time.

■ *Increase daily intake of fruits and vegetables, whole grains, and nonfat or low-fat milk and milk products.*

Fruits contain glucose, fructose, sucrose, and fiber, and most fruits are relatively low in calories. In addition, fruits are important sources of at least

FIGURE 3.16 2005 Dietary Guidelines for Americans.

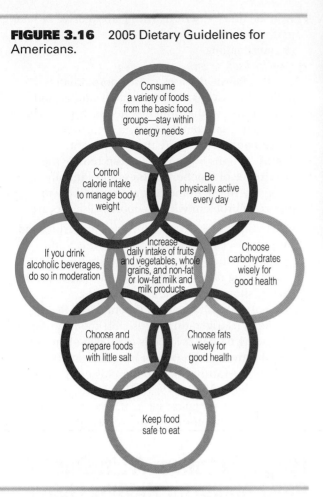

Consume a variety of foods from the basic food groups—stay within energy needs

Control calorie intake to manage body weight

Be physically active every day

If you drink alcoholic beverages, do so in moderation

Increase daily intake of fruits and vegetables, whole grains, and non-fat or low-fat milk and milk products

Choose carbohydrates wisely for good health

Choose and prepare foods with little salt

Choose fats wisely for good health

Keep food safe to eat

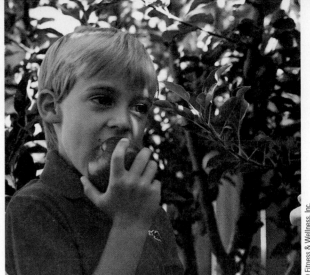

Positive nutrition habits should be taught and reinforced in early youth.

eight additional nutrients, including vitamin C, folate, and potassium. Many vegetables provide only small amounts of sugars and/or starch, some are high in starch, and all provide fiber. Vegetables are important sources of 19 or more nutrients, including potassium, folate, and vitamins A and E.

Moreover, increased consumption of fruits and vegetables may be a useful component of programs designed to achieve and sustain weight loss. Consuming a variety of fruits and vegetables daily is recommended (choose among citrus fruits, melons, and berries; other fruits; dark green leafy vegetables; bright orange vegetables; legumes; starchy vegetables; and other vegetables).

Whole grains are high in starch, and they are important sources of 14 nutrients including fiber. Important sources of whole grains include whole wheat, oatmeal, popcorn, bulgur, and brown rice. The goal is to eat at least three 1-ounce equivalents per day of whole-grain foods, preferably in place of refined grains.

Milk and milk products are important sources of at least 12 nutrients including calcium, magnesium, potassium, and vitamin D. Diets that provide

three cups or the equivalent of nonfat or low-fat milk and/or milk products per day can improve bone mass and is not associated with weight gain.

■ *Choose fats wisely for good health.*

Keeping intake of saturated fat, trans fat and cholesterol very low can help reduce the risk of coronary heart disease. The lower the combined intake of saturated and trans fat and the lower the dietary cholesterol intake, the greater the cardio-vascular benefit will be.

The major way to keep saturated fat low is to limit one's intake of animal fats (such as those in cheese, milk, butter, ice cream, and other full-fat dairy products; fatty meat; bacon and sausage; and poultry skin and fat). The major way to limit trans fat intake is to limit the intake of foods made with partially hydrogenated vegetable oils. To limit dietary intake of cholesterol, one needs to limit the intake of eggs and organ meats especially, as well as limit the intake of meat, shellfish, poultry, and dairy products that contain fat.

Total fat intake of 20 to 35 percent of calories is recommended for all Americans age 18 years or older. Intakes of fat outside of this range are not recommended for most Americans because of potential adverse effects on achieving recommended nutrient intakes and on risk factors for chronic diseases. The lower limit of fat intake is higher for children: 30 percent of calories from fat for children age 2 and 3 years, and 25 percent of calories from fat for those age 4 to 18 years.

■ *Choose carbohydrates wisely for good health.*

When selecting foods from the fruit, vegetable, and grains groups, it is beneficial to make fiber-rich choices often. This means, for example, choosing whole fruits rather than juices and whole grains rather than refined grains. Following guidance to increase one's intake of fruits, vegetables, whole grains, and nonfat or low-fat milk or milk products is a healthful way to obtain the recommended amounts of carbohydrates. Compared with individuals who consume small amounts of foods and beverages that are high in added sugars, those who consume large amounts tend to consume more calories but smaller amounts of vitamins and minerals. A reduced intake of added sugars (especially sugar-sweetened beverages) may be helpful in achieving the recommended intakes of nutrients and in weight control.

■ *Choose and prepare foods with little salt.*

Reducing salt (sodium chloride) intake is one of several ways that people can lower their blood pressure. Reducing blood pressure, ideally to the normal range, reduces the chance of developing a stroke, heart disease, heart failure, and kidney disease. The relationship between salt intake and blood pressure is direct and progressive without an apparent threshold. The goal is to consume less than 2,300 mg of sodium per day. On average, the higher a person's salt intake, the higher the blood pressure. Thus, reducing salt intake as much as possible is one way to lower blood pressure.

■ *If you drink alcoholic beverages, do so in moderation.*

Among middle-aged and older adults, the lowest all-cause mortality occurs at the level of one to two drinks per day. The mortality reduction is likely due to the protective effects of moderate alcohol consumption on coronary heart disease, primarily among males older than age 45 years and women older than age 55 years. Among younger people, alcohol consumption appears to provide little, if any, health benefit. Alcohol use among young adults is associated with an increased risk of traumatic injury and death. Heavy drinking is very hazardous, contributing to automobile injuries and deaths, assault, liver disease, and other health problems. Abstention is an important option.

The goal for adults who choose to drink is to do so in moderation. Moderation is defined as the consumption of up to one drink per day for women and two drinks per day for men. One drink is defined as 12 ounces of regular beer, 5 ounces of wine (12 percent alcohol), or 1.5 ounces of 80-proof distilled spirits.

Among the people who should not consume alcoholic beverages are those who cannot restrict their drinking to moderate levels, children and adolescents, and individuals taking medications that can interact with alcohol or who have specific medical conditions. Drinking alcoholic beverages should be avoided by women who may become pregnant or who are pregnant, by breastfeeding

women, and by persons who plan to drive or take part in other activities that require attention, skill, or coordination.

■ *Keep food safe to eat.*

Foodborne diseases cause approximately 76 million illnesses, 325,000 hospitalizations, and 5,000 deaths in the United States each year. Three pathogens (Salmonella, Listeria, and Toxoplasma) are responsible for more than 75 percent of these deaths. Actions by consumers can reduce the occurrence of foodborne illness substantially. The behaviors in the home that are most likely to prevent a problem with foodborne illnesses are

- Cleaning hands, contact surfaces, and fruits and vegetables (this does not apply to meat and poultry, which should not be washed)
- Separating raw, cooked, and ready-to-eat foods while shopping, preparing, or storing
- Cooking foods to a safe temperature
- Chilling (refrigerating) perishable foods promptly
- Avoiding higher-risk foods (e.g., deli meats and frankfurters that have not been reheated to a safe temperature [may contain Listeria]). This is especially important for high-risk groups (the very young, pregnant women, the elderly, and those who are immunocompromised).

Proper Nutrition: A Lifetime Prescription for Healthy Living

The three factors that do the most for health, longevity, and quality of life are proper nutrition, a sound exercise program, and quitting (or never starting) smoking. Achieving and maintaining a balanced diet is not as difficult as most people think. If parents were to do a better job of teaching and reinforcing proper nutrition habits in early youth, the current magnitude of nutrition-related health problems would be much smaller. Although treatment of obesity is important, we should place far greater emphasis on preventing obesity in youth and adults in the first place.

Children tend to eat the way their parents do. If parents adopt a healthy diet, children most likely will follow. The difficult part for most people is retraining themselves to follow a lifetime healthy nutrition plan—a diet that includes lots of grains, legumes, fruits, vegetables, and low-fat dairy products, with moderate use of animal protein, junk food, sodium, and alcohol.

In spite of the ample scientific evidence linking poor dietary habits to early disease

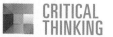

CRITICAL THINKING

What factors in your life and the environment have contributed to your current dietary habits? Do you need to make changes? What may prevent you from doing so?

and mortality rates, many people remain precontemplators: They are not willing to change their eating patterns. Even when faced with obesity, elevated blood lipids, hypertension, and other nutrition-related conditions, people do not change. The motivating factor to change one's eating habits seems to be a major health breakdown, such as a heart attack, a stroke, or cancer—by which time the damage has been done already. In many cases it is irreversible and, for some, fatal.

An ounce of prevention is worth a pound of cure. The sooner you implement the dietary guidelines presented in this chapter, the better are your chances of preventing chronic diseases and reaching a higher state of wellness.

ASSESS YOUR KNOWLEDGE

1. The science of nutrition studies the relationship of
   a. vitamins and minerals to health.
   b. foods to optimal health and performance.
   c. carbohydrates, fats, and proteins to the development and maintenance of good health.
   d. the macronutrients and micronutrients to physical performance.
   e. kilocalories to calories in food items.

2. Faulty nutrition often plays a crucial role in the development and progression of which disease?
   a. cardiovascular disease
   b. cancer
   c. osteoporosis
   d. diabetes
   e. All are correct choices.

3. According to MyPyramid, daily vegetable consumption is measured in
   a. servings.
   b. ounces.
   c. cups.
   d. calories.
   e. All of the above.

4. The recommended amount of fiber intake for adults 50 years and younger is
   a. 10 grams per day for women and 12 grams for men.
   b. 21 grams per day for women and 30 grams for men.
   c. 28 grams per day for women and 35 grams for men.
   d. 25 grams per day for women and 38 grams for men.
   e. 45 grams per day for women and 50 grams for men.

5. Unhealthy fats include
   a. unsaturated fatty acids.
   b. monounsaturated fats.
   c. polyunsaturated fatty acids.
   d. saturated fats.
   e. alpha-linolenic acid.

6. The daily recommended carbohydrate intake is:
   a. 45 to 65 percent of the total calories.
   b. 10 to 35 percent of the total calories.
   c. 20 to 35 percent of the total calories.
   d. 60 to 75 percent of the total calories.
   e. 35 to 50 percent of the total calories.

7. The amount of a nutrient that is estimated to meet the nutrient requirement of half the healthy people in specific age and gender groups is known as the
   a. Estimated Average Requirement.
   b. Recommended Dietary Allowance.
   c. Daily Values.
   d. Adequate Intake.
   e. Dietary Reference Intakes.

8. The percent fat intake for an individual who on a given day consumes 2,385 calories with 106 grams of fat is
   a. 44 percent of total calories.
   b. 17.7 percent of total calories.
   c. 40 percent of total calories.
   d. 31 percent of total calories.
   e. 22.5 percent of total calories.

9. Carbohydrate loading is beneficial for
   a. endurance athletes.
   b. diabetics.
   c. strength athletes.
   d. sprinters.
   e. all of the above.

10. Osteoporosis is
    a. a crippling disease.
    b. more prevalent in women.
    c. higher in people who were calcium-deficient at a young age.
    d. linked to heavy drinking and smoking.
    e. All are correct choices.

Correct answers can be found at the back of the book.

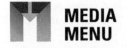

MEDIA MENU

PROFILE PLUS CD CONNECTIONS

■ Analyze your diet and plan for a healthy change.
■ Check how well you understand the chapter's concepts.

INTERNET CONNECTIONS

■ American Dietetic Association. This comprehensive site features daily food tips, frequently asked questions, nutrition resources, and links to other reliable Web sites on nutrition.

http://www.eatright.org

■ U.S. Department of Agriculture Center for Nutrition Policy and Promotion. The Center for Nutrition Policy and Promotion is the national organization where scientific research is linked with the nutritional needs of the American public. This site includes "The Interactive Health Eating Index," an online dietary assessment tool that includes nutrition messages. After providing a day's worth of dietary information, you will receive a "score" on the overall quality of your diet, based on the types and amounts of food compared with those recommended by the Food Guide Pyramid.

http://www.usda.gov/cnpp

■ Professional Nutrition Online Course sponsored by the United States Department of Agriculture. This site features a professional course outlining the ABC's of dietary guidelines (Aim, Build, and Choose). Registration is free to access this online automated self-study course (released in cooperation with East Carolina University) that describes the importance of physical fitness, the Food Guide Pyramid, and healthy food choices.

http://www.dga2000training.usda.gov

■ Cyberkitchen. This interactive site helps you discover how much you are really eating with an activity on comparing standard serving sizes vs. real serving sizes. You can also provide personal information regarding your age, gender, height, weight, and activity level, and the Cyberkitchen will provide you with a healthy diet plan to meet your weight management goals. It's fun and educational.

http://www.nhlbi.nih.gov/chd/Tipsheets/cyberkit.htm

Notes

1. National Academy of Sciences, Institute of Medicine. *Dietary Reference Intakes for Energy, Carbohydrates, Fiber, Fat, Protein and Amino Acids (Macronutrients)* (Washington, DC: National Academy Press, 2002).

2. "Is There Flaxseed In Your Fridge Yet?" *Tufts University Health & Nutrition Letter,* Sept. 2002.

3. Bowen, P. E. "Evaluating the Health Claim of Flaxseed and Cancer Prevention," *Nutrition Today* 36 (2001): 144–158.

   "Flax Facts," *University of California at Berkeley Wellness Letter* (May 2002).

4. See note 1.

5. A. Trichopoulou et al., "Adherence to a Mediterranean Diet and Survival in a Greek Population, "*New England Journal of Medicine* 348 (2003): 2599–2608.

6. "Should You Take Vitamin C and E Supplements?" *University of California at Berkeley Wellness Letter* (June 2001).

7. L. C. Clark et al., "Effects of Selenium Supplementation for Cancer Prevention in Patients with Carcinoma of the Skin: A Randomized Controlled Trial," *Journal of the American Medical Association* 276 (1996): 1957–1963.

8. "The Merits of Multivitamins: EN's Guide to Choosing a Supplement," *Environmental Nutrition* 24, no. 6 (2001): 1.

9. "New Advice About Bone Density Tests," *University of California at Berkeley Wellness Letter* 18, no. 10 (2002): 1–2.

10. M. T. Goodman et al. "Association of Dairy Products, Lactose, and Calcium with the Risk of Ovarian Cancer," *American Journal of Epidemiology* 156 (2002): 148–157.

11. "How to Build Better Bones: Overview of All the New Osteoporosis Options," *Environmental Nutrition* 24, no. 9 (2001): 1, 4–5.

12. Writing Group for the Women's Health Initiative, "Risks and Benefits of Combined Estrogen and Progestin in Healthy Postmenopausal Women: Principal Results from the Women's Health Initiative Randomized Controlled Trial," *Journal of the American Medical Association* 288 (2002): 321–333.

13. U.S. Department of Health and Human Services, Department of Agriculture, *Nutrition and Your Health: Dietary Guidelines for Americans,* Home and Garden Bulletin No. 232 (Washington, DC: DHHS, 2000).

Suggested Readings

Coleman, E. *Eating for Endurance.* Palo Alto, CA: Bull Publishing, 2003.

Clark, N. *Nancy Clark's Sports Nutrition Guidebook.* Champaign, IL: Human Kinetics, 2003.

McArdle, W. D., F. I. Katch, and V. L. Katch. *Sports & Exercise Nutrition.* Baltimore: Lippincott Williams & Wilkins, 1999.

National Academy of Sciences, Institute of Medicine. *Dietary Reference Intakes.* Washington, DC: National Academy Press, 1998.

National Academy of Sciences, Institute of Medicine. *Dietary Reference Intakes for Energy, Carbohydrates, Fiber, Fat, Protein and Amino Acids (Macronutrients).* Washington, DC: National Academy Press, 2002.

Sizer, F. S., and E. N. Whitney. *Nutrition: Concepts and Controversies.* Belmont, CA: Wadsworth/Thomson Learning, 2003.

Whitney, E. N., and S. R. Rolfes. *Understanding Nutrition.* Belmont, CA: Wadsworth/Thomson Learning, 2005.

Lab 3A

NUTRIENT ANALYSIS

Name: _____   Date: _____   Grade: _____

Instructor: _____   Course: _____   Section: _____

Necessary Lab Equipment

List of "Nutritive Value of Selected Foods" (Appendix A), and a small calculator or the computer software available with this book.

Objective

To evaluate your present diet using the Recommended Dietary Allowances (RDA).

Instructions

To conduct the following nutritional analysis, you need a record of all foods eaten during a 3-day period (use the list of "Nutritive Value of Selected Foods" given in Appendix A). Record this information prior to this lab session in the forms provided in Figure 3A.1 of this lab. After recording the nutritive values for each day, add up the values in each column and record the totals at the bottom of the form. During your lab, proceed to compute an average for the 3 days. The percentages for carbohydrates, fat, saturated fat, and the protein requirements can be computed by using the instructions at the bottom of Figure 3A.2. The results can then be compared against the Recommended Dietary Allowances.

The analysis can be simplified by using the computer software for this lab. Up to 7 days may be analyzed when using the software, and Figure 3A.3 should be used instead of 3A.1. Further, you have to record only the amount of servings eaten for each food (.5 for half a serving, 2 for twice the standard serving, and so forth).

Foods	Amount	Calories	Protein (gm)	Fat (total gm)	Sat. Fat (gm)	Chol- esterol (mg)	Carbo- hydrates (gm)	Cal- cium (mg)	Iron (mg)	Sodium (mg)	Vit. A (IU)	Vit. B$_1$ (mg)	Vit. B$_2$ (mg)	Niacin (mg)	Vit. C (mg)
Totals															

FIGURE 3A.1 Daily nutrient intake.

Date:

Foods	Amount	Calories	Protein (gm)	Fat (total gm)	Sat. Fat (gm)	Cholesterol (mg)	Carbohydrates (gm)	Calcium (mg)	Iron (mg)	Sodium (mg)	Vit. A (IU)	Vit. B$_1$ (mg)	Vit. B$_2$ (mg)	Niacin (mg)	Vit. C (mg)
Totals															

Name:

Day	Calories	Protein (gm)	Fat (gm)	Sat. Fat (gm)	Cholesterol (mg)	Carbohydrates (gm)	Calcium (mg)	Iron (mg)	Sodium (mg)	Vit. A (µg RE)	Thiamin Vit. B$_1$ (mg)	Riboflavin Vit. B$_2$ (mg)	Niacin (mg)	Vit. C (mg)
One														
Two														
Three														
Totals														
Average[a]														
Percentages[b]														

Recommended Dietary Allowances*

	Calories	Protein (gm)	Fat (gm)	Sat. Fat (gm)	Cholesterol (mg)	Carbohydrates (gm)	Calcium (mg)	Iron (mg)	Sodium (mg)	Vit. A (µg RE)	Thiamin Vit. B$_1$ (mg)	Riboflavin Vit. B$_2$ (mg)	Niacin (mg)	Vit. C (mg)
Men 14–18 yrs.	See below[c]	See below[d]	<30%[e]	<10%[e]	<300[e]	45–65%	1,300	12	2,400[e]	1,000	1.2	1.3	16	75
19–30 yrs.			<30%[e]	<10%[e]	<300[e]	45–65%	1,000	10	2,400[e]	1,000	1.2	1.3	16	90
31–50 yrs.			<30%[e]	<10%[e]	<300[e]	45–65%	1,000	10	2,400[e]	1,000	1.2	1.3	16	90
51+ yrs.			<30%[e]	<10%[e]	<300[e]	45–65%	1,200	10	2,400[e]	1,000	1.2	1.3	16	90
Women 14–18 yrs.			<30%[e]	<10%[e]	<300[e]	45–65%	1,300	15	2,400[e]	800	1.0	1.0	14	65
19–30 yrs.			<30%[e]	<10%[e]	<300[e]	45–65%	1,000	15	2,400[e]	800	1.1	1.1	14	75
31–50 yrs.			<30%[e]	<10%[e]	<300[e]	45–65%	1,000	15	2,400[e]	800	1.1	1.1	14	75
51+ yrs.			<30%[e]	<10%[e]	<300[e]	45–65%	1,200	10	2,400[e]	800	1.1	1.1	14	75
Pregnant			<30%[e]	<10%[e]	<300[e]	45–65%	1,200	30	2,400[e]	800	1.4	1.4	18	75
Lactating			<30%[e]	<10%[e]	<300[e]	45–65%	1,200	15	2,400[e]	1,300	1.5	1.5	17	95

[a] Divide totals by 3 or number of days assessed.
[b] Percentages: Protein and carbohydrates = multiply average by 4, divide by average calories, and multiply by 100.
   Fat and saturated fat = multiply average by 9, divide by average calories, and multiply by 100.
[c] Use Table 5.3 (page 141) for all categories.
[d] Protein intake should be .8 grams per kilogram of body weight. Pregnant women should consume an additional 15 grams of daily protein, and lactating women should have an extra 20 grams.
[e] Based on recommendations by nutrition experts.

* Adapted from *Recommended Dietary Allowances*, 10th Edition, and the Dietary Reference Intakes series, National Academy Press, © National Academy of Sciences 1989, 1997, 1998, 2000, 2001. Washington, DC.

FIGURE 3A.3 Daily nutrient intake form for computer software.

Name: _____ Date: _____

Gender: ☐ Male ☐ Female ☐ Pregnant ☐ Nursing

Activity: ☐ Sedentary ☐ Lightly active ☐ Moderately active ☐ Very active ☐ Extremely active

Height: ___ ft ___ in   Weight: ___ lbs   Age ___

Student ID #: _____   Instructor's Name: _____

Class Days: _____   Class Times: _____

No.	Item	Amount
1		
2		
3		
4		
5		
6		
7		
8		
9		
10		
11		
12		
13		
14		
15		
16		
17		
18		
19		
20		
21		
22		
23		
24		
25		
26		
27		
28		
29		
30		
31		

FIGURE 3A.3 Daily nutrient intake form for computer software.

Name: _____ Date: _____

Gender: ☐ Male ☐ Female ☐ Pregnant ☐ Nursing

Activity: ☐ Sedentary ☐ Lightly active ☐ Moderately active ☐ Very active ☐ Extremely active

Height: ___ ft ___ in   Weight: ___ lbs   Age ___

Student ID #: _____   Instructor's Name: _____

Class Days: _____   Class Times: _____

No.	Item	Amount
1		
2		
3		
4		
5		
6		
7		
8		
9		
10		
11		
12		
13		
14		
15		
16		
17		
18		
19		
20		
21		
22		
23		
24		
25		
26		
27		
28		
29		
30		
31		

Lab 3B

HEALTHY DIET PLAN

HOMEWORK ASSIGNMENT

Name: _____   Date: _____   Grade: _____

Instructor: _____   Course: _____   Section: _____

Assignment

This laboratory experience should be carried out as a homework assignment to be completed over the next few days.

Objective

To meet the minimum daily required servings of the basic food groups and monitor total daily fat intake.

Lab Resources

"MyPyramid" (Figure 3.1, page 51) and list of "Nutritive Value of Selected Foods" (Appendix A).

I. Instructions

Keep a 1- to 7-day record of your food consumption using MyPyramid and the form given in Figure 3B.1 (make additional copies of this form as needed—at least 3 days are recommended). Whenever you have something to eat, record the food from the Nutritive Value of Selected Foods list contained in Appendix A and the number of calories and amount in the corresponding spaces provided for each food group. If a food item is not listed in the Nutritive Value of Selected Foods list, the information can be obtained from the food container itself. Record all information immediately after each meal, because it will be easier to keep track of foods and amounts eaten.

At the end of the day, evaluate the diet by checking whether the minimum required amounts for each food group were met, and by the total amount of calories consumed. If you meet the required amounts, you are well on your way to achieving a well-balanced diet.

II. Nutrition Stage of Change

Using Figure 2.4 (page 41) and Table 2.3 (page 41) identify your stage of change for nutrition (healthy diet): _____

III. What I Learned and What I Can Do to Improve My Nutrition:

Based on the nutrient analysis conducted in Lab 3A and your daily diet analysis conducted in this lab, explain what these experiences have taught you and list specific changes and strategies that you can use to improve your present nutrition habits. Use an extra blank sheet of paper as needed.

I have learned the following about myself/my current diet: _____

_____

_____

Briefly state what you have learned from your online experience at http://mypyramid.gov: _____

_____

_____

Specific changes I plan to make: _____

_____

_____

Strategies I will use: _____

_____

_____

FIGURE 3B.1 Daily diet record form.

Name: _____

No.	Food*	Calories	Food Groups (amount)					
			Grains	Vegetables	Fruits	Oils	Milk	Meat and Beans
1								
2								
3								
4								
5								
6								
7								
8								
9								
10								
11								
12								
13								
14								
15								
16								
17								
18								
19								
20								
21								
22								
23								
24								
25								
26								
27								
28								
29								
30								
Totals								
Recommended amount based on age, sex, and activity level: Obtain online at http://mypyramid.gov								
Deficiencies								

*See "List of Nutritive Value of Selected Foods" in Appendix A.

Body Composition

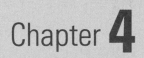

Objectives

- Define body composition and understand its relationship to assessment of recommended body weight.
- Explain the difference between essential fat and storage fat.
- Describe various techniques used to assess body composition.
- Be able to assess body composition using hydrostatic weighing, skinfold thickness, and girth measurement techniques.
- Understand the importance of body mass index (BMI) and waist circumference in the assessment of risk for disease.
- Be able to determine recommended weight according to recommended percent body fat values.

Profile Plus CD Connections

- Learn how to measure body composition.
- Assess your risks for potential disease.
- Check how well you understand the chapter's concepts.

Body composition consists of fat and nonfat components. The fat component is usually called fat mass or **percent body fat**. The non-fat component is termed **lean body mass**.

For many years people relied on simple height/weight charts to determine their **recommended body weight**. We know, however, that these tables can be highly inaccurate and fail to identify critical fat values associated with higher risk for disease. The proper way to determine recommended weight is to find out what percent of total body weight is fat and what amount is lean tissue—in other words, to determine body composition. Body composition should be assessed by a well-trained technician who understands the procedure that is being used.

Once the fat percentage is known, recommended body weight can be calculated from recommended body fat. Recommended body weight, also called "healthy weight," implies the absence of any medical condition that would improve with weight loss and a fat distribution pattern that is not associated with higher risk for illness.

Although various techniques for determining percent body fat were developed years ago, many people still are unaware of these procedures and continue to depend on height/weight charts to find out their recommended body weight. The standard height/weight tables, first published in 1912, were based on average weights (including shoes and clothing) for men and women who obtained life insurance policies between 1888 and 1905—a notably unrepresentative population. The recommended body weight on these tables is obtained according to sex, height, and frame size. Because no scientific guidelines are given to determine frame size, most people choose their frame size based on the column in which the weight comes closest to their own!

To determine whether people are truly **overweight** or falsely at recommended body weight, body composition must be established. **Obesity** is an excess of body fat. If body weight is the only criterion, an individual might easily appear to be overweight according to height/weight charts, yet not have too much body fat. Typical examples are football players, body builders, weight lifters, and other athletes with large muscle size. Some athletes who appear to be 20 or 30 pounds overweight really have little body fat.

The inaccuracy of height/weight charts was illustrated clearly when a young man who weighed about 225 pounds applied to join a city police force but was turned down without having been granted an interview. The reason? He was "too fat," according to the height/weight charts. When this young man's body composition was assessed at a preventive medicine clinic, it was determined that only 5 percent of his total body weight was in the form of fat—considerably lower than the recommended standard.

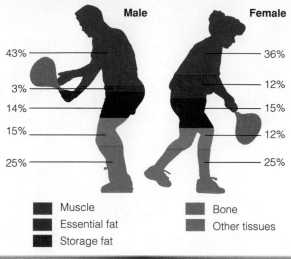

FIGURE 4.1 Typical body composition of an adult man and woman.

Male — 43%, 3%, 14%, 15%, 25%
Female — 36%, 12%, 15%, 12%, 25%

Muscle
Essential fat
Storage fat
Bone
Other tissues

In the words of the director of the clinic, "The only way this fellow could come down to the chart's target weight would have been through surgical removal of a large amount of his muscle tissue."

At the other end of the spectrum, some people who weigh very little (and may be viewed as skinny or underweight) can actually be classified as obese because of their high body fat content. People who weigh as little as 120 pounds but are more than 30 percent fat (about one-third of their total body weight) are not uncommon. These cases are found more readily in the sedentary population and among people who are always dieting. Physical inactivity and a constant negative caloric balance both lead to a loss in lean body mass (see Chapter 5). These examples illustrate that body weight alone clearly does not tell the whole story.

Essential and Storage Fat

Total fat in the human body is classified into two types: **essential fat** and **storage fat**. Essential fat is needed for normal physiological function. Without it, human health and physical performance deteriorate. This type of fat is found within tissues such as muscles, nerve cells, bone marrow, intestines, heart, liver, and lungs. This essential fat constitutes about 3 percent of the total weight in men and 12 percent in women (see Figure 4.1). The percentage is higher in women because it includes sex-specific fat, such as that found in the breast tissue, the uterus, and other sex-related fat deposits.

Storage fat is the fat stored in adipose tissue, mostly just beneath the skin (subcutaneous fat) and around major organs in the body. This fat serves three basic functions:

1. As an insulator to retain body heat.
2. As energy substrate for metabolism.
3. As padding against physical trauma to the body.

The amount of storage fat does not differ between men and women, except that men tend to store fat around the waist and women around the hips and thighs.

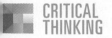

CRITICAL THINKING

Mary is a cross-country runner whose coach has asked her to decrease her total body fat to 7 percent. Can Mary's performance increase at this lower percent body fat? How would you respond to this coach?

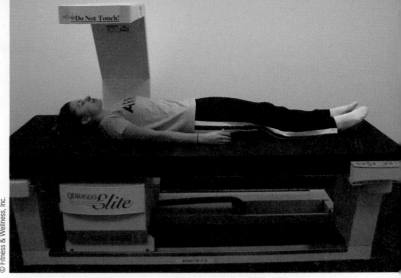

© Fitness & Wellness, Inc.

The dual energy X-ray absorptiometry (DEXA) technique is used to assess body composition and bone density.

Techniques to Assess Body Composition

Body composition can be determined through several procedures. These are described in the following pages.

Dual Energy X-Ray Absorptiometry (DEXA)

Dual energy X-ray absorptiometry (DEXA) is a method to assess body composition that is used most frequently in research and by medical facilities. A radiographic technique, DEXA uses very low-dose beams of X-ray energy (hundreds of times lower than a typical body X-ray) to measure total body fat mass, fat distribution pattern (see waist circumference on page 112), and bone density. Bone density is measured to assess the risk for osteoporosis.

The procedure itself is simple and takes only about 15 minutes to administer. Many exercise scientists consider DEXA to be the standard technique to assess body composition.

Because DEXA is not readily available to most fitness participants, other methods to estimate body composition are used. The most common of these are:

1. hydrostatic or underwater weighing
2. air displacement
3. skinfold thickness
4. girth measurements
5. bioelectrical impedance.

Because these procedures yield estimates of body fat, each technique may yield slightly different values. Therefore, when assessing changes in body composition, be sure to use the same technique for pre- and post-test comparisons.

Profile Plus

How do you determine your healthy body weight? Learn actual techniques used to measure body composition on your CD-ROM.

Hydrostatic weighing and air displacement are the two most accurate techniques presently available in fitness laboratories. Other techniques to assess body composition are available, but the equipment is costly and not easily accessible to the general population. In addition to percentages of lean tissue and body fat, some of these methods also provide information on total body water and bone mass. Besides DEXA, these techniques include magnetic resonance imaging (MRI), computed tomography (CT), and total body electrical conductivity (TOBEC). In terms of predicting percent body fat, these techniques do not seem to be more accurate than hydrostatic weighing or air displacement.

Body composition The fat and non-fat components of the human body; important in assessing recommended body weight.

Percent body fat Proportional amount of fat in the body based on the person's total weight; includes both essential fat and storage fat; also termed fat mass.

Lean body mass Body weight without body fat.

Recommended body weight Body weight at which there seems to be no harm to human health; healthy weight.

Overweight An excess amount of weight against a given standard, such as height or recommended percent body fat.

Obesity An excessive accumulation of body fat, usually at least 30 percent above recommended body weight.

Essential fat Minimal amount of body fat needed for normal physiological functions; constitutes about 3 percent of total weight in men and 12 percent in women.

Storage fat Body fat in excess of essential fat; stored in adipose tissue.

Dual energy X-ray absorptiometry (DEXA) Method to assess body composition that uses very low-dose beams of X-ray energy to measure total body fat mass, fat distribution pattern, and bone density.

FIGURE 4.2 Hydrostatic weighing procedure.

A small tank or pool, an autopsy scale, and a submersible chair are needed. The scale should measure up to about 10 kilograms (kg) and should be readable to the nearest .01 kilogram. The chair is suspended from the scale and submerged in a tank of water or pool measuring at least 5 × 5 × 5 feet. A swimming pool can be used in place of the tank.

The procedure for the technician is

1. Ask the person to be weighed to fast for approximately 6 to 8 hours and to have a bladder and bowel movement prior to underwater weighing.

2. Measure the individual's residual lung volume (RV, or amount of air left in the lungs following complete exhalation). If no equipment (spirometer) is available to measure the residual volume, estimate it using the following predicting equations* (to convert inches to centimeters, multiply inches by 2.54):

    Men: $RV = [(0.027 \times \text{height in centimeters}) + (0.017 \times \text{age})] - 3.447$

    Women: $RV = [(0.032 \times \text{height in centimeters}) + (0.009 \times \text{age})] - 3.9$

3. Have the person remove all jewelry prior to weighing. Weigh the person on land in a swimsuit and subtract the weight of the suit. Convert the weight from pounds to kilograms (divide pounds by 2.2046).

4. Record the water temperature in the tank in degrees Centigrade. Use that temperature to obtain the water density factor provided below, which is required in the formula to compute body density.

Temp (°C)	Water Density (gr/ml)	Temp (°C)	Water Density (gr/ml)
28	0.99626	35	0.99406
29	0.99595	36	0.99371
30	0.99567	37	0.99336
31	0.99537	38	0.99299
32	0.99505	39	0.99262
33	0.99473	40	0.99224
34	0.99440		

5. After the person is dressed in the swimsuit, have him or her enter the tank and completely wipe off all air clinging to the skin. Have the person sit in the chair with the water at chin level (raise or lower the chair as needed). Make sure the water and scale remain as still as possible during the entire procedure, because this allows for a more accurate reading. (During underwater weighing, you can decrease scale movement by

Hydrostatic Weighing

For decades, **hydrostatic weighing** has been the most common technique used in determining body composition in exercise physiology laboratories. In essence, a person's "regular" weight is compared with a weight taken underwater. Because fat is more buoyant than lean tissue, comparing the two weights can determine a person's percent of fat. Almost all other indirect techniques to assess body composition have been validated against hydrostatic weighing. The procedure requires a considerable amount of time, skill, space, and equipment and must be administered by a well-trained technician.

This technique has several drawbacks. First, because each individual assessment can take as long as

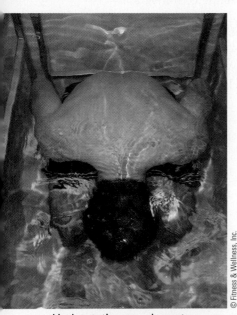

Hydrostatic or underwater weighing technique.

© Fitness & Wellness, Inc.

30 minutes, hydrostatic weighing is not feasible when testing a lot of people. Furthermore, the person's residual lung volume (amount of air left in the lungs following complete forceful exhalation) should be measured before testing. If residual volume cannot be measured, as is the case in some laboratories and health/fitness centers, it is estimated using the predicting equations—which may decrease the accuracy of hydrostatic weighing. Also, the requirement of being completely under water makes hydrostatic weighing difficult to administer to **aquaphobic** people. For accurate results, the individual must be able to perform the test properly.

As described in Figure 4.2 and in Lab 4A, for each underwater weighing trial, the person has to (a) force out all of the air in the lungs, (b) lean forward and completely submerge underwater for about 5 to 10 seconds (long enough to get the underwater weight), and (c) remain as calm as possible (chair movement makes reading the scale difficult). This procedure is repeated eight to ten times.

Forcing all of the air out of the lungs is not easy for everyone but is important for an accurate reading. Leaving additional air (beyond residual volume) in the lungs makes a person more buoyant. Because fat is less dense than water, overweight individuals weigh less in water. Additional air in the lungs makes holding and slowly releasing the neck of the scale until the subject is floating freely in the water.)

6. Place a clip on the person's nose and have him or her forcefully exhale all of the air out of the lungs. The individual then totally submerges underwater. Make sure that all the air is exhaled from the lungs prior to submerging. Record the reading on the scale. Repeat this procedure 8 to 10 times, because practice and experience increases the accuracy of the underwater weight. Use the average of the three heaviest underwater weights as the gross underwater weight.

7. Because tare weight (the weight of the chair and chain or rope used to suspend the chair) accounts for part of the gross underwater weight, subtract this weight to obtain the person's net underwater weight. To determine tare weight, place a clothespin on the chain or rope at the water level when the person is submerged completely. After the person comes out of the water, lower the chair into the water to the pin level. Now record tare weight. Determine the net underwater weight by subtracting the tare weight from the gross underwater weight.

8. Compute body density and percent fat using the following equations:

$$\text{Body density} = \frac{BW}{\dfrac{BW - UW}{WD} - RV - .1}$$

$$\text{Percent fat**} = \frac{495}{BD} - 450$$

WHERE:

BW = body weight in kg
UW = net underwater weight
WD = water density (determined by water temperature)
RV = residual volume
BD = body density

A sample computation for body fat assessment according to hydrostatic weighing is provided in Lab 4A.

---

*From: H. L. Goldman and M. R. Becklake, "Respiratory Function Tests: Normal Values at Medium Altitudes and the Prediction of Normal Results," in *American Review of Tuberculosis* 79 (1959): 457–467.

** From W. E. Siri, *Body Composition from Fluid Spaces and Density* (Berkeley: University of California, Donner Laboratory of Medical Physics, March 19, 1956).

---

a person lighter in water, yielding a false, higher body fat percentage.

Air Displacement

Air displacement is a new technique that holds considerable promise. With this method, an individual sits inside a small chamber, commercially known as the **Bod Pod**. Computerized pressure sensors determine the amount of air displaced by the person inside the chamber. Body volume is calculated by subtracting the air volume with the person inside the chamber from the volume of the empty chamber. The amount of air in the person's lungs is also taken into consideration when determining the actual body volume. Body density and percent body fat are then calculated from the obtained body volume.

Initial research has shown that this technique compares very favorably with hydrostatic weighing and it is less cumbersome to administer. The procedure takes only about 5 minutes. Additional research is needed, however, to determine its accuracy among different age groups, ethnic backgrounds, and athletic populations. Administering this assessment is a relatively easy procedure, but because of the high cost, the Bod Pod is not readily available in fitness centers and exercise laboratories.

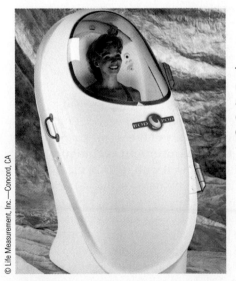

© Life Measurement, Inc.—Concord, CA

The Bod Pod, used for assessment of body composition.

Hydrostatic weighing Underwater technique to assess body composition; considered the most accurate of the body composition assessment techniques.

Aquaphobic Having a fear of water.

Air displacement Technique to assess body composition by calculating the body volume from the air displaced by an individual sitting inside a small chamber.

Bod Pod Commercial name of the equipment used for the assessment of body composition through the air displacement technique.

FIGURE 4.3 Anatomical landmarks for skinfold measurements.

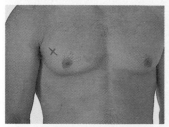
Chest (men)

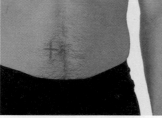
Abdomen (men)

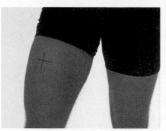
Thigh (men and women)

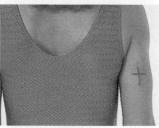
Triceps (women)

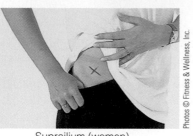
Suprailium (women)

Photos © Fitness & Wellness, Inc.

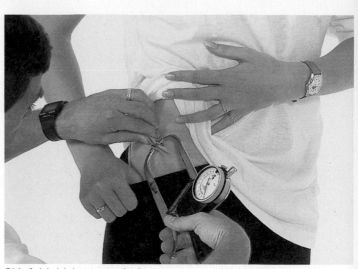
Skinfold thickness technique.

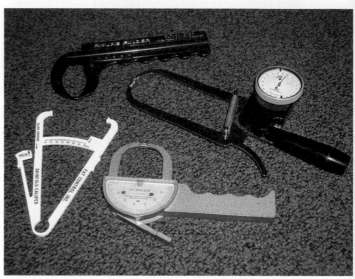
Various types of calipers used to assess skinfold thickness.

Skinfold Thickness

Because of the cost, time, and complexity of hydrostatic weighing and the expense of Bod Pod equipment, most health and fitness programs use **anthropometric measurement techniques**, which correlate quite well with hydrostatic weighing. These techniques, primarily skinfold thickness and girth measurements, allow quick, simple, and inexpensive estimates of body composition.

Assessing body composition using **skinfold thickness** is based on the principle that approximately half of the body's fatty tissue is directly beneath the skin. Valid and reliable measurements of this tissue give a good indication of percent body fat.

The skinfold test is done with the aid of pressure calipers. Several sites must be measured to reflect the total percentage of fat (see Figure 4.3):

women: triceps, suprailium, and thigh skinfolds
men: chest, abdomen, and thigh.

All measurements should be taken on the right side of the body.

Even with the skinfold technique, training is necessary to obtain accurate measurements. In addition, different technicians may produce slightly different measurements of the same person. Therefore, the same technician should take pre-test and post-test measurements.

Measurements should be done at the same time of the day—preferably in the morning—because changes in water hydration from activity and exercise can affect skinfold girth. The procedure is given in Figure 4.4. If skinfold calipers are available, you may assess your percent body fat with the help of your instructor or an experienced technician (also see Lab 4B). Then locate the percent fat estimates on the appropriate Table 4.1, 4.2, or 4.3.

FIGURE 4.4 Procedure for body fat assessment using skinfold thickness technique.

1. Select the proper anatomical sites. For men, use chest, abdomen, and thigh skinfolds. For women, use triceps, suprailium, and thigh skinfolds. Take all measurements on the right side of the body with the person standing. The correct anatomical landmarks for skinfolds are

Chest: a diagonal fold halfway between the shoulder crease and the nipple.

Abdomen: a vertical fold taken about one inch to the right of the umbilicus.

Triceps: a vertical fold on the back of the upper arm, halfway between the shoulder and the elbow.

Thigh: a vertical fold on the front of the thigh, midway between the knee and the hip.

Suprailium: a diagonal fold above the crest of the ilium (on the side of the hip).

2. Measure each site by grasping a double thickness of skin firmly with the thumb and forefinger, pulling the fold slightly away from the muscular tissue. Hold the calipers perpendicular to the fold and take the measurement ½ inch below the finger hold. Measure each site three times and read the values to the nearest .1 to .5 mm. Record the average of the two closest readings as the final value. Take the readings without delay to avoid excessive compression of the skinfold. Releasing and refolding the skinfold is required between readings.

3. When doing pre- and post-assessments, conduct the measurement at the same time of day. The best time is early in the morning to avoid hydration changes resulting from activity or exercise.

4. Obtain percent fat by adding the three skinfold measurements and looking up the respective values on Table 4.1 for women, Table 4.2 for men under age 40, and Table 4.3 for men over 40.

For example, if the skinfold measurements for an 18-year-old female are (a) triceps = 16, (b) suprailium = 4, and (c) thigh = 30 (total = 50), the percent body fat is 20.6%.

Anthropometric measurement techniques Measurement of body girths at different sites.

Skinfold thickness Technique to assess body composition by measuring a double thickness of skin at specific body sites.

TABLE 4.1 Skinfold Thickness Technique: Percent Fat Estimates for Women Calculated from Triceps, Suprailium, and Thigh

Sum of 3 Skinfolds	Age at Last Birthday								
	22 or Under	23 to 27	28 to 32	33 to 37	38 to 42	43 to 47	48 to 52	53 to 57	58 and Over
23– 25	9.7	9.9	10.2	10.4	10.7	10.9	11.2	11.4	11.7
26– 28	11.0	11.2	11.5	11.7	12.0	12.3	12.5	12.7	13.0
29– 31	12.3	12.5	12.8	13.0	13.3	13.5	13.8	14.0	14.3
32– 34	13.6	13.8	14.0	14.3	14.5	14.8	15.0	15.3	15.5
35– 37	14.8	15.0	15.3	15.5	15.8	16.0	16.3	16.5	16.8
38– 40	16.0	16.3	16.5	16.7	17.0	17.2	17.5	17.7	18.0
41– 43	17.2	17.4	17.7	17.9	18.2	18.4	18.7	18.9	19.2
44– 46	18.3	18.6	18.8	19.1	19.3	19.6	19.8	20.1	20.3
47– 49	19.5	19.7	20.0	20.2	20.5	20.7	21.0	21.2	21.5
50– 52	20.6	20.8	21.1	21.3	21.6	21.8	22.1	22.3	22.6
53– 55	21.7	21.9	22.1	22.4	22.6	22.9	23.1	23.4	23.6
56– 58	22.7	23.0	23.2	23.4	23.7	23.9	24.2	24.4	24.7
59– 61	23.7	24.0	24.2	24.5	24.7	25.0	25.2	25.5	25.7
62– 64	24.7	25.0	25.2	25.5	25.7	26.0	26.2	26.4	26.7
65– 67	25.7	25.9	26.2	26.4	26.7	26.9	27.2	27.4	27.7
68– 70	26.6	26.9	27.1	27.4	27.6	27.9	28.1	28.4	28.6
71– 73	27.5	27.8	28.0	28.3	28.5	28.8	29.0	29.3	29.5
74– 76	28.4	28.7	28.9	29.2	29.4	29.7	29.9	30.2	30.4
77– 79	29.3	29.5	29.8	30.0	30.3	30.5	30.8	31.0	31.3
80– 82	30.1	30.4	30.6	30.9	31.1	31.4	31.6	31.9	32.1
83– 85	30.9	31.2	31.4	31.7	31.9	32.2	32.4	32.7	32.9
86– 88	31.7	32.0	32.2	32.5	32.7	32.9	33.2	33.4	33.7
89– 91	32.5	32.7	33.0	33.2	33.5	33.7	33.9	34.2	34.4
92– 94	33.2	33.4	33.7	33.9	34.2	34.4	34.7	34.9	35.2
95– 97	33.9	34.1	34.4	34.6	34.9	35.1	35.4	35.6	35.9
98–100	34.6	34.8	35.1	35.3	35.5	35.8	36.0	36.3	36.5
101–103	35.2	35.4	35.7	35.9	36.2	36.4	36.7	36.9	37.2
104–106	35.8	36.1	36.3	36.6	36.8	37.1	37.3	37.5	37.8
107–109	36.4	36.7	36.9	37.1	37.4	37.6	37.9	38.1	38.4
110–112	37.0	37.2	37.5	37.7	38.0	38.2	38.5	38.7	38.9
113–115	37.5	37.8	38.0	38.2	38.5	38.7	39.0	39.2	39.5
116–118	38.0	38.3	38.5	38.8	39.0	39.3	39.5	39.7	40.0
119–121	38.5	38.7	39.0	39.2	39.5	39.7	40.0	40.2	40.5
122–124	39.0	39.2	39.4	39.7	39.9	40.2	40.4	40.7	40.9
125–127	39.4	39.6	39.9	40.1	40.4	40.6	40.9	41.1	41.4
128–130	39.8	40.0	40.3	40.5	40.8	41.0	41.3	41.5	41.8

Body density is calculated based on the generalized equation for predicting body density of women developed by A. S. Jackson, M. L. Pollock, and A. Ward and published in *Medicine and Science in Sports and Exercise* 12 (1980): 175–182. Percent body fat is determined from the calculated body density using the Siri formula.

TABLE 4.2 Skinfold Thickness Technique: Percent Fat Estimates for Men Under 40 Calculated from Chest, Abdomen, and Thigh

Sum of 3 Skinfolds	Age at Last Birthday							
	19 or Under	20 to 22	23 to 25	26 to 28	29 to 31	32 to 34	35 to 37	38 to 40
8– 10	.9	1.3	1.6	2.0	2.3	2.7	3.0	3.3
11– 13	1.9	2.3	2.6	3.0	3.3	3.7	4.0	4.3
14– 16	2.9	3.3	3.6	3.9	4.3	4.6	5.0	5.3
17– 19	3.9	4.2	4.6	4.9	5.3	5.6	6.0	6.3
20– 22	4.8	5.2	5.5	5.9	6.2	6.6	6.9	7.3
23– 25	5.8	6.2	6.5	6.8	7.2	7.5	7.9	8.2
26– 28	6.8	7.1	7.5	7.8	8.1	8.5	8.8	9.2
29– 31	7.7	8.0	8.4	8.7	9.1	9.4	9.8	10.1
32– 34	8.6	9.0	9.3	9.7	10.0	10.4	10.7	11.1
35– 37	9.5	9.9	10.2	10.6	10.9	11.3	11.6	12.0
38– 40	10.5	10.8	11.2	11.5	11.8	12.2	12.5	12.9
41– 43	11.4	11.7	12.1	12.4	12.7	13.1	13.4	13.8
44– 46	12.2	12.6	12.9	13.3	13.6	14.0	14.3	14.7
47– 49	13.1	13.5	13.8	14.2	14.5	14.9	15.2	15.5
50– 52	14.0	14.3	14.7	15.0	15.4	15.7	16.1	16.4
53– 55	14.8	15.2	15.5	15.9	16.2	16.6	16.9	17.3
56– 58	15.7	16.0	16.4	16.7	17.1	17.4	17.8	18.1
59– 61	16.5	16.9	17.2	17.6	17.9	18.3	18.6	19.0
62– 64	17.4	17.7	18.1	18.4	18.8	19.1	19.4	19.8
65– 67	18.2	18.5	18.9	19.2	19.6	19.9	20.3	20.6
68– 70	19.0	19.3	19.7	20.0	20.4	20.7	21.1	21.4
71– 73	19.8	20.1	20.5	20.8	21.2	21.5	21.9	22.2
74– 76	20.6	20.9	21.3	21.6	22.0	22.2	22.7	23.0
77– 79	21.4	21.7	22.1	22.4	22.8	23.1	23.4	23.8
80– 82	22.1	22.5	22.8	23.2	23.5	23.9	24.2	24.6
83– 85	22.9	23.2	23.6	23.9	24.3	24.6	25.0	25.3
86– 88	23.6	24.0	24.3	24.7	25.0	25.4	25.7	26.1
89– 91	24.4	24.7	25.1	25.4	25.8	26.1	26.5	26.8
92– 94	25.1	25.5	25.8	26.2	26.5	26.9	27.2	27.5
95– 97	25.8	26.2	26.5	26.9	27.2	27.6	27.9	28.3
98–100	26.6	26.9	27.3	27.6	27.9	28.3	28.6	29.0
101–103	27.3	27.6	28.0	28.3	28.6	29.0	29.3	29.7
104–106	27.9	28.3	28.6	29.0	29.3	29.7	30.0	30.4
107–109	28.6	29.0	29.3	29.7	30.0	30.4	30.7	31.1
110–112	29.3	29.6	30.0	30.3	30.7	31.0	31.4	31.7
113–115	30.0	30.3	30.7	31.0	31.3	31.7	32.0	32.4
116–118	30.6	31.0	31.3	31.6	32.0	32.3	32.7	33.0
119–121	31.3	31.6	32.0	32.3	32.6	33.0	33.3	33.7
122–124	31.9	32.2	32.6	32.9	33.3	33.6	34.0	34.3
125–127	32.5	32.9	33.2	33.5	33.9	34.2	34.6	34.9
128–130	33.1	33.5	33.8	34.2	34.5	34.9	35.2	35.5

Body density is calculated based on the generalized equation for predicting body density of men developed by A. S. Jackson and M. L. Pollock and published in the *British Journal of Nutrition* 40 (1978): 497–504. Percent body fat is determined from the calculated body density using the Siri formula.

TABLE 4.3 Skinfold Thickness Technique: Percent Fat Estimates for Men Over 40 Calculated from Chest, Abdomen, and Thigh

Sum of 3 Skinfolds	Age at Last Birthday							
	41 to 43	44 to 46	47 to 49	50 to 52	53 to 55	56 to 58	59 to 61	62 and Over
8– 10	3.7	4.0	4.4	4.7	5.1	5.4	5.8	6.1
11– 13	4.7	5.0	5.4	5.7	6.1	6.4	6.8	7.1
14– 16	5.7	6.0	6.4	6.7	7.1	7.4	7.8	8.1
17– 19	6.7	7.0	7.4	7.7	8.1	8.4	8.7	9.1
20– 22	7.6	8.0	8.3	8.7	9.0	9.4	9.7	10.1
23– 25	8.6	8.9	9.3	9.6	10.0	10.3	10.7	11.0
26– 28	9.5	9.9	10.2	10.6	10.9	11.3	11.6	12.0
29– 31	10.5	10.8	11.2	11.5	11.9	12.2	12.6	12.9
32– 34	11.4	11.8	12.1	12.4	12.8	13.1	13.5	13.8
35– 37	12.3	12.7	13.0	13.4	13.7	14.1	14.4	14.8
38– 40	13.2	13.6	13.9	14.3	14.6	15.0	15.3	15.7
41– 43	14.1	14.5	14.8	15.2	15.5	15.9	16.2	16.6
44– 46	15.0	15.4	15.7	16.1	16.4	16.8	17.1	17.5
47– 49	15.9	16.2	16.6	16.9	17.3	17.6	18.0	18.3
50– 52	16.8	17.1	17.5	17.8	18.2	18.5	18.8	19.2
53– 55	17.6	18.0	18.3	18.7	19.0	19.4	19.7	20.1
56– 58	18.5	18.8	19.2	19.5	19.9	20.2	20.6	20.9
59– 61	19.3	19.7	20.0	20.4	20.7	21.0	21.4	21.7
62– 64	20.1	20.5	20.8	21.2	21.5	21.9	22.2	22.6
65– 67	21.0	21.3	21.7	22.0	22.4	22.7	23.0	23.4
68– 70	21.8	22.1	22.5	22.8	23.2	23.5	23.9	24.2
71– 73	22.6	22.9	23.3	23.6	24.0	24.3	24.7	25.0
74– 76	23.4	23.7	24.1	24.4	24.8	25.1	25.4	25.8
77– 79	24.1	24.5	24.8	25.2	25.5	25.9	26.2	26.6
80– 82	24.9	25.3	25.6	26.0	26.3	26.6	27.0	27.3
83– 85	25.7	26.0	26.4	26.7	27.1	27.4	27.8	28.1
86– 88	26.4	26.8	27.1	27.5	27.8	28.2	28.5	28.9
89– 91	27.2	27.5	27.9	28.2	28.6	28.9	29.2	29.6
92– 94	27.9	28.2	28.6	28.9	29.3	29.6	30.0	30.3
95– 97	28.6	29.0	29.3	29.7	30.0	30.4	30.7	31.1
98–100	29.3	29.7	30.0	30.4	30.7	31.1	31.4	31.8
101–103	30.0	30.4	30.7	31.1	31.4	31.8	32.1	32.5
104–106	30.7	31.1	31.4	31.8	32.1	32.5	32.8	33.2
107–109	31.4	31.8	32.1	32.4	32.8	33.1	33.5	33.8
110–112	32.1	32.4	32.8	33.1	33.5	33.8	34.2	34.5
113–115	32.7	33.1	33.4	33.8	34.1	34.5	34.8	35.2
116–118	33.4	33.7	34.1	34.4	34.8	35.1	35.5	35.8
119–121	34.0	34.4	34.7	35.1	35.4	35.8	36.1	36.5
122–124	34.7	35.0	35.4	35.7	36.1	36.4	36.7	37.1
125–127	35.3	35.6	36.0	36.3	36.7	37.0	37.4	37.7
128–130	35.9	36.2	36.6	36.9	37.3	37.6	38.0	38.5

Body density is calculated based on the generalized equation for predicting body density of men developed by A. S. Jackson and M. L. Pollock and published in the *British Journal of Nutrition* 40 (1978): 497–504. Percent body fat is determined from the calculated body density using the Siri formula.

FIGURE 4.5 Procedure for body fat assessment according to girth measurements.

Girth Measurements for Women*

1. Using a regular tape measure, determine the following girth measurements in centimeters (cm):

   Upper arm: Take the measure halfway between the shoulder and the elbow.

   Hip: Measure at the point of largest circumference.

   Wrist: Take the girth in front of the bones where the wrist bends.

2. Obtain the person's age.

3. Using Table 4.4, find the subject's age, girth measurement for each site in the left column below, then look up the constant values for each. These values will allow you to derive body density (BD) by substituting the constants in the following formula:

   BD = A − B − C + D

4. Using the derived body density, calculate percent body fat (%F) according to the following equation:

   %F = (495 ÷ BD) − 450**

Example: Jane is 20 years old, and the following girth measurements were taken: biceps = 27 cm, hip = 99.5 cm, wrist = 15.4 cm.

Data		Constant		
Upper arm	= 27 cm	A	=	1.0813
Age	= 20	B	=	.0102
Hip	= 99.5 cm	C	=	.1206
Wrist	= 15.4 cm	D	=	.0971

BD = A − B − C + D

BD = 1.0813 − .0102 − .1206 + .0971 = 1.0476

%F = (495 ÷ BD) − 450

%F = (495 ÷ 1.0476) − 450 = 22.5

Girth Measurements for Men***

1. Using a regular tape measure, determine the following girth measurements in inches (the men's measurements are taken in inches, as opposed to centimeters for women):

   Waist: Measure at the umbilicus (belly button).

   Wrist: Measure in front of the bones where the wrist bends.

2. Subtract the wrist from the waist measurement.

3. Obtain the weight of the subject in pounds.

4. Look up the percent body fat (%F) in Table 4.5 by using the difference obtained in number 2 above and the person's body weight.

Example: John weighs 160 pounds, and his waist and wrist girth measurements are 36.5 and 7.5 inches, respectively.

Waist girth = 36.5 inches

Wrist girth = 7.5 inches

Difference − 29.0 inches

Body weight = 160.0 lbs.

%F = 22

---

* From R. B. Lambson, "Generalized Body Density Prediction Equations for Women Using Simple Anthropometric Measurements." Unpublished doctoral dissertation, Brigham Young University, Provo, UT, August 1987. Reproduced by permission.

** From W. E. Siri, *Body Composition from Fluid Spaces and Density* (Berkeley: University of California, Donner Laboratory of Medical Physics, 1956).

*** From A. G. Fisher and P. E. Allsen, *Jogging*, Dubuque, IA: Wm. C. Brown, 1987. This table was developed according to "Generalized Body Composition Equation for Men Using Simple Measurement Techniques," by K. W. Penrouse, A. G Nelson, and A G. Fisher, *Medicine and Science in Sports and Exercise* 17, no. 2 (1985): 189. © American College of Sports Medicine, 1985.

Girth Measurements

A simpler method to determine body fat is by measuring circumferences, or **girth measurements**, at various body sites. This technique requires only a standard measuring tape. Good accuracy can be achieved with little practice. The limitation is that it may not be valid for athletic individuals (men or women) who participate actively in strenuous physical activity or for people who can be classified visually as thin or obese.

The required procedure for girth measurements is given in Figure 4.5; conversion factors are listed in Tables 4.4 and 4.5. Measurements for women are the upper arm, hip, and wrist; for men, the waist and wrist.

Bioelectrical Impedance

The **bioelectrical impedance** technique is much simpler to administer, but its accuracy is questionable. In this technique, several sensors are applied to the skin and a weak (totally painless) electrical current is run through the body to estimate body fat, lean body mass, and body water. The technique is based on the principle that fat tissue is a less efficient conductor of electrical current than lean tissue

Girth measurements Technique to assess body composition by measuring circumferences at specific body sites.

Bioelectrical impedance Technique to assess body composition by running a weak electrical current through the body.

TABLE 4.4 Girth Measurement Technique: Conversion Constants to Calculate Body Density for Women

Upper Arm (cm)	Constant A	Age	Constant B	Hip (cm)	Constant C	Hip (cm)	Constant C	Wrist (cm)	Constant D
20.5	1.0966	17	.0086	79	.0957	114.5	.1388	13.0	.0819
21	1.0954	18	.0091	79.5	.0963	115	.1394	13.2	.0832
21.5	1.0942	19	.0096	80	.0970	115.5	.1400	13.4	.0845
22	1.0930	20	.0102	80.5	.0976	116	.1406	13.6	.0857
22.5	1.0919	21	.0107	81	.0982	116.5	.1412	13.8	.0870
23	1.0907	22	.0112	81.5	.0988	117	.1418	14.0	.0882
23.5	1.0895	23	.0117	82	.0994	117.5	.1424	14.2	.0895
24	1.0883	24	.0122	82.5	.1000	118	.1430	14.4	.0908
24.5	1.0871	25	.0127	83	.1006	118.5	.1436	14.6	.0920
25	1.0860	26	.0132	83.5	.1012	119	.1442	14.8	.0933
25.5	1.0848	27	.0137	84	.1018	119.5	.1448	15.0	.0946
26	1.0836	28	.0142	84.5	.1024	120	.1454	15.2	.0958
26.5	1.0824	29	.0147	85	.1030	120.5	.1460	15.4	.0971
27	1.0813	30	.0152	85.5	.1036	121	.1466	15.6	.0983
27.5	1.0801	31	.0157	86	.1042	121.5	.1472	15.8	.0996
28	1.0789	32	.0162	86.5	.1048	122	.1479	16.0	.1009
28.5	1.0777	33	.0168	87	.1054	122.5	.1485	16.2	.1021
29	1.0775	34	.0173	87.5	.1060	123	.1491	16.4	.1034
29.5	1.0754	35	.0178	88	.1066	123.5	.1497	16.6	.1046
30	1.0742	36	.0183	88.5	.1072	124	.1503	16.8	.1059
30.5	1.0730	37	.0188	89	.1079	124.5	.1509	17.0	.1072
31	1.0718	38	.0193	89.5	.1085	125	.1515	17.2	.1084
31.5	1.0707	39	.0198	90	.1091	125.5	.1521	17.4	.1097
32	1.0695	40	.0203	90.5	.1097	126	.1527	17.6	.1109
32.5	1.0683	41	.0208	91	.1103	126.5	.1533	17.8	.1122
33	1.0671	42	.0213	91.5	.1109	127	.1539	18.0	.1135
33.5	1.0666	43	.0218	92	.1115	127.5	.1545	18.2	.1147
34	1.0648	44	.0223	92.5	.1121	128	.1551	18.4	.1160
34.5	1.0636	45	.0228	93	.1127	128.5	.1558	18.6	.1172
35	1.0624	46	.0234	93.5	.1133	129	.1563		
35.5	1.0612	47	.0239	94	.1139	129.5	.1569		
36	1.0601	48	.0244	94.5	.1145	130	.1575		
36.5	1.0589	49	.0249	95	.1151	130.5	.1581		
37	1.0577	50	.0254	95.5	.1157	131	.1587		
37.5	1.0565	51	.0259	96	.1163	131.5	.1593		
38	1.0554	52	.0264	96.5	.1169	132	.1600		
38.5	1.0542	53	.0269	97	.1176	132.5	.1606		
39	1.0530	54	.0274	97.5	.1182	133	.1612		
39.5	1.0518	55	.0279	98	.1188	133.5	.1618		
40	1.0506	56	.0284	98.5	.1194	134	.1624		
40.5	1.0495	57	.0289	99	.1200	134.5	.1630		
41	1.0483	58	.0294	99.5	.1206	135	.1636		
41.5	1.0471	59	.0300	100	.1212	135.5	.1642		
42	1.0459	60	.0305	100.5	.1218	136	.1648		
42.5	1.0448	61	.0310	101	.1224	136.5	.1654		
43	1.0434	62	.0315	101.5	.1230	137	.1660		
43.5	1.0424	63	.0320	102	.1236	137.5	.1666		
44	1.0412	64	.0325	102.5	.1242	138	.1672		
		65	.0330	103	.1248	138.5	.1678		
		66	.0335	103.5	.1254	139	.1685		
		67	.0340	104	.1260	139.5	.1691		
		68	.0345	104.5	.1266	140	.1697		
		69	.0350	105	.1272	140.5	.1703		

(continued)

TABLE 4.4 (Continued)

Upper Arm (cm)	Constant A	Age	Constant B	Hip (cm)	Constant C	Hip (cm)	Constant C	Wrist (cm)	Constant D
		70	.0355	105.5	.1278	141	.1709		
		71	.0360	106	.1285	141.5	.1715		
		72	.0366	106.5	.1291	142	.1721		
		73	.0371	107	.1297	142.5	.1728		
		74	.0376	107.5	.1303	143	.1733		
		75	.0381	108	.1309	143.5	.1739		
				108.5	.1315	144	.1745		
				109	.1321	144.5	.1751		
				109.5	.1327	145	.1757		
				110	.1333	145.5	.1763		
				110.5	.1339	146	.1769		
				111	.1345	146.5	.1775		
				111.5	.1351	147	.1781		
				112	.1357	147.5	.1787		
				112.5	.1363	148	.1794		
				113	.1369	148.5	.1800		
				113.5	.1375	149	.1806		
				114	.1382	149.5	.1812		
						150	.1818		

is. The easier the conductance, the leaner the individual. Body weight scales with sensors on the surface are also available to perform this procedure.

The accuracy of equations used to estimate percent body fat with this technique is questionable. Research has shown that it does not approach the accuracy of hydrostatic weighing, air displacement, skinfold thickness, or girth measurement techniques. Following all manufacturers' instructions will ensure the most accurate result, but even then percent body fat may be off by as much as 10 percentage points (or even more on some scales).

Body Mass Index

Another technique to determine thinness and excessive fatness is the **body mass index** (**BMI**), which incorporates height and weight to estimate critical fat values at which the risk for disease increases. Scientific evidence indicates that there is a significant increase in the risk for disease when BMI exceeds 25.[1]

BMI is calculated by either (a) multiplying body weight in pounds by 705 and dividing this figure by the square of the height in inches, or (b) dividing the weight in kilograms by the square of the height in meters. For example, the BMI for an individual who weighs 172 pounds (78 kg) and is 67 inches (1.7 m) tall would be 27: [172 × 705 ÷ (67)^2] or [78 ÷ (1.7)^2]. You can also look up your BMI in Table 4.6 according to your height and weight; then see Table 4.7 for your resultant risk for disease.

According to BMI, the lowest risk for chronic disease is in the 22-to-25 range.[2] Individuals are classified as overweight if their indexes lie between 25 and 30. BMIs above 30 are defined as obese; those below 20 as **underweight**. Scientific evidence has shown that even though the risk for premature illness and death is greater for those who are overweight, the risk also increases for individuals who are underweight[3] (see Figure 4.6).

Compared to individuals with a BMI between 22 and 25, people with a BMI between 25 and 30 (overweight) exhibit mortality rates up to 25 percent higher; rates for those with a BMI above 30 (obese) are 50 to 100 percent higher.[4] Approximately 22 percent of U.S. adults have a body BMI of 30 or more. Overweight and obesity trends starting in 1960 according to BMI are given in Figure 4.7.

In research studies and surveys, BMI is the most widely used measure to determine overweight and obesity. For most people, though, percent body fat

Body mass index (BMI) A technique to determine thinness and excessive fatness that incorporates height and weight to estimate critical fat values at which the risk for disease increases.

Underweight Extremely low body weight.

TABLE 4.5 Girth Measurement Technique: Estimated Percent Body Fat for Men

Waist Minus Wrist Girth Measurement (inches)

Body Weight (pounds)	22	22.5	23	23.5	24	24.5	25	25.5	26	26.5	27	27.5	28	28.5	29	29.5	30	30.5	31	31.5	32	32.5	33	33.5	34	34.5	35	35.5	36	36.5	37	37.5	38	38.5	39	39.5	40	40.5	41	41.5	42	42.5	43	43.5	44	44.5	45	45.5	46	46.5	47	47.5	48	48.5	49	49.5	50
120	4	6	8	10	12	14	16	18	20	21	23	25	27	29	31	33	35	37	39	41	43	45	47	49	50	52	54	56	58																											
125	4	6	7	9	11	13	15	17	19	20	22	24	26	28	29	31	33	35	37	39	41	43	45	47	48	50	52	54	56	58																										
130	3	5	7	9	11	13	15	16	18	20	22	23	25	27	29	30	32	34	36	37	39	41	43	44	46	48	50	51	53	55	57																								
135	3	5	7	8	10	12	14	16	18	19	21	23	24	26	28	30	31	33	35	36	38	40	42	43	45	47	48	50	52	53	55	56																						
140	3	4	6	8	10	12	14	15	17	19	20	22	24	25	27	29	30	32	34	35	37	39	40	42	44	45	47	49	50	52	53	55	56																					
145	3	4	6	8	9	11	13	15	16	18	20	21	23	24	26	28	29	31	33	34	36	38	39	41	42	44	46	47	49	50	52	53	54	55																				
150	2	4	6	7	9	11	12	14	16	17	19	21	22	24	25	27	28	30	32	33	35	36	38	40	41	43	44	46	48	49	51	52	53	54	55																		
155	2	4	5	7	8	10	12	13	15	16	18	20	21	23	24	26	27	29	31	32	34	35	37	38	40	42	43	45	46	48	49	51	52	53	54	55																
160	2	3	5	7	8	10	11	13	15	16	18	19	21	22	24	25	27	28	30	32	33	35	36	38	39	41	42	44	45	47	48	50	51	52	53	54	54															
165	2	3	5	6	8	9	11	13	14	16	17	19	20	22	23	25	26	28	29	31	32	34	35	37	39	40	42	43	45	46	48	49	50	52	53	54	54	54													
170	2	3	4	6	7	9	10	12	14	15	17	18	20	21	23	24	25	27	28	30	31	33	34	36	37	39	40	42	43	45	46	48	49	50	51	52	53	54	53												
175	2	3	4	6	7	8	10	12	13	15	16	18	19	21	22	23	25	26	28	29	31	32	33	35	36	38	39	41	42	44	45	47	48	49	50	52	53	53	53	53										
180		3	4	6	7	8	10	11	13	14	16	17	18	20	21	23	24	25	27	28	30	31	32	34	35	37	38	39	41	42	44	45	47	48	49	50	51	52	53	53	53									
185		3	4	5	7	8	9	11	12	14	15	16	18	19	21	22	23	25	26	27	29	30	31	33	34	36	37	38	40	41	43	44	45	47	48	49	50	51	52	53	53	53							
190		2	4	5	6	8	9	11	12	13	15	16	17	19	20	21	22	24	25	26	28	29	30	32	33	35	36	37	39	40	41	43	44	45	47	48	49	50	51	52	52	52	52						
195		2	3	5	6	7	9	10	11	13	14	15	17	18	19	21	22	23	24	26	27	28	30	31	32	34	35	36	37	39	40	41	43	44	45	47	48	49	50	51	51	52	52	52					
200		2	3	5	6	7	8	10	11	12	14	15	16	18	19	20	21	23	24	25	26	28	29	30	32	33	34	35	37	38	39	40	42	43	44	45	47	48	49	50	51	51	52	52					
205		2	3	4	6	7	8	9	11	12	13	14	16	17	18	19	21	22	23	24	26	27	28	29	31	32	33	34	36	37	38	39	40	42	43	44	45	46	48	49	50	51	51	52	52				
210		2	3	4	5	7	8	9	10	11	13	14	15	16	18	19	20	21	22	24	25	26	27	28	30	31	32	33	35	36	37	38	39	41	42	43	44	45	46	47	49	50	51	51	51				
215		2	3	4	5	6	7	9	10	11	12	13	15	16	17	18	19	21	22	23	24	25	26	28	29	30	31	32	34	35	36	37	38	39	41	42	43	44	45	46	47	48	50	51	51	51			
220			3	4	5	6	7	8	9	11	12	13	14	15	16	18	19	20	21	22	23	24	26	27	28	29	30	31	32	34	35	36	37	38	39	40	42	43	44	45	46	47	48	49	50	51	51		
225			3	4	5	6	7	8	9	10	11	12	13	15	16	17	18	19	20	21	23	24	25	26	27	28	29	31	32	33	34	35	36	37	38	40	41	42	43	44	45	46	47	48	49	50	51	51	
230			3	4	5	5	7	8	9	10	11	12	13	14	15	16	17	18	20	21	22	23	24	25	26	27	28	30	31	32	33	34	35	36	37	38	40	41	42	43	44	45	46	47	48	49	50	51	51
235			3	4	4	5	6	7	9	10	11	12	13	14	15	16	17	18	19	20	21	22	23	24	25	27	28	29	30	31	32	33	34	35	36	37	38	40	41	42	43	44	45	46	46	47	48	49	50
240			2	3	4	5	6	7	8	9	10	11	12	13	14	15	17	18	19	20	21	22	23	24	25	26	27	28	29	30	31	32	33	34	35	37	38	39	40	41	42	43	44	45	46	46	47	48	50
245			2	3	4	5	6	7	8	9	10	11	12	13	14	15	16	17	18	19	20	21	22	23	24	25	26	27	28	29	30	31	32	33	34	36	37	38	39	40	41	42	43	44	45	45	46	47	50
250			2	3	4	5	6	7	8	9	10	11	12	13	14	14	15	16	17	18	19	20	21	22	23	24	25	26	27	28	29	30	31	32	33	34	35	36	37	38	39	40	41	42	43	44	45	46	50
255			2	3	4	5	6	6	7	8	9	10	11	12	13	14	14	15	16	17	18	19	20	21	22	23	24	25	26	27	28	29	30	31	32	33	34	35	36	37	38	39	40	41	42	43	44	45	50
260			2	3	3	4	5	6	7	8	9	10	11	12	12	13	14	15	16	17	18	19	20	21	22	23	23	24	25	26	27	28	29	30	31	32	33	34	35	36	37	38	39	40	41	42	43	44	50
265				2	3	4	5	6	7	8	8	9	10	11	12	13	14	15	16	16	17	18	19	20	21	22	23	24	25	26	27	27	28	29	30	31	32	33	34	35	36	37	38	39	40	41	42	43	49
270				2	3	4	5	6	6	7	8	9	10	11	12	13	14	14	15	16	17	18	19	20	21	21	22	23	24	25	26	27	28	29	30	30	31	32	33	34	35	36	37	38	39	40	41	42	48
275				2	3	4	5	5	6	7	8	9	10	11	11	12	13	14	15	16	16	17	18	19	20	21	22	23	23	24	25	26	27	28	29	30	31	31	32	33	34	35	36	37	38	39	40	41	47
280				2	3	4	4	5	6	7	8	9	10	10	11	12	13	14	14	15	16	17	18	18	19	20	21	22	23	24	24	25	26	27	28	29	30	31	32	33	33	34	35	36	37	38	39	40	46
285				2	3	3	4	5	6	7	8	8	9	10	11	12	12	13	14	15	16	16	17	18	19	20	20	21	22	23	24	25	26	27	27	28	29	30	31	32	33	34	35	36	36	37	38	39	45
290				2	2	3	4	5	6	6	7	8	9	10	11	11	12	13	14	14	15	16	17	18	18	19	20	21	22	22	23	24	25	26	27	27	28	29	30	31	32	33	34	35	36	36	37	38	44
295					2	3	4	5	5	6	7	8	9	9	10	11	12	13	13	14	15	16	16	17	18	19	19	20	21	22	23	23	24	25	26	26	27	28	29	30	31	31	32	33	34	35	36	37	43
300					2	3	4	5	5	6	7	8	8	9	10	11	12	12	13	14	15	15	16	17	18	18	19	20	21	21	22	23	24	24	25	26	27	28	28	29	30	31	32	33	34	35	36	37	43

TABLE 4.6 Determination of Body Mass Index (BMI)

Determine your BMI by looking up the number where your weight and height intersect on the table. According to your results, look up your disease risk in Table 4.7.

Height	110	115	120	125	130	135	140	145	150	155	160	165	170	175	180	185	190	195	200	205	210	215	220	225	230	235	240	245	250
5'0"	21	22	23	24	25	26	27	28	29	30	31	32	33	34	35	36	37	38	39	40	41	42	43	44	45	46	47	48	49
5'1"	21	22	23	24	25	26	26	27	28	29	30	31	32	33	34	35	36	37	38	39	40	41	42	43	43	44	45	46	47
5'2"	20	21	22	23	24	25	26	27	27	28	29	30	31	32	33	34	35	36	37	37	38	39	40	41	42	43	44	45	46
5'3"	19	20	21	22	23	24	25	26	27	27	28	29	30	31	32	33	34	35	35	36	37	38	39	40	41	42	43	43	44
5'4"	19	20	21	21	22	23	24	25	26	27	27	28	29	30	31	32	33	33	34	35	36	37	38	39	39	40	41	42	43
5'5"	18	19	20	21	22	22	23	24	25	26	27	27	28	29	30	31	32	32	33	34	35	36	37	37	38	39	40	41	42
5'6"	18	19	19	20	21	22	23	23	24	25	26	27	27	28	29	30	31	32	33	34	35	35	36	36	37	38	39	40	40
5'7"	17	18	19	20	20	21	22	23	23	24	25	26	27	27	28	29	30	31	31	32	33	34	34	35	36	37	38	38	39
5'8"	17	17	18	19	20	21	21	22	23	24	24	25	26	27	27	28	29	30	30	31	32	32	33	34	35	35	36	37	38
5'9"	16	17	18	18	19	20	21	21	22	23	24	24	25	26	27	27	28	29	30	30	31	32	32	33	34	35	35	36	37
5'10"	16	17	17	18	19	19	20	21	22	22	23	24	24	25	26	27	27	28	29	29	30	31	32	32	33	34	34	35	36
5'11"	15	16	17	17	18	19	20	20	21	22	22	23	24	24	25	26	26	27	28	29	29	30	31	31	32	33	33	34	35
6'0"	15	16	16	17	18	18	19	20	20	21	22	22	23	24	24	25	26	26	27	28	28	29	30	31	31	32	33	33	34
6'1"	15	15	16	16	17	18	18	19	20	20	21	22	22	23	24	24	25	26	26	27	28	28	29	30	30	31	32	32	33
6'2"	14	15	15	16	17	17	18	19	19	20	21	21	22	23	23	24	25	25	26	26	27	28	28	29	30	30	31	31	32
6'3"	14	14	15	16	16	17	17	18	19	19	20	21	21	22	22	23	24	24	25	26	26	27	27	28	29	29	30	31	31
6'4"	13	14	15	15	16	16	17	18	18	19	19	20	21	21	22	23	23	24	24	25	26	26	27	27	28	29	29	30	30

TABLE 4.7 Disease Risk According to Body Mass Index (BMI)

BMI	Disease Risk	Classification
<20.00	Moderate to Very High	Underweight
20.00 to 21.99	Low	Acceptable
22.00 to 24.99	Very Low	
25.00 to 26.99	Low	Overweight
27.00 to 29.99	Moderate	
30.00 to 39.99	High	Obese
≥40.00	Very High	

FIGURE 4.6 Mortality risk versus body mass index (BMI).

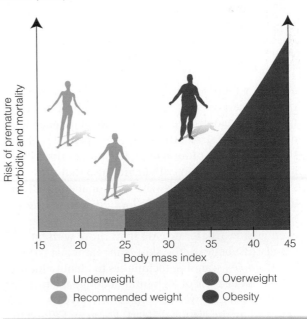

Underweight
Recommended weight
Overweight
Obesity

techniques are not readily available, nor do technicians have the necessary training and dependability to administer these procedures.

BMI is a useful tool to screen the general population, but its one weakness (similar to the original height/weight charts) is that it fails to differentiate fat from lean body mass or note where most of the fat is located (waist circumference—see discussion that follows). Using BMI, athletes with a large amount of muscle mass (such as body builders and football players) can easily fall in the moderate- or even high-risk categories.

FIGURE 4.7 Overweight and obesity trends in the United States, 1960–2000.

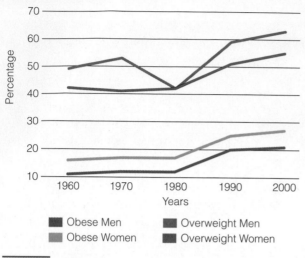

Obese Men
Obese Women
Overweight Men
Overweight Women

Adapted from the National Center for Health Statistics, Centers for Disease Control and Prevention, and the *Journal of the American Medical Association.*

TABLE 4.8 Disease Risk According to Waist Circumference (WC)

Men	Women	Disease Risk
<35.5	<32.5	Low
35.5–40.0	32.5–35.0	Moderate
>40.0	>35.0	High

TABLE 4.9 Disease Risk According to Waist-to-Hip Ratio

Waist-to-Hip Ratio		
Men	**Women**	**Disease Risk**
≤0.95	≤0.80	Very Low
0.96–0.99	0.81–0.84	Low
≥1.00	≥0.85	High

Waist Circumference

Scientific evidence suggests that the way people store fat affects their risk for disease. The total amount of body fat is not what increases the risk for disease but, rather, the location of the body fat. Some individuals tend to store fat in the abdominal area (which produces the "apple" shape). Others store it mainly around the hips and thighs, in gluteal and femoral fat (which creates the "pear" shape).

Research data show that obese individuals with a lot of abdominal fat are clearly at higher risk for heart disease, hypertension, type 2 diabetes (also called "adult-onset" or "non-insulin-dependent" diabetes), and stroke than are obese people with similar amounts of total body fat stored primarily in the hips and thighs.[5] Evidence also indicates that, among individuals with a lot of abdominal fat, those whose fat deposits are located around internal organs (intra-abdominal or visceral fat) have an even greater risk for disease than those with fat mainly just beneath the skin (subcutaneous fat).[6]

Complex scanning techniques to identify individuals at risk because of high intra-abdominal fatness are costly, so a simple waist circumference (WC) measure, designed by the National Heart, Lung, and Blood Institute, is used to assess this risk.[7] WC seems to predict abdominal visceral fat as accurately as the DEXA technique.[8] A waist circumference of more than 40 inches in men and 35 inches in women indicates a higher risk for cardiovascular disease, hypertension, and type 2 diabetes. Thus, weight loss is encouraged when individuals exceed these measurements. One study concluded that WC might be a better predictor of the risk for disease than BMI.[9] Table 4.8 helps you identify your disease risk according to WC.

A second procedure used for years to identify health risk based on the pattern of fat distribution is the **waist-to-hip ratio (WHR)** test. The waist measurement is taken at the umbilicus (belly button), and the hip measurement is taken at the point of greatest circumference. The waist measurement is then divided by the hip measurement.

The WHR differentiates the "apples" from the "pears." Men tend to be apples, and women tend to be pears. Men need to lose weight if the WHR is 1.0 or higher (that is, if the waist is even slightly larger than the hips). Women need to lose weight if the WHR is .85 or higher (see Table 4.9). For example, the WHR for a man with a 40-inch waist and a 38-inch hip would be 1.05 (40 ÷ 38)—which may indicate higher risk for disease.

During the last few years, several studies have found that WC is a better indicator than WHR of abdominal visceral obesity.[10] Thus, a combination of BMI and WC, rather than WHR, is now recommended by health care professionals to assess potential risk for disease.

Determining Recommended Body Weight

After finding out your percent body fat, you can determine your current body composition classification by consulting Table 4.10, which presents

TABLE 4.10 Body Composition Classification According to Percent Body Fat

MEN

Age	Underweight	Excellent	Good	Moderate	Overweight	Significantly Overweight
≤19	<3	12.0	12.1–17.0	17.1–22.0	22.1–27.0	≥27.1
20–29	<3	13.0	13.1–18.0	18.1–23.0	23.1–28.0	≥28.1
30–39	<3	14.0	14.1–19.0	19.1–24.0	24.1–29.0	≥29.1
40–49	<3	15.0	15.1–20.0	20.1–25.0	25.1–30.0	≥30.1
≥50	<3	16.0	16.1–21.0	21.1–26.0	26.1–31.0	≥31.1

WOMEN

Age	Underweight	Excellent	Good	Moderate	Overweight	Significantly Overweight
≤19	<12	17.0	17.1–22.0	22.1–27.0	27.1–32.0	≥32.1
20–29	<12	18.0	18.1–23.0	23.1–28.0	28.1–33.0	≥33.1
30–39	<12	19.0	19.1–24.0	24.1–29.0	29.1–34.0	≥34.1
40–49	<12	20.0	20.1–25.0	25.1–30.0	30.1–35.0	≥35.1
≥50	<12	21.0	21.1–26.0	26.1–31.0	31.1–36.0	≥36.1

High physical fitness standard   Health fitness standard

percentages of fat according to both the health fitness standard and the high physical fitness standard (see discussion in Chapter 1).

For example, the recommended health fitness fat percentage for a 20-year-old female is 28 percent or less. Although there are no clearly identified percent body fat levels at which the disease risk definitely increases (as is the case with BMI), the health fitness standard in Table 4.10 is currently the best estimate of the point at which there seems to be no harm to health.

According to Table 4.10, the high physical fitness range for this same 20-year-old woman would be between 18 and 23 percent. The high physical fitness standard does not mean you cannot be somewhat below this number. Many highly trained male athletes are as low as 3 percent, and some female distance runners have been measured at 6 percent body fat (which may not be healthy).

Although people generally agree that the mortality rate is higher for obese people, some evidence indicates that the same is true for underweight people. "Underweight" and "thin" do not necessarily mean the same thing. The body fat of a healthy thin person is around the high physical fitness standard, whereas an underweight person has extremely low body fat, even to the point of compromising the essential fat.

CRITICAL THINKING

Do you think you have a weight problem? Do your body composition results make you feel any different about the way you perceive your current body weight and image?

The 3 percent essential fat for men and 12 percent for women seem to be the lower limits for people to maintain good health. Below these percentages, normal physiological functions can be seriously impaired. Some experts point out that a little storage fat (in addition to the essential fat) is better than none at all. As a result, the health and high fitness standards for percent fat in Table 4.10 are set higher than the minimum essential fat requirements, at a point beneficial to optimal health and well-being. Finally, because lean tissue decreases with age, one extra percentage point is allowed for every additional decade of life.

Your recommended body weight is computed based on the selected health or high fitness fat percentage for your age and sex. Your decision to select a "desired" fat percentage should be based on your current percent body fat and your personal health/fitness objectives. Following are steps to compute your own recommended body weight:

1. Determine the pounds of body weight that are fat (FW) by multiplying your body weight (BW) by the current percent fat (%F) expressed in decimal form (FW = BW × %F).
2. Determine lean body mass (LBM) by subtracting the weight in fat from the total body weight (LBM = BW − FW). (Anything that is not fat must be part of the lean component.)
3. Select a desired body fat percentage (DFP) based on the health or high fitness standards given in Table 4.10.
4. Compute recommended body weight (RBW) according to the formula RBW = LBM ÷ (1.0 − DFP).

As an example of these computations, a 19-year-old female who weighs 160 pounds and is 30 percent fat would like to know what her recommended body weight would be at 22 percent:

Sex: female
Age: 19
BW: 160 lbs
%F: 30% (.30 in decimal form)
1. FW = BW × %F
   FW = 160 × .30 = 48 lbs
2. LBM = BW − FW
   LBM = 160 − 48 = 112 lbs
3. DFP: 22% (.22 in decimal form)

Waist-to-hip ratio (WHR) A measurement to assess potential risk for disease based on distribution of body fat.

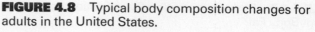

FIGURE 4.8 Typical body composition changes for adults in the United States.

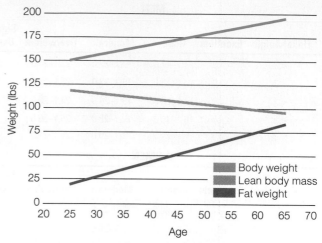

4. RBW = LBM ÷ (1.0 − .DFP)
   RBW = 112 ÷ (1.0 − .22)
   RBW = 112 ÷ .78 = 143.6 lbs

In Labs 4A and 4B, you will have the opportunity to determine your own body composition, recommended body weight, and disease risk according to waist-to-hip ratio and BMI. A second column is provided in both labs for a follow-up assessment at a future date.

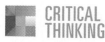

CRITICAL THINKING

How do you feel about your current body weight and what influence does society have on the way you perceive yourself in terms of your weight? Do your body composition results make you feel any different about the way you see your current body weight and image?

Other than hydrostatic weighing and air displacement, skinfold thickness seems to be the most practical and valid technique to estimate body fat. If skinfold calipers are available, use this technique to assess your percent body fat. If calipers are not available, estimate your percent fat according to the girth measurements technique or another technique available to you. You may also wish to use several techniques and compare the results.

Importance of Regular Body Composition Assessment

Children in the United States do not start with a weight problem. Although a small number struggle with weight throughout life, most are not overweight in the early years of life.

Trends indicate that, starting at age 25, the average person in the United States gains 1 pound of weight per year. Thus, by age 65, the average American will have gained 40 pounds. Because of the typical reduction in physical activity in our society, however, the average person also loses a half a pound of lean tissue each year. Therefore, this span of 40 years has produced an actual fat gain of 60 pounds accompanied by a 20-pound loss of lean body mass[11] (see Figure 4.8). These changes cannot be detected unless body composition is assessed periodically.

If you are on a diet/exercise program, you should repeat your percent body fat assessment and recommended weight computations about once a month. This is important because lean body mass is affected by weight-reduction programs and amount of physical activity. As lean body mass changes, so will your recommended body weight. To make valid comparisons, use the same technique for both pre- and post-program assessments. Knowing your percent body fat also is useful to identify fad diets that promote water loss and lean body mass, especially muscle mass (also see Diet Crazes in Chapter 5, page 125).

Changes in body composition resulting from a weight control/exercise program were illustrated in a co-ed aerobic dance course taught during a 6-week summer term. Students participated in a 60-minute aerobics routine 4 times a week. On the first and last days of class, several physiological parameters, including body composition, were assessed. Students also were given information on diet and nutrition, but they followed their own dietary program.

At the end of the 6 weeks, the average weight loss for the entire class was 3 pounds (see Figure 4.9). But, because body composition was assessed, class members were surprised to find that the average fat loss was actually 6 pounds, accompanied by a 3-pound increase in lean body mass.

When dieting, have your body composition reassessed periodically because of the effects of negative caloric balance on lean body mass. As discussed in Chapter 5, dieting does decrease lean body mass. This loss of lean body mass can be offset or eliminated by combining a sensible diet with exercise.

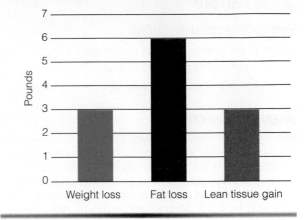

FIGURE 4.9 Effects of a 6-week aerobics exercise program on body composition.

ASSESS YOUR KNOWLEDGE

file
s

uate how
you
rstand
oncepts
ented in
chapter,
j the
ess Your
vledge"
"Practice
es"
ns
ur
OM.

1. Body composition incorporates
   a. a fat component.
   b. a non-fat component.
   c. percent body fat.
   d. lean body mass.
   e. all of the four components above.

2. The best way to determine recommended body weight is through
   a. height/weight charts.
   b. body composition analysis.
   c. lean body mass assessment.
   d. hip-to-waist ratio.
   e. body mass index.

3. Essential fat in women is
   a. 3 percent.
   b. 5 percent.
   c. 10 percent.
   d. 12 percent.
   e. 17 percent.

4. Which of the following is *not* a technique used in the assessment of body fat?
   a. body mass index
   b. skinfold thickness
   c. hydrostatic weighing
   d. circumference measurements
   e. air displacement

5. Which of the following sites is used in the assessment of percent body fat according to skinfold thickness in men?
   a. suprailium
   b. chest
   c. scapular
   d. triceps
   e. All four sites are used.

6. Which variable is *not* used in the assessment of percent body fat in women according to girth measurements?
   a. age
   b. hip
   c. wrist
   d. upper arm
   e. height

7. The waist-to-hip ratio is used to
   a. determine percent body fat.
   b. assess risk for disease.
   c. measure lean body mass.
   d. identify underweight people.
   e. do all of the above.

8. An acceptable BMI is between
   a. 15 and 19.99.
   b. 20 and 24.99.
   c. 25 and 29.99.
   d. 30 and 34.99.
   e. 35 and 39.99.

9. The health fitness percent body fat for women of various ages is in the range of
   a. 3 to 7 percent.
   b. 7 to 12 percent.
   c. 12 to 20 percent.
   d. 20 to 27 percent.
   e. 27 to 31 percent.

10. When a previously inactive individual starts an exercise program, the person may
    a. lose weight.
    b. gain weight.
    c. improve body composition.
    d. lose more fat pounds than total weight pounds.
    e. do all of the above.

Correct answers can be found at the back of the book.

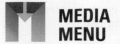

MEDIA MENU

PROFILE PLUS CD CONNECTIONS

■ Learn how to measure body composition.

■ Assess your risks for potential disease.

■ Check how well you understand the chapter's concepts.

INTERNET CONNECTIONS

■ Body Composition Laboratory. The Body Composition Laboratory at the Children's Nutrition Research Center in Houston, Texas, sponsors this informative Web site, which explains the techniques for and applications of body composition measurements in all populations, ranging from low–birth weight infants to adults. Learn how high-precision instruments are used to measure total body levels of body water, mineral, protein, and fat.

   http://www.bcm.tmc.edu/bodycomplab

■ The Exercise and Physical Fitness Laboratory at Georgia State University. This university site, from the Depart-

ment of Kinesiology and Health, describes six methods for measuring body composition and provides information regarding procedure description, accuracy, relative cost, as well as a list of advantages and disadvantages for each.

   http://www.gsu.edu/webprj01/coe/wwwfit/public_ html/bodycomp.html

■ Cornell University Research on Body Composition and Metabolic Rate. This instructional Web site describes methods used to calculate basal metabolic rate and body composition.

   http://instruct1.cit.cornell.edu/Courses/ns421/BMR.html

■ Body Fat Lab. An informative, interactive, and fun site from Shape Up, America describing body mass measurements, percent body fat, and the role body fat plays in overall health. You can check your level of knowledge with the "Body Fat IQ Test."

   http://www.shapeup.org/bodylab/frmst.htm

Notes

1. J. Stevens, J. Cai, E. R. Pamuk, D. F. Williamson, M. J. Thun, and J. L. Wood, "The Effect of Age on the Association Between Body Mass Index and Mortality," *New England Journal of Medicine* 338 (1998): 1–7.

2. E. E. Calle, M. J. Thun, J. M. Petrelli, C. Rodriguez, and C. W. Heath, "Body-Mass Index and Mortality in a Prospective Cohort of U.S. Adults," *New England Journal of Medicine* 341 (1999): 1097–1105.

3. American College of Sports Medicine, "Position Stand: Appropriate Intervention Strategies for Weight Loss and Prevention for Weight Regain for Adults," *Medicine and Science in Sports and Exercise* 33 (2001): 2145–2156.

4. K. M. Flegal, M. D. Carrol, R. J. Kuczmarski, and C. L. Johnson, "Overweight and Obesity in the United States: Prevalence and Trends, 1960–1994," *International Journal of Obesity and Related Metabolic Disorders* 22 (1998): 39–47.

5. "Comparing Apples and Pears," *University of California at Berkeley Wellness Letter* (Palm Coast, FL: The Editors, March 2004).

6. C. Bouchard, G. A. Bray, and V. S. Hubbard, "Basic and Clinical Aspects of Regional Fat Distribution," *American Journal of Clinical Nutrition* 52 (1990): 946–950.

   J. P. Després, I. Lemieux, and D. Prudhomme, "Treatment of Obesity: Need to Focus on High Risk Abdominally Obese Patients," *British Medical Journal* 322 (2001): 716–720.

M. C. Pouliot et al., "Waist Circumference and Abdominal Sagittal Diameter: Best Simple Anthropometric Indexes of Abdominal Visceral Adipose Tissue Accumulation and Related Cardiovascular Risk in Men and Women," *American Journal of Cardiology* 73 (1994): 460–468.

7. National Heart, Lung, and Blood Institute, National Institutes of Health, *The Practical Guide: Identification, Evaluation, and Treatment of Overweight and Obesity in Adults* (NIH Publication no. 00–4084) (Washington DC: Government Printing Office, 2000).

8. M. B. Snijder, et al., "The Prediction of Visceral Fat by Dual-Energy X-ray Absorptiometry in the Elderly: A Comparison with Computed Tomography and Anthropometry," *International Journal of Obesity* 26 (2002): 984–993.

9. I. Janssen, P. T. Katzmarzyk, and R. Ross, "Waist Circumference and Not Body Mass Index Explains Obesity-Related Health Risk," *American Journal of Clinical Nutrition* 79 (2004): 379–384.

10. P. M. Ribisl, "Toxic 'Waist' Dump: Our Abdominal Visceral Fat," *ACSM's Health & Fitness Journal* 8, no. 4 (2004): 22–25.

11. J. H. Wilmore, "Exercise and Weight Control: Myths, Misconceptions, and Quackery," lecture given at annual meeting of American College of Sports Medicine, Indianapolis, June 1994.

Suggested Readings

Heyward, V. H., and D. Wagner. *Applied Body Composition Assessment.* Champaign, IL: Human Kinetics, 2004.

Roche, A. F., T. G. Lohman, and S. B. Heymsfield. *Human Body Composition.* Champaign, IL: Human Kinetics, 1996.

Lab 4A

HYDROSTATIC WEIGHING FOR BODY COMPOSITION ASSESSMENT

Name: _____   Date: _____   Grade: _____

Instructor: _____   Course: _____   Section: _____

Necessary Lab Equipment

Hydrostatic or underwater weighing tank and residual volume spirometer (if no spirometer is available, predicting equations can be used to determine this volume—see Figure 4.2, pages 102–103).

Objective

To determine body density and percent body fat.

Lab Preparation

Bring a swimsuit and towel to this lab. A 6- to 8-hour fast and bladder and bowel movements are recommended prior to underwater weighing.

Instructions

Follow the procedure outlined in Figure 4.2. If time is a factor, assess only the body composition of one or two participants in the course and compute the results using the form provided below. A sample of the computations is provided on the back of this page.

I. Hydrostatic Weighing

Name: _____   Age: ____   Weight: ____ lbs

Height: ____ inches × 2.54 = ____ cm   Water temperature: ____ °C   Water density (WD): ____ gr/ml

Residual volume (RV): ____ lt   (See Figure 4.2)

Body weight (BW) in kg = weight in pounds ÷ 2.2046

BW in kg = ____ ÷ 2.2046 = ____ kg

Gross underwater weights:

1. ____ kg   2. ____ kg   3. ____ kg   4. ____ kg   5. ____ kg

6. ____ kg   7. ____ kg   8. ____ kg   9. ____ kg   10. ____ kg

Average of three heaviest underwater weights (AUW): ____ kg

Tare weight (TW): ____ kg

Net underwater weight (UW) = AUW − TW

Net underwater weight (UW) = ____ − ____ = ____ kg

Body density (BD):

$$BD = \frac{BW}{\dfrac{BW - UW}{WD} - RV - .1} \qquad BD = \frac{\rule{2cm}{0.4pt}}{\dfrac{\rule{1.5cm}{0.4pt}}{\rule{1.5cm}{0.4pt}} - \rule{1cm}{0.4pt} - .1} = \rule{1.5cm}{0.4pt}$$

Percent body fat (%Fat):

$$\%Fat = \frac{495}{BD} - 450 = \frac{495}{\rule{1.5cm}{0.4pt}} - 450 = \rule{1.5cm}{0.4pt} \%$$ **Follow-up** percent body fat: ____ %

FIGURE 4A.1 Sample computation for percent body fat according to hydrostatic weighing.

Name: Jane Doe Age: 20 Weight: 148.5 lbs

Height: 67 inches × 2.54 = 170.2 cm Water temperature: 33 °C Water density (WD): .99473 gr/ml

Residual volume (RV): 1.73 lt See Figure 4.2.

Body weight (BW) in kg = weight in pounds ÷ 2.2046

BW in kg = 148.5 ÷ 2.2046 = 67.36 kg

Gross underwater weights:

1. 6.15 kg 2. 6.12 kg 3. 6.24 kg 4. 6.26 kg 5. 6.21 kg

6. 6.26 kg 7. 6.29 kg 8. 6.28 kg 9. 6.24 kg 10. 6.27 kg

Average of three heaviest underwater weights (AUW): 6.28 kg

Tare weight (TW): 5.154 kg

Net underwater weight (UW) = AUW − TW

Net underwater weight (UW) = 6.28 − 5.154 = 1.126 kg

Body density (BD):

$$BD = \frac{BW}{\dfrac{BW - UW}{WD} - RV - .1}$$

$$BD = \frac{67.36}{\dfrac{67.36 - 1.126}{.99473} - 1.73 - .1} = 1.0402301$$

Percent body fat (%Fat):

$$\%Fat = \frac{495}{BD} - 450 = \frac{495}{1.0402301} - 450 = 25.9 \%$$

Follow-up percent body fat: ____ %

II. What I learned from the underwater weighing procedure.

Describe the experience of being weighed underwater. Do you feel that the results of the test were accurate?

LAB 4B

BODY COMPOSITION ASSESSMENT, DISEASE RISK ASSESSMENT, AND RECOMMENDED BODY WEIGHT DETERMINATION

Name: _____ Date: _____ Grade: _____

Instructor: _____ Course: _____ Section: _____

Necessary Lab Equipment
Skinfold calipers and standard measuring tapes.

Objective
To assess percent body fat using skinfold thickness or girth measurements, disease risk according to waist-to-hip ratio and body mass index, and recommended body weight.

Instructions
If skinfold calipers are available, use the skinfold thickness technique to assess your percent body fat (see Figure 4.4, page 104). If calipers are unavailable, estimate the percent fat according to the girth measurements technique (see Figure 4.5, page 107). You may wish to use both techniques and compare the results. Next, compute your recommended body weight according to your current percent body fat and the recommended percent body fat guidelines provided in Table 4.9, page 112. Determine also your waist-to-hip ratio, body mass index, and recommended weight using the guidelines provided in this lab.

I. Percent Body Fat According to Skinfold Thickness

Men

Chest (mm): _____

Abdomen (mm): _____

Thigh (mm): _____

Total (mm): _____

% Fat: _____

Women

Triceps (mm): _____

Suprailium (mm): _____

Thigh (mm): _____

Total (mm): _____

% Fat: _____

Follow-up

% Fat _____ %

II. Percent Fat According to Girth Measurements

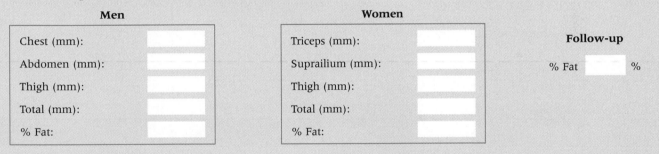

Men

Waist (inches): _____

Wrist (inches): _____

Difference: _____

Body Weight: _____

% Fat: _____

Women

Upper Arm (cm): _____   Constant A = _____

Age: _____   Constant B = _____

Hip (cm): _____   Constant C = _____

Wrist (cm): _____   Constant D = _____

BD* = A − B − C + D

BD = _____ − _____ − _____ + _____ = _____

% Fat = (495 ÷ BD) − 450 = (495 ÷ _____) − 450 = _____

*Body density

Follow-up

% Fat _____ %

III. Disease Risk According to Waist Circumference and Body Mass Index

Waist Circumference

Waist (inches): _____

Disease Risk: _____

Follow-up

_____

_____

Recommended Standards

Waist Circumference		
Men	Women	Disease Risk
<35.5	<32.5	Low
35.5–40.0	32.5–35.0	Moderate
>40.0	>35.0	High

Body Mass Index

Weight: [____] lbs [____] kg

Height: [____] inches [____] meters

BMI = Weight (lbs) × 705 ÷ Height (in) ÷ Height (in)

BMI = [____] (lbs) × 705 ÷ [____] (in) ÷ [____] (in) = [____]

Or BMI = Weight (kg) ÷ Height (m) ÷ Height (m)

BMI = [____] (kg) ÷ [____] (m) ÷ [____] (m) = [____]

Disease Risk: [____]

Follow-up BMI = [____]   Disease Risk: [____]

Recommended Standards

BMI	Disease Risk	Classification
<20.00	Moderate to Very High	Underweight
20.00 to 21.99	Low	Acceptable
22.00 to 24.99	Very Low	
25.00 to 26.99	Low	Overweight
27.00 to 29.99	Moderate	
30.00 to 39.99	High	Obese
≥40.00	Very High	

IV. Recommended Body Weight Determination

A. Body weight (BW): [____]

B. Current %F*: [____] %

C. Fat weight (FW) = BW × %F

   FW = [____] × [____] = [____]

D. Lean body mass (LBM) = BW − FW = [____] − [____] = [____]

E. Age: [____]

F. Desired fat percent (DFP − see Table 4.9, page 112): [____] %

G. Recommended body weight (RBW) = LBM ÷ (1.0 − DFP*)

   RBW = [____] ÷ (1.0 − [____]) = [____]

___
*Express percentages in decimal form (for example, 25% = .25)

Follow Up

A. BW: [____]

B. %F: [____] %

C. FW: [____]

D. LBM: [____]

E. Age: [____]

F. DFP: [____] %

G. RBW: [____]

V. Body Composition Conclusions and Goals

Briefly state your feelings about your body composition results and your recommended body weight. Do you need to reduce percent body fat and/or increase lean body mass? Write the goal(s) you want to achieve by the end of the term and indicate how you plan to achieve them.

Chapter 5

Weight Management

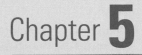

Objectives

- Describe the health consequences of obesity.
- Expose some popular fad diets and myths and fallacies regarding weight control.
- Describe eating disorders and their associated medical problems and behavior patterns, and the need for professional help in treating these conditions.
- Explain the physiology of weight loss, including setpoint theory and the effects of diet on basal metabolic rate.
- Explain the role of a lifetime exercise program as the key to a successful weight loss and weight maintenance program.
- Be able to implement a physiologically sound weight reduction and weight maintenance program.
- Describe behavior modification techniques that help a person adhere to a lifetime weight maintenance program.

Profile Plus CD Connections

- On your exercise log, check your progress.
- Check how well you understand the chapter's concepts.

Two terms commonly used to describe the condition of weighing more than recommended are *overweight* and *obesity*. The obesity level is the point at which excess body fat can lead to serious health problems. Obesity is a health hazard of epidemic proportions in most developed countries around the world. According to the World Health Organization, an estimated 35 percent of the adult population in industrialized nations is obese. **Obesity** has been defined as a body mass index (BMI) of 30 or higher.

During the last few years there has been a dramatic increase in the United States in the number of people who are overweight and obese, a direct result of physical inactivity and poor dietary habits. More than 60 percent of adults in the United States do not achieve the recommended amount of physical activity. According to the latest government statistics, American women consume 335 more calories daily than they did 20 years ago and men an additional 170 calories per day.[1]

Approximately 63 percent of men and 55 percent of women are **overweight** (having a BMI greater than 25), and 21 percent of men and 27 percent of women are obese (see Figure 5.1).[2] An estimated 120 million people are overweight and 30 million are obese. Between 1960 and 2000, the overall (men and women combined) prevalence of adult obesity increased from about 13 percent to 24 percent. Most of this increase occurred in the 1990s.

As illustrated in Figure 5.2, the obesity epidemic continues to escalate. Before 1990, not a single state reported an obesity rate above 15 percent of the state's total population (includes both adults and children). By the year 2003, all states reported a rate above 15 percent, 33 states had an obesity rate between 20 and 24 percent, and four states had reached a rate above 25 percent.

Most of the blame for the alarming increase in obesity lies in the amount of food that we eat and our lack of physical activity. According to the U.S. Department of Agriculture, the average daily caloric intake in the United States increased from 3,100 calories per person in the 1960s to 3,700 calories in the 1990s. Further, as the nation continues to evolve into a more mechanized and automated society (relying on escalators, elevators, remote controls, computers, electronic mail, cell phones, and automatic-sensor doors), the amount of required daily physical activity continues to decrease. We are being "lulled" into a high-risk sedentary lifestyle.

In the last decade alone, the average weight of American adults increased by about 15 pounds. The prevalence of obesity is even higher in ethnic groups, especially African Americans and Hispanic Americans.

About 44 percent of all women and 29 percent of all men are on a diet at any given moment.[3] People spend about $40 billion yearly attempting to

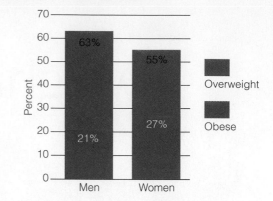

FIGURE 5.1 Percentage of adult population that is obese (BMI ≥ 30) and overweight (BMI = 25 to 29.9) in the United States.

Source: A. Must et al., "The Disease Burden Associated with Overweight and Obesity," *Journal of the American Medical Association* 282 (1999): 1523–1529.

lose weight. More than $10 billion goes to memberships in weight reduction centers and another $30 billion to diet food sales. Furthermore, the total cost attributable to treating obesity-related diseases is estimated at $100 billion per year.[4]

As the second leading cause of preventable death in the United States, overweight and obesity have been associated with several serious health problems and account for about 20 percent of the annual mortality rate. Within the next couple of years, obesity is expected to overcome tobacco as the leading cause of preventable deaths in the United States.

More than 400,000 deaths each year are caused by excessive body weight and physical inactivity[5] (only tobacco use causes more deaths, accounting for 435,000 deaths per year). Furthermore, obesity is more prevalent than smoking (19 percent), poverty (14 percent), and problem drinking (6 percent) and is associated with at least as much morbidity and poor quality of life as the latter three conditions.[6] Obesity and unhealthy lifestyle habits are the most critical public health problems that we face in the 21st century.

Excessive body weight and obesity are associated with poor health status and are risk factors for many physical ailments, including cardiovascular disease and cancer. Evidence indicates that health risks associated with increased body weight start at a BMI over 25 and are greatly enhanced at a BMI over 30.

The American Heart Association identifies obesity as one of the six major risk factors for coronary heart disease. Estimates also indicate that 14 percent of all cancer deaths in men and 20 percent in women

FIGURE 5.2 Obesity trends in the United States 1985–2003, based on BMI ≥ 30 or 30 pounds overweight.

Percentages of the total number of people in the respective state who are obese.

○ No data   ● 10%–14%   ● 20–24%
● <10%   ● 15%–19%   ● ≥25%

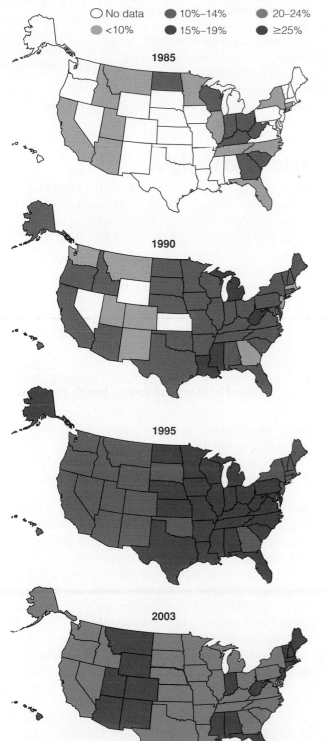

1985

1990

1995

2003

Source: *Obesity Trends Among U. S. Adults Between 1985 and 2003.* (Atlanta: Centers for Disease Control and Prevention, 2004).

HEALTH CONSEQUENCES OF EXCESSIVE BODY WEIGHT

Being overweight or obese increases the risk for

- high blood pressure
- elevated blood lipids (high blood cholesterol and triglycerides
- type 2 (non-insulin-dependent) diabetes
- insulin resistance, glucose intolerance
- coronary heart disease
- angina pectoris
- congestive heart failure
- stroke
- gallbladder disease
- gout
- osteoarthritis
- obstructive sleep apnea and respiratory problems
- some types of cancer (endometrial, breast, prostate, and colon)
- complications of pregnancy (gestational diabetes, gestational hypertension, preeclampsia, and complications during C-sections)
- poor female reproductive health (menstrual irregularities, infertility, irregular ovulation)
- bladder control problems (stress incontinence)
- psychological disorders (depression, eating disorders, distorted body image, discrimination, and low self-esteem)
- shortened life expectancy
- decreased quality of life

Source: Centers for Disease Control and Prevention, 2004.

are related to current overweight and obesity patterns in the United States.[7] Furthermore, excessive body weight is implicated in psychological maladjustment and a higher accidental death rate. Extremely obese people have worse mental health-related quality of life.

Overweight Versus Obesity

Overweight and obesity are not the same thing. Many overweight people (people who weigh about 10 to 20 pounds over the recommended weight) are not obese. Although a few pounds of excess weight may not be harmful to most people, this is not always the case. People with excessive body fat who have type 2 diabetes and other cardiovascular risk

Obesity A chronic disease characterized by body mass index (BMI) 30 or higher.

Overweight Excess weight characterized by a body mass index (BMI) greater than 25 but less than 30.

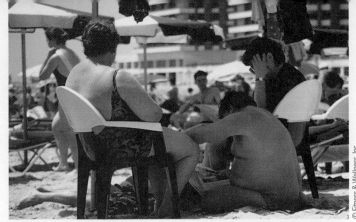

Obesity is a health hazard of epidemic proportions in industrialized nations.

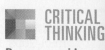

CRITICAL THINKING

Do you consider yourself overweight? If so how long have you had a weight problem what attempts have you made to lose weight, and what has worked best for you

the number of people who develop eating disorders (anorexia nervosa and bulimia, discussed under "Eating Disorders" on pages 128–131).

Extreme weight loss can lead to medical conditions such as heart damage, gastrointestinal problems, shrinkage of internal organs, immune system abnormalities, disorders of the reproductive system, loss of muscle tissue, damage to the nervous system, and even death. About 14 percent of people in the United States are underweight.

Tolerable Weight

Many people want to lose weight so they will look better. That's a noteworthy goal. The problem, however, is that they have a distorted image of what they would really look like if they were to reduce to what they think is their ideal weight. Hereditary factors play a big role, and only a small fraction of the population has the genes for a "perfect body."

The media have the greatest influence on people's perception of what constitutes ideal body weight. Most people use fashion, fitness, and beauty magazines to determine what they should look like. The "ideal" body shapes, physiques, and proportions seen in these magazines are rare and are achieved mainly through airbrushing and medical reconstruction.[11] Many individuals, primarily young women, go to extremes in an attempt to achieve these unrealistic figures. Failure to attain a "perfect body" may lead to eating disorders in some individuals.

When people set their own target weight, they should be realistic. Attaining the "Excellent" percent of body fat shown in Table 4.10 (page 113) is extremely difficult for some. It is even more difficult to maintain over time, unless the person makes a commitment to a vigorous lifetime exercise program and permanent dietary changes. Few people are willing to do that. The "Moderate" percent body fat category may be more realistic for many people.

The question you should ask yourself is: Am I happy with my weight? Part of enjoying a higher quality of life is being happy with yourself. If you are not, you either need to do something about it or learn to live with it.

If your percent of body fat is higher than those in the Moderate category of Table 4.10 (page 113), you should try to reduce it and stay in this category, for health reasons. This is the category that seems to pose no detriment to health.

If you are in the Moderate category but would like to reduce your percent of body fat further, you

factors (elevated blood lipids, high blood pressure, physical inactivity, and poor eating habits) benefit from weight loss. People who have a few extra pounds of weight but who are otherwise healthy and physically active, exercise regularly, and eat a healthy diet may not be at greater risk for early death. Such is not the case, however, with obese individuals.

Research data indicate that individuals who are 30 or more pounds overweight during middle age (30 to 49 years of age) lose about 7 years of life, whereas being 10 to 30 pounds overweight decreases lifespan by about three years.[8] These decreases are similar to those seen with tobacco use. Severe obesity (BMI greater than 45) at a young age, nonetheless, may cut up to 20 years off one's life.[9]

Although the loss of years of life is significant, the decreased life expectancy doesn't even begin to address the loss in quality of life and increased illness and disability throughout the years. Even a modest reduction of 5 to 10 percent can reduce the risk for chronic diseases including heart disease, high blood pressure, high cholesterol, and diabetes.[10]

A primary objective to achieve overall physical fitness and enhanced quality of life is to attain recommended body composition. Individuals at recommended body weight are able to participate in a wide variety of moderate-to-vigorous activities without functional limitations. These people have the freedom to enjoy most of life's recreational activities to their fullest potential. Excessive body weight does not afford an individual the fitness level to enjoy many lifetime activities such as basketball, soccer, racquetball, surfing, mountain cycling, or mountain climbing. Maintaining high fitness and recommended body weight gives a person a degree of independence throughout life that most people in developed nations no longer enjoy.

Scientific evidence also recognizes problems with being underweight. Although the social pressure to be thin has declined slightly in recent years, the pressure to attain model-like thinness is still with us and contributes to the gradual increase in

need to ask yourself a second question: How badly do I want it? Do I want it badly enough to implement lifetime exercise and dietary changes? If you are not willing to change, you should stop worrying about your weight and deem the Moderate category "tolerable" for you.

The Weight Loss Dilemma

Yo-yo dieting carries as great a health risk as being overweight and remaining overweight in the first place. Epidemiological data show that frequent fluctuations in weight (up or down) markedly increase the risk of dying of cardio-vascular disease.

Based on the findings that constant losses and regains can be hazardous to health, quick-fix diets should be replaced by a slow but permanent weight-loss program (as described under "Losing Weight the Sound and Sensible Way"). Individuals reap the benefits of recommended body weight when they get to that weight and stay there throughout life.

Unfortunately, only about 10 percent of all people who begin a traditional weight-loss program without exercise are able to lose the desired weight. Worse, only 5 in 100 are able to keep the weight off. The body is highly resistant to permanent weight changes through caloric restrictions alone.

Traditional diets have failed because few of them incorporate lifetime changes in food selection and an overall increase in physical activity and exercise as fundamental to successful weight loss and weight maintenance. When the diet stops, weight gain begins. The $40 billion diet industry tries to capitalize on the false idea that weight can be lost quickly without considering the consequences of fast weight loss or the importance of lifetime behavioral changes to ensure proper weight loss and maintenance.

In addition, various studies indicate that most people, especially obese people, underestimate their energy intake. Those who try to lose weight but apparently fail to do so are often described as "diet-resistant." One study found that, while on a "diet," a group of obese individuals with a self-reported history of diet resistance underreported their average daily caloric intake by almost 50 percent (1,028 self-reported versus 2,081 actual calories—see Figure 5.3).[12] These individuals also overestimated their amount of daily physical activity by about 25 percent (1,022 self-reported versus 771 actual calories). These differences represent an additional 1,304 calories of energy per day unaccounted for by the subjects in the study. The findings indicate that failing to lose weight often is related to misreports of actual food intake and level of physical activity.

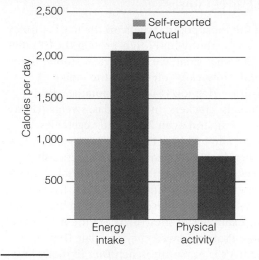

FIGURE 5.3 Differences between self-reported and actual daily caloric intake and exercise in obese individuals attempting to lose weight.

Source: S. W. Lichtman et al., "Discrepancy Between Self-Reported and Actual Caloric Intake and Exercise in Obese Subjects," *New England Journal of Medicine* 327 (1992): 1893–1898.

Diet Crazes

Capitalizing on hopes that the latest diet to hit the market will really work this time, fad diets continue to appeal to people of all shapes and sizes. These diets may work for awhile, but their success is usually short-lived. Regarding the effectiveness of these diets, Dr. Kelly Brownell, a foremost researcher in the field of weight management, has stated: "When I get the latest diet fad, I imagine a trick birthday cake candle that keeps lighting up and we have to keep blowing it out."

Fad diets deceive people and claim that dieters will lose weight by following all instructions. Most diets are very low in calories and deprive the body of certain nutrients, generating a metabolic imbalance. Under these conditions, a lot of the weight lost is in the form of water and protein, and not fat.

On a crash diet, close to half the weight loss is in lean (protein) tissue. When the body uses protein instead of a combination of fats and carbohydrates as a source of energy, weight is lost as much as 10 times faster. This is because a gram of protein produces half the amount of energy that fat does. In the case of muscle protein, one-fifth of protein is mixed with four-fifths water. Therefore, each pound of muscle yields only one-tenth the amount of energy of a pound of fat. As a result, most of the

Yo-yo dieting Constantly losing and gaining weight.

weight lost is in the form of water, which on the scale, of course, looks good.

Low-Carb Diets

Among the most popular diets on the market today are the low-carbohydrate/high-protein (LCHP) diet plans. Although small variations exist among them, in general, "low-carb" diets limit the intake of carbohydrate-rich foods—bread, potatoes, rice, pasta, cereals, crackers, juices, sodas, sweets (candy, cake, cookies), and even fruits and vegetables. Dieters are allowed to eat all the protein-rich foods they desire, including steak, ham, chicken, fish, bacon, eggs, nuts, cheese, tofu, high-fat salad dressings, butter, and small amounts of a few fruits and vegetables. Typically, these diets are also high in fat content. Examples of these diets are the Atkins Diet, The Zone, Protein Power, the Scarsdale Diet, The Carb Addict's Diet, South Beach Diet (initially low-carb), and Sugar Busters.

During digestion, carbohydrates are converted into glucose, a basic fuel used by every cell in the body. As blood glucose rises, insulin is released from the pancreas. Insulin is a hormone that facilitates the entry of glucose into the cells, thereby lowering the glucose level in the bloodstream. If the cells don't soon use the glucose for normal cell functions or to fuel physical activity, glucose is converted to, and stored as, body fat.

Not all carbohydrates cause a similar rise in blood glucose. The rise in glucose is based on the speed of digestion, which depends on a number of factors, including the size of the food particles. Small-particle carbohydrates break down rapidly and cause a quick, sharp rise in blood glucose. Thus, to gauge a food's effect on blood glucose, carbohydrates are classified by their **glycemic index**.

A high glycemic index signifies a food that causes a quick rise in blood glucose. At the top of the 100-point scale is glucose itself. This index is not directly related to simple and complex carbohydrates, and the glycemic values are not always what one might expect. Rather, the index is based on the actual laboratory-measured speed of absorption. Processed foods generally have a high glycemic index, whereas high-fiber foods tend to have a lower index (see Table 5.1).

The body functions best when blood sugar remains at a constant level. Although this is best accomplished with low-glycemic index foods, elimination of all high-glycemic index foods from the diet is not necessary (foods with a high glycemic index are especially useful to replenish depleted glycogen stores following prolonged or exhaustive exercise). Combining high- with low-glycemic index items or with some fat and protein brings the average index

TABLE 5.1 Glycemic Index of Selected Foods

Food Item	Index	Food Item	Index
Glucose	100	Muesli	56
Carrots	92	Frosted Flakes	55
Honey	87	Fruit cocktail	55
Baked potatoes	85	Sweet corn	55
Jelly beans	80	Sweet potato	51
White rice	72	Peas	51
White bread	69	White pasta	50
Whole-wheat bread	69	Whole-wheat pasta	42
Pineapple	66	Spaghetti	41
Table sugar	65	Oranges	40
Bananas	62	Apples	39
Boiled potatoes	62	Low-fat yogurt	33
Corn	59	Fructose	20
Oatmeal	59	Peanuts	13

BEHAVIOR MODIFICATION PLANNING

ARE LOW-CARB/HIGH-PROTEIN DIETS MORE EFFECTIVE?

A few studies suggest that, at least over the short-term, low-carb/high-protein (LCHP) diets are more effective in producing weight loss than carbohydrate-based diets. These results are preliminary and controversial. In LCHP diets:

▨ A large amount of weight loss is water and muscle protein, not body fat. Some of this weight is quickly regained when regular dietary habits are resumed.

▨ Few people are able to stay with LCHP diets for more than a few weeks at a time. The majority stop dieting before the targeted program completion.

▨ LCHP dieters are rarely found in a national weight-loss registry of people who have lost 30 pounds and kept them off for a minimum of six years.

▨ Food choices are severely restricted in LCHP diets. With less variety, individuals tend to eat less (800 to 1,200 calories/day) and thus lose more weight.

▨ LCHP diets may promote heart disease, cancer, and increase the risk for osteoporosis.

▨ LCHP diets are fundamentally high in fat (about 60 percent fat calories).

▨ LCHP diets are not recommended for people with diabetes, high blood pressure, heart disease, or kidney disease.

▨ LCHP diets do not promote long-term healthy eating patterns.

down. Regular consumption of high-glycemic foods, nonetheless, can increase the risk of cardiovascular disease, especially in people at risk for diabetes.

Proponents of LCHP diets indicate that if a person eats fewer carbohydrates and more protein, the pancreas will produce less insulin, and as insulin

BEHAVIOR MODIFICATION PLANNING

HOW TO RECOGNIZE FAD DIETS

Fad diets share common characteristics. These diets typically

- are nutritionally unbalanced.
- are based on testimonials.
- were developed according to "confidential research."
- promote rapid and "painless" weight loss.
- promise miraculous results.
- restrict food selection.
- require the use of selected products.
- use liquid formulas instead of foods.
- misrepresent salespeople as individuals qualified to provide nutrition counseling.
- fail to provide information on risks associated with weight loss and diet use.
- do not involve physical activity.
- do not encourage healthy behavioral changes.
- are not supported by the scientific community or national health organizations.
- fail to provide information for weight maintenance upon completion of diet phase.

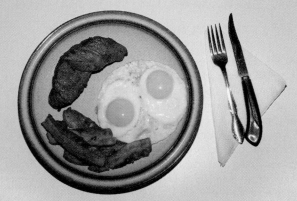

High-protein/low-carb diets create nutritional deficiencies and contribute to the development of cardiovascular disease, cancer, and osteoporosis.

drops, the body will turn to its own fat deposits for energy. There is no scientific proof, however, that high levels of insulin lead to weight gain. None of the authors of these diets have published any studies that validate their claims. Yet, these authors base their diets on the faulty premise that high insulin leads to obesity. In fact, we know the opposite to be true: Excessive body fat causes insulin levels to rise, thereby increasing the risk for developing diabetes.

The reason for rapid weight loss during LCHP diets is that a low carbohydrate intake forces the liver to produce glucose. The source for most of this glucose is body proteins—your lean body mass, including muscle. As indicated earlier, protein is mostly water; thus, weight is lost rapidly. When a person terminates the diet, the body rebuilds some of the protein tissue and quickly regains some weight.

A study in the *New England Journal of Medicine* indicated that individuals on a LCHP (Atkins) diet for 12 months lost about twice as much weight as those on a low-fat diet at the mid-point of the study.[13] The effectiveness of the diet, however, seemed to dwindle over time. At 12 months into the diet, the LCHP diet participants had regained more weight than those on the low-fat diet plan.

Years of research will be required to determine the extent to which long-term adherence to LCHP diets increase the risk for heart disease, cancer, and kidney or bone damage. Low-carb diets are contrary to the nutrition advice of most national leading health organizations (which recommend a diet low

in animal fat and saturated fat and high in complex carbohydrates). Without fruits, vegetables, and whole grains, high-protein diets lack many vitamins, minerals, and fiber—all dietary factors that protect against an array of ailments and diseases.

The major risk associated with long-term adherence to LCHP diets could be the increased risk of heart disease because high-protein foods are also high in fat content (see Chapter 11). A low carbohydrate intake also produces a loss of vitamin B, calcium, and potassium. Potential bone loss can further accentuate the risk for osteoporosis. Side effects commonly associated with these diets include weakness, nausea, bad breath, constipation, irritability, lightheadedness, and fatigue. Long-term adherence to a LCHP diet also can increase the risk of cancer. Phytochemicals found in fruits, vegetables, and whole grains protect against certain types of cancer. If you choose to go on a LCHP diet for longer than a few weeks, let your physician know so he or she may monitor your blood lipids, bone density, and kidney function.

Combo Diets

In addition to the low-carb diets, "combo diets" such as the Schwarzbein and Suzanne Sommers diets are also popular of late. The Schwarzbein diet claims that eating proteins and nonstarchy carbohydrates together will keep the food from being stored as fat. The Suzanne Sommers diet doesn't allow you to eat proteins within 3 hours of carbohydrates, and if

Glycemic index An index that is used to rate the plasma glucose response of carbohydrate-containing foods with the response produced by the same amount of carbohydrate from a standard source, usually glucose or white bread.

A very popular and controversial weight-loss supplement recently taken off the market was the herbal supplement ma huang, more commonly known as ephedra. Ma huang contains ephedra alkaloids, whose actions are similar to those of sympathetic nervous system hormones. The herb aids with weight loss but its use may pose a health risk to some people. The Food and Drug Administration, however, banned its use in early 2004 because "dietary supplements containing ephedra present an unreasonable risk of illness or injury." More than 155 deaths and 16,000 adverse effects were linked to ephedra use.

Serious side effects from using ephedra included heat stroke, dizziness, headaches, gastrointestinal distress, seizures, psychosis, irregular heartbeat, tachycardia (rapid heart rate), high blood pressure, stroke, heart attack, and even death. These side effects varied among individuals and were not directly related to the amount taken. The industry claimed that 30 mg per dose was safe. The government, however, did not recommend more than 8 mg per dose, a maximum of three times per day. The concentration of ephedra in commercially available products ranged from about 1 to 14 mg per suggested dose.

fruits are eaten, the dieter must wait at least 20 minutes before eating other carbohydrate foods. Both of these diets allow consumption of high-protein/high-fat food items, which can increase the risk for heart disease.

If people only would realize that no magic foods will provide all of the necessary nutrients, that a person has to eat a variety of foods to be well-nourished, the diet industry would not be as successful. Most of these diets create a nutritional deficiency, which at times may be fatal.

The reason many of these diets succeed is that they restrict a large number of foods. Thus, people tend to eat less food overall. With the extraordinary variety of foods available to us, it is unrealistic to think that people will adhere to these diets for very long. People eventually get tired of eating the same thing day in and day out and start eating less, leading to weight loss. If they happen to achieve the lower weight but do not make permanent dietary changes, they regain the weight quickly once they go back to their previous eating habits.

A few diets recommend exercise along with caloric restrictions—the best method for weight reduction, of course. People who adhere to these programs will succeed, so the diet has achieved its purpose. Unfortunately, if the people do not change their food selection and activity level permanently, they gain back the weight once they discontinue dieting and exercise.

Also, let's not forget that we eat for pleasure and for health. Two of the most essential components of a wellness lifestyle are healthy eating and regular physical activity, and they provide the best weight-management program available today.

Eating Disorders

Eating disorders are medical illnesses that involve critical disturbances in eating behaviors thought to stem from some combination of environmental pressures. These disorders are characterized by an intense fear of becoming fat, which does not disappear even when losing extreme amounts of weight. The two most common types of eating disorders are **anorexia nervosa** and bulimia nervosa. A third condition, binge-eating disorder, also known as compulsive overeating, is also recognized as an eating disorder.

Most people who have eating disorders are afflicted by significant family and social problems. They may lack fulfillment in many areas of their lives. The eating disorder then becomes the coping mechanism to avoid dealing with these problems. Taking control over their own body weight helps them feel that they are restoring some sense of control over their lives.

Anorexia nervosa and bulimia nervosa are common in industrialized nations where society encourages low-calorie diets and thinness. The female role in society is changing rapidly, which makes women more susceptible to eating disorders. Although frequently seen in young women, the majority seeking treatment are between the ages of 25 and 50. Surveys, nonetheless, indicate that as many as 40 percent of college-age women are struggling with an eating disorder.

Eating disorders are not limited to women. Every one in 10 cases exists in men. But because the role of men in society and their body image are viewed differently, these cases often go unreported.

Although genetics may play a role in the development of eating disorders, most cases are environmentally related. Individuals who have clinical depression and obsessive compulsive behavior are more susceptible. About half of all people with eating disorders have some sort of chemical dependency (alcohol and drugs), and a majority of them come

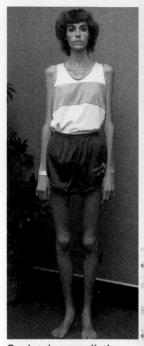

Society's unrealistic view of what constitutes recommended weight and "ideal" body image contributes to the development of eating disorders.

from families with alcohol and drug-related problems. Of reported cases of eating disorders, a large number are individuals who are, or have been, victims of sexual molestation.

Eating disorders develop in stages. Typically, individuals who are already dealing with significant issues in life start a diet. At first they feel in control and are happy about the weight loss even if they are not overweight. Encouraged by the prospect of weight loss and the control they can exert over their own weight, the dieting becomes extreme and often is combined with exhaustive exercise and the overuse of laxatives and diuretics.

Although a genetic predisposition may contribute, the syndrome typically emerges following emotional issues or a stressful life event and the uncertainty about the ability to cope efficiently. Life experiences that can trigger the syndrome might be gaining weight, starting the menstrual period, beginning college, losing a boyfriend, having poor self-esteem, being socially rejected, starting a professional career, or becoming a wife or a mother.

The eating disorder now takes on a life of its own and becomes the primary focus of attention for the individuals afflicted with it. Self-worth revolves around what the scale reads every day, their relationship with food, and their perception of how they look each day.

Anorexia Nervosa

An estimated 1 percent of the population in the United States is anorexic. Anorexic individuals seem to fear weight gain more than death from starvation. Furthermore, they have a distorted image of their body and think of themselves as being fat even when they are emaciated.

Anorexics commonly develop obsessive and compulsive behaviors and emphatically deny their condition. They are preoccupied with food, meal planning, and grocery shopping, and they have unusual eating habits. As they lose weight and their health begins to deteriorate, anorexics feel weak and tired. They might realize they have a problem, but they will not stop the starvation and refuse to consider the behavior as abnormal.

Once they have lost a lot of weight and malnutrition sets in, physical changes become more visible. Typical changes are amenorrhea (stopping menstruation), digestive problems, extreme sensitivity to cold, hair and skin problems, fluid and electrolyte abnormalities (which may lead to an irregular heartbeat and sudden stopping of the heart), injuries to nerves and tendons, abnormalities of immune function, anemia, growth of fine body hair, mental confusion, inability to concentrate,

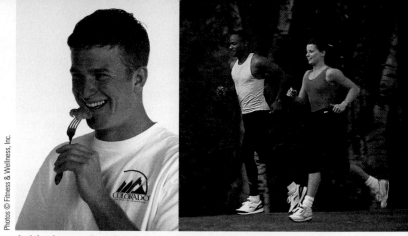

Photos © Fitness & Wellness, Inc.

Achieving and maintaining a high physical fitness percent body fat standard requires a lifetime commitment to regular physical activity and proper nutrition.

lethargy, depression, dry skin, lower skin and body temperature, and osteoporosis.

Diagnostic criteria for anorexia nervosa are:[14]

- Refusal to maintain body weight over a minimal normal weight for age and height (weight loss leading to maintenance of body weight less than 85 percent of that expected or failure to make expected weight gain during periods of growth, leading to body weight less than 85 percent of that expected).
- Intense fear of gaining weight or becoming fat, even though underweight.
- Disturbance in the way in which one's body weight, size, or shape is perceived, undue influences of body weight or shape on self-evaluation, or denial of the seriousness of the current low body weight.
- In postmenarcheal females, amenorrhea (absence of at least three consecutive menstrual cycles). (A woman is considered to have amenorrhea if her periods occur only following estrogen therapy).

Many of the changes induced by anorexia nervosa can be reversed. Individuals with this condition can get better with professional therapy, turn to bulimia nervosa, or die from the disorder. Twenty percent of anorexics die as a result of their condition. Anorexia nervosa has the highest mortality rate of all psychosomatic illnesses today. The disorder, however, is 100 percent curable. But treatment almost always requires professional help, and the sooner it is started, the better are the chances for reversibility and cure.

Therapy consists of a combination of medical and psychological techniques to restore proper nutrition, prevent medical complications, and

Anorexia nervosa An eating disorder characterized by self-imposed starvation to lose and maintain very low body weight.

modify the environment or events that triggered the syndrome.

Seldom can anorexics overcome the problem by themselves. They strongly deny their condition. They are able to hide it and deceive friends and relatives. Based on their behavior, many of them meet all of the characteristics of anorexia nervosa, but it goes undetected because both thinness and dieting are socially acceptable. Only a well-trained clinician is able to diagnose anorexia nervosa.

Bulimia Nervosa

Bulimia nervosa is more prevalent than anorexia nervosa. As many as one in every five women on college campuses may be bulimic, according to some estimates. Bulimia nervosa also is more prevalent than anorexia nervosa in males, although bulimia is still much more prevalent in females.

Bulimics usually are healthy-looking people, well-educated, and near recommended body weight. They seem to enjoy food and often socialize around it. In actuality, they are emotionally insecure, rely on others, and lack self-confidence and self-esteem. Recommended weight and food are important to them.

The binge–purge cycle usually occurs in stages. As a result of stressful life events or the simple compulsion to eat, bulimics engage periodically in binge eating that may last an hour or longer.

With some apprehension, bulimics anticipate and plan the cycle. Next they feel an urgency to begin, followed by large and uncontrollable food consumption, during which they may eat several thousand calories (up to 10,000 calories in extreme cases). After a short period of relief and satisfaction, feelings of deep guilt, shame, and intense fear of gaining weight ensue. Purging seems to be an easy answer, as the binging cycle can continue without fear of gaining weight.

The diagnostic criteria for bulimia nervosa are:[15]

- Recurrent episodes of binge eating. An episode of binge eating is characterized by both of the following:
  — Eating in a discrete period of time (for example, within any 2-hour period), an amount of food that is definitely more than most people would eat during a similar period and under similar circumstances.
  — A sense of lack of control over eating during the episode (a feeling that one cannot stop eating or control what or how much one is eating).
- Recurring inappropriate compensatory behaviors to prevent weight gain, such as self-induced vomiting; misuse of laxatives, diuretics, enemas, or other medications; fasting; or excessive exercise.

- The binge eating and inappropriate compensatory behaviors both occur, on average, at least twice a week for 3 months.
- Self-evaluation is unduly influenced by body shape and weight.

The most typical form of purging is self-induced vomiting. Bulimics, too, frequently ingest strong laxatives and emetics. Near-fasting diets and strenuous bouts of exercise are common. Medical problems associated with bulimia nervosa include cardiac arrhythmias, amenorrhea, kidney and bladder damage, ulcers, colitis, tearing of the esophagus or stomach, tooth erosion, gum damage, and general muscular weakness.

Unlike anorexics, bulimics realize their behavior is abnormal and feel great shame about it. Fearing social rejection, they pursue the binge–purge cycle in secrecy and at unusual hours of the day.

Bulimia nervosa can be treated successfully when the person realizes that this destructive behavior is not the solution to life's problems. A change in attitude can prevent permanent damage or death.

Binge-Eating Disorder

Binge-eating disorder is probably the most common of the three eating disorders. About 2 percent of American adults are afflicted with binge-eating disorder in a 6-month period. Although most people think they overeat from time to time, eating more than one should now and then does not mean the individual has a binge-eating disorder. The disorder is slightly more common in women than in men; three women for every two men have the disorder.

Binge-eating disorder is characterized by uncontrollable episodes of eating excessive amounts of food within a relatively short time. The causes of binge-eating disorder are unknown, although depression, anger, sadness, boredom, and worry can trigger an episode. Unlike bulimics, binge eaters do not purge; thus, most people with this disorder are either overweight or obese. Typical symptoms of binge-eating disorder include:

- Eating what most people think is an unusually large amount of food
- Eating until uncomfortably full
- Eating out of control
- Eating much faster than usual during binge episodes
- Eating alone because of embarrassment of how much food is being consumed
- Feeling disgusted, depressed, or guilty after overeating.

Treatment

Treatment for eating disorders is available on most school campuses through the school's counseling center or the health center. Local hospitals also offer treatment for these conditions. Many communities have support groups, frequently led by professional personnel and often free of charge. All information and the identity of the individual are kept confidential so the person need not fear embarrassment or repercussion when seeking professional help.

Physiology of Weight Loss

Traditional concepts related to weight control have centered on three assumptions:

1. Balancing food intake against output allows a person to achieve recommended weight.
2. All fat people just eat too much.
3. The human body doesn't care how much (or little) fat it stores.

Although these statements contain some truth, they are open to much debate and research. We now know that the causes of obesity are complex, including a combination of genetics, behavior, and lifestyle factors.

Energy-Balancing Equation

The principle embodied in the **energy-balancing equation** is simple: As long as caloric input equals caloric output, the person will not gain or lose weight. If caloric intake exceeds output, the person gains weight; when output exceeds input, the person loses weight. If daily energy requirements could be determined accurately, caloric intake could be balanced against output. This is not always the case, though, because genetic and lifestyle-related individual differences determine the number of calories required to maintain or lose body weight.

Table 5.3 (page 141) offers some general guidelines to determine the estimated energy requirement (EER) in calories per day according to lifestyle patterns. This is only an estimated figure and (as discussed under "Losing Weight the Sound and Sensible Way," pages 138–143) serves only as a starting point from which individual adjustments have to be made.

The total daily energy requirement has three basic components (see Figure 5.4):

1. resting metabolic rate (RMR)
2. the thermic effect of food (TEF)
3. physical activity

The **resting metabolic rate**—the energy requirement to maintain the body's vital processes in the resting state—accounts for approximately

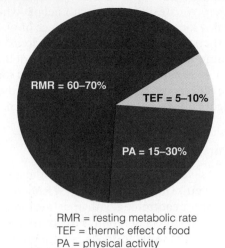

FIGURE 5.4 Components of Total Daily Energy Requirement

RMR = 60–70%
TEF = 5–10%
PA = 15–30%

RMR = resting metabolic rate
TEF = thermic effect of food
PA = physical activity

60 percent to 70 percent of the total daily energy requirement. The thermic effect of food, the energy required to digest, absorb, and store food, accounts for about 5 percent to 10 percent of the total daily requirement. Physical activity accounts for 15 percent to 30 percent of the daily total requirement.

One pound of fat is the equivalent of 3,500 calories. If a person's **estimated energy requirement (EER)** is 2,500 calories and that person were to decrease intake by 500 calories per day, it should result in a loss of 1 pound of fat in 7 days ($500 \times 7 = 3,500$). But research has shown—and many people have experienced—that even when dieters carefully balance caloric input against caloric output, weight loss does not always happen as predicted. Furthermore, two people with similar measured caloric intake and output seldom lose weight at the same rate.

Bulimia nervosa An eating disorder characterized by a pattern of binge eating and purging in an attempt to lose weight and maintain low body weight.

Binge-eating disorder An eating disorder characterized by uncontrollable episodes of eating excessive amounts of food within a relatively short time.

Energy-balancing equation A principle holding that as long as caloric input equals caloric output, the person will not gain or lose weight. If caloric intake exceeds output, the person gains weight; when output exceeds input, the person loses weight.

Resting metabolic rate (RMR) The energy requirement to maintain the body's vital processes in the resting state.

Estimated energy requirement (EER) The average dietary energy (caloric) intake that is predicted to maintain energy balance in a healthy adult of defined age, gender, weight, height, and level of physical activity, consistent with good health.

The most common explanation for individual differences in weight loss and weight gain has been the variation in human metabolism from one person to another. We are all familiar with people who can eat "all day long" and not gain an ounce of weight while others cannot even "dream about food" without gaining weight. Because experts did not believe that human metabolism alone could account for such extreme differences, they developed several theories that might better explain these individual variations.

Setpoint Theory

Results of several research studies point toward a **weight-regulating mechanism (WRM)** that has a **setpoint** for controlling both appetite and the amount of fat stored. Setpoint is hypothesized to work like a thermostat for body fat, maintaining fairly constant body weight, because it "knows" at all times the exact amount of adipose tissue stored in the fat cells. Some people have high settings; others have low settings.

If body weight decreases (as in dieting), the setpoint senses this change and triggers the WRM to increase the person's appetite or make the body conserve energy to maintain the "set" weight. The opposite also may be true. Some people have a hard time gaining weight. In this case, the WRM decreases appetite or causes the body to waste energy to maintain the lower weight.

SETPOINT AND CALORIC INPUT

Every person has his or her own certain body fat percentage (as established by the setpoint) that the body attempts to maintain. The genetic instinct to survive tells the body that fat storage is vital, and therefore it sets an acceptable fat level. This level may remain somewhat constant or may climb gradually because of poor lifestyle habits.

For instance, under strict calorie reduction, the body may make extreme metabolic adjustments in an effort to maintain its setpoint for fat. The **basal metabolic rate (BMR)**, the lowest level of caloric intake necessary to sustain life, may drop dramatically when operating under a consistent negative caloric balance, and that person's weight loss may plateau for days or even weeks. A low metabolic rate compounds a person's problems in maintaining recommended body weight.

These findings were substantiated by research conducted at Rockefeller University in New York.[16] The authors showed that the body resists maintaining altered weight. Obese and lifetime non-obese individuals were used in the investigation. Following a 10 percent weight loss, in an attempt to regain the lost weight, the body compensated by burning up to 15 percent fewer calories than expected for

the new reduced weight (after accounting for the 10 percent loss). The effects were similar in the obese and non-obese participants. These results imply that after a 10 percent weight loss, a person would have to eat even less or exercise even more to compensate for the estimated 15 percent slowdown (a difference of about 200 to 300 calories).

In this same study, when the participants were allowed to increase their weight to 10 percent above their "normal" body (pre-weight loss) weight, the body burned 10 to 15 percent *more* calories than expected—attempting to waste energy and maintain the pre-set weight. This is another indication that the body is highly resistant to weight changes unless additional lifestyle changes are incorporated to ensure successful weight management. (These methods are discussed under "Losing Weight the Sound and Sensible Way," pages 138–143.)

Dietary restriction alone will not lower the setpoint, even though the person may lose weight and fat. When the dieter goes back to the normal or even below-normal caloric intake (at which the weight may have been stable for a long time), he or she quickly regains the lost fat as the body strives to regain a comfortable fat store.

Let's use a practical illustration. A person would like to lose some body fat and assumes that his or her current, stable body weight has been reached at an average daily caloric intake of 1,800 calories (no weight gain or loss occurs at this daily intake). In an attempt to lose weight rapidly, this person now goes on a **very low-calorie diet** (defined as less than 800 calories per day) or, even worse, a near-fasting diet. This immediately activates the body's survival mechanism and re-adjusts the metabolism to a lower caloric balance. After a few weeks of dieting at fewer than 800 calories per day, the body can now maintain its normal functions at 1,300 calories per day. This new figure (1,300) represents a drop of 500 calories per day in the metabolic rate.

Having lost the desired weight, the person terminates the diet, but realizes that the original intake of 1,800 calories per day will have to be lower to maintain the new lower weight. To adjust to the new lower body weight, the person restricts intake to about 1,600 calories per day. The individual is surprised to find that, even at this lower daily intake (200 fewer calories), weight comes back at a rate of 1 pound every 1 to 2 weeks. After the diet is over, this new lowered metabolic rate may take several months to kick back up to its normal level.

CRITICAL THINKING

Is there a difference in the amount of food that you are now able to eat compared with the amount that you ate in your mid- to late-teen years? If so, to what do you attribute these differences? What actions are you taking to account for the difference?

Based on this explanation, individuals clearly should not go on very low-calorie diets. Not only will this slow down resting metabolic rate, but it will also deprive the body of basic daily nutrients required for normal function. Very low-calorie diets should be used only in conjunction with dietary supplements and under proper medical supervision.[17] Furthermore, people who use very low-calorie diets are not as effective in keeping the weight off once the diet is terminated.

Daily caloric intakes of 1,200 to 1,500 calories provide the necessary nutrients if they are distributed properly over the basic food groups (meeting the daily required servings from each group). Of course, the individual will have to learn which foods meet the requirements and yet are low in fat and sugar.

Under no circumstances should a person go on a diet that calls for less than 1,200 calories for women or 1,500 calories for men. Weight (fat) is gained over months and years, not overnight. Likewise, weight loss should be gradual, not abrupt.

A second way in which the setpoint may work is by keeping track of the nutrients and calories consumed daily. It is thought that the body, like a cash register, records the daily food intake and that the brain will not feel satisfied until the calories and nutrients have been "registered."

This setpoint for calories and nutrients seems to operate even when people participate in moderately intense exercise. Some evidence suggests that people do not become hungrier with moderate physical activity. Therefore, people can choose to lose weight either by going hungry or by combining a sensible calorie-restricted diet with an increase in daily physical activity. Burning more calories through physical activity helps to lower body fat.

LOWERING THE SETPOINT

The most common question regarding the setpoint is how it can be lowered so the body will feel comfortable at a reduced fat percentage. These factors seem to affect the setpoint directly by lowering the fat thermostat:

1. Exercise.
2. A diet high in complex carbohydrates.
3. Nicotine.
4. Amphetamines.

The last two are more destructive than the extra fat weight, so they are not reasonable alternatives (as far as the extra strain on the heart is concerned, smoking one pack of cigarettes per day is said to be the equivalent of carrying 50 to 75 pounds of excess body fat).

On the other hand, a diet high in fats and refined carbohydrates, near-fasting diets, and perhaps even artificial sweeteners seem to raise the setpoint. Therefore, the only practical and sensible way to lower the setpoint and lose fat weight is a combination of exercise and a diet high in complex carbohydrates and only moderate amounts of fat.

Because of the effects of proper food management on the body's setpoint, most of the successful dieter's effort should be spent in re-forming eating habits, increasing the intake of complex carbohydrates and high-fiber foods, and decreasing the consumption of processed foods that are high in refined carbohydrates (sugars) and fats. This change in eating habits will bring about a decrease in total daily caloric intake. Because 1 gram of carbohydrates provides only 4 calories, as opposed to 9 calories per gram of fat, you could eat twice the volume of food (by weight) when substituting carbohydrates for fat. Some fat, however, is recommended in the diet. Preferably use polyunsaturated and monounsaturated fats. These so called good fats do more than help protect the heart; they help delay hunger pangs.

A "diet" should not be viewed as a temporary tool to aid in weight loss but, instead, as a permanent change in eating behaviors to ensure weight management and better health. The role of increased physical activity also must be considered, because successful weight loss, maintenance, and recommended body composition seldom are attained without a moderate reduction in caloric intake combined with a regular exercise program.

Diet and Metabolism

Fat can be lost by selecting the proper foods, exercising, or restricting calories. When a person tries to lose weight by dietary restrictions alone, lean body mass (muscle protein, along with vital organ protein) always decreases. The amount of lean body mass lost depends entirely on caloric limitation.

When people go on a near-fasting diet, up to half of the weight loss is lean body mass and the other half is actual fat loss (see Figure 5.5).[18] When diet is combined with exercise, close to 100 percent of the weight loss is in the form of fat, and lean

Weight-regulating mechanism (WRM) A feature of the hypothalamus of the brain that controls how much the body should weigh.

Setpoint Weight control theory that the body has an established weight and strongly attempts to maintain that weight.

Basal metabolic rate (BMR) The lowest level of oxygen consumption necessary to sustain life.

Very low-calorie diet A diet that only allows an energy intake (consumption) of 800 or less calories per day.

FIGURE 5.5 Outcome of three forms of diet on fat loss.

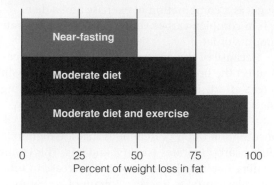

Adapted from R. J. Shephard, *Alive Man: The Physiology of Physical Activity.* (Springfield, IL: Charles C. Thomas, 1975): 484–488.

FIGURE 5.6 Body composition changes as a result of frequent dieting without exercise.

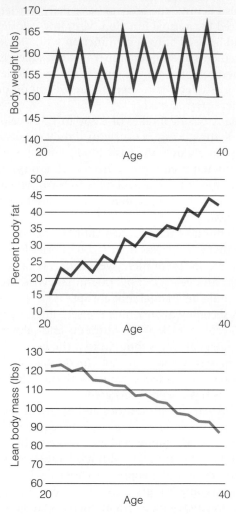

tissue actually may increase. Loss of lean body mass is never good, because it weakens the organs and muscles and slows metabolism. Large losses in lean tissue can cause disturbances in heart function and damage to other organs. Equally important is not to overindulge (binge) following a very low-calorie diet as this may cause changes in metabolic rate and electrolyte balance, which could trigger fatal cardiac arrhythmias.

Contrary to some beliefs, aging is not the main reason for the lower metabolic rate. It is not so much that metabolism slows down as that people slow down. As people age, they tend to rely more on the amenities of life (remote controls, cell telephones, intercoms, single-level homes, riding lawnmowers) that lull a person into sedentary living.

Basal metabolism is related directly to lean body weight. The more lean tissue, the higher is the metabolic rate. As a consequence of sedentary living and less physical activity, the lean component decreases and fat tissue increases. The human body requires a certain amount of oxygen per pound of lean body mass. Given that fat is considered metabolically inert from the point of view of caloric use, the lean tissue uses most of the oxygen, even at rest. As muscle and organ mass (lean body mass) decrease, so do the energy requirements at rest.

Diets with caloric intakes below 1,200 to 1,500 calories cannot guarantee the retention of lean body mass. Even at this intake level, some loss is inevitable, unless the diet is combined with exercise. Despite the claims of many diets that they do not alter the lean component, the simple truth is that, regardless of what nutrients may be added to the diet, severe

caloric restrictions always prompt the loss of lean tissue. Too many people go on very low-calorie diets constantly. Every time they do, their metabolic rate slows down as more lean tissue is lost.

People in their 40s and older who weigh the same as they did when they were 20 tend to think they are at recommended body weight. During this span of 20 years or more, they may have dieted many times without participating in an exercise program. After they terminate each diet, they regain the weight, and much of that gain is additional body fat. Maybe at age 20 they weighed 150 pounds, of which only 15 percent was fat. Now at age 40, even though they still weigh 150 pounds, they might be 30 percent fat (see Figure 5.6). At recommended body weight, they wonder why they are eating very little and still having trouble staying at that weight.

Exercise: The Key to Weight Management

A more effective way to tilt the energy-balancing equation in your favor is by burning calories through physical activity. Research shows that the combination of diet and exercise leads to greater weight loss. Further, maintenance of exercise appears to be the best predictor of long-term weight loss maintenance.[19]

Exercise seems to exert control over how much a person weighs. On the average, starting at age 25, the typical American gains 1 to 2 pounds of weight per year. A 1 pound weight gain represents a simple energy surplus of under 10 calories per day. The additional weight accumulated in middle age comes from people becoming less physically active and increasing caloric intake. Dr. Jack Wilmore, a leading exercise physiologist and expert weight management researcher, stated:

> Physical inactivity is certainly a major, if not the primary, cause of obesity in the United States today. A certain minimal level of activity might be necessary for us to accurately balance our caloric intake to our caloric expenditure. With too little activity, we appear to lose the fine control we normally have to maintain this incredible balance. This fine balance amounts to less than 10 calories per day, or the equivalent of one potato chip.[20]

Exercise enhances the rate of weight loss and is vital in maintaining the weight loss. Not only will exercise maintain lean tissue, but advocates of the setpoint theory say that exercise resets the fat thermostat to a new, lower level. This change may be rapid, or it may take time. Although a few individuals lose weight by participating in 30 minutes of exercise per day, many overweight people need 60 minutes of daily exercise to see significant weight loss. People with a "sticky" setpoint have to be patient and persistent.

If a person is trying to lose weight, a combination of aerobic and strength-training exercises works best. Aerobic exercise is the best to offset the setpoint, and the continuity and duration of these types of activities cause many calories to be burned in the process. The role of aerobic exercise in successful lifetime weight management cannot be overestimated. Strength training is critical in helping maintain lean body mass. Unfortunately, of those individuals who are attempting to lose weight, only 19 percent of women and 22 percent of men decrease their caloric intake and exercise above an average of 25 or more minutes per day.[21]

As illustrated in Figure 5.7, greater weight loss is achieved by combining a diet with an exercise program. Of even greater significance, only the individuals who remain physically active for 60 minutes

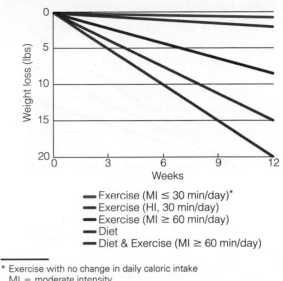

FIGURE 5.7 The roles of diet and exercise in weight loss.

Weeks

— Exercise (MI ≤ 30 min/day)*
— Exercise (HI, 30 min/day)
— Exercise (MI ≥ 60 min/day)
— Diet
— Diet & Exercise (MI ≥ 60 min/day)

* Exercise with no change in daily caloric intake
  MI = moderate intensity
  HI = high intensity
Diet: 1,200–1,500 calories/day   © Fitness & Wellness, Inc.

Based on data from American College of Sports Medicine, "Position Stand: Appropriate Intervention Strategies for Weight Loss and Prevention for Weight Regain for Adults," *Medicine and Science in Sports and Exercise* 33 (2001): 2145–2156.

or longer per day are able to keep the weight off[22] (see Figure 5.8). Those who are active for less than 60 minutes per day gradually regain lost weight, whereas individuals who completely stop physical activity regain almost 100 percent of the lost weight within 18 months of discontinuing the weight loss program. Thus, it appears that only those who remain physically active for about an hour per day are able to successfully maintain weight loss.

Weight loss might be more rapid when aerobic exercise is combined with a strength-training program. Each additional pound of muscle tissue may raise the basal metabolic rate by as many as 35 calories per day.[23] Thus, an individual who adds 5 pounds of muscle tissue as a result of strength training could increase the basal metabolic rate by 175 calories per day (35 × 5), which burns up the equivalent of 63,875 calories per year (175 × 365) eliminating the equivalent of 18.25 pounds of fat (63,875 ÷ 3,500).

Strength training is suggested especially for people who think they are at their recommended body weight, yet their body fat percentage is higher than recommended. The number of calories burned during a typical hour-long strength-training session is much less than during an hour of aerobic exercise. Because of the high intensity of strength training,

FIGURE 5.8 Effects of different amounts of daily energy expenditure on weight maintenance following a weight reduction program.

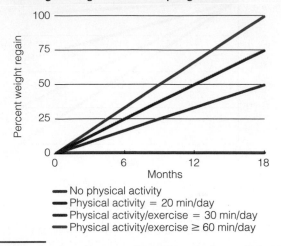

No physical activity
Physical activity = 20 min/day
Physical activity/exercise = 30 min/day
Physical activity/exercise ≥ 60 min/day

Based on data from American College of Sports Medicine, "Position Stand: Appropriate Intervention Strategies for Weight Loss and Prevention for Weight Regain for Adults," *Medicine and Science in Sports and Exercise* 33 (2001): 2145–2156.

the person needs frequent rest intervals to recover from each set of exercises. The average person actually lifts weights only 10 to 12 minutes during each hour of exercise. In the long run, however, the person enjoys the benefits of gains in lean tissue. Guidelines for developing aerobic and strength-training programs are given in Chapters 7 and 8.

Although size (inches) and percent body fat both decrease when sedentary individuals begin an exercise program, body weight often remains the same or may even increase during the first couple of weeks of the program. Exercise helps to increase muscle tissue, connective tissue, blood volume (as much as 500 ml, or the equivalent of 1 pound, following the first week of aerobic exercise), enzymes and other structures within the cell, and glycogen (which binds water). All of these changes lead to a higher functional capacity of the human body. With exercise, most of the weight loss becomes apparent after a few weeks of training, when the lean component has stabilized.

Although we know that a negative caloric balance of 3,500 calories does not always result in a loss of exactly 1 pound of fat, the role of exercise in achieving a negative balance by burning additional calories is significant in weight reduction and maintenance programs. Sadly, some individuals claim that the number of calories burned during exercise is hardly worth the effort. They think that cutting their daily intake by some 300 calories is easier than participating in some sort of exercise that would

burn the same amount of calories. The problem is that the willpower to cut those 300 calories lasts only a few weeks, and then the person goes right back to the old eating patterns.

If a person gets into the habit of exercising regularly, say 3 times a week, jogging 3 miles per exercise session (about 300 calories burned), this represents 900 calories in 1 week, about 3,600 calories in one month, or 46,800 calories per year. This minimal amount of exercise represents as many as 13.5 extra pounds of fat in one year, 27 in two, and so on.

We tend to forget that our weight creeps up gradually over the years, not just overnight. Hardly worth the effort? And we have not even taken into consideration the increase in lean tissue, possible resetting of the setpoint, benefits to the cardiovascular system, and, most important, the improved quality of life. The fundamental reasons for over-fatness and obesity, few could argue, are sedentary living and lack of a regular exercise program.

In terms of preventing disease, many of the health benefits people try to achieve by losing weight are reaped through exercise alone, even without weight loss. Exercise offers protection against premature morbidity and mortality for everyone, including people who already have risk factors for disease.

Low-Intensity Versus High-Intensity Exercise for Weight Loss

Some individuals promote low-intensity exercise over high-intensity for weight loss purposes. Compared with high intensity, a greater proportion of calories burned during low-intensity exercise are derived from fat. The lower the intensity of exercise, the higher the percentage of fat utilization as an energy source. In theory, if you are trying to lose fat, this principle makes sense, but in reality it is misleading. The bottom line when you are trying to lose weight is to burn more calories. When your daily caloric expenditure exceeds your intake, weight is lost. The more calories you burn, the more fat is lost.

During low-intensity exercise, up to 50 percent of the calories burned may be derived from fat (the other 50 percent from glucose [carbohydrates]). With intense exercise, only 30 to 40 percent of the caloric expenditure comes from fat. Overall, however, you can burn twice as many calories during high-intensity exercise and, subsequently, more fat as well.

Let's look at a practical illustration (also see Table 5.2). If you exercise for 30–40 minutes at moderate intensity and burn 200 calories, about

TABLE 5.2 Comparison of Energy Expenditure Between 30–40 Minutes of Low-Intensity vs. High-Intensity Exercise

Exercise Intensity	Total Energy Expenditure (Calories)	Percent Calories From Fat	Total Fat Calories	Percent Calories From CHO	Total CHO Calories	Calories Burned Per Minute	Calories Per Pound Per Minute
Low Intensity	200	50%	100	50%	100	6.67	0.045
High Intensity	400	30%	120	70%	280	13.5	0.090

* CHO = Carbohydrates

100 of those calories (50 percent) would come from fat. If you exercise at high intensity during those same 30–40 minutes, you can burn 400 calories with 120 to 160 of the calories (30 to 40 percent) coming from fat. Thus, even though it is true that the percentage of fat used is greater during low-intensity exercise, the overall amount of fat used is still less during low-intensity exercise. Plus, if you were to exercise at a low intensity, you would have to do so twice as long to burn the same amount of calories. Another benefit is that the metabolic rate remains at a slightly higher level longer after high-intensity exercise, so you continue to burn a few extra calories following exercise.

Moreover, high-intensity exercise by itself appears to trigger greater fat loss than low-intensity exercise. Research conducted at Laval University in Quebec, Canada, showed that subjects who performed a high-intensity intermittent-training program lost more body fat than participants in a low- to moderate-intensity continuous aerobic endurance group.[24] Even more surprisingly, this finding occurred despite the fact that the high-intensity group burned fewer total calories per exercise session. The results support the notion that vigorous exercise is more conducive to weight loss than low- to moderate-intensity exercise.

Before you start high-intensity exercise sessions, a word of caution is in order: Be sure that it is medically safe for you to participate in such activities and that you build up gradually to that level. If you are cleared to participate in high-intensity exercise, do not attempt to do too much too quickly, because you may incur injuries and become discouraged. You must allow your body a proper conditioning period of 8 to 12 weeks, or even longer for people with a moderate-to-serious weight problem. High intensity also does not mean high impact. High-impact activities are the most common cause of exercise-related injuries. Additional information on these topics is presented in Chapter 6.

The previous discussion on high- versus low-intensity exercise does not mean that low intensity is ineffective. Low-intensity exercise provides substantial health benefits, and people who initiate exercise programs are more willing to participate and stay with low-intensity programs. Low-intensity exercise does promote weight loss, but it is not as effective. You will need to exercise longer to obtain the same results.

Healthy Weight Gain

"Skinny" people, too, should realize that the only healthy way to gain weight is through exercise (mainly strength-training exercises) and a slight increase in caloric intake. Attempting to gain weight just by overeating will raise the fat component and not the lean component—which is not the path to better health. Exercise is the best solution to weight (fat) reduction and weight (lean) gain alike.

A strength-training program such as the one outlined in Chapter 7 is the best approach to add body weight. The training program should include at least two exercises of three sets for each major body part. Each set should consist of about 8 to 12 repetitions maximum.

Even though the metabolic cost of synthesizing a pound of muscle tissue is still unclear, consuming an estimated 500 additional calories per day is recommended to gain an average of 1 pound of muscle tissue per week. Your diet should include a daily total intake of about 1.5 grams of protein per kilogram of body weight. If your daily protein intake already exceeds 1.5 grams per day, the extra 500 calories should be primarily in the form of complex carbohydrates. The higher caloric intake must be accompanied by a strength-training program, otherwise, the increase in body weight will be in the form of fat, not muscle tissue.

Strength Training, Diet, and Muscle Mass

The time of day when carbohydrates and protein are consumed in relation to the strength-training workout also plays a role in promoting muscle growth. Studies suggest that consuming a pre-exercise snack consisting of a combination of carbohydrates and protein is beneficial to muscle development. The carbohydrates supply energy for training, and the availability of amino acids (the building blocks of protein) in the blood during training enhances the muscle building process. A peanut butter, turkey, or tuna fish sandwich; milk or yogurt and fruit; or nuts and fruit consumed 30 to 60 minutes before training are excellent choices for a pre-workout snack.

The consumption of a carbohydrate/protein snack immediately following strength training, as well as an hour thereafter, further promotes muscle growth and strength development. Post-exercise carbohydrates help restore muscle glycogen depleted during training, and, in combination with protein, induce an increase in blood insulin and growth hormone levels. These hormones are essential to the muscle-building process.

Muscle fibers also absorb a greater amount of amino acids up to 48 hours following strength-training. The first hour, nonetheless, seems to be the most critical. A higher level of circulating amino acids in the bloodstream immediately after training is believed to increase protein synthesis to a greater extent than amino acids made available later in the day. A ratio of 3-to-1 grams of carbohydrates to protein is recommended for a post-exercise snack.

Weight-Loss Myths

Cellulite and **spot reducing** are mythical concepts. **Cellulite** is nothing but enlarged fat cells that bulge out from accumulated body fat.

Doing several sets of daily sit-ups will not get rid of fat in the midsection of the body. When fat comes off, it does so throughout the entire body, not just the exercised area. The greatest proportion of fat may come off the biggest fat deposits, but the caloric output of a few sets of sit-ups has practically no effect on reducing total body fat. A person has to exercise much longer to really see results.

Other touted means toward quick weight loss, such as rubberized sweatsuits, steam baths, and mechanical vibrators, are misleading. When a person wears a sweatsuit or steps into a sauna, the weight lost is not fat, but merely a significant amount of water. Sure, it looks nice when you step on the scale immediately afterward, but this represents a false loss of weight. As soon as you replace body fluids, you gain back the weight quickly.

Wearing rubberized sweatsuits hastens the rate of body fluid that is lost—fluid that is vital during prolonged exercise—and raises core temperature at the same time. This combination puts a person in danger of dehydration, which impairs cellular function and, in extreme cases, can even cause death.

Similarly, mechanical vibrators are worthless in a weight-control program. Vibrating belts and turning rollers may feel good, but they require no effort whatsoever. Fat cannot be shaken off. It is lost primarily by burning it in muscle tissue.

Losing Weight the Sound and Sensible Way

Dieting never has been fun and never will be. People who are overweight and are serious about losing weight, however, have to include regular exercise in their lives along with proper food management and a sensible reduction in caloric intake.

Because excessive body fat is a risk factor for cardiovascular disease, some precautions are in order. Depending on the extent of the weight problem, a medical examination, and possibly a stress ECG (see "Abnormal Electrocardiograms" in Chapter 11), may be a good idea before undertaking the exercise program. A physician should be consulted in this regard.

Significantly overweight individuals may have to choose activities in which they will not have to support their own body weight but that still will be effective in burning calories. Injuries to joints and muscles are common in excessively overweight individuals who participate in weight-bearing exercises such as walking, jogging, and aerobics.

Swimming may not be a good weight loss exercise either. More body fat makes a person more buoyant, and many people are not at the skill level required to swim fast enough to get the best training effect; thus limiting the number of calories burned as well as the benefits to the cardiorespiratory system.

Better alternatives during the initial stages of exercise include riding a bicycle (either road or stationary), walking in a shallow pool, doing water aerobics, or running in place in deep water (treading water). The latter forms of water exercise are gaining popularity and have proven to be effective in reducing weight without fear of injuries.

How long should each exercise session last? The amount of exercise for successful weight loss and weight loss maintenance is different from the amount for improving fitness. For health fitness, accumulating 30 minutes of physical activity on most days of the week is recommended. To develop

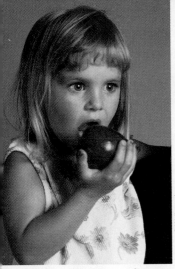

Establishing healthy eating patterns should start at a young age.

© Fitness & Wellness, Inc.

and maintain cardiorespiratory fitness, 20 to 30 minutes of exercise at the recommended target rate, three to five times per week, is suggested (see Chapter 6). For successful weight loss, however, 60 minutes of physical activity 5 to 6 times a week is recommended.

A person should not try to do too much too fast. Unconditioned beginners should start with about 15 minutes of aerobic activity 3 times a week, and during the next 3 to 4 weeks gradually increase the duration by approximately 5 minutes per week and the frequency by 1 day per week.

One final benefit of long-duration exercise for weight control is that it allows fat to be burned more efficiently. Carbohydrates and fats are both sources of energy. When the glucose levels begin to drop during prolonged exercise, more fat is used as energy substrate.

Equally important is that fat-burning enzymes increase with aerobic training. Fat is lost primarily by burning it in muscle. Therefore, as the concentration of the enzymes increases, so does the ability to burn fat.

In addition to exercise and adequate food management, a sensible reduction in caloric intake, and careful monitoring of this intake, are recommended. Most research finds that a negative caloric balance is required to lose weight because:

1. Most people underestimate their caloric intake and are eating more than they should be eating.
2. Developing new behaviors takes time, and most people have trouble changing and adjusting to new eating habits.
3. Many individuals are in such poor physical condition that they take a long time to increase their activity level enough to offset the setpoint and burn enough calories to aid in loss of body fat.
4. Most successful dieters carefully monitor their daily caloric intake.
5. A few people simply will not alter their food selection. For those who will not (which will still increase their risk for chronic diseases), the only solution to lose weight successfully is a large increase in physical activity, a negative caloric balance, or a combination of the two.

Perhaps the only exception to a decrease in caloric intake for weight loss purposes occurs in people who already are eating too few calories. A nutrient analysis (see Chapter 3) often reveals that long-term dieters are not consuming enough calories. These people actually need to increase their daily caloric intake and combine that with an exercise program to get their metabolism to kick back up to a normal level.

You must also learn to make wise food choices. Think in terms of long-term benefits (weight management) as opposed to instant gratification (unhealthy eating and subsequent weight gain). Making healthful choices allows you to eat a greater amount of food, more nutritious food, and ingest fewer calories. For example, instead of eating a high-fat, 700-calorie scone, you could eat as much as 1 orange, 1 cup of grapes, a hard-boiled egg, 2 slices of whole-wheat toast, 2 teaspoons of jam, 1/2 cup of honey-sweetened oatmeal, and 1 glass of skim milk (see Figure 5.9).

You can estimate your daily energy (caloric) requirement by consulting Tables 5.3 and 5.4 and completing Lab 5A. Given that this is only an estimated value, individual adjustments related to many of the factors discussed in this chapter may be necessary to establish a more precise value. Nevertheless, the estimated value does offer a beginning guideline for weight control or reduction.

The estimated energy requirement without exercise is based on typical lifestyle patterns, total body weight, and gender. Individuals who hold jobs that require heavy manual labor burn more calories during the day than those who have sedentary jobs (such as working behind a desk). To find your activity level, refer to Table 5.3 and rate yourself accordingly. The number given in Table 5.3 is per pound of body weight, so you multiply your current weight by that number. For example, the estimated energy requirement to maintain body weight for a moderately active male who weighs 160 pounds is 2,400 calories (160 lbs × 15 cal/lb).

To determine the average number of calories you burn daily as a result of exercise, figure out the total number of minutes you exercise weekly, then figure the daily average exercise time. For instance, a person cycling at 10 miles per hour five times a week, 60 minutes each time, exercises 300 minutes per week (5 × 60). The average daily exercise time is therefore 42 minutes (300 ÷ 7, rounded off to the lowest unit).

Next, from Table 5.4, find the energy expenditure for the activity (or activities) chosen for the

Spot reducing Fallacious theory that exercising a specific body part will result in significant fat reduction in that area.

Cellulite Term frequently used in reference to fat deposits that "bulge out"; these deposits are nothing but enlarged fat cells from excessive accumulation of body fat.

FIGURE 5.9 Making wise food choices.

These illustrations provide a comparison of how much more food you can eat when you make healthy choices. You also get more vitamins, minerals, phytochemicals, antioxidants, and fiber by making healthy choices.

Breakfast

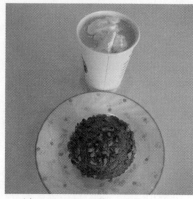

1 banana nut muffin, 1 cafe mocha
Calories: 940
Percent fat calories: 48%

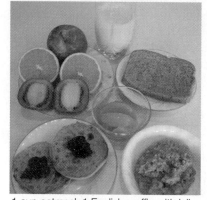

1 cup oatmeal, 1 English muffin with jelly,
1 slice whole wheat bread with honey,
½ cup peaches, 1 kiwi fruit, 1 orange,
1 apple, 1 cup skim milk
Calories: 900
Percent fat calories: 5%

Lunch

1 double-decker cheeseburger, 1 serving
medium French fries, 2 chocolate chip
cookies, 1 medium strawberry milkshake
Calories: 1790
Percent fat calories: 37%

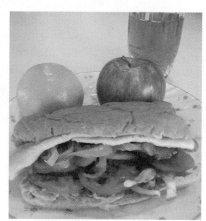

6-inch turkey breast/vegetable sandwich,
1 apple, 1 orange,
1 cup sweetened green tea
Calories: 500
Percent fat calories: 10%

Dinner

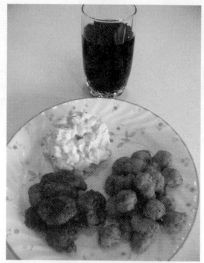

6 oz. popcorn chicken, 3 oz. barbecue
chicken wings, 1 cup potato salad,
1 12-oz. cola drink
Calories: 1250
Percent fat calories: 42%

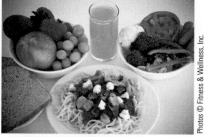

2 cups spaghetti with tomato sauce
and vegetables, a 2-cup salad bowl
with two tablespoons Italian dressing,
2 slices whole wheat bread, 1 cup
grapes, 3 large strawberries, 1 kiwi fruit,
1 peach, 1 12-oz fruit juice drink
Calories: 1240
Percent fat calories: 14%

exercise program. In the case of cycling (10 miles per hour), the expenditure is .05 calories per pound of body weight per minute of activity (cal/lb/min). With a body weight of 160 pounds, this man would burn 8 calories each minute (body weight × .05, or 160 × .05). In 42 minutes he burns approximately 336 calories (42 × 8).

Now you can obtain the daily energy requirement, with exercise, needed to maintain body weight. To do this, add the estimated energy requirement (without exercise) obtained from Table 5.3 and the average calories burned through exercise. In our example, it is 2,736 calories (2,400 + 336).

If a negative caloric balance is recommended to lose weight, this person has to consume fewer than 2,736 calories daily to achieve the objective. Because of the many factors that play a role in weight control, this 2,736-calorie value is only an estimated daily

TABLE 5.3 Estimated Energy Requirement (EER) per Pound of Body Weight Based on Lifestyle Patterns and Gender

	Calories Per Pound	
	Men	Women*
Sedentary—limited physical activity	13.0	12.0
Moderate physical activity	15.0	13.5
Hard labor—strenuous physical effort	17.0	15.0

* Pregnant or lactating women add 3 calories to these values.

TABLE 5.4 Caloric Expenditure of Selected Physical Activities

Activity*	Cal/lb/min	Activity*	Cal/lb/min
Aerobics		7.0 min/mile	0.102
Moderate	0.065	6.0 min/mile	0.114
Vigorous	0.095	Deep water**	0.100
Step aerobics	0.070	Skating (moderate)	0.038
Archery	0.030	Skiing	
Badminton		Downhill	0.060
Recreation	0.038	Level (5 mph)	0.078
Competition	0.065	Soccer	0.059
Baseball	0.031	Stairmaster	
Basketball		Moderate	0.070
Moderate	0.046	Vigorous	0.090
Competition	0.063	Stationary Cycling	
Bowling	0.030	Moderate	0.055
Calisthenics	0.033	Vigorous	0.070
Cycling (on a level surface)		Strength Training	0.050
5.5 mph	0.033	Swimming (crawl)	
10.0 mph	0.050	20 yds/min	0.031
13.0 mph	0.071	25 yds/min	0.040
Dance		45 yds/min	0.057
Moderate	0.030	50 yds/min	0.070
Vigorous	0.055	Table Tennis	0.030
Golf	0.030	Tennis	
Gymnastics		Moderate	0.045
Light	0.030	Competition	0.064
Heavy	0.056	Volleyball	0.030
Handball	0.064	Walking	
Hiking	0.040	4.5 mph	0.045
Judo/Karate	0.086	Shallow pool	0.090
Racquetball	0.065	Water Aerobics	
Rope Jumping	0.060	Moderate	0.050
Rowing (vigorous)	0.090	Vigorous	0.070
Running (on a level surface)		Wrestling	0.085
11.0 min/mile	0.070		
8.5 min/mile	0.090		

*Values are for actual time engaged in the activity.
**Treading water

Adapted from:
P. E. Allsen, J. M. Harrison, and B. Vance, *Fitness for Life: An Individualized Approach* (Dubuque, IA: Wm. C. Brown, 1989).
C. A. Bucher and W. E. Prentice, *Fitness for College and Life* (St. Louis: Times Mirror/Mosby College Publishing, 1989).
C. F. Consolazio, R. E. Johnson, and L. J. Pecora, *Physiological Measurements of Metabolic Functions in Man* (New York: McGraw-Hill, 1963).
R. V. Hockey, *Physical Fitness: The Pathway to Healthful Living* (St. Louis: Times Mirror/Mosby College Publishing, 1989).
W. W. K. Hoeger et al., Research conducted at Boise State University, 1986–1993.

requirement. Furthermore, we cannot predict that you will lose exactly 1 pound of fat in 1 week if you cut your daily intake by 500 calories (500 × 7 = 3,500 calories, or the equivalent of 1 pound of fat).

The daily energy requirement figure is only a target guideline for weight control. Periodic re-adjustments are necessary because individuals differ, and the daily requirement changes as you lose weight and modify your exercise habits.

To determine the target caloric intake to lose weight, multiply your current weight by 5 and subtract this amount from the total daily energy requirement (2,736 in our example) with exercise. For our moderately active male example, this would mean 1,936 calories per day to lose weight (160 × 5 = 800 and 2,736 − 800 = 1,936 calories).

This final caloric intake to lose weight should never be below 1,200 calories for women and 1,500 for men. If distributed properly over the various food groups, these figures are the lowest caloric intakes that provide the necessary nutrients the body needs. In terms of percentages of total calories, the daily distribution should be approximately 60 percent carbohydrates (mostly complex carbohydrates), less than 30 percent fat, and about 12 percent protein.

Many experts believe that a person can take off weight more efficiently by reducing the amount of daily fat intake to about 20 percent of the total daily caloric intake. Because 1 gram of fat supplies more than twice the amount of calories that carbohydrates and protein do, the general tendency when someone eats less fat is to consume fewer calories. With fat intake at 20 percent of total calories, the individual will have sufficient fat in the diet to feel satisfied and avoid frequent hunger pangs.

Further, it takes only 3 to 5 percent of ingested calories to store fat as fat, whereas it takes approximately 25 percent of ingested calories to convert carbohydrates to fat. Some evidence indicates that if people eat the same number of calories as carbohydrate or as fat, those on the fat diet will store more fat. Long-term successful weight-loss and weight-management programs are low in fat content.

TABLE 5.5 Grams of Fat at 10%, 20%, and 30% of Total Calories for Selected Energy Intakes

Caloric Intake	Grams of Fat		
	10%	20%	30%
1,200	13	27	40
1,300	14	29	43
1,400	16	31	47
1,500	17	33	50
1,600	18	36	53
1,700	19	38	57
1,800	20	40	60
1,900	21	42	63
2,000	22	44	67
2,100	23	47	70
2,200	24	49	73
2,300	26	51	77
2,400	27	53	80
2,500	28	56	83
2,600	29	58	87
2,700	30	60	90
2,800	31	62	93
2,900	32	64	97
3,000	33	67	100

Many people have trouble adhering to a low-fat-calorie diet. During times of weight loss, however, you are strongly encouraged to do so. Refer to Table 5.5 to aid you in determining the grams of fat at 20 percent of the total calories for selected energy intakes. Also, use the form provided in Lab 3B (Chapter 3, page 98) to monitor your daily fat intake. For weight maintenance, data from the National Weight Control Registry shows that individuals who have been successful in maintaining an average weight loss of 30 pounds for more than 5 years are consuming about 24 percent of calories from fat, 56 percent from carbohydrates, and 20 percent from protein.[25]

The time of day when food is consumed also may play a part in weight reduction. When a person is attempting to lose weight, intake should consist of a minimum of 25 percent of the total daily calories for breakfast, 50 percent for lunch, and 25 percent or less at dinner. Breakfast, in particular, is a critical meal. Many people skip breakfast because it's the easiest meal to skip. Evidence, however, indicates that people who skip breakfast are hungrier later in the day and end up consuming more total daily calories than those who eat breakfast. Furthermore, regular breakfast eaters have less of a weight problem, lose weight more effectively, and have less difficulty maintaining lost weight.

BEHAVIOR MODIFICATION PLANNING

CALCIUM AND WEIGHT MAINTENANCE

Eating calcium-rich foods—especially from dairy products—may help control or reduce body weight. Individuals with a high calcium intake gain less weight and body fat than those with a lower intake. Women on low-calcium diets more than double the risk of becoming overweight.

These data indicate that even in the absence of caloric restriction, obese people with high dietary calcium intake (the equivalent of 3 to 4 cups of milk per day) lose body fat and weight. Furthermore, dieters who consume calcium-rich dairy foods lose more fat and less lean body mass than those who consume less dairy products. Researchers believe that

- calcium regulates fat storage inside the cell.
- calcium helps the body break down fat or cause fat cells to produce less fat.
- high calcium intake converts more calories into heat rather than fat.
- adequate calcium intake contributes to a decrease in intra-abdominal (visceral) fat.

The data also seem to indicate that calcium from dairy sources is more effective in attenuating weight and fat gain and accelerating fat loss than calcium obtained from other sources. Most likely, other nutrients found in dairy products may enhance the weight-regulating action of calcium.

Although additional research is needed, the best recommendation at this point is that if you are attempting to lose or maintain weight loss, do not eliminate dairy foods from your diet. Substitute nonfat (skim milk) or low-fat dairy products for other drinks and foods in your diet to help you manage weight and total daily caloric intake.

Sources: M. B. Zemel. *Role of Dietary Calcium and Dairy Products in Modulating Adiposity.* Lipids 38 (2): 139–146, 2003.

A Nice Surprise from Calcium. *University of California Berkeley Wellness Letter*, 19, no. 11 (August 2003): 1.

If most of the daily calories are consumed during one meal (as in the typical evening meal), the body may perceive that something is wrong and will slow down the metabolism so it can store more calories in the form of fat. Also, eating most of the calories during one meal causes a person to go hungry the rest of the day, making it more difficult to adhere to the diet.

Consuming most of the calories earlier in the day seems helpful in losing weight and also in managing atherosclerosis. The time of day when most of the fats and cholesterol are consumed can influence blood lipids and coronary heart disease. Peak digestion time following a heavy meal is about 7 hours after that meal. If most lipids are consumed during the evening meal, digestion peaks while the person is sound asleep, when the metabolism is at its lowest rate. Consequently, the body may not metabolize fats and cholesterol as well, leading to a higher blood lipid count and increasing the risk for atherosclerosis and coronary heart disease.

Before you proceed with the development of a thorough weight-loss program, take a moment to identify, in Section II of Lab 5A, your current stage of change as it pertains to your recommended body weight. If applicable—that is, if you are not at recommended weight—list also the processes and techniques for change that you will use to accomplish your goal. In Section III of this lab, you can outline your exercise program for weight management.

Monitoring Your Diet with Daily Food Logs

To help you monitor and adhere to a weight-loss program, use the daily food logs provided in Lab 5B. If the goal is to maintain or increase body weight, use Lab 5C.

Evidence indicates that people who monitor daily caloric intake are more successful at weight loss than those who don't self-monitor. Before using the forms in Lab 5B, make a master copy for your files so you can make future copies as needed. Guidelines are provided for 1,200-, 1,500-, 1,800-, and 2,000-calorie diet plans. These plans have been developed based on the Food Guide Pyramid and the Dietary Guidelines for Americans to meet the Recommended Dietary Allowances.[26] The objective is to meet (not exceed) the number of servings allowed for each diet plan. Each time you eat a serving of a certain food, record it in the appropriate box.

To lose weight, you should use the diet plan that most closely approximates your target caloric intake. The plan is based on the following caloric allowances for each food group:

- Bread, cereal, rice, and pasta group: 80 calories per serving.
- Fruit group: 60 calories per serving.
- Vegetable group: 25 calories per serving.
- Milk, yogurt, and cheese group (use low-fat products): 120 calories per serving.
- Meat, poultry, fish, dry beans, eggs, and nuts group: Use low-fat (300 calories per serving) frozen entrees or an equivalent amount if you prepare your own main dish (see the following discussion).

As you start your diet plan, pay particular attention to food serving sizes. To find out what counts as one serving, refer to the Food Guide Pyramid (see Figure 3.1, page 51). Take care with cup and glass sizes. A standard cup is 8 ounces, but most glasses nowadays contain between 12 and 16 ounces. If you drink 12 ounces of fruit juice, in essence you are getting two servings of fruit because a standard serving is ¾ cup of juice.

Read food labels carefully to compare the caloric value of the serving listed on the label with the caloric guidelines provided above. Here are some examples:

- One slice of standard white bread has about 80 calories. A plain bagel may have 200 to 350 calories. Although it is low in fat, a 350-calorie bagel is equivalent to almost 4 servings in the bread, cereal, rice, and pasta group.
- The standard serving size listed on the food label for most cereals is 1 cup. As you read the nutrition information, however, you will find that for the same cup of cereal, one type of cereal has 120 calories and another cereal has 200 calories. Because a standard serving in the bread, cereal, rice, and pasta group is 80 calories, the first cereal would be 1½ servings and the second one 2½ servings.
- A medium-size fruit is usually considered to be 1 serving. A large fruit could provide as many as 2 or more servings.
- In the milk, yogurt, and cheese groups, 1 serving represents 120 calories. A cup of whole milk has about 160 calories, compared to a cup of skim milk, which contains 88 calories. A cup of whole milk, therefore, would provide 1⅓ servings in this food group.

Using Low-Fat Entrees

To be more accurate with caloric intake and to simplify meal preparation, use commercially prepared low-fat frozen entrees as the main dish for lunch and dinner meals (only one entree per meal for the 1,200-calorie diet plan see Lab 5B, page 151). Look for entrees that provide about 300 calories and no more than 6 grams of fat per entree. These two entrees can be used as selections for the meat, poultry, fish, dry beans, eggs, and nuts group and will provide most of your daily protein requirement. Along with each entree, supplement the meal with some of your servings from the other food groups. This diet plan has been used successfully in weight loss research programs.[27] If you choose not to use these low-fat entrees, prepare a similar meal using 3 ounces (cooked) of lean meat, poultry, or fish with additional vegetables, rice, or pasta, which will provide 300 calories with fewer than 6 grams of fat per dish.

In your daily logs, be sure to record the precise amount in each serving. You can also run a computerized nutrient analysis to verify your caloric intake and food distribution pattern (percent of total calories from carbohydrate, fat, and protein).

Behavior Modification and Adherence to a Weight Management Program

Achieving and maintaining recommended body composition is by no means impossible, but it does require desire and commitment. If weight management is to become a priority in life, people must realize that they have to transform their behavior to some extent.

Modifying old habits and developing new, positive behaviors take time. Individuals who apply the management techniques provided in the Behavior Modification box (below) are more successful at changing detrimental behavior and adhering to a positive lifetime weight-control program. In developing a retraining program, people are not expected to incorporate all of the strategies given, but should note the ones that apply to them. The form provided in Lab 5D will allow you to evaluate and monitor your own weight management behaviors.

CRITICAL THINKING

What behavioral strategies have you used to properly manage your body weight? How do you think those strategies would work for others?

BEHAVIOR MODIFICATION PLANNING

WEIGHT LOSS STRATEGIES

1. Make a commitment to change. The first necessary ingredient is the desire to modify your behavior. You need to stop precontemplating or contemplating change and get going! You must accept that you have a problem and decide by yourself whether you really want to change. Sincere commitment increases your chances for success.

2. Set realistic goals. The weight problem developed over several years. Similarly, new lifetime eating and exercise habits both take time to develop. A realistic long-term goal will also include short-term objectives that allow for regular evaluation and help maintain motivation and renewed commitment to attain the long-term goal.

3. Incorporate exercise into the program. Choosing enjoyable activities, places, times, equipment, and people to work out with will help you adhere to an exercise program. (See Chapters 6, 7, 8, and 9.)

4. Differentiate hunger and appetite. Hunger is the actual physical need for food. Appetite is a desire for food, usually triggered by factors such as stress, habit, boredom, depression, availability of food, or just the thought of food itself. Developing and sticking to a regular meal pattern will help control hunger.

5. Eat less fat. Each gram of fat provides 9 calories, and protein and carbohydrates provide only 4. In essence, you can eat more food on a low-fat diet because you consume fewer calories with each meal.

6. Pay attention to calories. Just because food is labeled "low-fat" does not mean you can eat as much as you want. When reading food labels—and when eating—don't just look at the fat content but pay attention to calories as well.

7. Cut unnecessary items from your diet. Substituting water for a daily can of soda would cut 51,100 (140 × 365) calories yearly from the diet—the equivalent of 14.6 (51,000 ÷ 3,500) pounds of fat.

8. Maintain daily intake of calcium-rich foods, especially low-fat or non-fat dairy products.

9. Add foods to your diet that reduce cravings, such as eggs; small amounts of red meat, fish, poultry, tofu, oils, fats; and nonstarchy vegetables such as lettuce, green beans, peppers, asparagus, broccoli, mushrooms, and Brussels sprouts. Consuming only carbohydrates increases cravings.

10. Avoid automatic eating. Many people associate certain daily activities with eating, for example, cooking, watching television, or reading. Most foods consumed in these situations lack nutritional value or are high in sugar and fat.

11. Stay busy. People tend to eat more when they sit around and do nothing. Occupying the mind and body with activities not associated with eating helps take away the desire to eat. Some options are walking; cycling; playing sports; gardening; sewing; or visiting a library, a museum, or a park. You might also develop other skills and interests not associated with food.

12. Plan meals and shop sensibly. Always shop on a full stomach, because hungry shoppers tend to buy unhealthy foods impulsively—and then snack on the way home. Always use a shopping list, which should include whole-grain breads and cereals, fruits and vegetables, low-fat milk and dairy products, lean meats, fish, and poultry.

13. Cook wisely:

   ■ Use less fat and fewer refined foods in food preparation.
   ■ Trim all visible fat from meats and remove skin from poultry before cooking.
   ■ Skim the fat off gravies and soups.
   ■ Bake, broil, boil, or steam instead of frying.
   ■ Sparingly use butter, cream, mayonnaise, and salad dressings.

The Simple Truth

There is no quick and easy way to take off excess body fat and keep it off for good. Weight management is accomplished by making a lifetime commitment to physical activity and proper food selection. When taking part in a weight (fat) reduction program, people also have to decrease their caloric intake moderately, be physically active, and implement strategies to modify unhealthy eating behaviors.

During the process, relapses into past negative behaviors are almost inevitable. The three most common reasons for relapse are:

1. Stress-related factors (such as major life changes, depression, job changes, illness).

2. Social reasons (entertaining, eating out, business travel).

3. Self-enticing behaviors (placing yourself in a situation to see how much you can get away with: "One small taste won't hurt" leads to "I'll eat just one slice" and finally to "I haven't done well, so I might as well eat some more").

Making mistakes is human and does not necessarily mean failure. Failure comes to those who give up and do not use previous experiences to build upon and, in turn, develop skills that will prevent self-defeating behaviors in the future. Where there's a will, there's a way, and those who persist will reap the rewards.

■ Avoid coconut oil, palm oil, and cocoa butter.
■ Prepare plenty of foods that contain fiber.
■ Include whole-grain breads and cereals, vegetables, and legumes in most meals.
■ Eat fruits for dessert.
■ Stay away from soda pop, fruit juices, and fruit-flavored drinks.
■ Use less sugar and cut down on other refined carbohydrates, such as corn syrup, malt sugar, dextrose, and fructose.
■ Drink plenty of water—at least six glasses a day.

14. Do not serve more food than you should eat. Measure the food in portions and keep serving dishes away from the table. Do not force yourself or anyone else to "clean the plate" after they are satisfied (including children after they already have had a healthy, nutritious serving).

15. Try "junior size" instead of "super size." People who are served larger portions eat more, whether they are hungry or not. Use smaller plates, bowls, cups, and glasses. Try eating half as much food as you commonly eat. Watch for portion sizes at restaurants as well: Supersized foods create supersized people.

16. Eat out infrequently. The more often people eat out, the more body fat they have. People who eat out 6 or more times per week consume an average of about 300 extra calories per day and 30 percent more fat than those who eat out less often.

17. Eat slowly and at the table only. Eating on the run promotes overeating because the body doesn't have enough time to "register" consumption, and people overeat before the body perceives the fullness signal. Eating at the table encourages people to take time out to eat and deters snacking between meals. After eating, do not sit around the table but, rather, clean up and put away the food to avoid snacking.

18. Avoid social binges. Social gatherings tend to entice self-defeating behavior. Use visual imagery to plan ahead. Do not feel pressured to eat or drink and don't rationalize in these situations. Choose low-calorie foods and entertain yourself with other activities, such as dancing and talking.

19. Do not place unhealthy foods within easy reach. Ideally, avoid bringing high-calorie, high-sugar, or high-fat foods into the house. If they are there already, store them where they are hard to get to or see—perhaps the garage or basement.

20. Avoid evening food raids. Most people do really well during the day but then "lose it" at night. Take control. Stop and think. To avoid excessive nighttime snacking, stay busy after your evening meal. Go for a short walk; floss and brush your teeth, and get to bed earlier.

21. Practice stress management techniques (discussed in Chapter 10). Many people snack and increase food consumption in stressful situations.

22. Get support. People who receive support from friends, relatives, and formal support groups are much more likely to lose and maintain weight loss than those without such support. The more support you receive, the better off you will be.

23. Monitor changes and reward accomplishments. Being able to exercise without interruption for 15, 20, 30, or 60 minutes; swimming a certain distance; running a mile—all these accomplishments deserve recognition. Create rewards that are not related to eating: new clothing, a tennis racquet, a bicycle, exercise shoes, or something else that is special and you would not have acquired otherwise.

24. Prepare for slips. Most people will slip and occasionally splurge. Do not despair and give up. Reevaluate and continue with your efforts. An occasional slip will not make much difference in the long run.

25. Think positive. Avoid negative thoughts about how difficult changing past behaviors might be. Instead, think of the benefits you will reap, such as feeling, looking, and functioning better, plus enjoying better health and improving the quality of life. Avoid negative environments and unsupportive people.

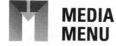

Profile Plus

Evaluate how well you understand the concepts presented in this chapter using the "Assess Your Knowledge" and "Practice Quizzes" options on your CD-ROM.

ASSESS YOUR KNOWLEDGE

1. During the last decade, the rate of obesity in the United States has
   a. been on the decline.
   b. increased at an alarming rate.
   c. increased slightly.
   d. remained steady.
   e. increased in men and decreased in women.

2. Obesity is defined as a body mass index equal to or above
   a. 10.
   b. 25.
   c. 30.
   d. 45.
   e. 50.

3. Obesity increases the risk for
   a. hypertension.
   b. congestive heart failure.
   c. atherosclerosis.
   d. Type 2 diabetes.
   e. all of the above.

4. Tolerable weight is a body weight
   a. that is not ideal but one that you can live with.
   b. that will tolerate the increased risk of chronic diseases.
   c. with a BMI range between 25 and 30.
   d. that meets both ideal values for percent body weight and BMI.
   e. All are correct choices.

5. When the body uses protein instead of a combination of fats and carbohydrates as a source of energy
   a. weight loss is very slow.
   b. a large amount of weight loss is in the form of water.
   c. muscle turns into fat.
   d. fat is lost very rapidly.
   e. fat cannot be lost.

6. Eating disorders
   a. are characterized by an intense fear of becoming fat.
   b. are physical and emotional conditions.
   c. almost always require professional help for successful treatment of the disease.
   d. are common in societies that encourage thinness.
   e. All are correct choices.

7. The mechanism that seems to regulate how much a person weighs is known as
   a. setpoint.
   b. weight factor.
   c. basal metabolic rate.
   d. metabolism.
   e. energy-balancing equation.

8. The key to successful weight loss maintenance is
   a. frequent dieting.
   b. very low-calorie diets when "normal" dieting doesn't work.
   c. a lifetime exercise program.
   d. regular high protein/low carbohydrate meals.
   e. All are correct choices.

9. The daily amount of physical activity recommended for weight-loss purposes is
   a. 15 to 20 minutes.
   b. 20 to 30 minutes.
   c. 30 to 40 minutes.
   d. 45 to 60 minutes.
   e. Any amount is sufficient as long as it is done daily.

10. A daily energy expenditure of 300 calories through physical activity is the equivalent of approximately _____ pounds of fat per year.
    a. 12
    b. 15
    c. 22
    d. 27
    e. 31

Correct answers can be found at the back of the book.

MEDIA MENU

PROFILE PLUS CD CONNECTIONS

- On your exercise log, check your progress.
- Check how well you understand the chapter's concepts.

INTERNET CONNECTIONS

- Shape Up America. This excellent fitness and weight management site is endorsed by former U.S. Surgeon General C. Everett Koop, M.D.
  http://www.shapeup.org

- Eating Disorders. This award-winning site, by Mental Health Net, features links describing symptoms, possible causes, consequences, treatment, online resources, organizations, online support, and research.
  http://eatingdisorders.mentalhelp.net

- Mayo Clinic Food & Nutrition Center. This site features a wealth of reliable nutrition information including information on different food pyramids and the benefits and dangers of herbs, vitamins, and mineral supplements.
  http://www.mayoclinic.com/home?id=4.1.5

- Count Your Calories Because Your Calories Count. This interactive site, sponsored by Wake Forest University Baptist Medical Center, features a four-step assessment of your diet—including "How's Your Diet?," "Fit or Not Quiz," Calorie Counter," and "Drive-Through Diet"—plus an "Eating Disorders" quiz.
  http://www.bgsm.edu/nutrition/in.html

Notes

1. "Wellness Facts," *University of California at Berkeley Wellness Letter* (Palm Coast, FL: The Editors, May 2004).

2. A. Must et al., "The Disease Burden Associated with Overweight and Obesity," *Journal of the American Medical Association* 282 (1999): 1523–1529.

3. M. K. Serdula et al., "Prevalence of Attempting Weight Loss and Strategies for Controlling Weight," *Journal of the American Medical Association* 282 (1999): 1353–1358.

4. A. M. Wolf and G. A. Colditz, "Current Estimates of the Economic Cost of Obesity in the United States," *Obesity Research* 6 (1998): 97–106.

5. A. H. Mokdad, J. S. Marks, D. F. Stroup, and J. L. Gerberding, "Actual Causes of Death in the United States, 2000," *Journal of the American Medical Association* 291 (2004): 1238–1241.

6. R. Sturm and K. B. Wells, "Does Obesity Contribute as much to Morbidity as Poverty or Smoking?" *Public Health* 115 (2001): 229–235.

7. E. E. Calle et. al., "Overweight, Obesity, and Mortality from Cancer in a Prospectively Studied Cohort of U.S. Adults," *New England Journal of Medicine* 348 (2003): 1625–1638.

8. A. Peeters et al., "Obesity in Adulthood and Its Consequences for Life Expectancy: A Life-Table Analysis," *Annals of Internal Medicine* 138 (2003): 2432.

9. K. R. Fontaine et al., "Years of Life Lost Due to Obesity," *Journal of the American Medical Association* 289 (2003): 187–193.

10. R. R. Wing, E. Venditti, J. M. Jakicic, B. A. Polley, and W. Lang, "Lifestyle Intervention in Overweight Individuals with a Family History of Diabetes," *Diabetes Care* 21 (1998): 350–359.

11. S. Thomsen, "A Steady Diet of Images," *BYU Magazine* 57, no. 3 (2003): 20–21.

12. S. Lichtman et al., "Discrepancy between Self-Reported and Actual Caloric Intake and Exercise in Obese Subjects," *New England Journal of Medicine* 327 (1992): 1893–1898.

13. G. D. Foster et al., "A Randomized Trial of a Low-Carbohydrate Diet for Obesity," *New England Journal of Medicine* 348 (2003): 2082–2090.

14. American Psychiatric Association, *Diagnostic and Statistical Manual of Mental Disorders* (Washington, DC: APA, 1994).

15. See note 14.

16. R. L. Leibel, M. Rosenbaum, and J. Hirsh, "Changes in Energy Expenditure Resulting from Altered Body Weight," *New England Journal of Medicine* 332 (1995): 621–628.

17. American College of Sports Medicine, "Position Stand: Appropriate Intervention Strategies for Weight Loss and Prevention for Weight Regain for Adults," *Medicine and Science in Sports and Exercise* 33 (2001): 2145–2156.

18. R. J. Shepard, *Alive Man: The Physiology of Physical Activity* (Springfield, IL: Charles C Thomas, 1975): 484–488.

19. W. C. Miller, D. M. Koceja, and E. J. Hamilton, "A Meta-Analysis of the Past 25 Years of Weight Loss Research Using Diet, Exercise, or Diet Plus Exercise Intervention," *International Journal of Obesity* 21 (1997): 941–947.

20. J. H. Wilmore, "Exercise, Obesity, and Weight Control," *Physical Activity and Fitness Research Digest* (Washington DC: President's Council on Physical Fitness & Sports, 1994).

21. See note 3.

22. National Academy of Sciences, Institute of Medicine, *Dietary Reference Intakes for Energy, Carbohydrates, Fiber, Fat, Protein and Amino Acids (Macronutrients).* Washington, DC: National Academy Press, 2002.

23. W. W. Campbell, M. C. Crim, V. R. Young, and W. J. Evans, "Increased Energy Requirements and Changes in Body Composition with Resistance Training in Older Adults," *American Journal of Clinical Nutrition* 60 (1994): 167–175.

24. A. Tremblay, J. A. Simoneau, and C. Bouchard. "Impact of Exercise Intensity on Body Fatness and Skeletal Muscle Metabolism," *Metabolism* 43 (1994): 814–818.

25. M. L. Klem, R. R. Wing, M. T. McGuire, H. M. Seagle, and J. O. Hill, "A Descriptive Study of Individuals Successful at Long-Term Maintenance of Substantial Weight Loss," *American Journal of Clinical Nutrition* 66 (1997): 239–246.

26. U.S. Department of Health and Human Services, Department of Agriculture, *Nutrition and Your Health: Dietary Guidelines for Americans* (Home and Garden Bulletin 232), 2000.

   U.S. Department of Agriculture, Human Nutrition Information Service, *The Food Guide Pyramid* (Home and Garden Bulletin 252), Dec. 1992.

   National Academy of Sciences, Institute of Medicine, *Dietary Reference Intakes for Energy, Carbohydrates, Fiber, Fat, Protein and Amino Acids (Macronutrients)* (Washington, DC: National Academy Press, 2002).

27. W. W. K. Hoeger, C. Harris, E. M. Long, and D. R. Hopkins, "Four-Week Supplementation with a Natural Dietary Compound Produces Favorable Changes in Body Composition," *Advances in Therapy* 15, no. 5 (1998): 305–313.

   W. W. K. Hoeger, C. Harris, E. M. Long, R. L. Kjorstad, M. Welch, T. L. Hafner, and D. R. Hopkins, "Dietary Supplementation with Chromium Picolinate/L-Carnitine Complex in Combination with Diet and Exercise Enhances Body Composition," *Journal of the American Nutraceutical Association* 2, no. 2 (1999): 40–45.

Suggested Readings

American College of Sports Medicine. "Effective Weight Management." *ACSM Fit Society Page* (http://acsm.org/health+fitness/fit_society.htm), Summer 2004.

American College of Sports Medicine. "Position Stand: Appropriate Intervention Strategies for Weight Loss and Prevention for Weight Regain for Adults." *Medicine and Science in Sports and Exercise* 33 (2001): 2145–2156.

American Diabetes Association and American Dietetic Association. *Exchange Lists for Meal Planning*. Chicago: American Dietetic Association and American Diabetes Association, 1995.

Brownell, K. *The Learn Program for Weight Control*. Dallas: American Health Publishing, 1997.

Clarkson, P. M. "The Skinny on Weight Loss Supplements and Drugs: Winning the War against Fat." *ACSM's Health and Fitness Journal* (1998): 18.

Mokdad, A. H., et al. "The Spread of the Obesity Epidemic in the United States, 1991–1998." *Journal of the American Medical Association* 282 (1999): 1519–1522.

National Academy of Sciences, Institute of Medicine. *Dietary Reference Intakes for Energy, Carbohydrates, Fiber, Fat, Protein and Amino Acids (Macronutrients)*. Washington, DC: National Academy Press, 2002.

National Institutes of Health. *Clinical Guidelines on the Identification, Evaluation, and Treatment of Overweight and Obesity in Adults* (NIH Publication No. 98-4083). Washington, DC: NIH, 1998.

Lab 5A

ESTIMATION OF DAILY CALORIC REQUIREMENT, STAGE OF CHANGE, AND EXERCISE PROGRAM SELECTION

Name: _____   Date: _____   Grade: _____

Instructor: _____   Course: _____   Section: _____

Necessary Lab Equipment

Tables 5.2 and 5.3.

Instructions

Complete all of the sections provided in this lab.

Objective

To estimate your daily caloric requirement for weight maintenance or reduction and to select fitness activities for your exercise program.

I. Computation Form for Daily Caloric Requirement and Weight Loss if Necessary

A. Current body weight in pounds . . . .

B. Caloric requirement per pound of body weight (use Table 5.3) . . . .

C. Estimated daily energy requirement without exercise to maintain body weight (A × B) . . . .

D. Selected physical activity (e.g., jogging)[a] . . . .

E. Number of exercise sessions per week . . . .

F. Duration of exercise session (in minutes) . . . .

G. Total weekly exercise time in minutes (E × F) . . . .

H. Average daily exercise time in minutes (G ÷ 7) . . . .

I. Caloric expenditure per pound per minute (cal/lb/min) of physical activity (use Table 5.4) . . . .

J. Total calories burned per minute of physical activity (A × I) . . . .

K. Average daily calories burned as a result of the exercise program (H × J) . . . .

L. Total daily energy requirement with exercise to maintain body weight (C + K) . . . .

Stop here if no weight loss is required, otherwise proceed to items M and N.

M. Number of calories to subtract from daily requirement to achieve a negative caloric balance
(multiply current body weight by 5). . . . .

N. Target caloric intake to lose weight (L − M)[b] . . . .

---

[a] If more than one physical activity is selected, you will need to estimate the average daily calories burned as a result of each additional activity (steps D through K) and add all of these figures to L above.

[b] This figure should never be below 1,200 calories for women or 1,500 calories for men. See Lab 5B for the 1,200-, 1,500-, 1,800-, and 2,000-calorie diet plans.

II. Stage of Change

1. Using Figure 2.4 (page 41) and Table 2.3 (41), identify your current stage of change regarding **recommended body weight:** _____

2. If weight loss is recommended, how much weight do you need to lose? _____   Is it a realistic goal? _____

3. Based on the processes and techniques of change discussed in Chapter 2, indicate what you can do to help yourself implement a weight management program.

_____

_____

III. Exercise Program Selection

1. How much effort are you willing to put into maintaining recommended weight or reaching your weight loss goal?

_____
_____
_____

2. Indicate your feelings about participating in an exercise program.

_____
_____
_____

3. Will you commit to participate in a combined aerobic and strength-training program?[c] Yes ☐ No ☐

   If your answer is "Yes," proceed to the next question; if you answered "No," please review Chapters 3, 4, and 5 again and read Chapters 6, 7, 8, and 9.

4. List aerobic activities you enjoy or may enjoy doing.

_____
_____

5. Select one or two aerobic activities in which you will participate regularly.

_____   _____

6. List facilities available to you where you can carry out the aerobic and strength-training programs.

_____
_____

7. Indicate days and times you will set aside for your aerobic and strength-training program (5 to 6 days per week should be devoted to aerobic exercise and 1 to 3 nonconsecutive days per week to strength training).

   Monday: _____

   Tuesday: _____

   Wednesday: _____

   Thursday: _____

   Friday: _____

   Saturday: _____

   Sunday: A complete day of rest once a week is recommended to allow your body to fully recover from exercise.

---

[c] Flexibility programs are necessary for injury prevention, adequate fitness, and good health but do not help with weight loss. Stretching exercises can be conducted regularly during the cool-down phase of your aerobic and strength-training programs (see Chapter 8).

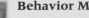

Behavior Modification

Briefly describe whether you think you can meet the goals of your aerobic and strength training programs. What obstacles will you have to overcome and how will you overcome them?

_____
_____

Lab 5B

CALORIE-RESTRICTED DIET PLANS

Name: _____ Date: _____ Grade: _____

Instructor: _____ Course: _____ Section: _____

Necessary Lab Equipment
None required.

Objective
To help you implement a calorie-restricted diet plan according to your target caloric intake obtained in Lab 5A.

Lab Preparation
Read Chapter 5 prior to this lab and make additional copies (as needed) of your selected diet plan.

1,200 Calorie Diet Plan

Instructions:

The objective of the diet plan is to meet (not exceed) the number of servings allowed for the food groups listed. Each time that you eat a particular food, record it in the space provided for each group along with the amount you ate. Refer to the Food Guide Pyramid to find out what counts as one serving for each group listed. Instead of the meat, poultry, fish, dry beans, eggs, and nuts group, you are allowed to have a commercially available low-fat frozen entree for your main meal (this entree should provide no more than 300 calories and less than 6 grams of fat). You can make additional copies of this form as needed.

Bread, Cereal, Rice, Pasta Group (80 calories/serving): 6 servings

1 _____
2 _____
3 _____
4 _____
5 _____
6 _____

Vegetable Group (25 calories/serving): 3 servings

1 _____
2 _____
3 _____

Fruit Group (60 calories/serving): 2 servings

1 _____
2 _____

Milk Group (120 calories/serving, use low-fat milk and milk products): 2 servings

1 _____
2 _____

Low-fat Frozen Entree (300 calories and less than 6 grams of fat): 1 serving

1 _____

Today's physical activity: _____ Intensity: _____ Duration: _____ min

1,500 Calorie Diet Plan

Instructions:

The objective of the diet plan is to meet (not exceed) the number of servings allowed for the food groups listed. Each time that you eat a particular food, record it in the space provided for each group along with the amount you ate. Refer to the Food Guide Pyramid to find out what counts as one serving for each group listed. Instead of the meat, poultry, fish, dry beans, eggs, and nuts group, you are allowed to have two commercially available low-fat frozen entrees for your main meal (these entrees should provide no more than 300 calories and less than 6 grams of fat). You can make additional copies of this form as needed.

Bread, Cereal, Rice, Pasta Group (80 calories/serving): 6 servings

1

2

3

4

5

6

Vegetable Group (25 calories/serving): 3 servings

1

2

3

Fruit Group (60 calories/serving): 2 servings

1

2

Milk Group (120 calories/serving, use low-fat milk and milk products): 2 servings

1

2

Two Low-fat Frozen Entrees (300 calories and less than 6 grams of fat): 2 servings

1

2

Today's physical activity: Intensity: Duration: min

1,800 Calorie Diet Plan

Instructions:

The objective of the diet plan is to meet (not exceed) the number of servings allowed for the food groups listed. Each time that you eat a particular food, record it in the space provided for each group along with the amount you ate. Refer to the Food Guide Pyramid to find out what counts as one serving for each group listed. Instead of the meat, poultry, fish, dry beans, eggs, and nuts group, you are allowed to have two commercially available low-fat frozen entrees for your main meal (these entrees should provide no more than 300 calories and less than 6 grams of fat). You can make additional copies of this form as needed.

Bread, Cereal, Rice, Pasta Group (80 calories/serving): 8 servings

1.
2.
3.
4.
5.
6.
7.
8.

Vegetable Group (25 calories/serving): 5 servings

1.
2.
3.
4.
5.

Fruit Group (60 calories/serving): 3 servings

1.
2.
3.

Milk Group (120 calories/serving, use low-fat milk and milk products): 2 servings

1.
2.

Two Low-fat Frozen Entrees (300 calories and less than 6 grams of fat): 2 servings

1.
2.

Today's physical activity: _____   Intensity: _____   Duration: _____ min

2,000 Calorie Diet Plan

Instructions:

The objective of the diet plan is to meet (not exceed) the number of servings allowed for the food groups listed. Each time that you eat a particular food, record it in the space provided for each group along with the amount you ate. Refer to the Food Guide Pyramid to find out what counts as one serving for each group listed. Instead of the meat, poultry, fish, dry beans, eggs, and nuts group, you are allowed to have two commercially available low-fat frozen entrees for your main meal (these entrees should provide no more than 300 calories and less than 6 grams of fat). You can make additional copies of this form as needed.

Bread, Cereal, Rice, Pasta Group (80 calories/serving): 10 servings

1
2
3
4
5
6
7
8
9
10

Vegetable Group (25 calories/serving): 5 servings

1
2
3
4
5

Fruit Group (60 calories/serving): 4 servings

1
2
3
4

Milk Group (120 calories/serving, use low-fat milk and milk products): 2 servings

1
2

Two Low-fat Frozen Entrees (300 calories and less than 6 grams of fat): 2 servings

1
2

Today's physical activity: _____ Intensity: _____ Duration: _____ min

Lab 5C

HEALTHY DIETARY PLAN FOR WEIGHT MAINTENANCE OR WEIGHT GAIN

Name: _____ Date: _____ Grade: _____

Instructor: _____ Course: _____ Section: _____

Necessary Lab Equipment
None.

Lab Preparation
Read Chapters 3, 4, and 5 prior to this lab.

Objective
To design a sample daily healthy diet plan to maintain current body weight or increase body weight.

I. Daily Caloric Requirement

A. Current body weight in pounds . . . . _____

B. Current percent body fat . . . . _____

C. Current body composition classification (Table 4.10, page 113) . . . . _____

D. Total daily energy requirement with exercise to maintain body weight (use item L from Lab 5A). Use this figure and stop further computations if the goal is to maintain body weight . . . . _____

E. Target body weight to increase body weight . . . . _____

F. Number of additional daily calories to increase body weight (combine this increased caloric intake with a strength-training program, see Chapter 7) 500

G. Total daily energy (caloric) requirement with exercise to increase body weight (D + 500) . . . . _____

II. Strength-Training Program

For weight gain purposes, indicate three days during the week and the time when you will engage in a strength-training program.

_____

_____

III. Healthy Diet Plan

Design a sample healthy daily diet plan according to the total daily energy requirement computed in D (maintenance) or G (weight gain) above. Using Appendix A, list all individual food items that you can consume on that day, along with their caloric, carbohydrate, fat, protein content. Be sure that the diet meets the recommended number of servings from the five food groups.

Breakfast

Food item	Serving Size	Calories	Carbohydrates (gr)	Fat (gr)	Protein (gr)
1.					
2.					
3.					
4.					
5.					

Breakfast

	Food item	Serving Size	Calories	Carbohydrates (gr)	Fat (gr)	Protein (gr)
6.						
7.						
8.						

Lunch

1.						
2.						
3.						
4.						
5.						
6.						
7.						
8.						

Snack

1.						

Dinner

1.						
2.						
3.						
4.						
5.						
6.						
7.						
8.						
Totals:						

IV. Percent of Macronutrients

Determine the percent of total calories that are derived from carbohydrates, fat, and protein.

A. Total calories = [   ]

B. Grams of carbohydrates [   ] × 4 ÷ [   ] (total calories) = [   ] %

C. Grams of fat [   ] × 9 ÷ [   ] (total calories) = [   ] %

D. Grams of protein [   ] × 4 ÷ [   ] (total calories) = [   ] %

Lab 5D

BEHAVIORAL GOALS FOR WEIGHT MANAGEMENT

Name: _____   Date: _____   Grade: _____

Instructor: _____   Course: _____   Section: _____

Necessary Lab Equipment
None.

Lab Preparation
Read Chapters 2, 3, 4, and 5 prior to this lab.

Objective
To prepare and monitor behavioral changes for weight management.

I. Please answer all of the following:

1. State your own feelings regarding your current body weight, your target body composition, and a completion date for this goal.

_____

_____

_____

_____

Completion date: _____

2. Do you have an eating disorder? If so, express your feelings about it. Can your instructor help you find professional advice so that you can work toward resolving this problem?

_____

_____

_____

_____

_____

3. Is your present diet adequate according to the nutrient analysis?   Yes _____   No _____

4. State dietary changes necessary to achieve a balanced diet and/or to lose weight (increase or decrease caloric intake, decrease fat intake, increase intake of complex carbohydrates, etc.). List specific foods that will help you improve in areas where you may have deficiencies and food items to avoid or consume in moderation to help you achieve better nutrition.

Changes to make: _____

_____

Foods that will help: _____

_____

Foods to avoid: _____

_____

II. Behavior Modification Progress Form

Instructions: Read the section on tips for behavior modification and adherence to a weight management program (page 144). On a weekly or bi-weekly basis, go through the list of strategies and provide a "Yes" or "No" answer to each statement. If you are able to answer "Yes" to most questions, you have been successful in implementing positive weight management behaviors. (Make additional copies of this page as needed.)

Strategy Date						
1. I have made a commitment to change.						
2. I set realistic goals.						
3. I exercise regularly.						
4. I have healthy eating patterns.						
5. I exercise control over my appetite.						
6. I am consuming less fat in my diet.						
7. I pay attention to the number of calories in food.						
8. I have eliminated unnecessary food items from my diet.						
9. I use craving-reducing foods in my diet.						
10. I avoid automatic eating.						
11. I stay busy.						
12. I plan meals ahead of time.						
13. I cook wisely.						
14. I do not serve more food than I should eat.						
15. I use portion control in my diet.						
16. I eat slowly and at the table only.						
17. I avoid social binges.						
18. I avoid food raids.						
19. I do not eat out more than once per week. When I do, I eat low-fat meals.						
20. I practice stress management.						
21. I have a strong support group.						
22. I monitor behavior changes.						
23. I prepare for lapses/relapses.						
24. I reward my accomplishments.						
25. I think positive.						

Chapter 6

Cardiorespiratory Endurance

Exercise is the closest thing we'll ever get to the miracle pill that everyone is seeking. It brings weight loss, appetite control, improved mood and self-esteem, an energy kick, and longer life by decreasing the risk of heart disease, diabetes, stroke, osteoporosis, and chronic disabilities.[1]

Objectives

- Define cardiorespiratory endurance and describe the benefits of cardiorespiratory endurance training in maintaining health and well-being.
- Define aerobic and anaerobic exercise, and give examples.
- Be able to assess cardiorespiratory fitness through five different test protocols (1.5-Mile Run Test, 1.0-Mile Walk Test, Step Test, Astrand-Ryhming Test, and 12-Minute Swim Test).
- Be able to interpret cardiorespiratory endurance assessment test results according to health fitness and physical fitness standards.
- Be able to estimate oxygen uptake and caloric expenditure from walking and jogging.
- Determine your readiness to start an exercise program.
- Explain the principles that govern cardiorespiratory exercise prescription: intensity, type, mode, duration, and frequency.
- Learn some ways to foster adherence to exercise.

Profile Plus CD Connections

- Assess your cardiorespiratory endurance.
- Maintain a log of all your fitness activities.
- Check how well you understand the chapter's concepts.

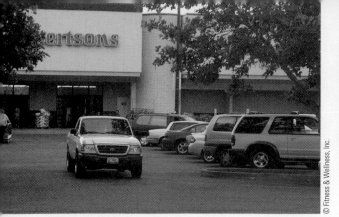

The epitome of physical inactivity: driving around a parking lot for several minutes in search of a parking spot 20 yards closer to the store's entrance.

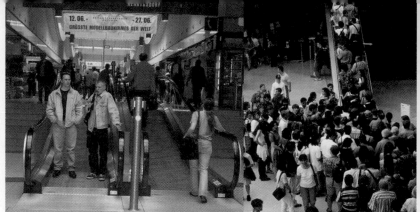

Advances in modern technology have almost completely eliminated the need for physical activity, significantly enhancing the deterioration rate of the human body.

The single most important component of health-related physical fitness is **cardiorespiratory endurance**. The exception occurs among older adults, for whom muscular strength is particularly important. A person does need a certain amount of muscular strength and flexibility to engage in normal daily activities. Nevertheless, one can get by without high levels of strength and flexibility but cannot do without a good cardiorespiratory system.

Aerobic exercise is especially important in preventing cardiovascular disease. A poorly conditioned heart, which has to pump more often just to keep a person alive, is subject to more wear and tear than a well-conditioned heart. In situations that place strenuous demands on the heart, such as doing yardwork, lifting heavy objects or weights, or running to catch a bus, the unconditioned heart may not be able to sustain the strain. Regular participation in cardiorespiratory endurance activities also helps a person achieve and maintain recommended body weight, the fourth component of health-related physical fitness.

Physical activity, unfortunately, is no longer a natural part of our existence. Technological developments have driven most people in developed countries into sedentary lifestyles. For instance, when many people go to a store only a couple of blocks away, most drive their automobiles and then spend a couple of minutes driving around the parking lot to find a spot 20 yards closer to the store's entrance. They do not even have to carry out the groceries, as an employee working at the store usually offers to take them out in a cart and place them in the vehicle.

Similarly, during a visit to a multi-level shopping mall, almost everyone chooses to ride the escalators instead of taking the stairs (which tend to be inaccessible). Automobiles, elevators, escalators, telephones, intercoms, remote controls, electric garage door openers—all are modern-day commodities that minimize the amount of movement and effort required of the human body.

One of the most harmful effects of modern-day technology is an increase in chronic conditions related to a lack of physical activity. These include hypertension, heart disease, chronic low-back pain, and obesity and are referred to as **hypokinetic diseases**. The term "hypo" means low or little, and "kinetic" implies motion. Lack of adequate physical activity is a fact of modern life that most people can avoid no longer. To enjoy modern-day conveniences and still expect to live life to its fullest, however, one needs to make a personalized lifetime exercise program a part of daily living.

Basic Cardiorespiratory Physiology: A Quick Survey

Before we begin to overhaul our bodies with an exercise program, we should understand the mechanisms that we propose to alter and survey the ways by which to measure their performance.

Cardiorespiratory endurance is a measure of how the pulmonary (lungs), cardiovascular (heart and blood vessels), and muscular systems work together during aerobic activities. As a person breathes, part of the oxygen in the air is taken up by the **alveoli** in the lungs. As blood passes through the alveoli, oxygen is picked up by **hemoglobin** and transported in the blood to the heart. The heart then is responsible for pumping the oxygenated blood through the circulatory system to all organs and tissues of the body.

At the cellular level, oxygen is used to convert food substrates (primarily carbohydrates and fats) through aerobic metabolism into **adenosine triphosphate (ATP)**. This compound provides the energy for physical activity, body functions, and maintenance of a constant internal equilibrium. During physical exertion, more ATP is needed to perform the activity. As a result, the lungs, heart, and blood vessels have to deliver more oxygen to

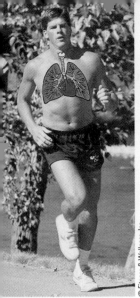

Cardiorespiratory endurance refers to the ability of the lungs, heart, and blood vessels to deliver adequate amounts of oxygen to the cells to meet the demands of prolonged physical activity.

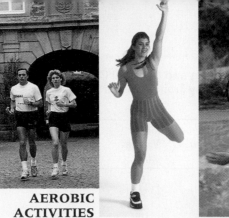

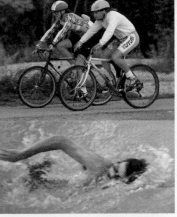

AEROBIC ACTIVITIES

Photos © Fitness & Wellness, Inc.

ANAEROBIC ACTIVITIES

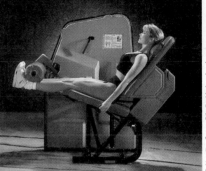

© Nautilus Sports/Medical Industries, Inc.

Photos © Fitness & Wellness, Inc.

the muscle cells to supply the required energy.

During prolonged exercise, an individual with a high level of cardiorespiratory endurance is able to deliver the required amount of oxygen to the tissues with relative ease. In contrast, the cardiorespiratory system of a person with a low level of endurance has to work much harder, the heart has to work at a higher rate, less oxygen is delivered to the tissues and, consequently, the individual fatigues faster. Hence, a higher capacity to deliver and utilize oxygen—called **oxygen uptake** or **VO₂**—indicates a more efficient cardiorespiratory system. Measuring oxygen uptake is therefore an important way to evaluate our cardiorespiratory health.

Aerobic and Anaerobic Exercise

Cardiorespiratory endurance activities often are called **aerobic** exercises; examples are walking, jogging, swimming, cycling, cross-country skiing, water aerobics, rope skipping, and aerobics. The intensity of **anaerobic** exercise is so high that oxygen cannot be delivered and utilized to produce energy. Because energy production is limited in the absence of oxygen, these activities can be carried out for only short periods—2 to 3 minutes. The higher the intensity of the activity, the shorter the duration.

Good examples of anaerobic activities are the 100, 200, and 400 meters in track and field, the 100 meters in swimming, gymnastics routines, and strength training. Anaerobic activities do not contribute much to development of the cardiorespiratory system. Only aerobic activities will help increase cardiorespiratory endurance. The basic guidelines for cardiorespiratory exercise prescription are set forth later in this chapter.

Cardiorespiratory endurance The ability of the lungs, heart, and blood vessels to deliver adequate amounts of oxygen to the cells to meet the demands of prolonged physical activity.

Hypokinetic diseases "Hypo" denotes "lack of"; therefore, lack of physical activity.

Alveoli Air sacs in the lungs where oxygen is taken up and carbon dioxide (produced by the body) is released from the blood.

Hemoglobin Iron-containing compound, found in red blood cells, that transports oxygen.

Adenosine triphosphate (ATP) A high-energy chemical compound that the body uses for immediate energy.

Oxygen uptake (VO₂) The amount of oxygen used by the human body.

Aerobic Exercise that requires oxygen to produce the necessary energy (ATP) to carry out the activity.

Anaerobic Exercise that does not require oxygen to produce the necessary energy (ATP) to carry out the activity.

TABLE 6.1 Average Resting and Maximal Cardiac Output, Stroke Volume, and Heart Rate for Sedentary, Trained, and Highly Trained Males*

	Resting			Maximal		
	Cardiac Output (l/min)	Stroke Volume (ml)	Heart Rate (bpm)	Cardiac Output (l/min)	Stroke Volume (ml)	Heart Rate (bpm)
Sedentary	5–6	68	74	20	100	200
Trained	5–6	90	56	30	150	200
Highly Trained	5–6	110	45	35	175	200

*Cardiac output and stroke volume in women are about 25 percent lower than in men.

Benefits of Aerobic Training

Everyone who participates in a cardiorespiratory or aerobic exercise program can expect a number of beneficial physiological adaptations from training. Among them are the following:

1. A higher **maximal oxygen uptake (VO$_{2max}$)**. The amount of oxygen the body is able to use during physical activity increases significantly. This allows the individual to exercise longer and more intensely before becoming fatigued. Depending on the initial fitness level, the increases in maximal oxygen uptake average 15 to 20 percent; although increases greater than 50 percent have been reported in people who have very low initial levels of fitness or who were significantly overweight prior to starting the aerobic exercise program.

2. An increase in the oxygen-carrying capacity of the blood. As a result of training, the red blood cell count goes up. Red blood cells contain hemoglobin, which transports oxygen in the blood.

3. A decrease in **resting heart rate** and an increase in cardiac muscle strength. During resting conditions, the heart ejects between 5 and 6 liters of blood per minute (a liter is slightly larger than a quart). This amount of blood, also referred to as **cardiac output**, meets the body's energy demands in the resting state.

   Like any other muscle, the heart responds to training by increasing in strength and size. As the heart gets stronger, the muscle can produce a more forceful contraction, which helps the heart to eject more blood with each beat. This **stroke volume** yields a lower heart rate. The lower heart rate also allows the heart to rest longer between beats. Average resting and maximal cardiac outputs, stroke volumes, and heart rates for sedentary, trained, and highly trained (elite) individuals are shown in Table 6.1.

   Resting heart rates frequently decrease by 10 to 20 beats per minute (bpm) after only 6 to 8 weeks of training. A reduction of 20 bpm saves the heart about 10,483,200 beats per year. The average heart beats between 70 and 80 bpm. As seen in the table, resting heart rates in highly trained athletes are often around 45 bpm.

4. A lower heart rate at given **workloads**. When compared with untrained individuals, a trained person has a lower heart rate response to a given task because of greater efficiency of the cardiorespiratory system. Individuals also are surprised to find that, following several weeks of training, a given workload (let's say a 10-minute mile) elicits a much lower heart rate response than the response when they first started training.

5. An increase in the number and size of the **mitochondria**. All energy necessary for cell function is produced in the mitochondria. As their size and numbers increase, so does the potential to produce energy for muscular work.

6. An increase in the number of functional **capillaries**. Capillaries allow for the exchange of oxygen and carbon dioxide between the blood and the cells. As more vessels open up, more gas exchange can take place, delaying the onset of fatigue during prolonged exercise. This increase in capillaries also speeds up the rate at which waste products of cell metabolism can be removed. This increased capillarization also occurs in the heart, which enhances the oxygen delivery capacity to the heart muscle itself.

7. A faster **recovery time**. Trained individuals recover more rapidly after exercising. A fit system is able to more quickly restore any internal equilibrium disrupted during exercise.

8. Lower blood pressure and blood lipids. A regular aerobic exercise program leads to lower blood pressure (thus reducing a major risk factor for stroke) and lower levels of fats (such as

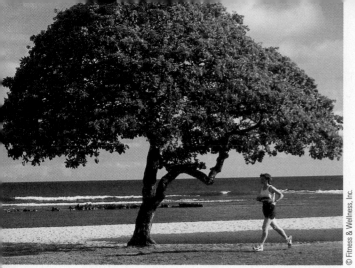

Aerobic fitness leads to better health and a higher quality of life.

cholesterol and triglycerides), all of which have been linked to the formation of atherosclerotic plaque, which obstructs the arteries. This decreases the risk of coronary heart disease (see Chapter 11).

9. An increase in fat-burning enzymes. These enzymes are significant because fat is lost primarily by burning it in muscle. As the concentration of the enzymes increases, so does the ability to burn fat.

Physical Fitness Assessment

The assessment of physical fitness serves several purposes:

- To educate participants regarding their present fitness levels and compare them to health fitness and physical fitness standards.
- To motivate individuals to participate in exercise programs.
- To provide a starting point for individualized exercise prescriptions.
- To evaluate improvements in fitness achieved through exercise programs and make adjustments in exercise prescriptions.
- To monitor changes in fitness throughout the years.

Responders versus Nonresponders

Individuals who follow similar training programs show a wide variation in physiological responses. Heredity plays a crucial role in how each person responds to and improves after beginning an exercise program. Several studies have documented that following exercise training, most individuals, called **responders**, readily show improvements, but a few, **nonresponders**, exhibit small or no improvements at all. This concept is referred to as the **principle of individuality**.

After several months of aerobic training, VO_{2max} increases are between 15 and 20 percent, on the average, although individual responses can range from 0 percent (in a few selected cases) to more than 50 percent improvement, even when all

Maximal oxygen uptake (VO_{2max}) Maximum amount of oxygen the body is able to utilize per minute of physical activity, commonly expressed in ml/kg/min; the best indicator of cardiorespiratory or aerobic fitness.

Resting heart rate (RHR) Heart rate after a person has been sitting quietly for 15–20 minutes.

Cardiac output Amount of blood pumped by the heart in one minute.

Stroke volume Amount of blood pumped by the heart in one beat.

Workload Load (or intensity) placed on the body during physical activity.

Mitochondria Structures within the cells where energy transformations take place.

Capillaries Smallest blood vessels carrying oxygenated blood to the tissues in the body.

Recovery time Amount of time the body takes to return to resting levels after exercise.

Responders Individuals who exhibit improvements in fitness as a result of exercise training.

Nonresponders Individuals who exhibit small or no improvements in fitness as compared to others who undergo the same training program.

Principle of individuality Training concept that states that genetics plays a major role in individual responses to exercise training and these differences must be considered when designing exercise programs for different people.

participants follow exactly the same training program. Non-fitness and low-fitness participants, however, should not label themselves as nonresponders based the previous discussion. Nonresponders constitute less than 5 percent of exercise participants. Although additional research is necessary, lack of improvement in cardiorespiratory endurance among nonresponders might be related to low levels of leg strength. A lower body strength-training program has been shown to help these individuals improve VO_{2max} through aerobic exercise.[2]

Following assessment of cardiorespiratory fitness, if your fitness level is less than adequate, do not let that discourage you, but make it a priority to be physically active every day. In addition to regular exercise; lifestyle behaviors such as walking, taking stairs, cycling to work, parking farther from the office, doing household tasks, gardening, and doing yardwork provide substantial benefits. In this regard, monitoring daily physical activity and exercise habits should be used in conjunction with fitness testing to evaluate compliance among nonresponders. After all, it is through increased daily activity that we reap the health benefits that improve quality of life.

Assessment of Cardiorespiratory Endurance

Cardiorespiratory endurance, cardiorespiratory fitness, or aerobic capacity is determined by the maximal amount of oxygen the human body is able to utilize (the oxygen uptake) per minute of physical activity (VO_{2max}). This value can be expressed in liters per minute (l/min) or milliliters per kilogram per minute (ml/kg/min). The relative value in ml/kg/min is used most often because it considers total body mass (weight) in kilograms. When comparing two individuals with the same absolute value, the one with the lesser body mass will have a higher relative value, indicating that more oxygen is available to each kilogram (2.2 pounds) of body weight. Because all tissues and organs of the body need oxygen to function, higher oxygen consumption indicates a more efficient cardiorespiratory system.

Profile Plus

Looking for a starting point? Assess your cardiorespiratory endurance by participating in the activities on your CD-ROM.

Components of Oxygen Uptake (VO_2)

The amount of oxygen that the body actually uses at rest or during submaximal (VO_2) or maximal (VO_{2max}) physical activity is determined by the heart rate, the stroke volume, and the amount of oxygen removed from the vascular system (for use by all organs and tissues of the body, including the muscular system).

HEART RATE
Normal heart rate may range from about 40 bpm during resting conditions in trained athletes to 200 bpm or higher during maximal exercise. The **maximal heart rate** that a person can achieve starts to drop by about one beat per year beginning at about 12 years of age. Maximal heart rate in trained endurance athletes is sometimes slightly lower than in untrained individuals. This adaptation to training is thought to allow the heart more time to effectively fill with blood so as to produce a greater stroke volume.

STROKE VOLUME
Stroke volume ranges from 50 ml per beat (stroke) during resting conditions in untrained individuals to 200 ml at maximum in endurance-trained athletes (see Table 6.1). Following endurance training, stroke volume increases significantly. Some of the increase is the result of a stronger heart muscle, but it is also related to an increase in total blood volume and a greater filling capacity of the ventricles during the resting phase (diastole) of the heart cycle. As more blood enters the heart, a greater amount can be ejected with each heartbeat (systole). The increase in stroke volume is primarily responsible for the increase in VO_{2max} seen with endurance training.

AMOUNT OF OXYGEN REMOVED FROM BLOOD
The amount of oxygen removed from the vascular system is known as the **arterial-venous oxygen difference (a-$\bar{v}O_2$diff)**. The oxygen content in the arteries at sea level is typically 20 ml of oxygen per 100 cc of blood. (This value decreases at higher altitudes because of the drop in barometric pressure which affects the amount of oxygen picked up by hemoglobin.) The oxygen content in the veins during a resting state is about 15 ml per 100 cc. Thus, the a-$\bar{v}O_2$diff—that is, the amount of oxygen in the arteries minus the amount in the veins—at rest is 5 ml per 100 cc. The arterial value remains constant during both resting and exercise conditions but, during maximal exercise, the venous oxygen content drops to about 5 ml per 100 cc, yielding an a-$\bar{v}O_2$diff of 15 ml per 100 cc. The latter value may be slightly higher in endurance athletes.

These three factors are used to compute VO_2 using the following equation:

$$VO_2 \text{ in l/min} = (HR \times SV \times \text{a-}\bar{v}O_2\text{diff}) \div 100,000$$

where

HR = heart rate
SV = stroke volume

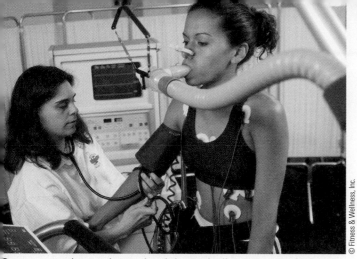

Oxygen uptake, as determined through direct gas analysis.

For example, the resting VO_2 (also known as "resting metabolic rate") of an individual with a resting heart rate of 76 bpm and a stroke volume of 79 ml would be

$$VO_2 \text{ in l/min} = (76 \times 79 \times 5) \div 100,000 = .3 \text{ l/min}$$

Likewise, the VO_{2max} of a person exercising maximally who achieves a heart rate of 190 bpm and a maximal stroke volume of 120 ml would be

$$VO_{2max} \text{ in l/min} = (190 \times 120 \times 15) \div 100,000 = 3.42 \text{ l/min}$$

To convert l/min to ml/kg/min, multiply the l/min value by 1,000 and divide by body weight in kilograms. In the above example, if the person weighed 70 kilograms, the VO_{2max} in ml/kg/min would be 48.9 ($3.42 \times 1000 \div 70$)

Because the actual measurement of the stroke volume and the a-$\overline{v}O_2$diff is impractical in the fitness setting, VO_2 is also determined through gas (air) analysis. The person being tested breathes into a metabolic cart that measures the difference in oxygen content between the person's exhaled air and the atmosphere. (The air we breathe contains 21 percent oxygen; thus, VO_2 can be assessed by establishing the difference between 21 percent, the percent of oxygen left in the air the person exhales, and the total amount of air taken into the lungs.) This type of equipment, however, is expensive. Consequently, several alternative methods of estimating VO_{2max} using limited equipment have been developed. These methods are discussed in the next section.

VO_{2max} is affected by genetics, training, gender, age, and body composition. Although aerobic training can help people attain good or excellent cardiorespiratory fitness, only those with a strong genetic component are able to reach an "elite" level of aerobic capacity (60 to 80 ml/kg/min). Further, VO_{2max} is 15 to 30 percent higher in men. This is related to a greater hemoglobin content, lower body fat (see "Essential and Storage Fat" in Chapter 4),

and larger heart size in men (a larger heart pumps more blood, thus producing a greater stroke volume). VO_{2max} also decreases by about 1 percent per year starting at age 25. This decrease, however, is only 0.5 percent per year in physically active individuals.

Tests to Estimate VO_{2max}

Even though most cardiorespiratory endurance tests probably are safe to administer to apparently healthy individuals (those with no major coronary risk factors or symptoms), the American College of Sports Medicine recommends that a physician be present for all maximal exercise tests on apparently healthy men over age 45 and women over age 55. A maximal test is any test that requires the participant's all-out or nearly all-out effort. For submaximal exercise tests, a physician should be present when testing higher risk/symptomatic individuals or diseased people, regardless of the participant's current age.

Five exercise tests used to assess cardiorespiratory fitness are introduced in this chapter: the 1.5-Mile Run Test, the 1.0-Mile Walk Test, the Step Test, the Astrand–Ryhming Test, and the 12-Minute Swim Test. The test procedures are explained in detail in Figures 6.1, 6.2, 6.3, 6.4, and 6.5, respectively.

Multiple tests are provided in this chapter so you may choose one test depending on time, equipment, and individual physical limitations. For example, people who can't jog or walk could take the bike or swim test. You may perform more than one of these tests, but because these are different tests and they estimate maximal oxygen uptake, they will not necessarily yield the same results. Therefore, to make valid comparisons, you should take the same test when doing pre- and post-assessments. You may record the results of your test(s) in Lab 6A.

1.5-MILE RUN TEST

The 1.5-Mile Run Test is used most frequently to predict maximal oxygen uptake according to the time the person takes to run or walk a 1.5-mile course (see Figure 6.1). Maximal oxygen uptake is estimated based on the time the person takes to cover the distance (see Table 6.2).

The only equipment necessary to conduct this test is a stopwatch and a track or premeasured 1.5-mile course. This perhaps is the easiest test to administer, but a note of caution is in order when

Maximal heart rate (MHR) Highest heart rate for a person, related primarily to age.

Arterial-venous oxygen difference (a-vO_2diff) The amount of oxygen removed from the blood as determined by the difference in oxygen content between arterial and venous blood.

FIGURE 6.1 Procedure for the 1.5-Mile Run Test.

1. Make sure you qualify for this test. This test is contra-indicated for unconditioned beginners, individuals with symptoms of heart disease, and those with known heart disease or risk factors.
2. Select the testing site. Find a school track (each lap is one-fourth of a mile) or a premeasured 1.5-mile course.
3. Have a stopwatch available to determine your time.
4. Conduct a few warm-up exercises prior to the test. Do some stretching exercises, some walking, and slow jogging.
5. Initiate the test and try to cover the distance in the fastest time possible (walking or jogging). Time yourself during the run to see how fast you have covered the distance. If any unusual symptoms arise during the test, do not continue. Stop immediately and retake the test after another 6 weeks of aerobic training.
6. At the end of the test, cool down by walking or jogging slowly for another 3 to 5 minutes. Do not sit or lie down after the test.
7. According to your performance time, look up your estimated maximal oxygen uptake(VO_{2max}) in Table 6.2.

Example: A 20-year-old female runs the 1.5-mile course in 12 minutes and 40 seconds. Table 6.2 shows a VO_{2max} of 39.8 ml/kg/min for a time of 12:40. According to Table 6.8, this VO_{2max} would place her in the "good" cardio-respiratory fitness category.

TABLE 6.2 Estimated Maximal Oxygen Uptake (VO_{2max}) for the 1.5-Mile Run Test

Time	VO_{2max} (ml/kg/min)	Time	VO_{2max} (ml/kg/min)	Time	VO_{2max} (ml/kg/min)
6:10	80.0	10:30	48.6	14:50	34.0
6:20	79.0	10:40	48.0	15:00	33.6
6:30	77.9	10:50	47.4	15:10	33.1
6:40	76.7	11:00	46.6	15:20	32.7
6:50	75.5	11:10	45.8	15:30	32.2
7:00	74.0	11:20	45.1	15:40	31.8
7:10	72.6	11:30	44.4	15:50	31.4
7:20	71.3	11:40	43.7	16:00	30.9
7:30	69.9	11:50	43.2	16:10	30.5
7:40	68.3	12:00	42.3	16:20	30.2
7:50	66.8	12:10	41.7	16:30	29.8
8:00	65.2	12:20	41.0	16:40	29.5
8:10	63.9	12:30	40.4	16:50	29.1
8:20	62.5	12:40	39.8	17:00	28.9
8:30	61.2	12:50	39.2	17:10	28.5
8:40	60.2	13:00	38.6	17:20	28.3
8:50	59.1	13:10	38.1	17:30	28.0
9:00	58.1	13:20	37.8	17:40	27.7
9:10	56.9	13:30	37.2	17:50	27.4
9:20	55.9	13:40	36.8	18:00	27.1
9:30	54.7	13:50	36.3	18:10	26.8
9:40	53.5	14:00	35.9	18:20	26.6
9:50	52.3	14:10	35.5	18:30	26.3
10:00	51.1	14:20	35.1	18:40	26.0
10:10	50.4	14:30	34.7	18:50	25.7
10:20	49.5	14:40	34.3	19:00	25.4

Source: Adapted from K. H. Cooper, "A Means of Assessing Maximal Oxygen Intake," *Journal of the American Medical Association*, 203 (1968): 201–204; M. L. Pollock, J. H. Wilmore, and S. M. Fox III, *Health and Fitness Through Physical Activity*, (New York: John Wiley & Sons, 1978); and J. H. Wilmore and D. L. Costill, *Training for Sport and Activity* (Dubuque, IA: Wm. C. Brown Publishers, 1988).

conducting the test: Given that the objective is to cover the distance in the shortest time, it is considered a maximal exercise test. The 1.5-Mile Run Test should be limited to conditioned individuals who have been cleared for exercise. The test is not recommended for unconditioned beginners, men over age 45, and women over age 55 without proper medical clearance, symptomatic individuals, and those with known disease or risk factors for coronary heart disease. A program of at least 6 weeks of aerobic training is recommended before unconditioned individuals take this test.

1.0-MILE WALK TEST

This test can be used by individuals who are unable to run because of low fitness levels or injuries. All that is required is a brisk 1.0-mile walk that will elicit an exercise heart rate of at least 120 beats per minute at the end of the test.

You will need to know how to take your heart rate by counting your pulse. This can be done by gently placing the middle and index fingers over the radial artery on the wrist (inside the wrist on the side of the thumb) or over the carotid artery in the neck just below the jaw, next to the voice box. The thumb should not be used to check the pulse because it has a strong pulse of its own, which can make you miscount. When checking the carotid pulse, do not press too hard, because it may cause a reflex action that slows the heart. Some exercise leaders recommend that when you check the pulse over the carotid artery, the hand on the same side of the neck (left hand over left carotid artery) be used to avoid excessive pressure on the artery. With minimum experience, however, you can be accurate using either hand as long as only gentle

FIGURE 6.2 Procedure for the 1.0-Mile Walk Test.

1. Select the testing site. Use a 440-yard track (4 laps to a mile) or a premeasured 1.0-mile course.
2. Determine your body weight in pounds prior to the test.
3. Have a stopwatch available to determine total walking time and exercise heart rate.
4. Walk the 1.0-mile course at a brisk pace (the exercise heart rate at the end of the test should be above 120 beats per minute).
5. At the end of the 1.0-mile walk, check your walking time and immediately count your pulse for 10 seconds. Multiply the 10-second pulse count by 6 to obtain the exercise heart rate in beats per minute.
6. Convert the walking time from minutes and seconds to minute units. Because each minute has 60 seconds, divide the seconds by 60 to obtain the fraction of a minute. For instance, a walking time of 12 minutes and 15 seconds would equal 12 + (15 ÷ 60), or 12.25 minutes.
7. To obtain the estimated maximal oxygen uptake (VO_{2max}) in ml/kg/min, plug your values in the following equation: VO_{2max} = 88.768 − (0.0957 × W) + (8.892 × G) − (1.4537 × T) − (0.1194 × HR)

WHERE:

- W = Weight in pounds
- G = Gender (use 0 for women and 1 for men)
- T = Total time for the one-mile walk in minutes (see item 6)
- HR = Exercise heart rate in beats per minute at the end of the 1.0-mile walk

Example: A 19-year-old female who weighs 140 pounds completed the 1.0-mile walk in 14 minutes 39 seconds and with an exercise heart rate of 148 beats per minute. The estimated VO_{2max} would be:

- W = 140 lbs
- G = 0 (female gender = 0)
- T = 14:39 = 14 + (39 ÷ 60) = 14.65 min
- HR = 148 bpm
- VO_{2max} = 88.768 − (0.0957 × 140) + (8.892 × 0) − (1.4537 × 14.65) − (0.1194 × 148)
- VO_{2max} = 36.4 ml/kg/min

Source: F. A. Dolgener, L. D. Hensley, J. J. Marsh, and J. K. Fjelstul, "Validation of the Rockport Fitness Walking Test in College Males and Females," *Research Quarterly for Exercise and Sport* 65 (1994): 152–158.

---

pressure is applied. If available, heart rate monitors can be used to increase the accuracy of heart rate assessment.

Maximal oxygen uptake is estimated according to a prediction equation that requires the following data: 1.0-mile walk time, exercise heart rate at the end of the walk, gender, and body weight in pounds. The procedure for this test and the equation are given in Figure 6.2.

STEP TEST

The Step Test requires little time and equipment and can be administered to almost anyone, because a submaximal workload is used to estimate maximal oxygen uptake. Symptomatic and diseased individuals should not take this test. Significantly overweight individuals and those with joint problems in the lower extremities may have difficulty performing the test.

The actual test takes only 3 minutes. A 15-second recovery heart rate is taken between 5 and 20 seconds following the test (see Figure 6.3 and Table 6.3). The equipment required consists of a bench or gymnasium bleacher 16¼ inches high, a stopwatch, and a metronome.

You also will need to know how to take your heart rate by counting your pulse (explained under the 1.0-Mile Walk Test). Once people learn to take

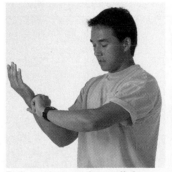

Pulse taken at the radial artery.

Pulse taken at the carotid artery.

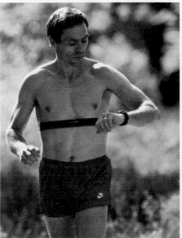

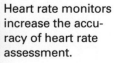

Heart rate monitors increase the accuracy of heart rate assessment.

FIGURE 6.3 Procedure for the Step Test.

1. Conduct the test with a bench or gymnasium bleacher 16¼ inches high.
2. Perform the stepping cycle to a four-step cadence (up-up-down-down). Men should perform 24 complete step-ups per minute, regulated with a metronome set at 96 beats per minute. Women perform 22 step-ups per minute, or 88 beats per minute on the metronome.
3. Allow a brief practice period of 5 to 10 seconds to familiarize yourself with the stepping cadence.
4. Begin the test and perform the step-ups for exactly 3 minutes.
5. Upon completing the 3 minutes, remain standing and take your heart rate for a 15-second interval from 5 to 20 seconds into recovery. Convert recovery heart rate to beats per minute (multiply 15-second heart rate by 4).
6. Maximal oxygen uptake (VO_{2max}) in ml/kg/min is estimated according to the following equations:

Men:

$VO_{2max} =$

$111.33 - (0.42 \times \text{recovery heart rate in bpm})$

Women:

$VO_{2max} =$

$65.81 - (0.1847 \times \text{recovery heart rate in bpm})$

Example: The recovery 15-second heart rate for a male following the 3-minute step test is found to be 39 beats. VO_{2max} is estimated as follows:

15-second heart rate = 39 beats

Minute heart rate = $39 \times 4 = 156$ bpm

$VO_{2max} = 111.33 - (0.42 \times 156) = 45.81$ ml/kg/min

VO_{2max} also can be obtained according to recovery heart rates in Table 6.3.

Source: From W. D. McArdle et al., *Exercise Physiology: Energy, Nutrition, and Human Performance* (Philadelphia: Lea & Febiger, 1986).

TABLE 6.3 Predicted Maximal Oxygen Uptake for the Step Test

15-Sec Heart Rate	Heart Rate (bpm)	VO₂max (ml/kg/min)	
		Men	Women
30	120	60.9	43.6
31	124	59.3	42.9
32	128	57.6	42.2
33	132	55.9	41.4
34	136	54.2	40.7
35	140	52.5	40.0
36	144	50.9	39.2
37	148	49.2	38.5
38	152	47.5	37.7
39	156	45.8	37.0
40	160	44.1	36.3
41	164	42.5	35.5
42	168	40.8	34.8
43	172	39.1	34.0
44	176	37.4	33.3
45	180	35.7	32.6
46	184	34.1	31.8
47	188	32.4	31.1
48	192	30.7	30.3
49	196	29.0	29.6
50	200	27.3	28.9

their own heart rate, a large group of people can be tested at once, using gymnasium bleachers for the steps.

ASTRAND–RYHMING TEST

Because of its simplicity and practicality, the Astrand–Ryhming test is one of the most popular tests used to estimate maximal oxygen uptake in the laboratory setting. The test is conducted on a bicycle ergometer, and, similar to the Step Test, it requires only sub-maximal workloads and little time to administer.

The cautions given for the Step Test also apply to the Astrand–Ryhming Test. Nevertheless, because the participant does not have to support his or her own body weight while riding the bicycle, overweight individuals and those with limited joint problems in the lower extremities can take this test.

The bicycle ergometer to be used for this test should allow for the regulation of workloads (see the test procedure in Figure 6.4). Besides the bicycle ergometer, a stopwatch and an additional technician to monitor the heart rate are needed to conduct the test.

The heart rate is taken every minute for 6 minutes. At the end of the test, the heart rate should be in the range given for each workload in Table 6.5 (generally between 120 and 170 bpm).

When administering the test to older people, good judgment is essential. Low workloads should be used, because if the higher heart rates (around 150 to 170 bpm) are reached, these individuals could be working near or at their maximal capacity, making it an unsafe test without adequate medical supervision. When testing older people, choose workloads so the final exercise heart rates do not exceed 130 to 140 bpm.

CRITICAL THINKING

Should fitness testing be a part of a fitness program? Why or why not? Are there benefits to pre-participation fitness testing or should fitness testing be done at a later date?

FIGURE 6.4 Procedure for the Astrand–Ryhming Test.

1. Adjust the bike seat so the knees are almost completely extended as the foot goes through the bottom of the pedaling cycle.
2. During the test, keep the speed constant at 50 revolutions per minute. Test duration is 6 minutes.
3. Select the appropriate workload for the bike based on age, weight, health, and estimated fitness level. For unconditioned individuals: women, use 300 kpm (kilopounds per meter) or 450 kpm; men, 300 kpm or 600 kpm. Conditioned adults: women, 450 kpm or 600 kpm; men, 600 kpm or 900 kpm.*
4. Ride the bike for 6 minutes and check the heart rate every minute, during the last 10 seconds of each minute. Determine heart rate by recording the time it takes to count 30 pulse beats and then converting to beats per minute using Table 6.4.
5. Average the final two heart rates (5th and 6th minutes). If these two heart rates are not within 5 beats per minute of each other, continue the test for another few minutes until this is accomplished. If the heart rate continues to climb significantly after the 6th minute, stop the test and rest for 15 to 20 minutes. You may then retest, preferably at a lower workload. The final average heart rate should also fall between the ranges given for each workload in Table 6.5 (men: 300 kpm = 120 to 140

beats per minute; 600 kpm = 120 to 170 beats per minute).
6. Based on the average heart rate of the final 2 minutes and your workload, look up the maximal oxygen uptake (VO_{2max}) in Table 6.5 (for example: men: 600 kpm and average heart rate = 145, VO_{2max} = 2.4 liters/minute).
7. Correct VO_{2max} using the correction factors found in Table 6.6 (if VO_{2max} = 2.4 and age 35, correction factor = .870. Multiply 2.4 × .870 and final corrected VO_{2max} = 2.09 liters/minute).
8. To obtain VO_{2max} in ml/kg/min, multiply the VO_{2max} by 1,000 (to convert liters to milliliters) and divide by body weight in kilograms (to obtain kilograms, divide your body weight in pounds by 2.2046).

Example: Corrected VO_{2max} = 2.09 liters/minute
Body weight = 132 pounds or 60 kilograms
   (132 ÷ 2.2046 = 60)

$$VO_{2max} \text{ in ml/kg/min} = \frac{2.09 \times 1,000}{60} = 34.8 \text{ ml/kg/min}$$

2,090 divided by 60 = 34.8 ml/kg/min

---

* On the Monarch bicycle ergometer, at a speed of 50 revolutions per minute, a load of 1 kp = 300 kpm, 1.5 kp = 450, 2 kp = 600 kpm, and so forth, with increases of 150 kpm to each half kp.

TABLE 6.4 Conversion of Time for 30 Pulse Beats to Pulse Rate Per Minute

Sec.	bpm	Sec.	bpm	Sec.	bpm	Sec.	bpm	Sec.	bpm	Sec.	bpm
22.0	82	19.6	92	17.2	105	14.8	122	12.4	145	10.0	180
21.9	82	19.5	92	17.1	105	14.7	122	12.3	146	9.9	182
21.8	83	19.4	93	17.0	106	14.6	123	12.2	148	9.8	184
21.7	83	19.3	93	16.9	107	14.5	124	12.1	149	9.7	186
21.6	83	19.2	94	16.8	107	14.4	125	12.0	150	9.6	188
21.5	84	19.1	94	16.7	108	14.3	126	11.9	151	9.5	189
21.4	84	19.0	95	16.6	108	14.2	127	11.8	153	9.4	191
21.3	85	18.9	95	16.5	109	14.1	128	11.7	154	9.3	194
21.2	85	18.8	96	16.4	110	14.0	129	11.6	155	9.2	196
21.1	85	18.7	96	16.3	110	13.9	129	11.5	157	9.1	198
21.0	86	18.6	97	16.2	111	13.8	130	11.4	158	9.0	200
20.9	86	18.5	97	16.1	112	13.7	131	11.3	159	8.9	202
20.8	87	18.4	98	16.0	113	13.6	132	11.2	161	8.8	205
20.7	87	18.3	98	15.9	113	13.5	133	11.1	162	8.7	207
20.6	87	18.2	99	15.8	114	13.4	134	11.0	164	8.6	209
20.5	88	18.1	99	15.7	115	13.3	135	10.9	165	8.5	212
20.4	88	18.0	100	15.6	115	13.2	136	10.8	167	8.4	214
20.3	89	17.9	101	15.5	116	13.1	137	10.7	168	8.3	217
20.2	89	17.8	101	15.4	117	13.0	138	10.6	170	8.2	220
20.1	90	17.7	102	15.3	118	12.9	140	10.5	171		
20.0	90	17.6	102	15.2	118	12.8	141	10.4	173		
19.9	90	17.5	103	15.1	119	12.7	142	10.3	175		
19.8	91	17.4	103	15.0	120	12.6	143	10.2	176		
19.7	91	17.3	104	14.9	121	12.5	144	10.1	178		

TABLE 6.5 Maximal Oxygen Uptake (VO_{2max}) Estimates for the Astrand–Ryhming Test

	Men Workload					Women Workload				
Heart Rate	300	600	900	1200	1500	300	450	600	750	900
120	2.2	3.4	4.8			2.6	3.4	4.1	4.8	
121	2.2	3.4	4.7			2.5	3.3	4.0	4.8	
122	2.2	3.4	4.6			2.5	3.2	3.9	4.7	
123	2.1	3.4	4.6			2.4	3.1	3.9	4.6	
124	2.1	3.3	4.5	6.0		2.4	3.1	3.8	4.5	
125	2.0	3.2	4.4	5.9		2.3	3.0	3.7	4.4	
126	2.0	3.2	4.4	5.8		2.3	3.0	3.6	4.3	
127	2.0	3.1	4.3	5.7		2.2	2.9	3.5	4.2	
128	2.0	3.1	4.2	5.6		2.2	2.8	3.5	4.2	4.8
129	1.9	3.0	4.2	5.6		2.2	2.8	3.4	4.1	4.8
130	1.9	3.0	4.1	5.5		2.1	2.7	3.4	4.0	4.7
131	1.9	2.9	4.0	5.4		2.1	2.7	3.4	4.0	4.6
132	1.8	2.9	4.0	5.3		2.0	2.7	3.3	3.9	4.5
133	1.8	2.8	3.9	5.3		2.0	2.6	3.2	3.8	4.4
134	1.8	2.8	3.9	5.2		2.0	2.6	3.2	3.8	4.4
135	1.7	2.8	3.8	5.1		2.0	2.6	3.1	3.7	4.3
136	1.7	2.7	3.8	5.0		1.9	2.5	3.1	3.6	4.2
137	1.7	2.7	3.7	5.0		1.9	2.5	3.0	3.6	4.2
138	1.6	2.7	3.7	4.9		1.8	2.4	3.0	3.5	4.1
139	1.6	2.6	3.6	4.8		1.8	2.4	2.9	3.5	4.0
140	1.6	2.6	3.6	4.8	6.0	1.8	2.4	2.8	3.4	4.0
141		2.6	3.5	4.7	5.9	1.8	2.3	2.8	3.4	3.9
142		2.5	3.5	4.6	5.8	1.7	2.3	2.8	3.3	3.9
143		2.5	3.4	4.6	5.7	1.7	2.2	2.7	3.3	3.8
144		2.5	3.4	4.5	5.7	1.7	2.2	2.7	3.2	3.8
145		2.4	3.4	4.5	5.6	1.6	2.2	2.7	3.2	3.7
146		2.4	3.3	4.4	5.6	1.6	2.2	2.6	3.2	3.7
147		2.4	3.3	4.4	5.5	1.6	2.1	2.6	3.1	3.6
148		2.4	3.2	4.3	5.4	1.6	2.1	2.6	3.1	3.6
149		2.3	3.2	4.3	5.4		2.1	2.6	3.0	3.5
150		2.3	3.2	4.2	5.3		2.0	2.5	3.0	3.5
151		2.3	3.1	4.2	5.2		2.0	2.5	3.0	3.4
152		2.3	3.1	4.1	5.2		2.0	2.5	2.9	3.4
153		2.2	3.0	4.1	5.1		2.0	2.4	2.9	3.3
154		2.2	3.0	4.0	5.1		2.0	2.4	2.8	3.3
155		2.2	3.0	4.0	5.0		1.9	2.4	2.8	3.2
156		2.2	2.9	4.0	5.0		1.9	2.3	2.8	3.2
157		2.1	2.9	3.9	4.9		1.9	2.3	2.7	3.2
158		2.1	2.9	3.9	4.9		1.8	2.3	2.7	3.1
159		2.1	2.8	3.8	4.8		1.8	2.2	2.7	3.1
160		2.1	2.8	3.8	4.8		1.8	2.2	2.6	3.0
161		2.0	2.8	3.7	4.7		1.8	2.2	2.6	3.0
162		2.0	2.8	3.7	4.6		1.8	2.2	2.6	3.0
163		2.0	2.8	3.7	4.6		1.7	2.2	2.6	2.9
164		2.0	2.7	3.6	4.5		1.7	2.1	2.5	2.9
165		2.0	2.7	3.6	4.5		1.7	2.1	2.5	2.9
166		1.9	2.7	3.6	4.5		1.7	2.1	2.5	2.8
167		1.9	2.6	3.5	4.4		1.6	2.1	2.4	2.8
168		1.9	2.6	3.5	4.4		1.6	2.0	2.4	2.8
169		1.9	2.6	3.5	4.3		1.6	2.0	2.4	2.8
170		1.8	2.6	3.4	4.3		1.6	2.0	2.4	2.7

From Astrand, I. *Acta Physiologica Scandinavica* 49 (1960). Supplementum 169: 45–60.

TABLE 6.6 Age-Based Correction Factors for Maximal Oxygen Uptake

Age	Correction Factor	Age	Correction Factor	Age	Correction Factor
14	1.11	32	.909	50	.750
15	1.10	33	.896	51	.742
16	1.09	34	.883	52	.734
17	1.08	35	.870	53	.726
18	1.07	36	.862	54	.718
19	1.06	37	.854	55	.710
20	1.05	38	.846	56	.704
21	1.04	39	.838	57	.698
22	1.03	40	.830	58	.692
23	1.02	41	.820	59	.686
24	1.01	42	.810	60	.680
25	1.00	43	.800	61	.674
26	.987	44	.790	62	.668
27	.974	45	.780	63	.662
28	.961	46	.774	64	.656
29	.948	47	.768	65	.650
30	.935	48	.762		
31	.922	49	.756		

Adapted from Astrand, I. *Acta Physiologica Scandinavica* 49 (1960). Supplementum 169: 45–60.

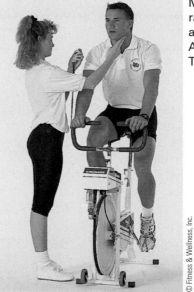

Monitoring heart rate on the carotid artery during the Astrand–Ryhming Test.

12-MINUTE SWIM TEST

Similar to the 1.5-Mile Run test, the 12-Minute Swim Test is considered a maximal exercise test, and the same precautions apply. The objective is to swim as far as possible during the 12-minute test.

Unlike land-based tests, predicting maximal oxygen uptake through a swimming test is difficult.

FIGURE 6.5 Procedure for the 12-Minute Swim Test.

1. Enlist a friend to time the test. The only other requisites are a stopwatch and a swimming pool. Do not attempt to do this test in an unsupervised pool.
2. Warm up by swimming slowly and doing a few stretching exercises before taking the test.
3. Start the test and swim as many laps as possible in 12 minutes. Pace yourself throughout the test and do not swim to the point of complete exhaustion.
4. After completing the test, cool down by swimming another 2 or 3 minutes at a slower pace.
5. Determine the total distance you swam during the test and look up your fitness category in Table 6.7.

TABLE 6.7 12-Minute Swim Test Fitness Categories

Distance (yards)	Fitness Category
≥700	Excellent
500–700	Good
400–500	Average
200–400	Fair
≤200	Poor

Adapted from K. H. Cooper, *The Aerobics Program for Total Well-Being* (New York: Bantam Books, 1982).

TABLE 6.8 Cardiorespiratory Fitness Category According to Maximal Oxygen Uptake (VO_{2max})

		FITNESS CLASSIFICATION (based on VO_{2max} in ml/kg/min)				
Gender	Age	Poor	Fair	Average	Good	Excellent
Men	<29	<24.9	25–33.9	34–43.9	44–52.9	>53
	30–39	<22.9	23–30.9	31–41.9	42–49.9	>50
	40–49	<19.9	20–26.9	27–38.9	39–44.9	>45
	50–59	<17.9	18–24.9	25–37.9	38–42.9	>43
	60–69	<15.9	16–22.9	23–35.9	36–40.9	>41
	≥70	≤12.9	13–20.9	21–32.9	33–37.9	≥38
Women	<29	<23.9	24–30.9	31–38.9	39–48.9	>49
	30–39	<19.9	20–27.9	28–36.9	37–44.9	>45
	40–49	<16.9	17–24.9	25–34.9	35–41.9	>42
	50–59	<14.9	15–21.9	22–33.9	34–39.9	>40
	60–69	<12.9	13–20.9	21–32.9	33–36.9	>37
	≥70	≤11.9	12–19.9	20–30.9	31–34.9	≥35

■ Health fitness standard   ■ High physical fitness standard

See the Chapter 1 discussion on health fitness versus physical fitness.

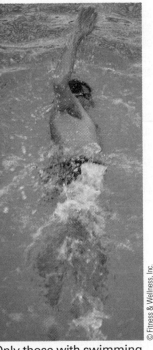

Only those with swimming skill and proper conditioning should take the 12-minute swim test.

A swimming test (Figure 6.5) is practical only for those who are planning to take part in a swimming program or who cannot perform any of the other tests. Differences in skill level, swimming conditioning, and body composition greatly affect the energy requirements (oxygen uptake) of swimming.

Unskilled and unconditioned swimmers can expect lower cardiorespiratory fitness ratings than those obtained with a land-based test. A skilled swimmer is able to swim more efficiently and expend much less energy than an unskilled swimmer. Improper breathing patterns cause premature fatigue. Overweight individuals are more buoyant in the water, and the larger surface area (body size) produces greater friction against movement in the water medium.

Lack of conditioning affects swimming test results as well. An unconditioned skilled swimmer who is in good cardiorespiratory shape because of a regular jogging program will not perform as effectively in a swimming test. Swimming conditioning is important for adequate performance on this test.

Because of these limitations, maximal oxygen uptake cannot be estimated for a swimming test and the fitness categories given in Table 6.7 are only estimated ratings.

Interpreting Your Maximal Oxygen Uptake Results

After obtaining your maximal oxygen uptake, you can determine your current level of cardiorespiratory fitness by consulting Table 6.8. Locate the maximal oxygen uptake in your age category, and on the top row you will find your present level of cardiorespiratory fitness. For example, a 19-year-old male with a maximal oxygen uptake of 35 ml/kg/min would be classified in the "Average" cardiorespiratory fitness category. After you initiate your personal cardiorespiratory

CRITICAL THINKING

Your relative maximal oxygen uptake can be improved without engaging in an aerobic exercise program. How do you accomplish this? Would you benefit from doing so?

exercise program (see Lab 6D), you may wish to retest yourself periodically to evaluate your progress.

Predicting Oxygen Uptake and Caloric Expenditure from Walking and Jogging

As indicated earlier in the chapter, oxygen uptake can be expressed in liters per minute (l/min) or milliliters per kilogram per minute (ml/kg/min). The latter is used to classify individuals into the various cardio-respiratory fitness categories (see Table 6.8).

Oxygen uptake expressed in l/min is valuable in determining the caloric expenditure of physical activity. The human body burns about 5 calories for each liter of oxygen consumed. During aerobic exercise the average person trains between 60 and 75 percent of maximal oxygen uptake.[3]

A person with a maximal oxygen uptake of 3.5 l/min who trains at 60 percent of maximum uses 2.1 (3.5 × .60) liters of oxygen per minute of physical activity. This indicates that 10.5 calories are burned each minute of exercise (2.1 × 5). If the activity is carried out for 30 minutes, 315 calories (10.5 × 30) have been burned.

For individuals concerned about weight management, these computations are valuable in determining energy expenditure. Because a pound of body fat represents 3,500 calories, this individual would have to exercise for a total of 333 minutes (3,500 ÷ 10.5) to burn the equivalent of a pound of body fat. At 30 minutes per exercise session, approximately 11 sessions would be required to expend the 3,500 calories.

Applying the principle of 5 calories burned per liter of oxygen consumed, you can determine with reasonable accuracy your own caloric output for walking and jogging. Table 6.9 contains the oxygen requirement (uptake) for walking speeds between 50 and 100 meters per minute and for jogging speeds in excess of 80 meters per minute.

There is a transition period from walking to jogging for speeds in the range of 80 to 134 meters per minute. Consequently, the person must be truly jogging at these lower speeds to use the estimated oxygen uptakes for jogging in Table 6.9. Because these uptakes are expressed in ml/kg/min, you will have to convert this figure to l/min to predict caloric output. This is done by multiplying the oxygen uptake in ml/kg/min by your body weight in kilograms (kg) and then dividing by 1,000.

For example, let's estimate the caloric cost for an individual who weighs 145.5 pounds and runs 3 miles in 21 minutes. Each mile is about 1,600 meters, or four laps around a 400-meter (440-yard) track. Three miles then would be 4,800 meters

TABLE 6.9 Oxygen Requirement Estimates for Selected Walking and Jogging Speeds

Walking		Jogging			
Speed (m/min)	VO₂ (ml/kg/min)	Speed (m/min)	VO₂ (ml/kg/min)	Speed (m/min)	VO₂ (ml/kg/min)
50	8.5	80	19.5	210	45.5
52	8.7	85	20.5	215	46.5
54	8.9	90	21.5	220	47.5
56	9.1	95	22.5	225	48.5
58	9.3	100	23.5	230	49.5
60	9.5	105	24.5	235	50.5
62	9.7	110	25.5	240	51.5
64	9.9	115	26.5	245	52.5
66	10.1	120	27.5	250	53.5
68	10.3	125	28.5	255	54.5
70	10.5	130	29.5	260	55.5
72	10.7	135	30.5	265	56.5
74	10.9	140	31.5	270	57.5
76	11.1	145	32.5	275	58.5
78	11.3	150	33.5	280	59.5
80	11.5	155	34.5		
82	11.7	160	35.5		
84	11.9	165	36.5		
86	12.1	170	37.5		
88	12.3	175	38.5		
90	12.5	180	39.5		
92	12.7	185	40.5		
94	12.9	190	41.5		
96	13.1	195	42.5		
98	13.3	200	43.5		
100	13.5	205	44.5		

m/min = meters per minute

ml/kg/min = milliliters per kilogram per minute

Table developed using the metabolic calculations contained in *Guidelines for Exercise Testing and Exercise Prescription*, by the American College of Sports Medicine (Baltimore: Williams & Wilkins, 2000).

(1,600 × 3). Therefore, 3 miles (4,800 meters) in 21 minutes represents a pace of 228.6 meters per minute (4,800 ÷ 21).

Table 6.9 indicates an oxygen requirement (uptake) of about 49.5 ml/kg/min for a speed of 228.6 meters per minute. A weight of 145.5 pounds equals 66 kilograms (145.5 ÷ 2.2046). The oxygen uptake in l/min now can be calculated by multiplying the value in ml/kg/min by body weight in kg and dividing by 1,000. In our example, it is (49.5 × 66) ÷ 1,000 = 3.3 l/min. This oxygen uptake in 21 minutes represents a total of 347 calories (3.3 × 5 × 21).

In Lab 6B you have an opportunity to determine your own oxygen uptake and caloric expenditure for walking and jogging. Using your oxygen uptake information in conjunction with exercise heart rates allows you to estimate your caloric expenditure for almost any activity, as long as the heart rate ranges from 110 to 180 beats per minute.

To make an accurate estimate, you have to be skilled in assessing exercise heart rate. Also, as your level of fitness improves, you will need to reassess your exercise heart rate because it will drop (given the same workload) with improved physical condition.

Principles of Cardiorespiratory Exercise Prescription

Before proceeding with the principles of exercise prescription, you should ask yourself if you are willing to give exercise a try. A low percentage of the U.S. population is truly committed to exercise. Further, more than half of the people who start exercising drop out during the first 3 to 6 months of the program. Sports psychologists are trying to find out why some people exercise habitually and many do not. All of the benefits of exercise cannot help unless people commit to a lifetime program of physical activity.

Readiness for Exercise

The first step is to answer the question: Am I ready to start an exercise program? The information provided in Lab 6C can help you answer this question. You are evaluated in four categories: mastery (self-control), attitude, health, and commitment. The higher you score in any category—mastery, for example—the more important that reason is for you to exercise.

Scores can vary from 4 to 16. A score of 12 and above is a strong indicator that that factor is important to you, whereas 8 and below is low. If you score 12 or more points in each category, your chances of initiating and sticking to an exercise program are good. If you do not score at least 12 points each in any three categories, your chances of succeeding at exercise may be slim. You need to be better informed about the benefits of exercise, and a retraining process might be helpful. More tips on how you can become committed to exercise are provided in the section "Getting Started and Adhering to a Lifetime Exercise Program" (pages 180–181).

Next, you will have to decide positively that you will try. Using Lab 6C, you can list the advantages and disadvantages of incorporating exercise into your lifestyle. Your list might include advantages such as the following:

- It will make me feel better.
- I will lose weight.
- I will have more energy.
- It will lower my risk for chronic diseases.

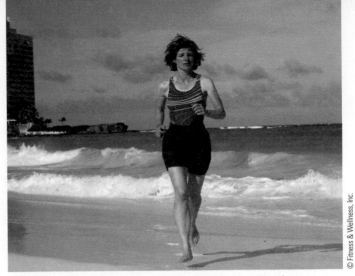

Aerobic exercise promotes cardiorespiratory development and helps decrease the risk for disease.

Your list of disadvantages might include the following:

- I don't want to take the time.
- I'm too out of shape.
- There's no good place to exercise.
- I don't have the willpower to do it.

When your reasons for exercising outweigh your reasons for not exercising, you will find it easier to try. In Lab 6C you will also determine your stage of change for aerobic exercise. Using the information learned in Chapter 2, you can outline specific processes and techniques for change.

Guidelines for Cardiorespiratory Exercise Prescription

In spite of the release of the U.S. Surgeon General statement on physical activity and health in 1996 (see Chapter 1, pages 5–6) and the overwhelming amount of evidence on the benefits of exercise on health and longevity, current estimates indicate that only about 19 percent of adults in the United States meet minimum recommendations of the American College of Sports Medicine (ACSM) for the improvement and maintenance of cardiorespiratory fitness.[4]

Most people are not familiar with the basic principles of cardiorespiratory exercise prescription. Thus, although they exercise regularly, they do not reap significant improvements in cardiorespiratory endurance.

To develop the cardiorespiratory system, the heart muscle has to be overloaded—like any other muscle in the human body. Just as the biceps muscle in the upper arm is developed through strength-training exercises, the heart muscle has to be exercised to increase in size, strength, and efficiency. To better understand how the cardiorespiratory system can be developed, you have to be familiar with the four variables that govern exercise prescription: intensity, mode, duration, and frequency.[5] The acronym FITT is sometimes used to describe these variables: *Frequency, Intensity, Type* (mode), and *Time* (duration).

First, however, you should be aware that the ACSM recommends that a medical exam and a diagnostic exercise stress test be administered prior to **vigorous exercise** to apparently healthy men over age 45 and women over age 55.[6] The ACSM has defined vigorous exercise as an exercise intensity above 60 percent of maximal capacity. For people initiating an exercise program, this intensity is the equivalent of exercise that provides a "substantial challenge" to the participant or one that cannot be maintained for 20 continuous minutes.

Intensity of Exercise

When trying to develop the cardiorespiratory system, many people often ignore **intensity** of exercise. For muscles to develop, they have to be overloaded to a given point. The training stimulus to develop the biceps muscle, for example, can be accomplished with arm curl-up exercises with increasing weights. Likewise, the cardiorespiratory system is stimulated by making the heart pump faster for a specified period.

Cardiorespiratory development occurs when the heart is working between 40 and 85 percent of heart rate reserve (see the section below on calculating intensity).[7] Individuals who are not fit should start at a 40 to 50 percent training intensity. Active and fit people can train at higher intensities. Increases in VO_{2max} are accelerated when the heart is working closer to 85 percent of **heart rate reserve (HRR)**. For this reason, many experts prescribe exercise between 60 and 85 percent. Intensity of exercise can be calculated easily, and training can be monitored by checking your pulse.

To determine the intensity of exercise or **cardiorespiratory training zone** according to heart rate reserve, follow these steps:

1. Estimate your maximal heart rate (MHR) according to the following formula:

   MHR = 220 minus age (220 − age)

2. Check your resting heart rate (RHR) some time after you have been sitting quietly for 15 to 20 minutes. You may take your pulse for 30 seconds and multiply by 2, or take it for a full minute. As explained on pages 166–167, you can check your pulse on the wrist, by placing two or three fingers over the radial artery or in the neck, using the carotid artery.

3. Determine the heart rate reserve (HRR) by subtracting the resting heart rate from the maximal heart rate (HRR = MHR − RHR).

4. Calculate the training intensities (TI) at 40, 50, 60, and 85 percent. Multiply the heart rate reserve by the respective .40, .50, .60, and .85, and then add the resting heart rate to all four of these figures (for example, 85% TI = HRR × .85 + RHR).

Example. The 40, 50, 60, and 85 percent training intensities for a 20-year-old with a resting heart rate of 68 beats per minute (bpm) would be as follows:

MHR: 220 − 20 = 200 bpm

RHR: = 68 bpm

HRR: 200 − 68 = 132 beats

40% TI = (132 × .40) + 68 = 121 bpm

50% TI = (132 × .50) + 68 = 134 bpm

60% TI = (132 × .60) + 68 = 147 bpm

85% TI = (132 × .85) + 68 = 180 bpm

Low-intensity cardiorespiratory training zone: 121 to 134 bpm

Moderate-intensity cardiorespiratory training zone: 134 to 147 bpm

Optimal cardiorespiratory training zone: 147 to 180 bpm

When you exercise to improve the cardiorespiratory system, maintain your heart rate between the 60 and 85 percent training intensities to obtain adequate development (see Figure 6.6). If you have been physically inactive, you should train around the 40 to 60 percent intensity during the first 6 to 8 weeks of the exercise program. After that, you should exercise between 60 and 85 percent training intensity.

Following a few weeks of training, you may have a considerably lower resting heart rate (10 to 20 beats fewer in 8 to 12 weeks). Therefore, you should recompute your target zone periodically. You can compute your own cardiorespiratory training zone using Lab 6D, or you can also use the computer software available with this book to obtain a printout of your personalized cardiorespiratory exercise prescription (see Figure 9.5, page 290). You can also use this software to create and regularly update an exercise log to keep a record of your activity program (see Figure 9.6, page 291). Once you have reached an ideal level of cardiorespiratory endurance, continued training in the 60 to 85 percent range will allow you to maintain your fitness level.

Profile Plus

You can keep a computerized exercise record by regularly entering your exercise sessions into the exercise log in the activities on the CD-ROM. This exercise log will generate a summary of caloric expenditure, exercise heart rate, exercise time, and body weight on a weekly or monthly basis.

COUNTING THE PULSE

During the first few weeks of an exercise program, you should monitor your exercise heart rate

FIGURE 6.6 Recommended cardiorespiratory or aerobic training pattern.

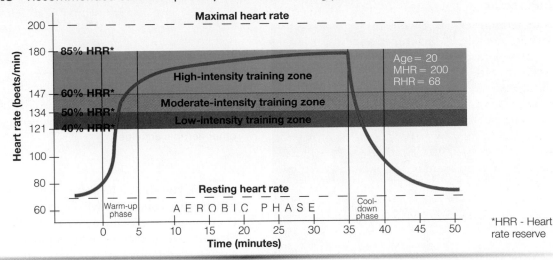

To develop the cardiorespiratory system, you do not have to exercise above the 85 percent rate. From a fitness standpoint, training above this percentage will not give extra benefits and actually may be unsafe for some individuals. Unconditioned people and older adults should train around the 50 percent rate to discourage potential problems associated with high-intensity exercise.

regularly to make sure you are training in the proper zone. Wait until you are about 5 minutes into the aerobic phase of your exercise session before taking your first reading. When you check your heart rate, count your pulse for 10 seconds, then multiply by 6 to get the per-minute pulse rate. The exercise heart rate will remain at the same level for about 15 seconds following aerobic exercise, then drop rapidly. Do not hesitate to stop during your exercise bout to check your pulse. If the rate is too low, increase the intensity of exercise. If the rate is too high, slow down.

To develop the cardiorespiratory system, you do not have to exercise above the 85 percent rate. From a fitness standpoint, training above this percentage will not give extra benefits and actually may be unsafe for some individuals. Unconditioned people and older adults should train around the 50 percent rate to discourage potential problems associated with high-intensity exercise.

When determining the training intensity for your own program, you need to consider your personal fitness goals. Individuals who exercise at around the 50 percent training intensity will reap significant health benefits—in particular, improvements in the metabolic profile (see "Health Fitness Standards" in Chapter 1). Training at this lower percentage, however, may place you in only the "average" (moderate fitness) category (see Table 6.8 on page 171). Exercising at this lower intensity does lower the risk for cardiovascular mortality (the health fitness standard), but will not allow you to achieve a "good" or "excellent" cardiorespiratory fitness rating (the physical fitness standard). The latter ratings are obtained by exercising closer to the 85 percent threshold.

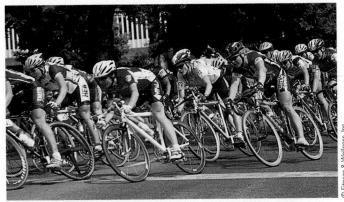

High-intensity exercise is required to achieve the high physical fitness standard (excellent category) for cardiorespiratory endurance.

RATE OF PERCEIVED EXERTION

Because many people do not check their heart rate during exercise, an alternative method of prescribing intensity of exercise was created using the **rate of perceived exertion (RPE)** scale. Using the scale in

Vigorous exercise Cardiorespiratory exercise that requires an intensity level above 60 percent of maximal capacity.

Intensity In cardiorespiratory exercise, how hard a person has to exercise to improve or maintain fitness.

Heart rate reserve (HRR) The difference between the maximal heart rate and the resting heart rate.

Cardiorespiratory training zone The recommended training intensity range, in terms of exercise heart rate, to obtain adequate cardiorespiratory endurance development.

Rate of perceived exertion (RPE) A perception scale to monitor or interpret the intensity of aerobic exercise.

FIGURE 6.7 Rate of perceived exertion (RPE) scale.

6	
7	Very, very light
8	
9	Very light
10	
11	Fairly light
12	
13	Somewhat hard
14	
15	Hard
16	
17	Very Hard
18	
19	Very, very hard
20	

From G. Borg, "Perceived Exertion: A Note on History and Methods," *Medicine and Science in Sports and Exercise,* 5 (1983): 90–93.

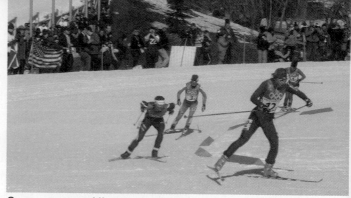

Cross-country skiing uses more oxygen and energy than most other aerobic activities.

Figure 6.7, a person subjectively rates the perceived exertion or difficulty of exercise when training in the appropriate target zone. The exercise heart rate then is associated with the corresponding RPE value.

For example, if the training intensity requires a heart rate between 150 and 170 bpm, the person may associate this with training between "hard" and "very hard." Some individuals perceive less exertion than others when training in the correct zone. Therefore, you have to associate your own inner perception of the task with the phrases given on the scale. You then may proceed to exercise at that rate of perceived exertion.

The numbers on the scale can also be used in reference to exercise heart rates. If you multiply each number by 10, it will approximate the exercise heart rate at the perceived exertion phase. For example, when you are exercising "somewhat hard," your heart rate will be around 130 bpm (13 × 10). When you exercise "hard," the heart rate will be about 150 bpm.

You must be sure to cross-check your target zone with your perceived exertion during the first weeks of your exercise program. To help you develop this association, you should regularly keep a record of your activities, using the form provided in Figure 6.10 (pages 185–186). After several weeks of training, you should be able to predict your exercise heart rate just by your own perceived exertion of the intensity of exercise.

Whether you monitor the intensity of exercise by checking your pulse or through rate of perceived exertion, you should be aware that changes in normal exercise conditions will affect the training zone. For example, exercising on a hot, humid day or at high altitude increases the heart rate response to a given task, requiring adjustments in the intensity of your exercise.

Mode of Exercise

The **mode** of exercise that develops the cardiorespiratory system has to be aerobic in nature. Once you have established your cardiorespiratory training zone, any activity or combination of activities that will get your heart rate up to that training zone and keep it there for as long as you exercise will give you adequate development. Examples of these activities are walking, jogging, aerobics, swimming, water aerobics, cross-country skiing, rope skipping, cycling, racquetball, stair climbing, and stationary running or cycling.

Aerobic exercise has to involve the major muscle groups of the body, and it has to be rhythmic and continuous. As the amount of muscle mass involved during exercise increases, so do the demands on the cardiorespiratory system. The activity you choose should be based on your personal preferences, what you most enjoy doing, and your physical limitations. Low-impact activities greatly reduce the risk for injuries. Most injuries to beginners result from high-impact activities. General strength conditioning (see Chapter 7) is also recommended prior to initiating an aerobic exercise program for individuals who have been inactive. Strength conditioning can significantly reduce the incidence of injuries.

The amount of strength or flexibility you develop through various activities differs. In terms of cardiorespiratory development, though, the heart doesn't know whether you are walking, swimming, or cycling. All the heart knows is that it has to pump at a certain rate, and as long as that rate is in the desired range, your cardiorespiratory fitness will improve. From a health fitness point of view, training in the lower end of the cardiorespiratory zone will yield optimal health benefits. The closer the heart rate is to the higher end of the cardiorespiratory training zone, however, the greater will be the improvements in maximal oxygen uptake (high physical fitness).

Duration of Exercise

The general recommendation is that a person train between 20 and 60 minutes per session. The duration of exercise is based on how intensely a person trains. If the training is done at around 85 percent, 20 to 30 minutes are sufficient. At 50 percent intensity, the person should train between 30 and 60 minutes. As mentioned under "Intensity of Exercise" on page 174, unconditioned people and older adults should train at lower percentages; therefore, the activity should be carried out over a longer time.

Although most experts recommend 20 to 30 minutes of aerobic exercise per session, accumulating 30 minutes or more of moderate-intensity physical activity throughout the day does provide substantial health benefits.[8] Three 10-minute exercise sessions per day (separated by at least 4 hours), at approximately 70 percent of maximal heart rate, also produce training benefits.[9] Although the increases in maximal oxygen uptake with the latter program were not as large (57 percent) as those found in a group performing a continuous 30-minute bout of exercise per day, the researchers concluded that moderate-intensity physical activity, conducted for 10 minutes, three times per day, benefits the cardiorespiratory system significantly.

Results of this study are meaningful because people often mention lack of time as the reason for not taking part in an exercise program. Many think they have to exercise at least 20 continuous minutes to get any benefits at all. Even though a duration of 20 to 30 high-intensity minutes is ideal, short, intermittent exercise bouts are beneficial to the cardiorespiratory system.

From a weight management point of view, the National Institute of Medicine recommends that people accumulate 60 minutes of moderate-intensity physical activity most days of the week.[10] This recommendation is based on evidence that people who maintain healthy weight typically accumulate one hour of daily physical activity. If lack of time is a concern, you should exercise at a high intensity for 30 minutes, which can burn as many calories as 60 minutes of moderate intensity (see Low-Intensity Versus High-Intensity Exercise for Weight Loss, Chapter 5, pages 136–137), but only 19 percent of adults in the United States typically exercise at a high intensity level.

Exercise sessions should always be preceded by a 5-minute **warm-up** and be followed by a 5-minute **cool-down** period (see Figure 6.6, page 175). The warm-up should consist of general calisthenics, stretching exercises, or exercising at a lower intensity

FIGURE 6.8 Cardiorespiratory exercise prescription guidelines.

Activity: Aerobic (examples: walking, jogging, cycling, swimming, aerobics, racquetball, soccer, stair climbing)

Intensity: 40/50%–85% of heart rate reserve

Duration: 20–60 minutes of continuous aerobic activity

Frequency: 3 to 5 days per week

Source: Based on American College of Sports Medicine, "Position Stand: The Recommended Quantity and Quality of Exercise for Developing and Maintaining Cardiorespiratory and Muscular Fitness, and Flexibility in Healthy Adults," *Medical Science Sports Exercise*, 30 (1998): 975–991.

level than the actual target zone. In the cool-down, the intensity of exercise is decreased gradually. Stopping abruptly causes blood to pool in the exercised body parts, diminishing the return of blood to the heart. Less blood return can cause dizziness and faintness or even bring on cardiac abnormalities.

FREQUENCY OF EXERCISE

When you start an exercise program, a **frequency** of three to five 20- to 30-minute training sessions per week is recommended to improve maximal oxygen uptake. When training is conducted more than 5 days a week, further improvements are minimal.

For individuals on a weight-loss program, the recommendation is 60-minute exercise sessions of low to moderate intensity, on most days of the week. Longer exercise sessions increase caloric expenditure for faster weight reduction (see Chapter 5, "Exercise: The Key to Weight Management," pages 135–137). Three 20- to 30-minute training sessions per week, on nonconsecutive days, will maintain cardiorespiratory fitness as long as the heart rate is in the appropriate target zone. A summary of the cardiorespiratory exercise prescription guidelines according to the American College of Sports Medicine is provided in Figure 6.8.

Although three exercise sessions per week will maintain cardiorespiratory fitness, the importance of regular physical activity in preventing disease and enhancing quality of life has been pointed out

Mode Form or type of exercise.

Warm-up Starting a workout slowly.

Cool-down Tapering off an exercise session slowly.

Frequency How many times per week a person engages in an exercise session.

FIGURE 6.9 The Physical Activity Pyramid.

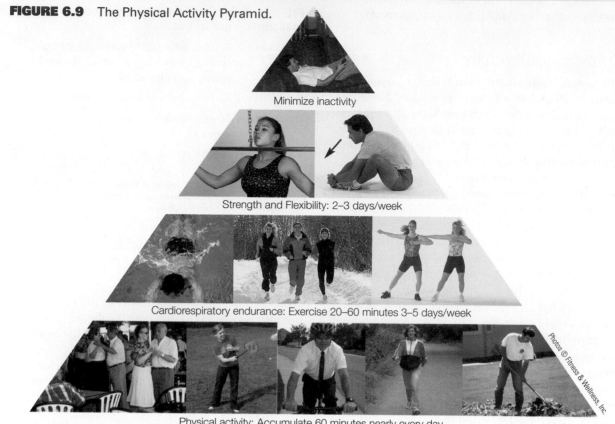

Minimize inactivity

Strength and Flexibility: 2–3 days/week

Cardiorespiratory endurance: Exercise 20–60 minutes 3–5 days/week

Physical activity: Accumulate 60 minutes nearly every day

Photos © Fitness & Wellness, Inc.

clearly by the American College of Sports Medicine, by the U.S. Centers for Disease Control and Prevention, and by the President's Council on Physical Fitness and Sports.[11] These organizations advocate at least 30 minutes of moderate-intensity physical activity almost daily. This routine has been promoted as an effective way to improve health.

These recommendations were subsequently upheld by the U.S. Surgeon General in the 1996 "Report on Physical Activity and Health"[12] and later in the 2005 Dietary Guidelines for Americans.[13] The Surgeon General's report states that people can improve their health and quality of life substantially by including moderate amounts of physical activity on most, preferably all, days of the week. Further, it states that no one, including older adults, is too old to enjoy the benefits of regular physical activity.

If you want to enjoy better health and fitness, physical activity must be pursued on a regular basis. According to Dr. William Haskell of Stanford University: "Most of the health-related benefits of exercise are relatively short-term, so people should think of exercise as medication and take it on a daily basis."[14] Many of the benefits of exercise and

activity diminish within 2 weeks of substantially decreased physical activity. These benefits are completely lost within 2 to 8 months of inactivity.[15]

To sum up: Ideally, a person should engage in physical activity six to seven times per week. Based on the previous discussion, to reap both the high-fitness and health-fitness benefits of exercise, a person needs to exercise a minimum of three times per week in the appropriate target zone for high fitness maintenance and three to four additional times per week in moderate-intensity activities (see Figure 6.9). Depending on the intensity of the activity, all aerobic exercise/activity sessions should last from 20 to 60 minutes.

Fitness Benefits of Aerobic Activities

The contributions of different aerobic activities to the health-related components of fitness vary. Although an accurate assessment of the contributions to each fitness component is difficult to establish, a summary of likely benefits of several activities is provided in Table 6.10. Instead of a single rating or

TABLE 6.10 Ratings for Selected Aerobic Activities

Activity	Recommended Starting Fitness Level[1]	Injury Risk[2]	Potential Cardiorespiratory Endurance Development (VO_{2max})[3,5]	Upper Body Strength Development[3]	Lower Body Strength Development[3]	Upper Body Flexibility Development[3]	Lower Body Flexibility Development[3]	Weight Control[3]	MET Level[4,5,6]	Caloric Expenditure (cal/hour)[5,6]
Aerobics										
High-Impact Aerobics	A	H	3–4	2	4	3	2	4	6–12	450–900
Moderate-Impact Aerobics	I	M	2–4	2	3	3	2	3	6–12	450–900
Low-Impact Aerobics	B	L	2–4	2	3	3	2	3	5–10	375–750
Step Aerobics	I	M	2–4	2	3–4	3	2	3–4	5–12	375–900
Cross-Country Skiing	B	M	4–5	4	4	2	2	4–5	10–16	750–1,200
Cross-Training	I	M	3–5	2–3	3–4	2–3	1–2	3–5	6–15	450–1,125
Cycling										
Road	I	M	2–5	1	4	1	1	3	6–12	450–900
Stationary	B	L	2–4	1	4	1	1	3	6–10	450–750
Hiking	B	L	2–4	1	3	1	1	3	6–10	450–750
In-Line Skating	I	M	2–4	2	4	2	2	3	6–10	450–750
Jogging	I	M	3–5	1	3	1	1	5	6–15	450–1,125
Jogging, Deep Water	A	L	3–5	2	2	1	1	5	8–15	600–1,125
Racquet Sports	I	M	2–4	3	3	3	2	3	6–10	450–750
Rope Skipping	I	H	3–5	2	4	1	2	3–5	8–15	600–1,125
Rowing	B	L	3–5	4	2	3	1	4	8–14	600–1,050
Spinning	I	L	4–5	1	4	1	1	4	8–15	600–1,125
Stair Climbing	B	L	3–5	1	4	1	1	4–5	8–15	600–1,125
Swimming (front crawl)	B	L	3–5	4	2	3	1	3	6–12	450–900
Walking	B	L	1–2	1	2	1	1	3	4–6	300–450
Walking, Water, Chest-Deep	I	L	2–4	2	3	1	1	3	6–10	450–750
Water Aerobics	B	L	2–4	3	3	3	2	3	6–12	450–900

[1] B = Beginner, I = Intermediate, A = Advanced

[2] L = Low, M = Moderate, H = High

[3] 1 = Low, 2 = Fair, 3 = Average, 4 = Good, 5 = Excellent

[4] One MET represents the rate of energy expenditure at rest (3.5 ml/kg/min). Each additional MET is a multiple of the resting value. For example, 5 METs represents an energy expenditure equivalent to five times the resting value, or about 17.5 ml/kg/min.

[5] Varies according to the person's effort (intensity) during exercise.

[6] Varies according to body weight.

number, ranges are given for some of the categories. The benefits derived are based on the person's effort while participating in the activity.

The nature of the activity often dictates the potential aerobic development. For example, jogging is much more strenuous than walking. The effort during exercise also affects the amount of physiological development. During a low-impact aerobics routine, accentuating all movements (instead of just going through the motions) increases training benefits by orders of magnitude.

Table 6.10 indicates a starting fitness level for each aerobic activity. Attempting to participate in high-intensity activities without proper conditioning often leads to injuries and discouragement. Beginners should start with low-intensity activities that carry a minimum risk for injuries.

In some cases, such as high-impact aerobics and rope skipping, the risk for injuries remains high even if the participants are adequately conditioned. These activities should be supplemental only and are not recommended as the sole mode of exercise.

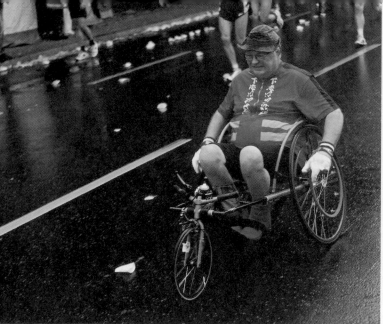

Physically challenged people can participate in and derive health and fitness benefits from a high-intensity exercise program.

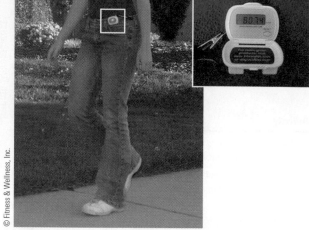
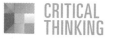

A pedometer can be used to monitor daily physical activity. The recommendation is a total of 10,000 steps daily.

Most exercise-related injuries occur as a result of high-impact activities, not high intensity of exercise.

Physicians who work with cardiac patients frequently use **METs** as an alternative method of prescribing exercise intensity. One **MET** represents the rate of energy expenditure at rest. METs, short for metabolic equivalents, are used to measure the intensity of physical activity and exercise in multiples of the resting metabolic rate. At an intensity level of 10 METs, the activity requires a tenfold increase in the resting energy requirement (or approximately 35 ml/kg/min). MET levels for a given activity vary according to the effort expended. The MET range for various activities is included in Table 6.10 on page 179. The harder a person exercises, the higher is the MET level.

The effectiveness of various aerobic activities in weight management is also provided in Table 6.10. As a general rule, the greater the muscle mass involved in exercise, the better the results. Rhythmic and continuous activities that involve large amounts of muscle mass are most effective in burning calories.

Higher-intensity activities increase caloric expenditure as well. Exercising longer, however, compensates for lower intensities. If carried out long enough (45 to 60 minutes five to six times per week), even walking is a good exercise mode for weight management. Additional information on a comprehensive weight management program is given in Chapter 5.

Getting Started and Adhering to a Lifetime Exercise Program

Following the guidelines provided in Lab 6D, you may proceed to initiate your cardiorespiratory endurance program. If you have not been exercising regularly, you might begin by attempting to train five or six times a week for 30 minutes at a time. You might find this discouraging, however, and drop out before getting too far, because you will probably develop some muscle soreness and stiffness and possibly incur minor injuries. Muscle soreness and stiffness and the risk for injuries can be lessened or eliminated by increasing the intensity, duration, and frequency of exercise progressively, as outlined in Lab 6D.

Once you have determined your exercise prescription, the difficult part begins: starting and sticking to a lifetime exercise program. Although you may be motivated after reading the benefits to be gained from

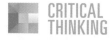

CRITICAL THINKING

Your friend Joe is not physically active and doesn't exercise. He manages to keep his weight down by dieting and tells you that because he feels and looks good, he doesn't need to exercise. How do you respond to your friend?

CRITICAL THINKING

Mary started an exercise program last year as a means to lose weight and enhance her body image. She now runs more than 6 miles every day, works out regularly on stair climbers and elliptical machines, strength-trains daily, participates in step-aerobics three times per week, and plays tennis or racquetball twice a week. Will you evaluate her program and make suggestions for improvements?

1. Set aside a regular time for exercise. If you don't plan ahead, it is a lot easier to skip. On a weekly basis, using red ink, schedule your exercise time into your day planner. Next, hold your exercise hour "sacred." Give exercise priority equal to the most important school or business activity of the day.

   If you are too busy, attempt to accumulate 30 to 60 minutes of daily activity by doing separate 10-minute sessions throughout the day. Try reading the mail while you walk, taking stairs instead of elevators, walking the dog, or riding the stationary bike as you watch the evening news.

2. Exercise early in the day, when you will be less tired and the chances of something interfering with your workout are minimal; thus you will be less likely to skip your exercise session.

3. Select aerobic activities you enjoy. Exercise should be as much fun as your favorite hobby. If you pick an activity you don't enjoy, you will be unmotivated and less likely to keep exercising. Don't be afraid to try out a new activity, even if that means learning new skills.

4. Combine different activities. You can train by doing two or three different activities the same week. This cross-training may reduce the monotony of repeating the same activity every day. Try lifetime sports. Many endurance sports, such as racquetball, basketball, soccer, badminton, roller skating, cross-country skiing, and body surfing (paddling the board), provide a nice break from regular workouts.

5. Use the proper clothing and equipment for exercise. A poor pair of shoes, for example, can make you more prone to injury, discouraging you from the beginning.

6. Find a friend or group of friends to exercise with. Social interaction will make exercise more fulfilling. Besides, it's harder to skip if someone is waiting to go with you.

7. Set goals and share them with others. Quitting is tougher when someone else knows what you are trying to accomplish. When you reach a targeted goal, reward yourself with a new pair of shoes or a jogging suit.

8. Purchase a pedometer (step counter) and build up to 10,000 steps per day. These 10,000 steps may include all forms of daily physical activity combined. Pedometers motivate people toward activity because they track daily activity, provide feedback on activity level, and remind the participant to enhance daily activity.

9. Don't become a chronic exerciser. Overexercising can lead to chronic fatigue and injuries. Exercise should be enjoyable, and in the process you should stop and smell the roses.

10. Exercise in different places and facilities. This will add variety to your workouts.

11. Exercise to music. People who listen to fast-tempo music tend to exercise more vigorously and longer. Using headphones when exercising outdoors, however, can be dangerous. Even indoors, it is preferable not to use headphones, so that you can still be aware of your surroundings.

12. Keep a regular record of your activities. Keeping a record allows you to monitor your progress and compare it against previous months and years (see Figure 6.10, pages 185 and 186).

13. Conduct periodic assessments. Improving to a higher fitness category is often a reward in itself, and creating your own rewards is even more motivating.

14. Listen to your body. Stop exercising if you experience pain or unusual discomfort. Pain and aches are an indication of potential injury. If you do suffer an injury, do not return to your regular workouts until you are fully recovered. You may cross-train using activities that do not aggravate your injury (for instance, swimming instead of jogging).

15. If a health problem arises, see a physician. When in doubt, it's better to be safe than sorry.

physical activity, lifelong dedication and perseverance are necessary to reap and maintain good fitness.

The first few weeks will probably be the most difficult, but where there's a will, there's a way. Once you begin to see positive changes, it won't be as hard. Soon you will develop a habit of exercising that will be deeply satisfying and will bring about a sense of self-accomplishment. The suggestions provided in the accompanying Behavior Modification Planning box have been used successfully to help change behavior and adhere to a lifetime exercise program.

A Lifetime Commitment to Fitness

The benefits of fitness can be maintained only through a regular lifetime program. Exercise is not like putting money in the bank. It doesn't help

METs Short for metabolic equivalents, an alternative method of prescribing exercise intensity in multiples of the resting metabolic rate.

MET Represents the rate of resting energy expenditure at rest; MET is the equivalent of 3.5 ml/kg/min.

much to exercise 4 or 5 hours on Saturday and not do anything else the rest of the week. If anything, exercising only once a week is unsafe for unconditioned adults.

Even the greatest athletes on earth, if they were to stop exercising, would be, after just a few years, at a risk for disease similar to someone who never has done any physical activity. Staying with a physical fitness program long enough brings about positive physiological and psychological changes. Once you are there, you will not want to have it any other way.

The time involved in losing the benefits of exercise varies among the different components of physical fitness and also depends on the person's condition before the interruption. In regard to

cardiorespiratory endurance, it has been estimated that 4 weeks of aerobic training are completely reversed in 2 consecutive weeks of physical inactivity. On the other hand, if you have been exercising regularly for months or years, 2 weeks of inactivity will not hurt you as much as it will someone who has exercised only a few weeks. As a rule, after 48 to 72 hours of aerobic inactivity, the cardiorespiratory system starts to lose some of its capacity.

To maintain fitness, you should keep up a regular exercise program, even during vacations. If you have to interrupt your program for reasons beyond your control, you should not attempt to resume training at the same level you left off but, rather, build up gradually again.

Profile Plus

Evaluate how well you understand the concepts presented in this chapter using the "Assess Your Knowledge" and "Practice Quizzes" options on your CD-ROM.

ASSESS YOUR KNOWLEDGE

1. Cardiorespiratory endurance is determined by
   a. the amount of oxygen the body is able to utilize per minute of physical activity.
   b. the length of time it takes the heart rate to return to 120 bpm following the 1.5-mile run test.
   c. the difference between the maximal heart rate and the resting heart rate.
   d. the product of the heart rate and blood pressure at rest versus exercise.
   e. the time it takes a person to reach a heart rate between 120 and 170 bpm during the Astrand–Ryhming test.

2. Which of the following is not a benefit of aerobic training?
   a. a higher maximal oxygen uptake
   b. an increase in red blood cell count
   c. a decrease in resting heart rate
   d. an increase in heart rate at a given workload
   e. an increase in functional capillaries

3. The oxygen uptake for a person with an exercise heart rate of 130, a stroke volume of 100, and an a-$\overline{v}O_2$diff of 10 is
   a. 130,000 ml/kg/min.
   b. 1300 l/min.
   c. 1.3 l/min.
   d. 130 ml/kg/min.
   e. 13 ml/kg/min.

4. The oxygen uptake in ml/kg/min for a person with a VO_2 of 2.0 l/min who weighs 60 kilograms is
   a. 120.
   b. 26.5.
   c. 33.3.
   d. 30.
   e. 120,000.

5. The step test estimates maximal oxygen uptake according to
   a. how long a person is able to sustain the proper step test cadence.
   b. the lowest heart rate achieved during the test.
   c. the recovery heart rate following the test.

   d. the difference between the maximal heart rate achieved and the resting heart rate.
   e. the exercise heart rate and the total stepping time.

6. An "excellent" cardiorespiratory fitness rating, in ml/kg/min, for young male adults is about
   a. 10.
   b. 20.
   c. 30.
   d. 40.
   e. 50.

7. A person exercising at 2 l/min burns approximately _____ calories per minute of physical activity.
   a. 2
   b. 5
   c. 10
   d. 12
   e. 20

8. The optimal or high-intensity cardiorespiratory training zone for a 22-year-old individual with a resting heart rate of 68 bpm is
   a. 120 to 148.
   b. 132 to 156.
   c. 138 to 164.
   d. 146 to 179.
   e. 154 to 188.

9. Which of the following activities does not contribute to the development of cardiorespiratory endurance?
   a. low-impact aerobics
   b. jogging
   c. 400-yard dash
   d. racquetball
   e. All of these activities contribute to its development.

10. The recommended duration for each cardiorespiratory training session is
    a. 10 to 20 minutes.
    b. 15 to 30 minutes.
    c. 20 to 60 minutes.
    d. 45 to 70 minutes.
    e. 60 to 120 minutes.

Correct answers can be found at the back of the book.

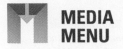
MEDIA MENU

PROFILE PLUS CD CONNECTIONS

■ Assess your cardiorespiratory endurance.

■ Maintain a log of all your fitness activities.

■ Check how well you understand the chapter's concepts.

INTERNET CONNECTIONS

■ FitFacts. This site features information about a variety of cardiovascular forms of exercise, including walking, running, jumping rope, swimming, spinning, cross-training, interval training, and others.

   http://www.acefitness.org/default.aspx

■ Fitness Fundamentals: Guidelines for Personal Exercise Programs. This site, developed by the President's Council on Physical Fitness and Sports, features information about starting an exercise program, including tips on how to select the right kinds of exercise to improve cardiovascular health, flexibility, and muscle strength and endurance.

   http://www.hoptechno.com/book1/1.htm

■ Exercise Physiology: The Methods and Mechanisms Underlying Performance. This site features information on the principles of training, gender differences in performance and training, cardiovascular benefits, and much more.

   http://home.hia.no/~stephens/exphys.htm

■ Check Your Physical Activity and Heart IQ. This site, sponsored by the National Heart, Lung, and Blood Institute, provides a true/false quiz to allow you to assess what you know about how physical activity affects your heart. The answers provided will uncover exercise myths and give you information on ways to improve your heart health.

   **http://www.nhlbi.nih.gov/health/public/heart/
   obesity/pa_iq_ab.htm**

Notes

1. H. Atkinson, "Exercise for Longer Life: The Physician's Perspective," *HealthNews* 7:3 (1997), 3.

2. R. B. O'Hara et al., "Increased Volume Resistance Training: Effects upon Predicted Aerobic Fitness in a Select Group of Air Force Men," *ACSM's Health and Fitness Journal* 8, no. 4 (2004): 16–25.

3. R. K. Dishman, "Prescribing Exercise Intensity for Healthy Adults Using Perceived Exertion," *Medicine and Science in Sports and Exercise* 26 (1994): 1087–1094.

4. U.S. Department of Health and Human Services, Centers for Disease Control and Prevention, National Center for Health Statistics, *Physical Activity among Adults: United States, 2000*, no. 15 (May 14, 2003).

5. American College of Sports Medicine, "Position Stand: The Recommended Quantity and Quality of Exercise for Developing and Maintaining Cardiorespiratory and Muscular Fitness, and Flexibility in Healthy Adults," *Medicine and Science in Sports and Exercise* 30 (1998): 975–991.

6. American College of Sports Medicine, *Guidelines for Exercise Testing and Prescription* (Philadelphia: Lippincott Williams & Wilkins, 2000).

7. See note 6.

8. S. Blair, "Surgeon General's Report on Physical Fitness: The Inside Story," *ACSM's Health & Fitness Journal* 1 (1997): 14–18.

9. R. F. DeBusk, U. Stenestrand, M. Sheehan, and W. L. Haskell, "Training Effects of Long Versus Short Bouts of Exercise in Healthy Subjects," *American Journal of Cardiology* 65 (1990): 1010–1013.

10. National Academy of Sciences, Institute of Medicine, *Dietary Reference Intakes for Energy, Carbohydrates, Fiber, Fat, Protein and Amino Acids (Macronutrients)*. Washington, DC: National Academy Press, 2002.

11. "Summary Statement: Workshop on Physical Activity and Public Health," *Sports Medicine Bulletin* 28 (1993): 7.

12. See note 5.

13. U.S. Department of Agriculture and U.S. Department of Health and Human Services, "Nutrition and Your Health: Dietary Guidelines for Americans," *Home and Garden Bulletin* 232 (2000).

14. "Scanning Sports," *Physician and Sportsmedicine* 21, no. 11 (1993): 34.

15. See note 6.

Suggested Readings

ACSM's Guidelines for Exercise Testing and Prescription. Philadelphia: Lippincott Williams & Wilkins, 2000.

ACSM's Resource Manual for Guidelines for Exercise Testing and Prescription. Philadelphia: Lippincott Williams & Wilkins, 2001.

Akalan, C., L. Kravitz, and R. Robergs. "VO$_{2max}$: Essentials of the Most Widely Used Test in Exercise Physiology." *ACSM's Health & Fitness Journal* 8, no. 3 (2004): 5–9.

Borg, G. "Perceived Exertion: A Note on History and Methods." *Medicine and Science in Sports and Exercise* 5 (1993): 90–93.

Hoeger, W. W. K., and S. A. Hoeger. *Lifetime Fitness & Wellness: A Personalized Program*. Belmont, CA: Wadsworth/ Thomson Learning, 2005.

Karvonen, M. J., E. Kentala, and O. Mustala. "The Effects of Training on the Heart Rate, a Longitudinal Study." *Annales Medicinae Experimetalis et Biologiae Fenniae* 35 (1957): 307–315.

McArdle, W. D., F. I. Katch, and V. L. Katch. *Exercise Physiology: Energy, Nutrition, and Human Performance*. Philadelphia: Lippincott Williams & Wilkins, 2004.

Nieman, D. C. *Exercise Testing and Prescription: A Health-Related Approach*. Boston: McGraw–Hill, 2003.

Wilmore, J. H., and D. L. Costill. *Physiology of Sport and Exercise*. Champaign, IL: Human Kinetics, 2004.

FIGURE 6.10 Cardiorespiratory exercise record form.

Month _____

Date	Body Weight	Exercise Heart Rate	Type of Exercise	Distance In Miles	Time Hrs/Min	RPE*
1						
2						
3						
4						
5						
6						
7						
8						
9						
10						
11						
12						
13						
14						
15						
16						
17						
18						
19						
20						
21						
22						
23						
24						
25						
26						
27						
28						
29						
30						
31						
Total						

*Rate of perceived exertion.

Month _____

Date	Body Weight	Exercise Heart Rate	Type of Exercise	Distance In Miles	Time Hrs/Min	RPE*
1						
2						
3						
4						
5						
6						
7						
8						
9						
10						
11						
12						
13						
14						
15						
16						
17						
18						
19						
20						
21						
22						
23						
24						
25						
26						
27						
28						
29						
30						
31						
Total						

*Rate of perceived exertion.

FIGURE 6.10 Cardiorespiratory exercise record form.

Month _____

Date	Body Weight	Exercise Heart Rate	Type of Exercise	Distance In Miles	Time Hrs/Min	RPE*
1						
2						
3						
4						
5						
6						
7						
8						
9						
10						
11						
12						
13						
14						
15						
16						
17						
18						
19						
20						
21						
22						
23						
24						
25						
26						
27						
28						
29						
30						
31						
Total						

*Rate of perceived exertion.

Month _____

Date	Body Weight	Exercise Heart Rate	Type of Exercise	Distance In Miles	Time Hrs/Min	RPE*
1						
2						
3						
4						
5						
6						
7						
8						
9						
10						
11						
12						
13						
14						
15						
16						
17						
18						
19						
20						
21						
22						
23						
24						
25						
26						
27						
28						
29						
30						
31						
Total						

*Rate of perceived exertion.

Lab 6A

CARDIORESPIRATORY ENDURANCE ASSESSMENT

Name: [   ]   Date: [   ]   Grade: [   ]

Instructor: [   ]   Course: [   ]   Section: [   ]

Necessary Lab Equipment

1.5-Mile Run: School track or premeasured course and a stopwatch.

1.0-Mile Walk Test: School track or premeasured course and a stopwatch.

Step Test: A bench or gymnasium bleachers 16¼ inches high, a metronome, and a stopwatch.

Astrand–Ryhming Test: A bicycle ergometer that allows for regulation of workloads in kilopounds per meter (or watts) and a stopwatch.

12-Minute Swim Test: Swimming pool and a stopwatch.

Objective

To estimate maximal oxygen uptake (VO_{2max}) and cardiorespiratory endurance classification.

Lab Preparation

Wear appropriate exercise clothing including jogging shoes and a swimsuit if required. Be prepared to take the 1.0-Mile Walk Test, the Step Test, the Astrand–Ryhming Test, the 1.5-Mile Run Test, and/or the 12-Minute Swim Test. If more than one test will be conducted, perform them in the order just listed and allow at least 15 minutes between tests. Avoid vigorous physical activity 24 hours prior to this lab.

I. 1.5-Mile Run Test

1.5-Mile Run Time: [   ] min and [   ] sec VO_{2max} (see Table 6.2, page 166): [   ] ml/kg/min

Cardiorespiratory Fitness Category (Table 6.8, page 171): [   ]

II. 1.0-Mile Walk Test

Weight (W) = [   ] lbs   Gender (G) = [   ] (female = 0, male = 1)   Time = [   ] min and [   ] sec

Heart Rate (HR) = [   ] bpm

Time in minutes (T) = min + (sec ÷ 60) or T = [   ] + ([   ] ÷ 60) = [   ] min

VO_{2max} = 88.768 − (0.0957 × W) + (8.892 × G) − (1.4537 × T) − (0.1194 × HR)

VO_{2max} = 88.768 − (0.0957 × [   ]) + (8.892 × [   ]) − (1.4537 × [   ]) − (0.1194 × [   ])

VO_{2max} = 88.768 − ([   ]) + ([   ]) − ([   ]) − ([   ]) = [   ] ml/kg/min

Cardiorespiratory Fitness Category (Table 6.8, page 171): [   ]

III. Step Test

15-second recovery heart rate: [   ] beats VO_{2max} (Table 6.3, page 168): [   ] ml/kg/min

Cardiorespiratory Fitness Category (Table 6.8, page 171): [   ]

IV. Astrand–Ryhming Test

Weight (W) = [_____] lbs   Weight (BW) in kilograms = (W ÷ 2.2046) = [_____] kg   Workload = [_____] kpm

Exercise Heart Rates	Time to count 30 beats	Heart Rate (bpm) (from Table 6.4, page 169)		Time to count 30 beats	Heart Rate (bpm) (from Table 6.4, page 169)
First minute:	[_____]	[_____]	Fourth minute:	[_____]	[_____]
Second minute:	[_____]	[_____]	Fifth minute:	[_____]	[_____]
Third minute:	[_____]	[_____]	Sixth minute:	[_____]	[_____]

Average heart rate for the fifth and sixth minutes = [_____] bpm

VO_{2max} in l/min (Table 6.5, page 170) = [_____] l/min   Correction factor (from Table 6.6, page 170) = [_____]

Corrected VO_{2max} = VO_{2max} in l/min × correction factor = [_____] × [_____] = [_____] l/min

VO_{2max} in ml/kg/min = corrected VO_{2max} in l/min × 1000 ÷ BW in kg = [_____] × 1000 ÷ [_____] = [_____] ml/kg/min

Cardiorespiratory Fitness Category (Table 6.8, page 171): [_____]

V. 12-Minute Swim Test

Distance swum in 12 minutes: [_____] yards

Cardiorespiratory Fitness Category (Table 6.7, page 171): [_____]

VI. What I Learned and Where I Go From Here:

1. Interpret the results of your cardiorespiratory endurance test(s). Indicate the cardiorespiratory fitness classification you would like to achieve by the end of the term and explain how you are planning to achieve this goal.

2. Briefly discuss the advantages and disadvantages of the cardiorespiratory endurance tests used in this lab.

Lab 6B

EXERCISE HEART RATE AND CALORIC COST OF PHYSICAL ACTIVITY

Name: _____ Date: _____ Grade: _____

Instructor: _____ Course: _____ Section: _____

Necessary Lab Equipment

A school track (or premeasured course) and a stopwatch. Each student also should bring a watch with a second hand.

Objective

To monitor exercise heart rate and determine the caloric cost of physical activity based on exercise heart rate.

Lab Preparation

Wear exercise clothing, including jogging shoes. Do not engage in vigorous physical activity prior to this lab. Read the information on predicting oxygen uptake and caloric expenditure in this Chapter, pages 172–173.

Procedure

1. **Cardiorespiratory Training Zone.** Look up your cardiovascular training zone at 60 percent and 85 percent of heart rate reserve in Lab 6D. Record this information in beats per minute (bpm) and in 10-second pulse counts in the blank spaces provided below.

	Beats/minute	10-sec count
60% intensity =		
85% intensity =		

2. **Resting Heart Rate (HR) and Body Weight (BW).** Determine your resting HR prior to exercise and your body weight in kilograms (divide pounds by 2.2046).

Resting HR: _____ bpm

BW: _____ lbs ÷ 2.2046 = _____ kg

3. **Walking HR, Oxygen Uptake (VO$_2$), and Caloric Expenditure.** Walk two laps around a 400-meter (440-yard) track at an average speed of 75 to 100 meters per minute. Try to maintain a constant speed around the track. You can monitor your speed by starting the walk at the beginning of the 100-meter straightway and making sure you have walked at least 75 meters and no more than 100 meters in one minute. As soon as you complete the two laps (800 meters), notice the time required to walk this distance and immediately check your exercise HR by taking a 10-second pulse count. Record this information in the spaces provided below. Do not record the time until after you have checked your pulse. Exercise HR will remain at the same rate for about 15 seconds following cessation of exercise. Therefore, you need to check your pulse as soon as you finish the walk, after noticing the 800-meter walk time.

10-sec. pulse count: _____ beats (from question 1 above)

800-meter time: _____ min _____ sec

HR in bpm = 10-sec pulse count × 6

HR in bpm = _____ × 6 = _____ bpm

800-meter time in minutes = min + (sec ÷ 60)

800-meter time in minutes = _____ + (_____ ÷ 60) = _____ min

Speed in meters per minute (mts/min) = 800 ÷ 800-meter time in min

Speed in mts/min = 800 ÷ _____ = _____ mts/min

VO$_2$ in ml/kg/min at this walking speed (Use Table 6.9, page 172) = [____] ml/kg/min

VO$_2$ in l/min = VO$_2$ in ml/kg/min × BW in kg ÷ 1,000

VO$_2$ in l/min = [____] × [____] ÷ 1000 = [____] l/min

Caloric expenditure for 800-meter walk = VO$_2$ in l/min × 5 × 800-meter time in min

Caloric expenditure for 800-meter walk = [____] × 5 × [____] = [____] calories

4. **Slow-Jogging HR, VO$_2$, and Caloric Expenditure.** Slowly jog 800 meters (two laps) around the track. Try to maintain the same slow-jogging pace throughout the two laps. Do NOT jog fast or sprint. This is not a speed test and is intended to be a slow jog only. As soon as you complete the 800 meters, notice the time required to complete the distance and check your exercise HR immediately by taking another 10-second pulse count. Record this information below.

10-sec pulse count: [____] beats

800-meter time: [____] min [____] sec.

HR in bpm = 10-sec pulse count × 6

HR in bpm = [____] × 6 = [____] bpm

800-meter time in minutes = min + (sec ÷ 60)

800-meter time in minutes = [____] + ([____] ÷ 60) = [____] min

Speed in mts/min = 800 ÷ 800-meter time in min

Speed in mts/min = 800 ÷ [____] = [____] mts/min.

VO$_2$ in ml/kg/min at this slow-jogging speed (Use Table 6.9, page 172) = [____] ml/kg/min

VO$_2$ in l/min = VO$_2$ in ml/kg/min × BW in kg ÷ 1,000

VO$_2$ in l/min = [____] × [____] ÷ 1000 = [____] l/min

Caloric expenditure for 800-meter slow jog = VO$_2$ in l/min × 5 × 800-meter time in min

Caloric expenditure for 800-meter slow jog = [____] × 5 × [____] = [____] calories

5. **Fast-Jogging HR, VO$_2$, Caloric Expenditure, and Recovery HR.** Jog another 800 meters at a faster speed around the track. Again try to maintain the same jogging pace throughout the two laps. Do NOT sprint. Your HR should not exceed 180 bpm on this test. As soon as you complete the 800 meters, notice your time for the two laps and check your 10-second pulse count. Record this information below. You also should check your 2- and 5-minute recovery HRs after the run and record these rates below.

10-sec pulse count: [____] beats

800-meter time: [____] min [____] sec

HR in bpm = 10-sec pulse count × 6

HR in bpm = [____] × 6 = [____] bpm

800-meter time in minutes = min + (sec ÷ 60)

800-meter time in minutes = [____] + ([____] ÷ 60) = [____] min

Speed in mts/min = 800 ÷ 800-meter time in min

Speed in mts/min = 800 ÷ [____] = [____] mts/min

VO$_2$ in ml/kg/min at this fast-jogging speed (Use Table 6.9, page 172) = [____] ml/kg/min

VO_2 in l/min = VO_2 in ml/kg/min $\times$ BW in kg $\div$ 1,000

VO_2 in l/min = [____] $\times$ [____] $\div$ 1,000 = [____] l/min

Caloric expenditure for 800-meter fast jog = VO_2 in l/min $\times$ 5 $\times$ 800-meter time in min

Caloric expenditure for 800-meter fast jog = [____] $\times$ 5 $\times$ [____] = [____] calories

Recovery HRs

	10-sec count	bpm
2 minutes	[____]	[____]
5 minutes*	[____]	[____]

6. **Resting, Exercise, and Recovery HRs.** Plot your resting, exercise, and recovery HRs on the graph provided below.

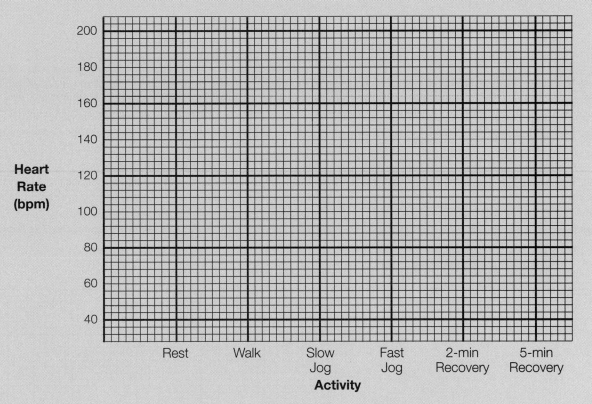

7. **Training Exercise HR and Equivalent Caloric Expenditure.** This part of the lab should be completed outside your regular lab time, during the next 2 or 3 days prior to turning in the assignment. According to the previous exercise HRs (items 3, 4, and 5), try to select a walking or jogging speed that will allow you to maintain your exercise HR in the appropriate cardiorespiratory training zone. Using a 400-meter track, walk or jog for 20 minutes at the selected speed and again try to maintain a constant speed throughout the exercise time. At the end of the 20 minutes, check your 10-second pulse count and estimate the distance covered in meters. Record this information below and estimate the VO_2 and caloric expenditure.

10-sec pulse count: [____] beats

HR in bpm = 10-sec pulse count $\times$ 6

HR in bpm = [____] $\times$ 6 = [____] bpm

Approximate distance covered in 20 minutes: [____] meters

---

* Your 5-minute recovery HR should be below 120 bpm. If it is above 120, you most likely have overexerted yourself and, therefore, need to decrease the intensity of exercise (and/or duration when exercising for long periods of time). If your 5-minute recovery HR is still above 120 after decreasing the intensity of exercise, you should consult a physician regarding this condition.

Speed in mts/min = distance in meters ÷ 20 minutes

Speed in mts/min = ⬚ ÷ 20 = ⬚ mts/min

VO_2 at this speed (see Table 6.9, page 172) = ⬚ ml/kg/min

VO_2 in l/min = VO_2 in ml/kg/min × BW in kg ÷ 1,000

VO_2 in l/min = ⬚ × ⬚ ÷ 1,000 = ⬚ l/min

Caloric expenditure for 20-min walk/jog = VO_2 in l/min × 5 × 20 min

Caloric expenditure for 20-min walk/jog = ⬚ × 5 × 20 = ⬚ calories

Using the previous information, how many calories would you have burned if you had maintained this pace for:

10 minutes (VO_2 in l/min × 5 × 10) = ⬚ × 5 × 10 = ⬚ calories

30 minutes (VO_2 in l/min × 5 × 30) = ⬚ × 5 × 30 = ⬚ calories

60 minutes (VO_2 in l/min × 5 × 60) = ⬚ × 5 × 60 = ⬚ calories

PREDICTING CALORIC EXPENDITURE ACCORDING TO EXERCISE HR

Research indicates that there is a linear relationship between HR and VO_2, as long as the HR ranges from about 110 to 180 bpm. If you obtain two exercise HRs in this range and the equivalent oxygen uptakes (in l/min), you can easily predict your VO_2 and caloric expenditure for any given HR in the specified range. Plot your two exercise HRs and the corresponding VO_2 values on the graph provided below. Next, draw a line between these two points on the graph and extend the line to 110 and 180 bpm. You now may look up the VO_2 for any HR by finding the desired HR on the Y axis, then going across to the reference line and straight down to the X axis, where you will find the corresponding VO_2 in l/min. To obtain the caloric expenditure in calories per minute, simply multiply the VO_2 by 5. You also may predict your maximal VO_2 (in l/min) by extending the line up to your estimated maximal HR. The maximal HR is estimated by subtracting your age from 220. To convert the maximal VO_2 to ml/kg/min, multiply the l/min value by 1,000 and divide by body weight in kilograms.

Using the results from your lab and the graph below, indicate the VO_2 in l/min and the caloric expenditure at the following HRs:

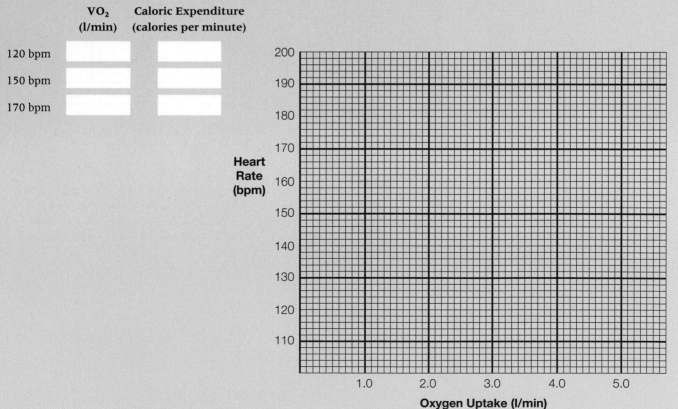

	VO₂ (l/min)	Caloric Expenditure (calories per minute)
120 bpm		
150 bpm		
170 bpm		

Lab 6C

EXERCISE READINESS QUESTIONNAIRE

Name: _____ Date: _____ Grade: _____

Instructor: _____ Course: _____ Section: _____

Necessary Lab Equipment
None required.

Objective
To determine your preparedness to start an exercise program.

Instructions
Read each statement carefully and circle the number that best describes your feelings in each statement. Please be completely honest with your answers. Interpret the results of this questionnaire using the guidelines provided on the next page.

I.

	Strongly Agree	Mildly Agree	Mildly Disagree	Strongly Disagree
1. I can walk, ride a bike (or a wheelchair), swim, or walk in a shallow pool.	4	3	2	1
2. I enjoy exercise.	4	3	2	1
3. I believe exercise can help decrease the risk for disease and premature mortality.	4	3	2	1
4. I believe exercise contributes to better health.	4	3	2	1
5. I have previously participated in an exercise program.	4	3	2	1
6. I have experienced the feeling of being physically fit.	4	3	2	1
7. I can envision myself exercising.	4	3	2	1
8. I am contemplating an exercise program.	4	3	2	1
9. I am willing to stop contemplating and give exercise a try for a few weeks.	4	3	2	1
10. I am willing to set aside time at least three times a week for exercise.	4	3	2	1
11. I can find a place to exercise (the streets, a park, a YMCA, a health club).	4	3	2	1
12. I can find other people who would like to exercise with me.	4	3	2	1
13. I will exercise when I am moody, fatigued, and even when the weather is bad.	4	3	2	1
14. I am willing to spend a small amount of money for adequate exercise clothing (shoes, shorts, leotards, swimsuit).	4	3	2	1
15. If I have any doubts about my present state of health, I will see a physician before beginning an exercise program.	4	3	2	1
16. Exercise will make me feel better and improve my quality of life.	4	3	2	1

Scoring Your Test:

This questionnaire allows you to examine your readiness for exercise. You have been evaluated in four categories: mastery (self-control), attitude, health, and commitment. Mastery indicates that you can be in control of your exercise program. Attitude examines your mental disposition toward exercise. Health provides evidence of the wellness benefits of exercise. Commitment shows dedication and resolution to carry out the exercise program. Write the number you circled after each statement in the corresponding spaces below. Add the scores on each line to get your totals. Scores can vary from 4 to 16. A score of 12 and above is a strong indicator that that factor is important to you, and 8 and below is low. If you score 12 or more points in each category, your chances of initiating and adhering to an exercise program are good. If you fail to score at least 12 points in three categories, your chances of succeeding at exercise may be slim. You need to be better informed about the benefits of exercise, and a retraining process may be required.

Mastery: 1. _____ + 5. _____ + 6. _____ + 9. _____ = _____

Attitude: 2. _____ + 7. _____ + 8. _____ + 13. _____ = _____

Health: 3. _____ + 4. _____ + 15. _____ + 16. _____ = _____

Commitment: 10. _____ + 11. _____ + 12. _____ + 14. _____ = _____

II. Stage of Change for Cardiorespiratory Endurance Exercise

Using Figure 2.4 (page 41) and Table 2.3 (page 41), identify your current stage of change in regard to participation in a cardiorespiratory endurance exercise program:

_____

III. Advantages and Disadvantages for Adding Aerobic Exercise to Your Lifestyle

Advantages: _____

_____

_____

_____

_____

_____

_____

_____

Disadvantages: _____

_____

_____

_____

_____

_____

_____

_____

Lab 6D

CARDIORESPIRATORY EXERCISE PRESCRIPTION

Name: _____ Date: _____ Grade: _____

Instructor: _____ Course: _____ Section: _____

Necessary Lab Equipment
None required.

Objective
To write your own cardiorespiratory exercise prescription.

I. Intensity of Exercise

1. Estimate your own maximal heart rate (MHR)

   MHR = 220 minus age (220 − age)

   MHR = 220 − _____ = _____ bpm

2. Resting Heart Rate (RHR) = _____ bpm

3. Heart Rate Reserve (HRR) = MHR − RHR

   HRR = _____ − _____ = _____ beats

4. Training Intensities (TI) = HRR × TI + RHR

   40 Percent TI = _____ × .40 + _____ = _____ bpm

   50 Percent TI = _____ × .50 + _____ = _____ bpm

   60 percent TI = _____ × .60 + _____ = _____ bpm

   85 Percent TI = _____ × .85 + _____ = _____ bpm

5. Cardiorespiratory Training Zone. The optimum cardiorespiratory training zone is found between the 60 percent and 85 percent training intensities. Older adults, individuals who have been physically inactive or are in the poor or fair cardiorespiratory fitness categories, however, should follow a 40 percent to 50 percent training intensity during the first few weeks of the exercise program.

   Cardiorespiratory Training Zone: _____ (60% TI) to _____ (85% TI)

   Rate of Perceived Exertion (see Figure 6.7, page 176): _____ to _____

II. Mode of Exercise

Select any activity or combination of activities that you enjoy doing. The activity has to be continuous in nature and must get your heart rate up to the cardiorespiratory training zone and keep it there for as long as you exercise. Indicate your preferred mode(s) of exercise:

1. _____ 2. _____ 3. _____

4. _____ 5. _____ 6. _____

III. Cardiorespiratory Exercise Program

The following is your weekly program for development of cardiorespiratory endurance. If you are in the average, good, or excellent fitness category, you may start at week 5. After completing this 12-week program, for you to maintain your fitness level, you should exercise in the 60 percent to 85 percent training zone for about 20 to 30 minutes, a minimum of three times per week, on non-consecutive days. You should also recompute your target zone periodically because you will experience a significant reduction in resting heart rate with aerobic training (approximately 10 to 20 beats in about 8 to 12 weeks).

Week	Duration (min)	Frequency	Training Intensity	Heart Rate (bpm)		10-Sec Pulse Count*		
1	15	3	Between 40% and 50%		to		to	beats
2	15	4	Between 40% and 50%					
3	20	4	Between 40% and 50%					
4	20	5	Between 40% and 50%					
5	20	4	Between 50% and 60%		to		to	beats
6	20	5	Between 50% and 60%					
7	30	4	Between 50% and 60%					
8	30	5	Between 50% and 60%					
9	30	4	Between 60% and 85%		to		to	beats
10	30	5	Between 60% and 85%					
11	30–40	5	Between 60% and 85%					
12	30–40	5	Between 60% and 85%					

*Fill out your own 10-second pulse count under this column.

IV. Briefly State Your Experiences and Feelings Regarding Aerobic Exercise:

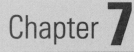

Chapter **7**

Muscular Strength and Endurance

Objectives

- Explain the importance of adequate strength levels in maintaining good health and well-being.
- Clarify misconceptions about strength fitness.
- Define muscular strength and muscular endurance.
- Be able to assess muscular strength and endurance and learn to interpret test results according to health fitness and physical fitness standards.
- Identify the factors that affect strength.
- Understand the principles of overload and specificity of training for strength development.
- Become acquainted with two distinct strength-training programs—core strength training and Pilates.

Profile Plus CD Connections

- Chart your achievements for strength tests.
- Check how well you understand the chapter's concepts.

The benefits of **strength training** (also referred to as resistance training) to enhance health and well-being are well-documented. Some people, nonetheless, have the impression that strength is necessary only for highly trained athletes, fitness enthusiasts, and individuals who have jobs that require heavy muscular work. In fact, a well-planned strength training program leads to increased muscle strength and endurance, muscle tone, tendon and ligament strength, and bone density—all of which help to improve functional physical capacity.

Benefits of Strength Training

Strength is a basic component of fitness and wellness and is crucial for optimal performance in daily activities such as sitting, walking, running, lifting and carrying objects, doing housework, and enjoying recreational activities. Strength also is of great value in improving posture, personal appearance, and self-image; in developing sports skills; in promoting joint stability; and in meeting certain emergencies in life. From a health standpoint, increasing strength helps to increase or maintain muscle and a higher resting metabolic rate, encourages weight loss and maintenance, lessens the risk for injury, prevents osteoporosis, reduces chronic low-back pain, alleviates arthritic pain, aids in childbearing, improves cholesterol levels, promotes psychological well-being, and may also help to lower blood pressure and control blood sugar.

An important adaptation to strength training is that, with time, the heart rate and blood pressure response to lifting a heavy resistance (that is, a weight) decreases. This adaptation reduces the demands on the cardiovascular system when performing activities such as carrying a child, the groceries, or a suitcase.

Regular strength training also can help control blood sugar. Much of the blood glucose from food consumption goes to the muscles, where it is stored as glycogen. When muscles are not used, muscle cells become insulin-resistant and glucose cannot enter the cells, thus increasing the risk for diabetes. Following 16 weeks of strength-training, a group of diabetic men and women improved their blood sugar control, gained strength, increased lean body mass, lost body fat, and lowered blood pressure.[1]

Muscular Strength and Aging

In the older adult population, muscular strength may be the most important health-related component of physical fitness. Though proper cardiorespiratory endurance is necessary to help maintain a healthy heart, good strength contributes more to independent living than any other fitness component. Older adults with good strength levels can successfully perform most **activities of daily living**.

Sarcopenia, or loss of lean body mass, strength, and function, is a common occurrence as people age. How much of this loss is related to the aging process itself or to actual physical inactivity and faulty nutrition is unknown. And while thinning of the bones from osteoporosis renders the bones prone to fractures, the gradual loss of muscle mass and ensuing frailty is what leads to falls and subsequent loss of function in older adults. Strength training helps to slow the age-related loss of muscle function. Protein deficiency, seen in some older adults, also contributes to loss of lean tissue.

More than anything else, older adults want to enjoy good health and to function independently. Many of them, however, are confined to nursing homes because they lack sufficient strength to move about. They cannot walk very far, and many have to be helped in and out of beds, chairs, and tubs.

A strength-training program can enhance quality of life tremendously, and nearly everyone can benefit from it. Only people with advanced heart disease are advised to refrain from strength training. Inactive adults between the ages of 56 and 86 who participated in a 12-week strength-training program increased their lean body mass by about 3 pounds, lost about 4 pounds of fat, and increased their resting metabolic rate by almost 7 percent.[2] In other research, leg strength improved by as much as 200 percent in previously inactive adults over age 90.[3] As strength improves, so does the ability to move about, the capacity for independent living, and enjoyment of life during the "golden years." More specifically, good strength enhances quality of life in the following ways:

- It improves balance and restores mobility.
- It makes lifting and reaching easier.
- It decreases the risk for injuries and falls.
- It stresses the bones and preserves bone mineral density, thus decreasing the risk for osteoporosis.

The Relationship Between Strength and Metabolism

Perhaps one of the most significant benefits of maintaining a good strength level is its relationship to human **metabolism**. A primary outcome of a strength-training program is an increase in muscle mass or size (lean body mass), known as muscle **hypertrophy**.

Muscle tissue uses energy even at rest. By contrast, fatty tissue uses little energy and may be considered metabolically inert from the standpoint of caloric use (that is, your body expends calories to maintain muscle and very few calories to maintain fat). As muscle size increases, so does **resting metabolism**. Even small increases in muscle mass may improve resting metabolism.

Each additional pound of muscle tissue increases resting metabolism by as much as 35 calories per day.[4] All other factors being equal, if two individuals both weigh 150 pounds but have different amounts of muscle mass, the one with more muscle mass will have a higher resting metabolic rate, allowing this person to ingest more calories (which will be used to maintain the muscle tissue, not to create fat). Briefly, the higher your metabolic rate, the more you can eat without gaining fat.

Effect of Aging on Metabolism

Loss of lean tissue is also thought to be the main reason for the decrease in metabolism as people grow older. Contrary to some beliefs, metabolism does not have to slow down significantly with aging. It is not so much that metabolism slows down. It's that we slow down.

Lean body mass decreases with sedentary living, which, in turn, slows down the resting metabolic rate. If people continue eating at the same rate, body fat increases. Daily requirements decrease an average of 360 calories between age 26 and age 60.[5] Hence, participating in a strength-training program is important in preventing and reducing excess body fat.

Gender Differences

One of the most common misconceptions about physical fitness concerns women in strength training. Because of the increase in muscle mass typically seen in men, some women think that a strength-training program will result in their developing large musculature. Even though the quality of muscle in men and women is the same, endocrinological differences do not allow women to achieve the same amount of muscle hypertrophy (size) as men. Men also have more muscle fibers and, because of the sex-specific male hormones, each individual fiber has more potential for hypertrophy. On the average, following 6 months of training, women can achieve up to a 50 percent increase in strength but only a 10 percent increase in muscle size.

The idea that strength training allows women to develop muscle hypertrophy to the same extent as men do is as false as the notion that playing basketball will turn women into giants. Masculinity and femininity are established by genetic inheritance, not by the amount of physical activity. Variations in the extent of masculinity and femininity are determined by individual differences in hormonal secretions of androgen, testosterone, estrogen, and progesterone. Women with a bigger-than-average

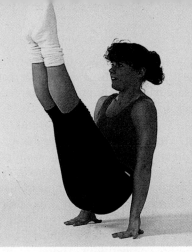

A female gymnast performs a strength skill.

build often are inclined to participate in sports because of their natural physical advantage. As a result, many people have associated women's participation in sports and strength training with large muscle size.

As the number of females who participate in sports increased steadily during the last few years, the myth of strength training in women leading to large increases in muscle size abated somewhat. For example, per pound of body weight, female gymnasts are among the strongest athletes in the world. These athletes engage regularly in serious strength-training programs. Yet, female gymnasts have some of the most well-toned and graceful figures of all women.

In recent years, improved body appearance has become the rule rather than the exception for women who participate in strength-training programs. Some of the most attractive female movie stars also train with weights to further improve their personal image.

Nonetheless, you may ask, "If weight training does not masculinize women, why do so many women body builders develop such heavy musculature?" In the sport of body building, the athletes

Strength training A program designed to improve muscular strength and/or endurance through a series of resistance (weight) training exercises that overload the muscular system and cause physiological development.

Activities of daily living Everyday behaviors that people normally do to function in life (cross the street, carry groceries, lift objects, do laundry, sweep floors).

Sarcopenia Age-related loss of lean body mass, strength, and function.

Metabolism All energy and material transformations that occur within living cells; necessary to sustain life.

Hypertrophy An increase in the size of the cell, as in muscle hypertrophy.

Resting metabolism Amount of energy (expressed in milliliters of oxygen per minute or total calories per day) an individual requires during resting conditions to sustain proper body function.

follow intense training routines consisting of two or more hours of constant weight lifting with short rest intervals between sets. Many body-building training routines call for back-to-back exercises using the same muscle groups. The objective of this type of training is to pump extra blood into the muscles. This additional fluid makes the muscles appear much bigger than they do in a resting condition. Based on the intensity and the length of the training session, the muscles can remain filled with blood, appearing measurably larger for several hours after completing the training session. Performing such routines is a common practice before competitions. Therefore, in real life, these women are not as muscular as they seem when they are participating in a contest.

In the sport of body building (among others), a big point of controversy is the use of **anabolic steroids** and human growth hormones. These hormones, however, produce detrimental and undesirable side effects in women (such as hypertension, fluid retention, decreased breast size, deepening of the voice, whiskers, and other atypical body hair growth), which some women deem tolerable. Anabolic steroid use in general—except for medical reasons and when carefully monitored by a physician—can lead to serious health consequences.

Anabolic steroid use among female body builders and female track and field athletes around the world is widespread. These athletes use anabolic steroids to remain competitive at the highest level. During the 2004 Olympic Games in Athens, Greece, two women shot putters, including the gold medal winner (later stripped of the medal), were expelled from the games for steroid use. Women who take steroids undoubtedly will build heavy musculature and, if they take the steroids long enough, the steroids will produce masculinizing effects.

As a result, the International Federation of Body Building instituted a mandatory steroid-testing program for females participating in the Miss Olympia contest. When drugs are not used to promote development, improved body image is the rule rather than the exception among females who participate in body building, strength training, or sports in general.

Changes in Body Composition

A benefit of strength training, accentuated even more when combined with aerobic exercise, is a decrease in adipose or fatty tissue around muscle

CRITICAL THINKING

What role should strength-training have in a fitness program? Should people be motivated for the health fitness benefits, or should they participate to enhance their body image? What are your feelings about individuals (male or female) with large body musculature?

SELECTED DETRIMENTAL EFFECTS OF ANABOLIC STEROID USE

- Liver tumors
- Hepatitis
- Hypertension
- Reduction of high-density lipoprotein (HDL) cholesterol
- Elevation of low-density lipoprotein (LDL) cholesterol
- Hyperinsulinism
- Impaired pituitary function
- Impaired thyroid function
- Mood swings
- Aggressive behavior
- Increased irritability
- Acne
- Fluid retention
- Decreased libido
- HIV infection (via injectable steroids)
- Prostate problems (men)
- Testicular atrophy (men)
- Reduced sperm count (men)
- Clitoral enlargement (women)
- Decreased breast size (women)
- Increased body and facial hair (nonreversible in women)
- Deepening of the voice (nonreversible in women)

fibers themselves. This decrease is often greater than the amount of muscle hypertrophy (see Figure 7.1). Therefore, losing inches but not body weight is common.

Because muscle tissue is more dense than fatty tissue (and despite the fact that inches are lost during a combined strength-training and aerobic program), people, especially women, often become discouraged because they cannot see the results readily on the scale. They can offset this discouragement by determining body composition regularly to monitor changes in percent body fat rather than simply measuring changes in total body weight (see Chapter 4).

Assessment of Muscular Strength and Endurance

Although muscular strength and endurance are interrelated, they do differ. **Muscular strength** is the ability to exert maximum force against resistance. **Muscular endurance** is the ability of a muscle to exert submaximal force repeatedly over time.

Muscular endurance (also referred to as "localized muscular endurance") depends to a large extent on muscular strength. Weak muscles cannot repeat an action several times or sustain it. Based upon these principles, strength

Profile Plus
Chart your achievements for strength tests on your CD–ROM.

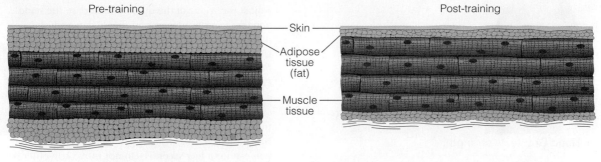

Pre-training   Post-training

Skin

Adipose
tissue
(fat)

Muscle
tissue

tests and training programs have been designed to measure and develop absolute muscular strength, muscular endurance, or a combination of the two.

Muscular strength is usually determined by the maximal amount of resistance (weight)—**one repetition maximum**, or **1 RM**—an individual is able to lift in a single effort. Although this assessment yields a good measure of absolute strength, it does require considerable time, because the 1 RM is determined through trial and error. For example, strength of the chest muscles is frequently measured through the bench press exercise. If an individual has not trained with weights, he may try 100 pounds and lift this resistance quite easily. After adding 50 pounds, he fails to lift the resistance. The resistance then is decreased by 10 or 20 pounds. Finally, after several trials, the 1 RM is established.

Using this method, a true 1 RM might be difficult to obtain the first time an individual is tested, because fatigue becomes a factor. By the time the 1 RM is established, the person has already made several maximal or near-maximal attempts.

Muscular endurance is typically established by the number of repetitions an individual can perform against a submaximal resistance or by the length of time a given contraction can be sustained. For example: How many push-ups can an individual do? Or how many times can a 30-pound resistance be lifted? Or how long can a person hold a chin-up?

If time is a factor and only one test item can be done, the Hand Grip Test, described in Figure 7.2, is commonly used to assess strength. This test, though, provides only a weak correlation with overall body strength. Two additional strength tests are provided in Figures 7.3 and 7.4. Lab 7A also provides the opportunity to assess your own level of muscular strength or endurance with all three tests. You may take one or more of these tests according to your time and the facilities available.

Muscular strength and muscular endurance are both highly specific. A high degree of strength or

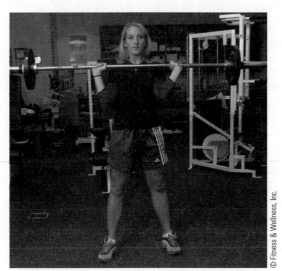

© Fitness & Wellness, Inc.

The maximal amount of resistance that an individual is able to lift in one single effort (one repetition maximum or 1 RM) is a measure of absolute strength.

endurance in one body part does not necessarily indicate similarity in other parts. Accordingly, exercises for the strength tests were selected to include the upper body, lower body, and abdominal regions.

In strength testing, several body sites should be assessed. Because different body parts have different strength levels, no single strength test provides a

Anabolic steroids Synthetic versions of the male sex hormone testosterone, which promotes muscle development and hypertrophy.

Muscular strength The ability of a muscle to exert maximum force against resistance (for example, 1 repetition maximum [or 1 RM] of the bench press exercise).

Muscular endurance The ability of a muscle to exert submaximal force repeatedly over time.

One repetition maximum (1 RM) The maximum amount of resistance an individual is able to lift in a single effort.

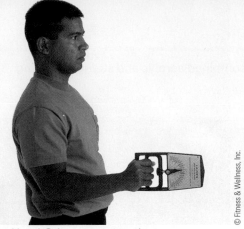

The Hand Grip tests strength.

good assessment of overall body strength. As a minimum, a strength profile should include the upper body, the lower body, and the abdominal muscles.

Before taking the strength test, you should become familiar with the procedures for the respective tests. For safety reasons, always take at least one friend with you whenever you train with weights or undertake any type of strength assessment. Also, these are different tests, so to make valid comparisons, the same test should be used for pre- and post-assessments. The following are your options.

Muscular Strength: Hand Grip Test

As indicated previously, when time is a factor, the Hand Grip Test can be used to provide a rough estimate of strength. Unlike the next two tests, this is an isometric (static contraction, discussed later in the chapter) test. If the proper grip is used, no finger motion or body movement is visible during the test. The test procedure is given in Figure 7.2, and percentile ranks based on your results are provided in Table 7.1. You can record the results of this test in Lab 7A.

Changes in strength may be more difficult to evaluate with this test. Most strength-training programs are dynamic in nature (body segments are moved through a range of motion, discussed later in the chapter), whereas this test provides an isometric assessment. Further, grip strength exercises are seldom used in strength training, and increases in strength are specific to the body parts exercised. This test, however, also can be used to supplement the following strength tests.

Muscular Endurance Test

Three exercises were selected to assess the endurance of the upper body, lower body, and mid-body muscle groups (see Figure 7.3). The advantage of

FIGURE 7.2 Procedure for the Hand Grip Strength Test.

1. Adjust the width of the dynamometer* so the middle bones of your fingers rest on the distant end of the dynamometer grip.
2. Use your dominant hand for this test. Place your elbow at a 90° angle and about 2 inches away from the body.

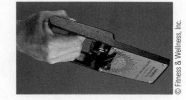

3. Now grip as hard as you can for a few seconds. Do not move any other body part as you perform the test (do not flex or extend the elbow, do not move the elbow away or toward the body, and do not lean forward or backward during the test).
4. Record the dynamometer reading in pounds (if reading is in kilograms, multiply by 2.2046).
5. Three trials are allowed for this test. Use the highest reading for your final test score. Look up your percentile rank for this test in Table 7.1.
6. Based on your percentile rank, obtain the hand grip strength fitness category according to the following guidelines:

Percentile Rank	Fitness Category
≥90	Excellent
70–80	Good
50–60	Average
30–40	Fair
≤20	Poor

* A Lafayette model 78010 dynamometer is recommended for this test (Lafayette Instruments Co., Sagamore and North 9th Street, Lafayette, IN 47903).

TABLE 7.1 Scoring Table for Hand Grip Strength Test

Percentile Rank	Men	Women
99	153	101
95	145	94
90	141	91
80	139	86
70	132	80
60	124	78
50	122	74
40	114	71
30	110	66
20	100	64
10	91	60
5	76	58

▮ High physical fitness standard

▮ Health fitness standard

FIGURE 7.3 Muscular Endurance Test.

Three exercises are conducted on this test: bench-jumps, modified dips (men) or modified push-ups (women), and bent-leg curl-ups or abdominal crunches. All exercises should be conducted with the aid of a partner. The correct procedure for performing each exercise is as follows:

Bench-jump. Using a bench or gymnasium bleacher 16¼" high, attempt to jump up and down the bench as many times as possible in 1 minute. If you cannot jump the full minute, you may step up and down. A repetition is counted each time both feet return to the floor.

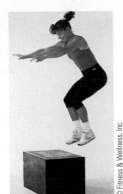

Figure 7.3a Bench jump

Modified dip. Men only: Using a bench or gymnasium bleacher, place the hands on the bench with the fingers pointing forward. Have a partner hold your feet in front of you. Bend the hips at approximately 90° (you also may use three sturdy chairs: Put your hands on two chairs placed by the sides of your body and place your feet on the third chair in front of you). Lower your body by flexing the elbows until they reach a 90° angle, then return to the starting position (also see Exercise 6, page 223). Perform the repetitions to a two-step cadence (down-up) regulated with a metronome set at 56 beats per minute. Perform as many continuous repetitions as possible. Do not count any more repetitions if you fail to follow the metronome cadence.

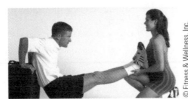

Figure 7.3b Modified dip

Modified push-up. Women: Lie down on the floor (face down), bend the knees (feet up in the air), and place the hands on the floor by the shoulders with the fingers pointing forward. The lower body will be supported at the knees (as opposed to the feet) throughout the test (see Figure 7.3c). The chest must touch the floor on each repetition. As with the modified-dip exercise (above), perform the repetitions to a two-step cadence (up-down) regulated with a metronome set at 56 beats per minute. Perform as many continuous repetitions as possible. Do not count any more repetitions if you fail to follow the metronome cadence.

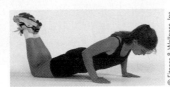

Figure 7.3c Modified push-up

Bent-leg curl-up. Lie down on the floor (face up) and bend both legs at the knees at approximately 100°. The feet should be on the floor, and you must hold them in place yourself throughout the test. Cross the arms in front of the chest, each hand on the opposite shoulder. Now raise the head off the floor, placing the chin against the chest. This is the starting and finishing position for each curl-up (see Figure 7.3d). **The back of the head may not come in contact with the floor, the hands cannot be removed from the shoulders, nor may the feet or hips be raised off the floor at any time during the test. The test is terminated if any of these four conditions occur.**

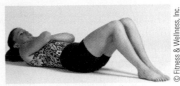

Figure 7.3d Bent-leg curl-up

When you curl up, the upper body must come to an upright position before going back down (see Figure 7.3e). The repetitions are performed to a two-step cadence (up-down) regulated with the metronome set at 40 beats per minute. For this exercise, you should allow a brief practice

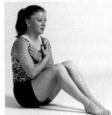

Figure 7.3e Bent-leg curl-up

period of 5 to 10 seconds to familiarize yourself with the cadence (the *up* movement is initiated with the first beat, then you must wait for the next beat to initiate the *down* movement; one repetition is accomplished every two beats of the metronome). Count as many repetitions as you are able to perform following the proper cadence. The test is also terminated if you fail to maintain the appropriate cadence or if you accomplish 100 repetitions. Have your partner check the angle at the knees throughout the test to make sure to maintain the 100° angle as close as possible.

Abdominal crunch. This test is recommended only for individuals who are unable to perform the bent-leg curl-up test because of susceptibility to low-back injury. Exercise form must be carefully monitored during the test. Several authors and researchers have indicated that proper form during this test is extremely difficult to control. Subjects often slide their bodies, bend their elbows, or shrug their shoulders during the test. Such actions facilitate the performance of the test and misrepresent the actual test results. Biomechanical factors also limit the ability to perform this test. Further, lack of spinal flexibility keeps some individuals from being able to move the full 3½" range of motion. Others are unable to keep their heels on the floor during the test. The validity of this test as an effective measure of abdominal strength or abdominal endurance has also been questioned in recent research.

Tape a 3½" × 30" strip of cardboard onto the floor. Lie down on the floor in a supine position (face up) with the knees bent at approximately 100° and the legs slightly apart. The feet should be on the floor, and you must hold them in place yourself throughout the test. Straighten out your arms and place them on the floor alongside the trunk with the palms down and the fingers fully extended. The fingertips of both hands should barely touch the closest

(Continued)

FIGURE 7.3 (Continued)

edge of the cardboard (see Figure 7.3f). Bring the head off the floor until the chin is 1" to 2" away from your chest. Keep the head in this position during the entire test (do not

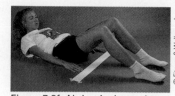

Figure 7.3f Abdominal crunch test

move the head by flexing or extending the neck). You are now ready to begin the test.

Perform the repetitions to a two-step cadence (up-down) regulated with a metronome set at 60 beats per minute. As

you curl up, slide the fingers over the cardboard until the fingertips reach the far edge (3½") of the board (see Figure 7.3g), then return to the starting position.

Allow a brief practice period of 5 to 10 seconds

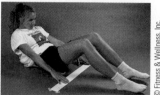

Figure 7.3g Abdominal crunch test

to familiarize yourself with the cadence. Initiate the *up* movement with the first beat and the *down* movement with the next beat. Accomplish one repetition every two beats of the metronome. Count as many repetitions as you are able to perform following the proper cadence. You may not count a repetition if the fingertips fail to reach the distant edge of the cardboard.

Terminate the test if you (a) fail to maintain the appropriate cadence, (b) bend the elbows, (c) shrug the shoulders, (d) slide the body, (e) lift heels off the floor, (f) raise the chin off the chest, (g) accomplish 100 repetitions, or (h) no longer can perform the test. Have your partner check the angle at the knees throughout the test to make sure that the 100° angle is maintained as close as possible.

For this test you may also use a Crunch-Ster Curl-Up Tester, available from Novel Products.* An illustration of the

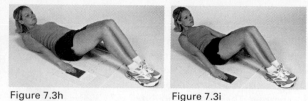

Figure 7.3h Figure 7.3i
Abdominal crunch test performed with a Crunch-Ster Curl-Up Tester.

test performed with this equipment is provided in Figures 7.3h and 7.3i.

According to the results, look up your percentile rank for each exercise in the far left column of Table 7.2 and determine your muscular endurance fitness category according to the following classification:

Average Score	Fitness Category	Points
≥ 90	Excellent	5
70–80	Good	4
50–60	Average	3
30–40	Fair	2
" 20	Poor	1

Look up the number of points assigned for each fitness category above. Total the number of points and determine your overall strength endurance fitness category according to the following ratings:

Total Points	Strength Endurance Category
≥ 13	Excellent
10–12	Good
7–9	Average
4–6	Fair
" 3	Poor

*Novel Products, Inc. Figure Finder Collection, P.O. Box 408, Rockton, IL 61072-0408. 1-800-323-5143, Fax 815-624-4866.

TABLE 7.2 Muscular Endurance Scoring Table

Percentile Rank	Men				Women			
	Bench Jumps	Modified Dips	Bent-Leg Curl-Ups	Abdominal Crunches	Bench Jumps	Modified Push-ups	Bent-Leg Curl-Ups	Abdominal Crunches
99	66	54	100	100	58	95	100	100
95	63	50	81	100	54	70	100	100
90	62	38	65	100	52	50	97	69
80	58	32	51	66	48	41	77	49
70	57	30	44	45	44	38	57	37
60	56	27	31	38	42	33	45	34
50	54	26	28	33	39	30	37	31
40	51	23	25	29	38	28	28	27
30	48	20	22	26	36	25	22	24
20	47	17	17	22	32	21	17	21
10	40	11	10	18	28	18	9	15
5	34	7	3	16	26	15	4	0

▇ High physical fitness standard   ▏Health fitness standard

FIGURE 7.4 Muscular Strength and Endurance Test.

1. Familiarize yourself with the six lifts used for this test: lat pull-down, leg extension, bench press, bent-leg curl-up or abdominal crunch,* leg curl, and arm curl. Graphic illustrations for each lift are given on pages 229, 230, 226, 222, 228, and 227, respectively. For the leg curl exercise, the knees should be flexed to 90°. A description and illustration of the bent-leg curl-up and the abdominal crunch exercises are provided in Figure 7.3. For the lateral pull-down exercise, use a sitting position and have your partner hold you down by the waist or shoulders. On the leg extension lift, maintain the trunk in an upright position.
2. Determine your body weight in pounds.
3. Determine the amount of resistance to be used on each lift. To obtain this number, multiply your body weight by the percent given below for each lift.

Lift	Percent of Body Weight	
	Men	**Women**
Lat Pull-Down	.70	.45
Leg Extension	.65	.50
Bench Press	.75	.45
Bent-Leg Curl-Up or Abdominal Crunch*	NA**	NA**
Leg Curl	.32	.25
Arm Curl	.35	.18

* The abdominal crunch exercise should be used only by individuals who suffer or are susceptible to low-back pain.

** NA = not applicable—see Figure 7.3

4. Perform the maximum continuous number of repetitions possible.
5. Based on the number of repetitions performed, look up the percentile rank for each lift in the left column of Table 7.3.
6. The individual strength fitness category is determined according to the following classification:

Percentile Rank	Fitness Category	Points
≥90	Excellent	5
70–80	Good	4
50–60	Average	3
30–40	Fair	2
≤20	Poor	1

7. Look up the number of points assigned for each fitness category under item 6 above, Total the number of points and determine your overall strength fitness category according to the following ratings:

Total Points	Strength Category
≥25	Excellent
19–24	Good
13–18	Average
7–12	Fair
≤6	Poor

8. Record your results in Lab 7A.

this test is that it does not require strength-training equipment—only a stopwatch, a metronome, a bench or gymnasium bleacher 16¼" high, a cardboard strip 3½" wide by 30" long, and a partner. A percentile rank is given for each exercise according to the number of repetitions performed (see Table 7.2). An overall endurance rating can be obtained by totaling the number of points obtained on each exercise. Record the results of this test in Lab 7A.

Muscular Strength and Endurance Test

In this test you will lift a submaximal resistance as many times as possible using the six strength-training exercises listed in Figure 7.4. The resistance for each lift is determined according to selected percentages of body weight (see Figure 7.4 and Lab 7A).

With this test, if an individual does only a few repetitions, the test will primarily measure absolute strength. For those who are able to do a lot of repetitions, the test will be an indicator of muscular endurance. If you are not familiar with the different lifts, illustrations are provided at the end of this chapter.

A strength/endurance rating is determined according to the maximum number of repetitions you are able to perform on each exercise. Fixed-resistance, Universal Gym units are necessary to administer all but the abdominal curls exercise on this test (see Dynamic Training on pages 208–209 for an explanation of fixed-resistance equipment).

A percentile rank for each exercise is given based on the number of repetitions performed (see Table 7.3). As with the muscular endurance test, an overall muscular strength/endurance rating is obtained by totaling the number of points obtained on each exercise.

If no fixed resistance Universal Gym equipment is available, you can still perform the test using different equipment. In that case, though, the percentile rankings and strength fitness categories may not be completely accurate because a certain resistance (for example, 50 pounds) is seldom the

TABLE 7.3 Muscular Strength and Endurance Scoring Table

Percentile Rank	Men							Women						
	Lat Pull-Down	Leg Extension	Bench Press	Bent-Leg Curl-Up	Abdominal Crunch	Leg Curl	Arm Curl	Lat Pull-Down	Leg Extension	Bench Press	Bent-Leg Curl-Up	Abdominal Crunch	Leg Curl	Arm Curl
99	30	25	26	100	100	24	25	30	25	27	100	100	20	25
95	25	20	21	81	100	20	21	25	20	21	100	100	17	21
90	19	19	19	65	100	19	19	21	18	20	97	69	12	20
80	16	15	16	51	66	15	15	16	13	16	77	49	10	16
70	13	14	13	44	45	13	12	13	11	13	57	37	9	14
60	11	13	11	31	38	11	10	11	10	11	45	34	7	12
50	10	12	10	28	33	10	9	10	9	10	37	31	6	10
40	9	10	7	25	29	8	8	9	8	5	28	27	5	8
30	7	9	5	22	26	6	7	7	7	3	22	24	4	7
20	6	7	3	17	22	4	5	6	5	1	17	21	3	6
10	4	5	1	10	18	3	3	3	3	0	9	15	1	3
5	3	3	0	3	16	1	2	2	1	0	4	0	0	2

■ High physical fitness standard   ■ Health fitness standard

same on two different weight machines (for example, Universal Gym versus Nautilus). The industry has no standard calibration procedure for strength equipment. Consequently, if you lift a certain resistance on one machine, you may or may not be able to lift the same amount on a different machine.

Even though the percentile ranks may not be valid when using different equipment, test results can be used to evaluate changes in fitness. For example, you may be able to do 7 repetitions during the initial test, but if you can perform 14 repetitions after 12 weeks of training, that's a measure of improvement. The results for the Muscular Strength and Endurance Test can be recorded in Lab 7A.

Strength-Training Prescription

The capacity of muscle cells to exert force increases and decreases according to the demands placed upon the muscular system. If muscle cells are overloaded beyond their normal use, such as in strength-training programs, the cells increase in size (hypertrophy) and strength. If the demands placed on the muscle cells decrease, such as in sedentary living or required rest because of illness or injury, the cells **atrophy** and lose strength. A good level of muscular strength is important to develop and maintain fitness, health, and total well-being.

Factors That Affect Strength

Several physiological factors combine to create muscle contraction and subsequent strength gains: neural stimulation, type of muscle fiber, overload, and specificity of training. Basic knowledge of these concepts is important to understand the principles involved in strength training.

Neural Stimulation

Within the neuromuscular system, single **motor neurons** branch and attach to multiple muscle fibers. The motor neuron and the fibers it innervates (supplies with nerves) form a **motor unit**. The number of fibers a motor neuron can innervate varies from just a few in muscles that require precise control (eye muscles, for example) to as many as 1,000 or more in large muscles that do not perform refined or precise movements.

Stimulation of a motor neuron causes the muscle fibers to contract maximally or not at all. Variations in the number of fibers innervated and the frequency of their stimulation determine the strength of the muscle contraction. As the number of fibers innervated and frequency of stimulation increases, so does the strength of the muscular contraction.

Types of Muscle Fiber

The human body has two basic types of muscle fibers: (a) slow-twitch or red fibers and (b) fast-twitch or white fibers. **Slow-twitch fibers** have a greater capacity for aerobic work. **Fast-twitch fibers** have a greater capacity for anaerobic work and produce more overall force. The latter are important for quick and powerful movements commonly used in strength-training activities.

The proportion of slow- and fast-twitch fibers is determined genetically, and consequently varies from one person to another. Nevertheless, training increases the functional capacity of both types of fiber and, more specifically, strength training increases their ability to exert force.

During muscular contraction, slow-twitch fibers always are recruited first. As the force and speed of muscle contraction increase, the relative importance of the fast-twitch fibers increases. To activate the fast-twitch fibers, an activity must be intense and powerful.

Overload

Strength gains are achieved in two ways:

1. Through increased ability of individual muscle fibers to generate a stronger contraction.
2. By recruiting a greater proportion of the total available fibers for each contraction.

These two factors combine in the **overload principle**. The demands placed on the muscle must be increased systematically and progressively over time, and the resistance must be of a magnitude significant enough to cause physiological adaptation. In simpler terms, just like all other organs and systems of the human body, to increase in physical capacity, muscles have to be taxed repeatedly beyond their accustomed loads. Because of this principle, strength training also is called "progressive resistance training."

Several procedures can be used to overload in strength-training:[6]

1. Increasing the resistance.
2. Increasing the number of repetitions.
3. Increasing the speed of the repetitions.
4. Decreasing rest interval for endurance improvements or lengthening the rest interval for strength gains.
5. Increasing volume (sum of the repetitions performed multiplied by the resistance used).
6. Using any combination of the above.

Specificity of Training

The principle of **specificity of training** states that, for a muscle to increase in strength or endurance, the training program must be specific to obtain the desired effects (also see discussion on Resistance on page 210).

The principle of specificity also applies to activity or sport-specific development and is commonly

referred to as **SAID training,** or **specific adaptation to imposed demand**. The SAID principle implies that if an individual is attempting to improve specific sport skills, the strength-training exercises performed should resemble as closely as possible the movement patterns encountered in that particular activity or sport.

For example, a soccer player who wishes to become stronger and faster would emphasize exercises that will develop leg strength and power. In contrast, an individual recovering from a lower-limb fracture initially exercises to increase strength and stability, and subsequently muscle endurance. Additional information on the principle of specificity is provided under "Sport-Specific Conditioning" on page 286 in Chapter 9.

Understanding all four concepts (neural stimulation, muscle fiber types, overload, and specificity) is required to design an effective strength-training program.

Principles Involved in Strength Training

Because muscular strength and endurance are important in developing and maintaining overall fitness and well-being, the principles necessary to develop a strength-training program have to be understood, just as in the prescription for cardio-respiratory endurance. These principles are mode, resistance, sets, frequency, and volume of training. The key factor to successful muscular strength development, however, is the individualization of the program according to these principles and the

Atrophy Decrease in the size of a cell.

Motor neurons Nerves connecting the central nervous system to the muscle.

Motor unit The combination of a motor neuron and the muscle fibers that neuron innervates.

Slow-twitch fibers Muscle fibers with greater aerobic potential and slow speed of contraction.

Fast-twitch fibers Muscle fibers with greater anaerobic potential and fast speed of contraction.

Overload principle Training concept that the demands placed on a system (cardiorespiratory or muscular) must be increased systematically and progressively over time to cause physiological adaptation (development or improvement).

Specificity of training Principle that training must be done with the specific muscle the person is attempting to improve.

Specific adaptation to imposed demand (SAID) training Training principle stating that, for improvements to occur in a specific activity, the exercises performed during a strength-training program should resemble as closely as possible the movement patterns encountered in that particular activity.

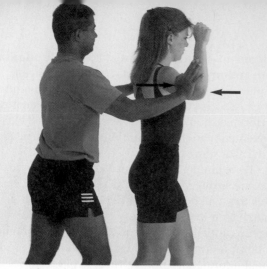

In isometric training, muscle contraction produces little or no movement.

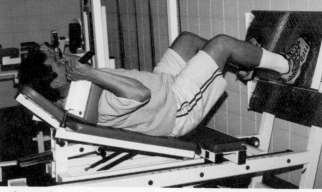

In dynamic training, muscle contraction produces movement in the respective joint.

person's goals, as well as the magnitude of the individual's effort during training itself.[7]

Mode of Training

Two types of training methods are used to improve strength: isometric (static) and dynamic (previously called "isotonic"). In isometric training, muscle contractions produce little or no movement, such as pushing or pulling against an immovable object. In dynamic training, the muscle contractions produce movement, such as extending the knees with resistance on the ankles (leg extension). The specificity of training principle applies here, too. To increase isometric versus dynamic strength, an individual must use static instead of dynamic training to achieve the desired results.

ISOMETRIC TRAINING

Isometric training does not require much equipment, but its popularity of several years ago has waned. Because strength gains with isometric training are specific to the angle of muscle contraction, this type of training is beneficial in a sport such as gymnastics, which requires regular static contractions during routines. As presented in Chapter 8, however, isometric training is a critical component of back health conditioning programs (see Preventing and Rehabilitating Low Back Pain, pages 249–254).

DYNAMIC TRAINING

Dynamic training is the most popular mode for strength training. The primary advantage is that strength is gained through the full **range of motion**. Most daily activities are dynamic in nature. We are constantly lifting, pushing, and pulling objects, and strength is needed through a complete range of motion. Another advantage is that improvements are measured easily by the amount lifted.

Dynamic training consists of two action phases when an exercise is performed: **concentric** or **positive resistance** and **eccentric** or **negative resistance**. In the concentric phase, the muscle shortens as it contracts to overcome the resistance; in the eccentric phase, it lengthens to overcome the resistance. For example, during a bench press exercise, when the person lifts the resistance from the chest to full-arm extension, the triceps muscle on the back of the upper arm shortens to extend the elbow. During the eccentric phase, the same triceps muscle must lengthen to lower the weight during elbow flexion, but the muscle lengthens slowly to avoid dropping the resistance. Both motions work the same muscle against the same resistance.

Eccentric muscle contractions allow us to lower weights in a smooth, gradual, and controlled manner. Without eccentric contractions, weights would be dropped on the way down. Because the same muscles work when you lift and lower a resistance, always be sure to execute both actions in a controlled manner. Failure to do so diminishes the benefits of the training program and increases the risk for injuries.

Dynamic training programs can be conducted without weights, with exercise bands, **free weights**, **fixed-resistance** machines, **variable-resistance** machines, or isokinetic equipment. When you perform dynamic exercises without weights (for example, pull-ups and push-ups), with free weights, or with fixed-resistance machines, you move a constant resistance through a joint's full range of motion. The greatest resistance that can be lifted equals the maximum weight that can be moved at the weakest angle of the joint. This is because of changes in muscle length and angle of pull as the joint moves through its range of motion.

As strength training became more popular, new strength-training machines were developed. This technology brought about **isokinetic training** and variable-resistance training programs, which require special machines equipped with mechanical devices that provide differing amounts of resistance, with

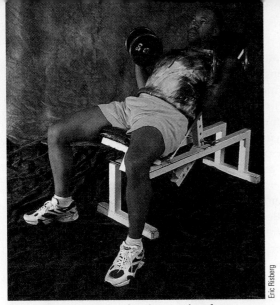

Strength training can be done using free weights.

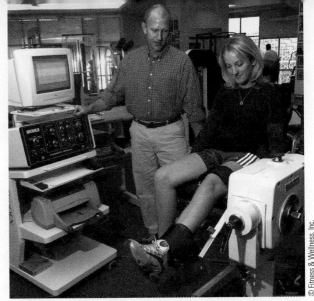

In isokinetic training, the speed of muscle contraction is constant.

the intent of overloading the muscle group maximally through the entire range of motion. A distinction of isokinetic training is that the speed of the muscle contraction is kept constant because the machine provides resistance to match the user's force through the range of motion. The mode of training an individual selects depends mainly on the type of equipment available and the specific objective the training program is attempting to accomplish.

The benefits of isokinetic and variable-resistance training are similar to the other dynamic training methods. Theoretically, strength gains should be better because maximum resistance is applied at all angles. Research, however, has not shown this type of training to be more effective than other modes of dynamic training.

FREE WEIGHTS VERSUS MACHINES IN DYNAMIC TRAINING

The most popular weight-training devices available during the first half of the twentieth century were plate-loaded barbells (free weights). Strength-training machines were developed in the middle of the century but did not become popular until the 1970s. With subsequent technological improvements to these machines, a stirring debate surfaced over which of the two training modalities was better.

Free weights require that the individual balance the resistance through the entire lifting motion. Thus, one could logically assume that free weights are a better training modality because additional stabilizing muscles are needed to balance the resistance as it is moved through the range of motion. Research, however, has not shown any differences in strength development between the two exercise modalities.[8]

Although each modality has pros and cons, muscles do not know whether the source of a

resistance is a barbell, a dumbbell, a Universal Gym machine, a Nautilus machine, or a simple cinder block. What determines the degree of a person's strength development is the quality of the program and the individual's effort during the training program itself—not the type of equipment used.

ADVANTAGES OF FREE WEIGHTS

Following are the advantages of using free weights instead of machines in a strength-training program.

1. *Cost:* Free weights are much less expensive than most exercise machines. On a limited budget, free weights are a better option.

Isometric training Strength-training method referring to a muscle contraction that produces little or no movement, such as pushing or pulling against an immovable object.

Range of motion Entire arc of movement of a given joint.

Dynamic training Strength-training method referring to a muscle contraction with movement.

Concentric Shortening of a muscle during muscle contraction.

Positive resistance The lifting, pushing, or concentric phase of a repetition during a strength-training exercise.

Eccentric Lengthening of a muscle during muscle contraction.

Negative resistance The lowering or eccentric phase of a repetition during a strength training exercise.

Free weights Barbells and dumbbells.

Fixed resistance Type of exercise in which a constant resistance is moved through a joint's full range of motion.

Isokinetic training Strength-training method in which the speed of the muscle contraction is kept constant because the equipment (machine) provides an accommodating resistance to match the user's force (maximal) through the range of motion.

Variable resistance Training using special machines equipped with mechanical devices that provide differing amounts of resistance through the range of motion.

2. *Variety:* A bar and a few plates can be used to perform many exercises to strengthen most muscles in the body.
3. *Portability:* Free weights are portable and can be easily moved from one area or station to another.
4. *Balance:* Free weights require that a person balance the weight through the entire range of motion. This feature involves additional stabilizing muscles to keep the weight moving properly.
5. *One size fits all:* Free weights can be used by people of almost all ages. A drawback of machines is that individuals who are at the extremes in terms of height or limb length often do not fit into the machines. In particular, small women and adolescents are at a disadvantage.

ADVANTAGES OF MACHINES

Strength training machines have the following advantages over free weights:

1. *Safety:* Machines are safer because spotters are rarely needed to monitor exercises.
2. *Selection:* A few exercises—such as hip flexion, hip abduction, leg curls, lat pulldowns, and neck exercises—can be performed only with machines.
3. *Variable resistance:* Most machines provide variable resistance. Free weights provide only fixed resistance.
4. *Isolation:* Individual muscles are better isolated with machines because stabilizing muscles are not used to balance the weight during the exercise.
5. *Time:* Exercising with machines requires less time because the resistance is quickly set using a selector pin instead of having to manually change dumbbells or weight plates on both sides of a barbell.
6. *Flexibility:* Most machines can provide resistance over a greater range of movement during the exercise, thereby contributing to greater flexibility in the joints. For example, a barbell pull-over exercise provides resistance over a range of 100 degrees, whereas a weight machine may allow for as much as 260 degrees.
7. *Rehabilitation:* Machines are more useful during injury rehabilitation. A knee injury, for instance, is practically impossible to rehab using free weights, whereas small loads can be easily selected through a limited range of motion with a weight machine.
8. *Skill acquisition:* Learning a new exercise movement—and performing it correctly—is faster because the machine controls the direction of the movement.

Resistance

Resistance in strength training is the equivalent of intensity in cardiorespiratory exercise prescription.

The amount of resistance, load, or weight lifted depends on whether the individual is trying to develop muscular strength or muscular endurance.

To stimulate strength development, a resistance of approximately 80 percent of the maximum capacity (1 RM) is recommended.[9] For example, a person with a 1 RM of 150 pounds should work with at least 120 pounds (150 × .80). Less than 80 percent will help increase muscular endurance rather than strength.

Because of the time factor involved in constantly determining the 1 RM on each lift to ensure that the person is indeed working above 80 percent, the rule is that individuals should be able to perform more than 3 but no more than 12 repetitions (3 to 12 RM) for adequate strength gains. For example, if a person is training with a resistance of 120 pounds and cannot lift it more than 12 times, the training stimulus (weight) is adequate for development of strength.

Once the person can lift the resistance more than 12 times, the resistance should be increased by 5 to 10 pounds and the person again should build up to 12 repetitions. This is referred to as **progressive resistance training**.

Research on strength indicates that the closer a person trains to the 1 RM, the greater are the strength gains. A disadvantage of working constantly at or near the 1 RM is that it increases the risk for injury.

Highly trained athletes seeking maximum strength development often use 1 to 6 repetitions maximum. Working around 10 repetitions maximum seems to produce the best results in terms of muscular hypertrophy (information on dietary guidelines to optimize muscle strength and hypertrophy is provided under the section "Healthy Weight Gain" in Chapter 5, page 137). Eccentric contractions are also more effective in producing muscle hypertrophy but result in greater muscle soreness.[10] If training is conducted with more than 12 repetitions, primarily muscular endurance will be developed.

Body builders tend to work with moderate resistance levels (60 to 85 percent of the 1 RM) and perform 8 to 20 repetitions to near fatigue. A foremost objective of body building is to increase muscle size. Moderate resistance promotes blood flow to the muscles, "pumping up the muscles" (also known as "the pump") and making them look much larger than they do in a resting state.

From a health-fitness point of view, 8 to 12 repetitions maximum are recommended for adequate development. We live in a dynamic world in which muscular strength and endurance are both required to lead an enjoyable life. Therefore, working near a 10-repetition threshold seems to improve overall performance most effectively.

Sets

In strength training, a **set** is the number of repetitions performed for a given exercise. For example, a person lifting 120 pounds eight times has performed one set of 8 repetitions (1 × 8 × 120).

When you work with 8 to 12 repetitions maximum, the recommendation is three sets per exercise. Because of the characteristics of muscle fiber, the number of sets that can be done is limited. As the number of sets increases, so does the amount of muscle fatigue and subsequent recovery time. Therefore, strength gains may be lessened by performing too many sets.

A recommended program for beginners in their first year of training is one or two light warm-up sets per exercise using about 50 percent of the 1 RM (no warm-up sets are necessary for subsequent exercises that use the same muscle group) followed by three heavy sets. At least one of these three sets should be performed to exhaustion or near exhaustion (up to the maximum number of repetitions selected). Maintaining a resistance and effort that will exhaust a muscle in 8 to 12 repetitions in at least one of these three heavy sets is critical to achieve optimal progress. Because of the lower resistances used in body building, four to eight sets can be done for each exercise.

To avoid muscle soreness and stiffness, new participants ought to build up gradually to the three sets of maximal repetitions. This can be done by performing only one set of each exercise with a lighter resistance on the first day, two sets of each exercise on the second day—the first light and the second with the regular resistance—and three sets on the third day—one light and two heavy. After that, a person should be able to do all three heavy sets.

The time necessary to recover between sets depends mainly on the resistance used during each set. In strength training, the energy to lift heavy weights is derived primarily from the ATP-CP or phosphagen system (see Chapter 3, "Energy (ATP) Production," pages 78–79). Ten seconds of maximal exercise nearly depletes the CP stores in the exercised muscle(s). These stores are replenished in about 3 minutes of recovery.

Based on this principle, a rest period of about 3 minutes between sets is necessary for people who are trying to maximize their strength gains. Individuals training for health-fitness purposes might allow 2 minutes of rest between sets. Body builders should rest no more than 1 minute to maximize the "pumping" effect. The exercise program will be more time-effective by alternating two or three exercises that require different muscle groups, called **circuit training**. In this way, an individual will not have to wait 2 to 3 minutes before proceeding to a new set on a different exercise. For example, the bench press, leg extension, and abdominal curl-up exercises may be combined so the person can go almost directly from one set to the next.

Men and women alike should observe the guidelines given previously. Many women, however, do not follow these guidelines. They erroneously believe that training with low resistances and many repetitions is best to enhance body composition and maximize energy expenditure. Unless a person is seeking to increase muscular endurance for a specific sport-related activity, the use of low resistances and high repetitions is not recommended to achieve optimal strength-fitness goals and maximize long-term energy expenditure (also see "Exercise: The Key to Weight Management" in Chapter 5, pages 135–137).

Frequency

Strength training should be done either through a total body workout two to three times a week, or more frequently if using a split-body routine (upper body one day, lower body the next). After a maximum strength workout, the muscles should be rested for about 2 to 3 days to allow adequate recovery. If not completely recovered in 2 to 3 days, the person most likely is overtraining and therefore not reaping the full benefits of the program. In that case, the person should do fewer sets of exercises than in the previous workout. A summary of strength training guidelines for health-fitness purposes is provided in Figure 7.5.

To achieve significant strength gains, a minimum of 8 weeks of consecutive training is necessary. After an individual has achieved a recommended strength level, from a health-fitness standpoint, one training session per week will be sufficient to maintain the new strength level. Highly trained athletes will need to train two times per week to maintain their strength level.

Frequency of strength training for body builders varies from person to person. Because they use moderate resistance, daily or even two-a-day workouts are common. The frequency depends on the amount of resistance, number of sets performed per session, and the person's ability to recover from the

---

Resistance Amount of weight that is lifted.

Progressive resistance training A gradual increase of resistance over a period of time.

Set A fixed number of repetitions; one set of bench presses might be 10 repetitions.

Circuit training Alternating exercises by performing them in a sequence of three to six or more.

FIGURE 7.5 Strength-training guidelines.

Mode: 8 to 10 dynamic strength-training exercises involving the body's major muscle groups

Resistance: Enough resistance to perform 8 to 12 repetitions to near-fatigue (10 to 15 repetitions for older and more frail individuals)

Sets: A minimum of 1 set

Frequency: At least two times per week

Based on "The Recommended Quantity and Quality of Exercise for Developing and Maintaining Cardiorespiratory and Muscular Fitness, and Flexibility in Healthy Adults," *Medicine and Science in Sports and Exercise* 30 (1998): 975–991.

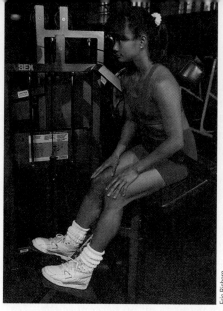

From a health fitness standpoint, one strength-training session per week is sufficient to maintain strength.

Eric Risberg

TABLE 7.4 Guidelines for Various Strength-Training Programs

Strength-Training Program	Resistance	Sets	Rest Between Sets*	Frequency (workouts per week)**
Health fitness	8–12 reps max	3	2 min	2–3
Maximal strength	1–6 reps max	3–6	3 min	2–3
Muscular endurance	10–30 reps	3–6	2 min	3–6
Body building	8–20 reps near max	3–8	0–1 min	4–12

* Recovery between sets can be decreased by alternating exercises that use different muscle groups.

** Weekly training sessions can be increased by using a split-body routine.

previous exercise bout (see Table 7.4). The latter often is dictated by level of conditioning.

Training Volume

Volume refers to the sum of all the repetitions performed multiplied by the resistances used during a strength-training session.[11] Volume is frequently used to quantify the amount of work performed in a given training session—in the example under "Sets" on page 211, the volume of a single set was calculated to be 960. The volume of training done in a strength-training session can be modified by changing the total number of exercises performed—either by changing the number of sets done per exercise or the number of repetitions performed per set. High initial training volumes and low intensities are used for muscle hypertrophy, whereas low volumes and high intensities are used to increase strength and power.

Altering training volume and intensity is known as **periodization**, a training approach frequently used by athletes to achieve peak fitness and prevent **overtraining**. Periodization means cycling of one's training objectives (hypertrophy, strength, and endurance), with each phase of the program lasting anywhere from 2 to 12 weeks. To prevent overtraining during periodization, the volume should not increase by more than 5 percent from one phase to the next.

Periodization is also used by fitness participants who want to achieve higher levels of fitness. A more thorough discussion on periodization is provided in Chapter 9 (pages 287–288).

Plyometrics

Strength, speed, and explosiveness are all crucial for success in athletics. All three of these factors are enhanced with a progressive resistance training program, but greater increases in speed and explosiveness are thought possible with **plyometric exercise**. The objective is to generate the greatest amount of force in the shortest amount of time. A sound strength base is necessary before attempting plyometric exercises.

Plyometric training is popular in sports that require powerful movements, such as basketball, volleyball, sprinting, jumping, and gymnastics. A typical plyometric exercise involves jumping off and back onto a box, attempting to rebound as quickly as possible on each jump. Box heights are increased progressively from about 12 to 22 inches.

The bounding action attempts to take advantage of the stretch-recoil and stretch reflex characteristics of muscle. The rapid stretch applied to the muscle during contact with the ground is thought to augment muscle contraction, leading to more explosiveness. Plyometrics can be used, too, for strengthening upper body muscles. An example is doing push-ups so the extension of the arms is forceful enough to drive the hands (and body) completely off the floor during each repetition.

A drawback of plyometric training is its higher risk for injuries compared to conventional modes of progressive resistance training. For instance, the potential for injury in rebound exercise escalates with the increase in box height or the number of repetitions.

Strength Gains

A common question by many strength-training participants is: How quickly can strength gains be observed? Strength-training studies have revealed that most of the strength gains are seen in the first 8 weeks of training. The amount of improvement, however, is related to previous training status. Increases of 40 percent are seen in individuals with no previous strength-training experience, 16 percent in previously strength-trained people, and 10 percent in advanced individuals.[12] Adhering to a periodized strength-training program will yield further improvements (see Chapter 9, pages 287–288).

Strength-Training Exercises With and Without Weights

The two strength-training programs introduced on pages 221–234 provide a complete body workout. The major muscles of the human body referred to in the exercises are pointed out in Figure 7.6, page 218.

Only a minimum of equipment is required for the first program, Strength-Training Exercises without Weights (Exercises 1 through 14). This program can be conducted in your own home. Your body weight is used as the primary resistance for most exercises. A few exercises call for a friend's help or some basic implements from around your house to provide greater resistance.

Strength-Training Exercises with Weights (Exercises 15 through 35), require machines (shown in the accompanying photographs). These exercises can be conducted on either fixed-resistance or variable-resistance equipment. Many of these exercises can also be performed with free weights. The first twelve exercises (15 to 26) are recommended to get a complete workout. You can do these exercises as circuit training. If time is a factor, as a minimum, perform the first eight (15 through 22) exercises. Exercises 27 to 35 are supplemental or can be used to replace some of the basic twelve (for instance, substitute Exercise 27 or 28 for 15; 29 for 16; 30 for 19; 31 for 20; 32 for 23; 33 or 34 for 25).

Core Strength Training

The trunk (spine) and pelvis are referred to as the "core" of the body. Core muscles include the abdominal muscles (rectus, transversus, and internal and external obliques), hip muscles (front and back), and spinal muscles (lower and upper back muscles). These muscle groups are responsible for maintaining the stability of the spine and pelvis.

Many of the major muscle groups of the legs, shoulder, and arms attach to the core. A strong core allows a person to perform activities of daily living with greater ease, improve sports performance through a more effective energy transfer from large to small body parts, and decrease the incidence of low-back pain.

Interest in **core strength training** programs has increased recently. A major objective of core training is to exercise the abdominal and lower back muscles in unison. Furthermore, individuals should spend as much time training the back muscles as they do the abdominal muscles. Besides enhancing stability, core training improves dynamic balance, which is often required during physical activity and sports participation.

Key core-training exercises include the abdominal crunch and bent-leg curl-up, reverse crunch, pelvic tilt, lateral bridge, prone bridge, leg press, seated back, lat pull-down, back extension, supine bridge, and pelvic clock (Exercises 4, 11, 12, 13, 14, 16, 21, 23, and 35 in this chapter and Exercises 26 and 27 in Chapter 8, respectively).

When core training is used in athletic conditioning programs, athletes attempt to mimic the dynamic

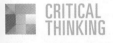

CRITICAL THINKING

Your roommate started a strength training program last year and has seen good results. He is now strength-training on a nearly daily basis and taking performance-enhancing supplements hoping to accelerate results. What are your feelings about his program? What would you say (and not say) to him?

Volume (in strength training) The sum of all the repetitions performed multiplied by the resistances used during a strength-training session.

Periodization A training approach that divides the season into cycles using a systematic variation in intensity and volume of training to enhance fitness and performance.

Overtraining An emotional, behavioral, and physical condition marked by increased fatigue, decreased performance, persistent muscle soreness, mood disturbances, and feelings of "staleness" or "burnout" as a result of excessive physical training.

Plyometric exercise Explosive jump training, incorporating speed and strength training to enhance explosiveness.

Core strength training A training program designed to strengthen the abdominal, hip, and spinal muscles (the core of the body).

skills they use in their sport. To do so, they use special equipment such as balance boards, stability balls, and foam pads. The use of this equipment allows the athletes to train the core while seeking balance and stability in a sport-specific manner.[13]

Pilates Exercise System

Pilates exercises have become increasingly popular in recent years. Previously, Pilates training was used primarily by dancers, but now this exercise modality is embraced by a large number of fitness participants, rehab patients, models, actors, and even professional athletes. Pilates studios, college courses, and classes at health clubs are available nationwide.

The Pilates training system was originally developed in the 1920s by German physical therapist Joseph Pilates. The exercises are designed to help strengthen the body's core by developing pelvic stability and abdominal control—coupled with focused breathing patterns.

Pilates exercises are performed either on a mat (floor) or specialized equipment to help increase strength and flexibility of deep postural muscles. The intent is to improve muscle tone and length (a limber body), instead of increasing muscle size (hypertrophy).

Pilates mat classes focus on body stability and correct body mechanics. The exercises are performed in a slow, controlled, and precise manner. Properly performed, these exercises require intense concentration. Initial Pilates training should be conducted under the supervision of certified instructors with extensive Pilates teaching experience.

Fitness goals of Pilates programs include better flexibility, muscle tone, posture, spinal support, body balance, low-back health, sports performance, and mind–body awareness. Individuals with loose or unstable joints benefit from Pilates because the exercises are designed to enhance joint stability. The Pilates program is also used to help lose weight, increase lean tissue, and manage stress. Although Pilates programs are quite popular, research is required to corroborate the benefits attributed to this training system.

Exercise Guidelines

As you prepare to design your strength training program, keep the following guidelines in mind:

1. Select exercises that will involve all major muscle groups: chest, shoulders, back, legs, arms, hip, and trunk.
2. Select exercises that will strengthen the core. Use controlled movements and start with light to moderate resistances (athletes may later use explosive movements with heavier resistances).
3. Never lift weights alone. Always have someone work out with you in case you need a spotter or help with an injury. When you use free weights, one to two spotters are recommended for certain exercises (for example, bench press, squats, overhead press).
4. Warm up properly prior to lifting weights by performing a light- to moderate-intensity aerobic activity (5 to 7 minutes) and some gentle stretches for a few minutes.
5. Use proper lifting technique for each exercise. Correct lifting technique will involve only those muscles and joints intended for a specific exercise. Involving other muscles and joints to "cheat" during the exercise to complete a repetition or to be able to lift a greater resistance decreases the long-term effectiveness of the exercise and can lead to injury (such as arching the back during the push-up, squat, or bench press exercises).

   Proper lifting technique also implies performing the exercises in a controlled manner and throughout the entire range of motion. Avoid fast and jerky movements and do not throw the entire body into the lifting motion. Do not arch the back when lifting a weight.
6. Maintain proper body balance while lifting. Proper balance involves good posture, a stable body position, and correct seat and arm/leg settings on exercise machines. Loss of balance places undue strain on smaller muscles and leads to injuries because of the heavy resistances suddenly placed on them.

   In the early stages of a program, first-time lifters often struggle with bar control and balance when using free weights. This problem is quickly overcome with practice following a few training sessions.
7. Exercise larger muscle groups (such as those in the chest, back, and legs) before exercising smaller muscle groups (arms, abdominals, ankles, neck). For example, the bench press exercise works the chest, shoulders, and back of the upper arms (triceps), whereas the triceps extension works the back of the upper arms only.
8. Exercise opposing muscle groups for a balanced workout. When you work the chest (bench press), also work the back (rowing torso). If you work the biceps (arm curl), also work the triceps (triceps extension).
9. Breathe naturally. Inhale during the eccentric phase (bringing the weight down) and exhale during the concentric phase (lifting or pushing the weight up). Practice proper breathing with lighter weights when you are learning a new exercise.

10. Avoid holding your breath while straining to lift a weight. Holding your breath greatly increases the pressure inside the chest and abdominal cavity, making it practically impossible for the blood in the veins to return to the heart. Although rare, a sudden high intrathoracic pressure may lead to dizziness, a blackout, a stroke, a heart attack, or a hernia.

11. Based on the program selected, allow adequate recovery time between sets of exercises (see Table 7.4, page 212).

12. Discontinue training if you experience unusual discomfort or pain. High tension loads used in strength training can exacerbate potential injuries. Discomfort and pain are signals to stop and determine what's wrong. Be sure to properly evaluate your condition before you continue training.

13. Use common sense on days when you feel fatigued or when you are performing sets to complete fatigue. Excessive fatigue affects lifting technique, body balance, muscles involved, and range of motion—all of which increase the risk for injury. A spotter is recommended when sets are performed to complete fatigue. The spotter's help through the most difficult part of the repetition will relieve undue stress on muscles, ligaments, and tendons—and help ensure you perform the exercise correctly.

14. Stretch out for a few minutes at the end of each strength-training workout to help your muscles return to their normal resting length and to minimize muscle soreness and risk for injury.

Setting Up Your Own Strength-Training Program

The same pre-exercise guidelines outlined for cardiorespiratory endurance training apply to strength training (see Clearance for Exercise Participation on page 25). If you have any concerns about your present health status or ability to participate safely in strength training, consult a physician before you start. Strength training is not advised for people with advanced heart disease.

Before you proceed to write your strength-training program, you should determine your stage of change for this fitness component in Lab 7B. Next, if you are prepared to do so, and depending on the facilities available, you can choose one of the training programs outlined in this chapter (use Lab 7B). Once you begin your strength-training program, you may use the form provided in Figure 7.7 (pages 219–220) to keep a record of your training sessions.

The resistance and the number of repetitions you use with your program should be based on whether you want to increase muscular strength or muscular endurance as follows:

■ For strength gains, do up to 12 repetitions maximum, and, for muscular endurance, more than 12. For most people, three training sessions per week on nonconsecutive days is an ideal arrangement for proper development.

■ For both strength and endurance gains, the recommendation is three sets of about 12 repetitions maximum for each exercise. In doing this, you will obtain good strength gains and yet be close to the endurance threshold.

■ If you are training for reasons other than health fitness, review Table 7.4, page 212, for a summary of the guidelines.

Perhaps the only exercise that calls for more than 12 repetitions is the abdominal group of exercises. The abdominal muscles are considered primarily antigravity or postural muscles. Hence, a little more endurance may be required. When doing abdominal work, most people perform about 20 repetitions.

If time is a concern in completing a strength training exercise program, the American College of Sports Medicine[14] recommends as a minimum (a) one set of 8 to 12 repetitions performed to near fatigue, and (b) 8 to 10 exercises involving the major muscle groups of the body, conducted twice a week. The recommendation is based on research showing that this training generates 70 to 80 percent of the improvements reported in other programs using three sets of about 10 RM.

Pilates A training program that uses exercises designed to help strengthen the body's core by developing pelvic stability and abdominal control; exercises are coupled with focused breathing patterns.

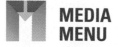

ASSESS YOUR KNOWLEDGE

1. The ability of a muscle to exert submaximal force repeatedly over time is known as:
   a. muscular strength.
   b. plyometric training.
   c. muscular endurance.
   d. isokinetic training.
   e. isometric training.

2. Each additional pound of muscle tissue increases resting metabolism by:
   a. 10 calories.
   b. 17 calories.
   c. 23 calories.
   d. 35 calories.
   e. 50 calories.

3. The Hand Grip Strength Test is an example of
   a. an isometric test.
   b. an isotonic test.
   c. a dynamic test.
   d. an isokinetic test.
   e. a plyometric test.

4. A 70 percentile rank places an individual in the _____ fitness category.
   a. excellent
   b. good
   c. average
   d. fair
   e. poor

5. During an eccentric muscle contraction
   a. the muscle shortens as it overcomes the resistance.
   b. there is little or no movement during the contraction.
   c. a joint has to move through the entire range of motion.
   d. the muscle lengthens as it contracts.
   e. the speed is kept constant throughout the range of motion.

6. The training concept stating that the demands placed on a system must be increased systematically and progressively over time to cause physiological adaptation is referred to as
   a. the overload principle.
   b. positive-resistance training.
   c. specificity of training.
   d. variable-resistance training.
   e. progressive resistance.

7. A set in strength training implies
   a. the starting position for an exercise.
   b. the recovery time required between exercises.
   c. a given number of repetitions.
   d. the starting resistance used in an exercise.
   e. the sequence in which exercises are performed.

8. For health-fitness, a person should perform between
   a. 1 and 6 reps max.
   b. 4 and 10 reps max.
   c. 8 and 12 reps max.
   d. 8 and 20 reps max.
   e. 10 and 30 reps max.

9. Plyometric training is frequently used to help with performance in
   a. gymnastics.
   b. basketball.
   c. volleyball.
   d. sprinting.
   e. all of these sports.

10. The posterior deltoid, rhomboids, and trapezius muscles can be developed with the following exercise:
    a. bench press
    b. lat pull-down
    c. rotary torso
    d. squat
    e. rowing torso

Correct answers can be found at the back of the book.

MEDIA MENU

PROFILE PLUS CD CONNECTIONS

■ Chart your achievements for strength tests.

■ Check how well you understand the chapter's concepts.

INTERNET CONNECTIONS

■ Muscle and Fitness. This comprehensive site features information on intermediate and advanced training techniques, with photographs and informative articles on the use of dietary supplements as well as the importance of mind-body activities to enhance your workout.

   http://www.muscleandfitness.com/training/25

■ Washington State University Department of Athletics Strength and Conditioning. This site features a series of articles dedicated to strength and conditioning exercises, including research topics such as biomechanics, nutrition, body composition, creatine supplementation, plyometrics, and more.

   http://www.wsu.edu/athletics/strength

■ Strength Training Muscle Map & Explanation. This site provides an anatomical map of the body's muscles. Click on the muscle for exercises designed to specifically strengthen that particular muscle, complete with a video and safety information.

   http://www.global-fitness.com/strength/s_muscle map.html

■ Strengthcoach.com. This comprehensive site features articles on a variety of strength-training topics. The virtual weight room features written descriptions of muscles used and proper movements as well as a video demonstration illustrating proper workout techniques that will improve muscle strength of abdominals, back, biceps, chest, and legs, plus information about plyometrics and speed development.

http://www.strengthcoach.com

Notes

1. C. Castaneda, et al., "A Randomized Controlled Trial of Resistance Exercise Training to Improve Glycemic Control in Older Adults with Type 2 Diabetes," *Diabetes Care* 25 (2202): 2335–2341.

2. W. W. Campbell, M. C. Crim, V. R. Young, and W. J. Evans, "Increased Energy Requirements and Changes in Body Composition with Resistance Training in Older Adults," *American Journal of Clinical Nutrition* 60 (1994): 167–175.

3. W. J. Evans, "Exercise, Nutrition and Aging," *Journal of Nutrition* 122 (1992): 796–801.

4. See note 2.

5. P. E. Allsen, *Strength Training: Beginners, Body Builders and Athletes* (Dubuque, IA: Kendall/Hunt, 2003).

6. American College of Sports Medicine. "Progression Models in Resistance Training for Healthy Adults," *Medicine and Science in Sports and Exercise* 34 (2002): 364–380.

7. J. K. Kraemer, and N. A. Ratamess, "Fundamentals of Resistance Training: Progression and Exercise Prescription," *Medicine and Science in Sports and Exercise* 36 (2004): 674–688.

8. S. P. Messier, and M. Dill, "Alterations in Strength and Maximal Oxygen Uptake Consequent to Nautilus Circuit Weight Training," *Research Quarterly for Exercise and Sport* 56 (1985): 345–351.

T. V. Pipes, "Variable Resistance Versus Constant Resistance Strength Training in Adult Males," *European Journal of Applied Physiology* 39 (1978): 27–35.

9. W. W. K. Hoeger, D. R. Hopkins, S. L. Barette, and D. F. Hale, "Relationship Between Repetitions and Selected Percentages of One Repetition Maximum: A Comparison Between Untrained and Trained Males and Females," *Journal of Applied Sport Science Research* 4, no. 2 (1990): 47–51.

10. B. M. Hather, P. A. Tesch, P. Buchanan, and G. A. Dudley, "Influence of Eccentric Actions on Skeletal Muscle Adaptations to Resistance Training," *Acta Physiologica Scandinavica* 143 (1991): 177–185.

C. B. Ebbeling and P. M. Clarkson, "Exercise-Induced Muscle Damage and Adaptation," *Sports Medicine* 7 (1989): 207–234.

11. See note 6.

12. See note 6.

13. Gatorade Sports Science Institute, "Core Strength Training," *Sports Science Exchange Roundtable* 13, no. 1 (2002): 1–4.

14. "The Recommended Quantity and Quality of Exercise for Developing and Maintaining Cardiorespiratory and Muscular Fitness and Flexibility in Healthy Adults," *Medicine and Science in Sports and Exercise* 30 (1998): 975–991.

Suggested Readings

American College of Sports Medicine. "Progression Models in Resistance Training for Healthy Adults." *Medicine and Science in Sports and Exercise* 34 (2002): 364–380.

Hesson, J. L. *Weight Training for Life*. Belmont, CA: Wadsworth/Thomson Learning, 2005.

Heyward, V. H. *Advanced Fitness Assessment and Exercise Prescription*. Champaign, IL: Human Kinetic Press, 2002.

Hoeger, W. W. K., and S. A. Hoeger. *Lifetime Physical Fitness and Wellness: A Personalized Program*. Belmont, CA: Wadsworth/Thomson Learning, 2005.

Kraemer, J. K., and N. A. Ratamess. "Fundamentals of Resistance Training: Progression and Exercise Prescription." *Medicine and Science in Sports and Exercise* 36 (2004): 674–688.

Liemohn, W. and G. Pariser. "Core Strength: Implications for Fitness and Low Back Pain." *ACSM's Health and Fitness Journal* 6, no. 5 (2002): 10–16.

Mannie, K. "Barbells Versus Machines: Balancing a Weighty Issue." *Coach and Athletic Director* 67 (1998): 6–7.

Wescott, W. L., and T. R. Baechle. *Strength Training for Seniors*. Champaign, IL: Human Kinetic Press, 1999.

Volek, J. "Influence of Nutrition on Responses to Resistance Training" *Medicine and Science in Sports and Exercise* 36 (2004): 689–696.

FIGURE 7.6 Major muscles of the human body.

THE MUSCULAR SYSTEM

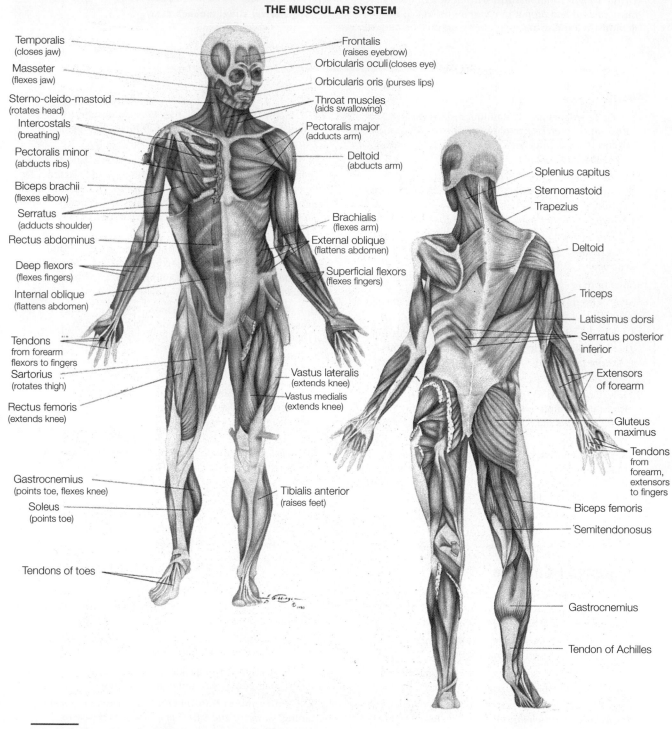

Temporalis
(closes jaw)

Masseter
(flexes jaw)

Sterno-cleido-mastoid
(rotates head)

Intercostals
(breathing)

Pectoralis minor
(abducts ribs)

Biceps brachii
(flexes elbow)

Serratus
(adducts shoulder)

Rectus abdominus

Deep flexors
(flexes fingers)

Internal oblique
(flattens abdomen)

Tendons
from forearm
flexors to fingers

Sartorius
(rotates thigh)

Rectus femoris
(extends knee)

Gastrocnemius
(points toe, flexes knee)

Soleus
(points toe)

Tendons of toes

Frontalis
(raises eyebrow)

Orbicularis oculi (closes eye)

Orbicularis oris (purses lips)

Throat muscles
(aids swallowing)

Pectoralis major
(adducts arm)

Deltoid
(abducts arm)

Brachialis
(flexes arm)

External oblique
(flattens abdomen)

Superficial flexors
(flexes fingers)

Vastus lateralis
(extends knee)

Vastus medialis
(extends knee)

Tibialis anterior
(raises feet)

Splenius capitus

Sternomastoid

Trapezius

Deltoid

Triceps

Latissimus dorsi

Serratus posterior
inferior

Extensors
of forearm

Gluteus
maximus

Tendons
from
forearm,
extensors
to fingers

Biceps femoris

Semitendonosus

Gastrocnemius

Tendon of Achilles

From E. Chaffee and F. Lytle, *Basic Physiology and Anatomy* (Philadelphia: Lippincott Co., 1980).

FIGURE 7.7 Strength training record form.

Name _____

Date											
Exercise	St/Reps/Res*	St/Reps/Res*	St/Reps/Res*	St/Reps/Res*	St/Reps/Res*	St/Reps/Res*	St/Reps/Res*	St/Reps/Res*	St/Reps/Res*	St/Reps/Res*	St/Reps/Res*

*Sets, Repetitions, and Resistance (e.g., 1/6/125 = 1 set of 6 repetitions with 125 pounds)

(continued)

FIGURE 7.7   Strength training record form.

Name

Date										
Exercise	St/Reps/Res*	St/Reps/Res*	St/Reps/Res*	St/Reps/Res*	St/Reps/Res*	St/Reps/Res*	St/Reps/Res*	St/Reps/Res*	St/Reps/Res*	St/Reps/Res*

*Sets, Repetitions, and Resistance (e.g., 1/6/125 = 1 set of 6 repetitions with 125 pounds)

Strength-Training Exercises without Weights

Exercise 1
Step-Up

Action Step up and down using a box or chair approximately 12 to 15 inches high (a). Conduct one set using the same leg each time you go up, and then conduct a second set using the other leg. You also could alternate legs on each step-up cycle. You may increase the resistance by holding an object in your arms (b). Hold the object close to the body to avoid increased strain in the lower back.

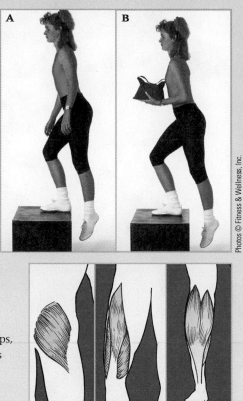

Photos © Fitness & Wellness, Inc.

Muscles Developed
Gluteal muscles, quadriceps, gastrocnemius, and soleus

Back   Front   Back

Exercise 2
Rowing Torso

Action Raise your arms laterally (abduction) to a horizontal position and bend your elbows to 90°. Have a partner apply enough pressure on your elbows to gradually force your arms forward (horizontal flexion) while you try to resist the pressure. Next, reverse the action, horizontally forcing the arms backward as your partner applies sufficient forward pressure to create resistance.

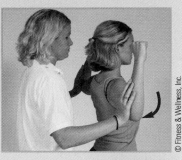

© Fitness & Wellness, Inc.

Muscles Developed
Posterior deltoid, rhomboids, and trapezius

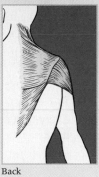

Back

Exercise 3
Push-Up

Action Maintaining your body as straight as possible (a), flex the elbows, lowering the body until you almost touch the floor (b), then raise yourself back up to the starting position. If you are unable to perform the push-up as indicated, decrease the resistance by supporting the lower body with the knees rather than the feet (c) or using an incline plane and supporting your hands at a higher point than the floor (d). If you wish to increase the resistance, have someone else add resistance to your shoulders as you are coming back up (e).

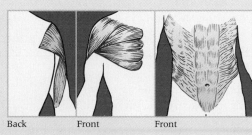

Back   Front   Front

Muscles Developed
Triceps, deltoid, pectoralis major, abdominals, and erector spinae

Back

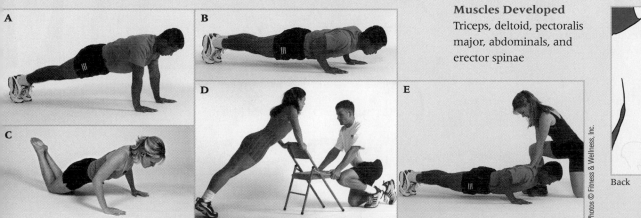

Photos © Fitness & Wellness, Inc.

MUSCULAR STRENGTH AND ENDURANCE   221

Exercise 4
Abdominal Crunch and Bent-Leg Curl-Up

Action Start with your head and shoulders off the floor, arms crossed on your chest, and knees slightly bent (a). The greater the flexion of the knee, the more difficult the curl-up. Now curl up to about 30° (abdominal crunch—illustration b) or curl up all the way (abdominal curl-up— illustration c), then return to the starting position without letting the head or shoulders touch the floor or allowing the hips to come off the floor. If you allow the hips to raise off the floor and the head and shoulders to touch the floor, you most likely will "swing up" on the next crunch or curl-up, which minimizes the work of the abdominal muscles. If you cannot curl up with the arms on the chest, place the hands by the side of the hips or even help yourself up by holding on to your thighs (d and e). Do not perform the sit-up exercise with your legs completely extended, because this will strain the lower back. For additional resistance during the abdominal crunch, have a partner add slight resistance to your shoulders as you "crunch up" (f).

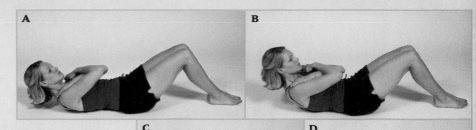

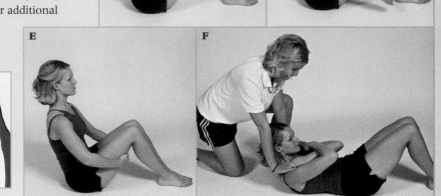

Muscles Developed
Abdominal muscles and hip flexors

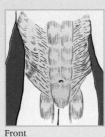

Front

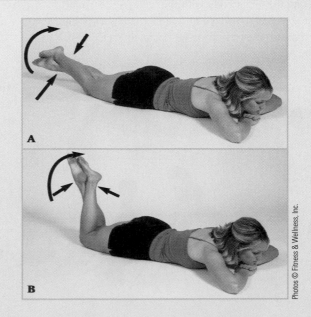

Note: The abdominal curl-up exercise should be used only by individuals of at least average fitness without a history of lower back problems. New participants and those with a history of lower back problems should use the abdominal crunch exercise in its place.

Exercise 5
Leg Curl

Action Lie on the floor face down. Cross the right ankle over the left heel (a). Apply resistance with your right foot while you bring the left foot up to 90° at the knee joint (b). Apply enough resistance so the left foot can only be brought up slowly. Repeat the exercise, crossing the left ankle over the right heel.

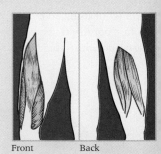

Front   Back

Muscles Developed
Hamstrings (and quadriceps)

Photos © Fitness & Wellness, Inc.

Exercise 6
Modified Dip

Action After making sure that the chairs are well stabilized, place your hands on two facing chairs and your feet on the third chair with knees slightly bent (a). Dip down at least to a 90° angle at the elbow joint (b), then return to the initial position. To increase the resistance, have someone hold you down by the shoulders as you press up (c). You may also perform this exercise using a gymnasium bleacher or box and with the help of a partner (d).

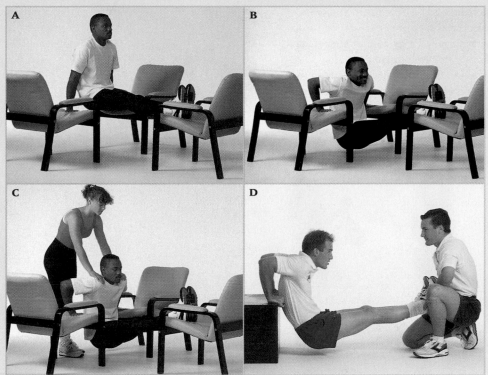

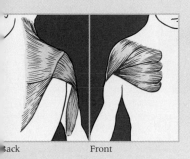

Back   Front

Muscles Developed Triceps, deltoid, and pectoralis major

Exercise 7
Pull-Up

Action Suspend yourself from a bar with a pronated (thumbs-in) grip (a). Pull your body up until your chin is above the bar (b), then lower yourself slowly to the starting position. If you are unable to perform the pull-up as described, either have a partner hold your feet to help you push off and facilitate the movement upward (c and d) or use a lower bar and support your feet on the floor (e).

Muscles Developed
Biceps, brachioradialis, brachialis, trapezius, and latissimus dorsi

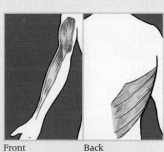

Front   Back

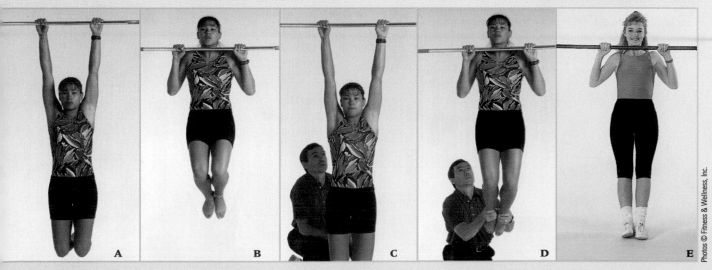

Exercise 8
Arm Curl

Action   Using a palms-up grip, start with the arm completely extended and, with the aid of a sandbag or bucket filled (as needed) with sand or rocks (a), curl up as far as possible (b), then return to the initial position. Repeat the exercise with the other arm.

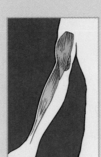

Front

Muscles Developed
Biceps, brachioradialis, and brachialis

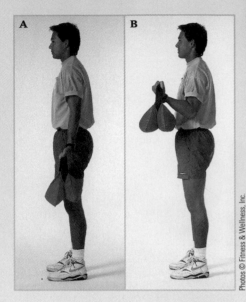

Photos © Fitness & Wellness, Inc.

Exercise 9
Heel Raise

Action   From a standing position with feet flat on the floor (a), raise and lower your body weight by moving at the ankle joint only (b). For added resistance, have someone else hold your shoulders down as you perform the exercise.

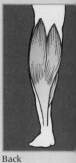

Back

Muscles Developed
Gastrocnemiu and soleus

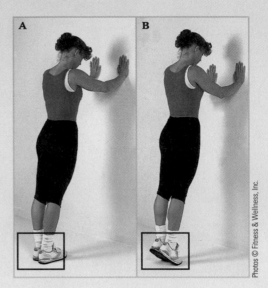

Photos © Fitness & Wellness, Inc.

Exercise 10
Leg Abduction and Adduction

Action   Both participants sit on the floor. The person on the left places the feet on the inside of the other person's feet. Simultaneously, the person on the left presses the legs laterally (to the outside —abduction), while the person on the right presses the legs medially (adduction). Hold the contraction for 5 to 10 seconds. Repeat the exercise at all three angles, and then reverse the pressing sequence: The person on the left places the feet on the outside and presses inward, while the person on the right presses outward.

Muscles Developed   Hip abductors (rectus femoris, sartori, gluteus medius and minimus) and adductors (pectineus, gracilis, adductor magnus, adductor longus, and adductor brevis)

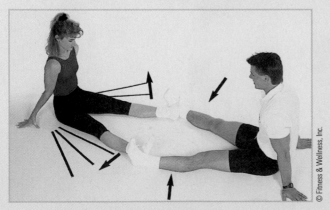

© Fitness & Wellness, Inc.

Exercise 11
Reverse Crunch

Action   Lie on your back with arms to the sides and knees and hips flexed at about 90° (a). Now attempt to raise the pelvis off the floor by lifting vertically from the knees and lower legs (b). This is a challenging exercise that may be difficult for beginners to perform.

Muscles Developed
Abdominals

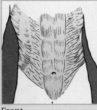

Front

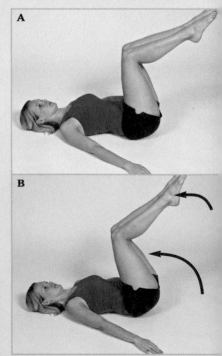

Exercise 12
Pelvic Tilt

Action Lie flat on the floor with the knees bent at about a 90° angle (a). Tilt the pelvis by tightening the abdominal muscles, flattening your back against the floor, and raising the lower gluteal area ever so slightly off the floor (b). Hold the final position for several seconds. The exercise can also be performed against a wall (c).

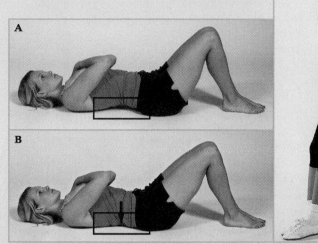

A

B

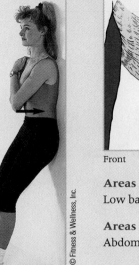

C

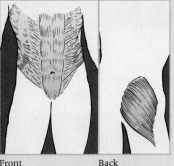

Front   Back

Areas Stretched
Low back muscles and ligaments

Areas Strengthened
Abdominal and gluteal muscles

Photos © Fitness & Wellness, Inc.

Exercise 13
Lateral Bridge

Action Lie on your side with legs bent (a: easier version) or straight (b: harder version) and support the upper body with your arm. Straighten out your body by raising the hip off the floor and hold the position for several seconds. Repeat the exercise with the other side of the body.

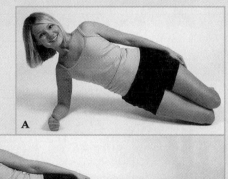

A

B

Photos © Fitness & Wellness, Inc.

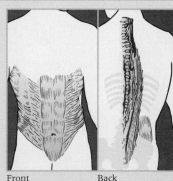

Muscles Developed
Abdominals (obliques and transversus abdominus) and quadratus lumborum (lower back)

Front   Back

Exercise 14
Prone Bridge

Action Starting in a prone position on a floor mat, balance yourself on the tips of your toes and elbows while attempting to maintain a straight body from head to toes (do not arch the lower back). You can increase the difficulty of this exercise by placing your hands in front of you and straightening out the arms (elbows off the floor).

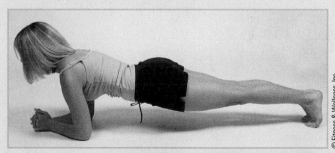

© Fitness & Wellness, Inc.

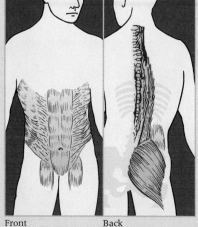

Muscles Developed
Anterior and posterior muscle groups of the trunk and pelvis

Front   Back

Strength-Training Exercises with Weights

Exercise 15
Bench Press

Machine   Lie down on the bench with the head by the weight stack, the bench press bar above the chest, and the knees bent so the feet rest on the far end of the bench (a). Grasp the bar handles and press upward until the arms are completely extended (b), then return to the original position. Do not arch the back during this exercise.

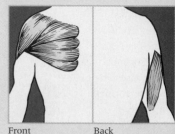

Muscles Developed
Pectoralis major, triceps, and deltoid

Front   Back

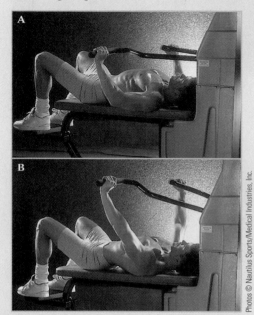

Photos © Nautilus Sports/Medical Industries, Inc.

Free Weights
Lie on the bench with arms extended and have one or two spotters help you place the barbell directly over your shoulders (a). Lower the weight to your chest (b) and then push it back up until you achieve full extension of the arms. Do not arch the back during this exercise.

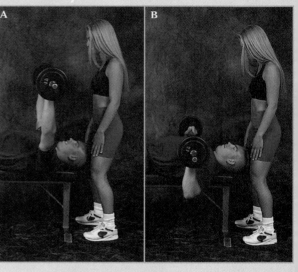

Exercise 16
Leg Press

Action   From a sitting position with the knees flexed at about 90° and both feet on the footrest (a), extend the legs fully (b), then return slowly to the starting position.

Muscles Developed
Quadriceps and gluteal muscles

Front   Back

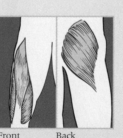

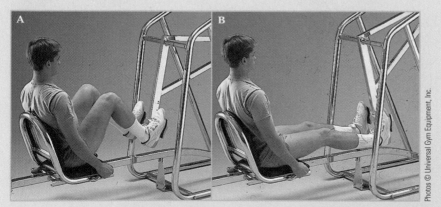

Photos © Universal Gym Equipment, Inc.

Exercise 17
Abdominal Crunch

Action   Sit in an upright position. Grasp the handles over your shoulders and crunch forward. Return slowly to the original position.

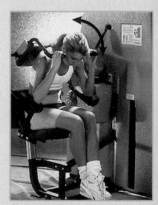

Muscles Developed
Abdominals

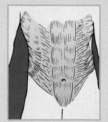

Front

Exercise 18
Rowing Torso

Action   Sit in the machine with your arms in front of you, elbows bent and resting against the padded bars (a). Press back as far as possible, drawing the shoulder blades together (b). Return to the original position.

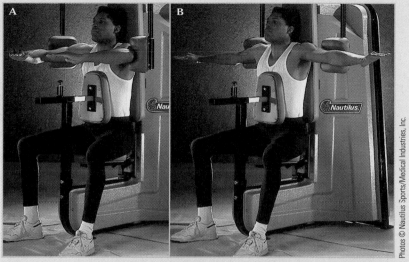

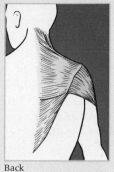

Back

Muscles Developed
Posterior deltoid, rhomboids, and trapezius

Photos © Nautilus Sports/Medical Industries, Inc.

Bent-Over Lateral Raise

Action   Bend over with your back straight and knees bent at about 5 to 10° (a). Hold one dumbbell in each hand. Raise the dumbbells laterally to about shoulder level (b) and then slowly return them to the starting position.

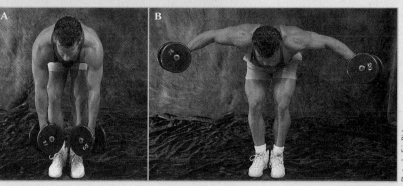

Photos by Eric Risberg

Exercise 19
Arm Curl

Machine   Using a supinated (palms-up) grip, start with the arms almost completely extended (a). Curl up as far as possible (b), then return to the starting position.

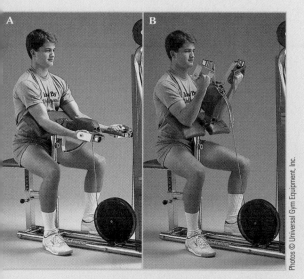

Photos © Universal Gym Equipment, Inc.

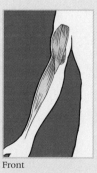

Front

Muscles Developed
Biceps, brachioradialis, and brachialis

Free Weights   Standing upright, hold a barbell in front of you at about shoulder width with arms extended and the hands in a thumbs-out position (supinated grip) (a). Raise the barbell to your shoulders (b) and slowly return it to the starting position.

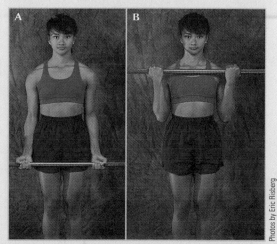

Photos by Eric Risberg

Exercise 20
Leg Curl

Action Lie with the face down on the bench, legs straight, and place the back of the feet under the padded bar (a). Curl up to at least 90° (b), and return to the original position.

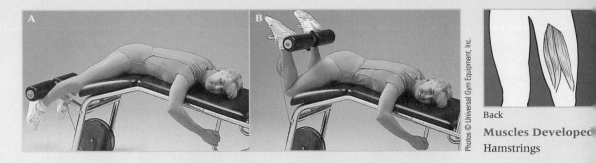

Photos © Universal Gym Equipment, Inc.

Back

Muscles Developed
Hamstrings

Exercise 21
Seated Back

Action Sit in the machine with your trunk flexed and the upper back against the shoulder pad. Place the feet under the padded bar and hold on with your hands to the bars on the sides (a). Start the exercise by pressing backward, simultaneously extending the trunk and hip joints (b). Slowly return to the original position.

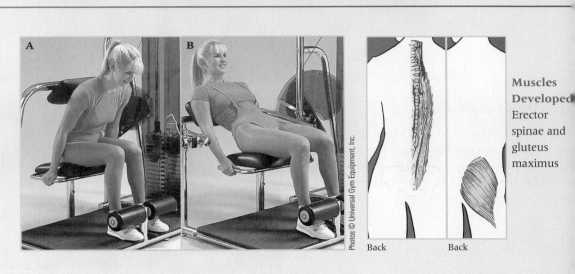

Photos © Universal Gym Equipment, Inc.

Back   Back

Muscles Developed
Erector spinae and gluteus maximus

Exercise 22
Heel Raise

Machine Start with your feet either flat on the floor or the front of the feet on an elevated block (a), then raise and lower yourself by moving at the ankle joint only (b). If additional resistance is needed, you can use a squat strength-training machine.

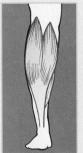

Back

Muscles Developed
Gastrocnemius, soleus

Free Weights In a standing position, place a barbell across the shoulders and upper back. Grip the bar away from the shoulders as far out as needed (a). Place the ball of your feet over a weight plate or a small board so that your heels are lower than the front of your feet. Raise your heels off the floor as far as possible (b) and then slowly return them to the starting position.

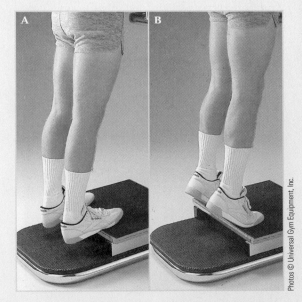

Photos © Universal Gym Equipment, Inc.

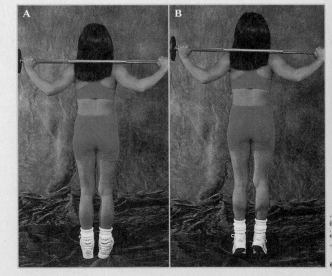

Exercise 23
Lat Pull-Down

Action   Starting from a sitting position, hold the exercise bar with a wide grip (a). Pull the bar down in front of you until it reaches the base of the neck (b), then return to the starting position.

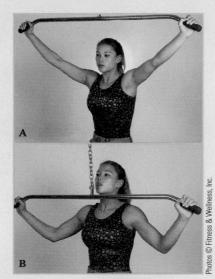

A

B

Photos © Fitness & Wellness, Inc.

Muscles Developed Latissimus dorsi, pectoralis major, and biceps

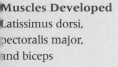

Back   Front

Exercise 24
Rotary Torso

Machine   Sit upright in the machine and place the elbows behind the padded bars. Rotate the torso as far as possible to one side and then return slowly to the starting position. Repeat the exercise to the opposite side.

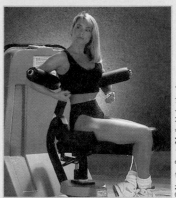

© Nautilus Sports/Medical Industries, Inc.

Free Weights Stand with your feet slightly apart. Place a barbell across your shoulders and upper back, holding on to the sides of the barbell. Now gently, and in a controlled manner, twist your torso to one side as far as possible and then do so in the opposite direction.

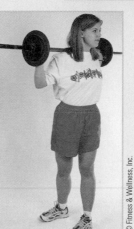

© Fitness & Wellness, Inc.

Front

Muscles Developed Internal and external obliques (abdominal muscles)

Exercise 25
Triceps Extension

Machine   Sit in an upright position, arms up, elbows bent, and place the little finger side of the hands and wrists against the pads, palms of the hands facing each other (a). Fully extend one arm at a time (b), and then return to the original position. Repeat with the other arm.

Muscles Developed Triceps

Back

Free Weights   In a standing position, hold a barbell with both hands overhead and with the arms in full extension (a). Slowly lower the barbell behind your head (b) and then return it to the starting position.

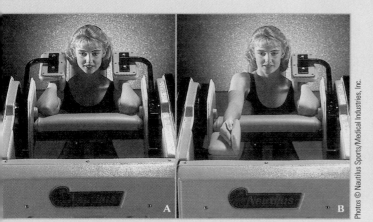

A   B

Photos © Nautilus Sports/Medical Industries, Inc.

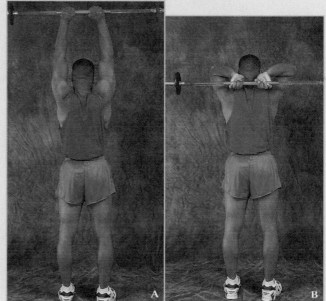

A   B

Photos by Eric Risberg

Exercise 26
Leg Extension

Action　Sit in an upright position with the feet under the padded bar and grasp the handles at the sides (a). Extend the legs until they are completely straight (b), then return to the starting position.

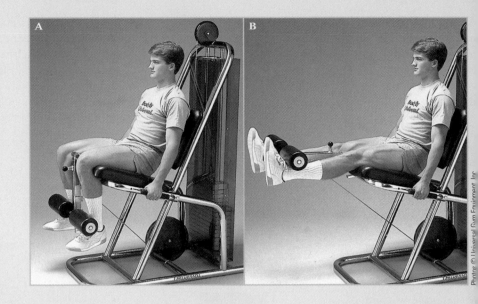

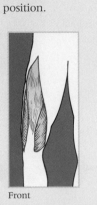

Muscles Developed
Quadriceps

Front

Exercise 27
Shoulder Press

Machine　Sit in an upright position and grasp the bar wider than shoulder width (a). Press the bar all the way up until the arms are fully extended (b), then return to the initial position.

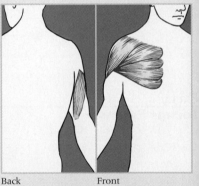

Muscles Developed
Triceps, deltoid, and pectoralis major

Back　　　　Front

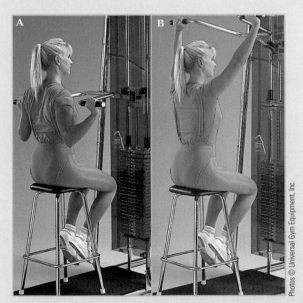

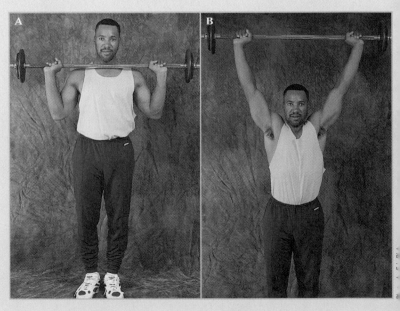

Free Weights　Place a barbell on your shoulders in front of the body (a) and press the weight overhead until complete extension of the arms is achieved (b). Then return the weight to the original position. Be sure not to arch the back or lean back during this exercise.

Exercise 28
Chest Press

Action   Start with the arms up to the side, hands resting against the handle bars and elbows bent at 90° (a). Press the movement arms forward as far as possible, leading with the elbows (b). Slowly return to the starting position.

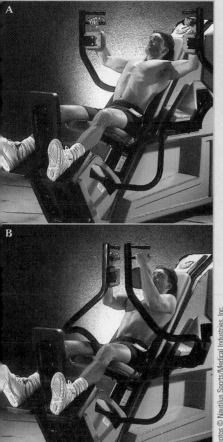

Photos © Nautilus Sports/Medical Industries, Inc.

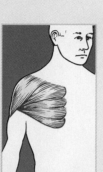

Front

Muscles Developed
Pectoralis major and deltoid

Bent-Arm Flyes

Action   Lie down on your back on a bench and hold a dumbbell in each hand directly overhead (a). Keeping your elbows slightly bent, lower the weights laterally to a horizontal position (b) and then bring them back up to the starting position.

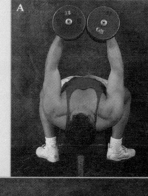

Photos by Eric Risberg

Exercise 29
Squat

Machine   Place the shoulders under the padded bars by bending the knees to about 120° (A). Completely extend the legs (B), then return to the original position.

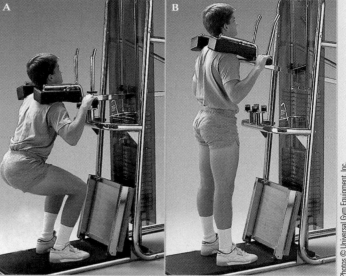

Photos © Universal Gym Equipment, Inc.

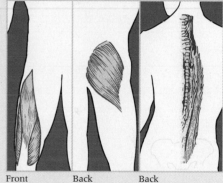

Front   Back   Back

Muscles Developed
Quadriceps, gluteus maximus, erector spinae

Free Weights   From a standing position, and with a spotter to each side, support a barbell over your shoulders and upper back (a). Keeping your head up and back straight, bend at the knees and the hips until you achieve an approximate 120° angle at the knees (b). Then return to the starting position. *Do not perform this exercise alone.* If no spotters are available, use a squat rack to ensure that you will not get trapped under a heavy weight.

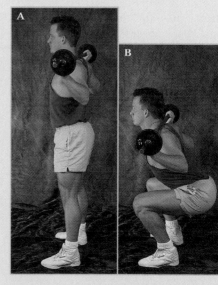

Photos by Eric Risberg

Exercise 30
Upright Rowing

Machine   Start with the arms extended and grip the handles with the palms down (a). Pull all the way up to the chin (b), then return to the starting position.

Free Weights   Hold a barbell in front of you, with the arms fully extended and hands in a thumbs-in (pronated) grip less than shoulder-width apart (a). Pull the barbell up until it reaches shoulder level (b) and then slowly return it to the starting position.

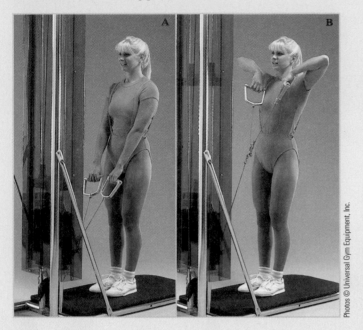

Photos © Universal Gym Equipment, Inc.

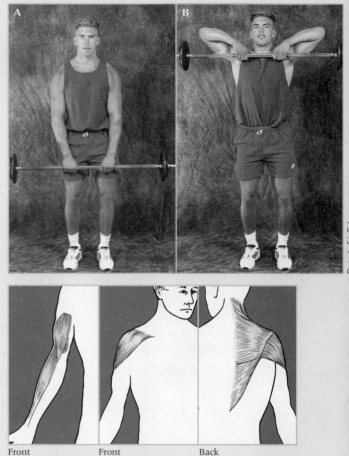

Muscles Developed
Biceps, brachioradialis, brachialis, deltoid, and trapezius

Front   Front   Back

Exercise 31
Seated Leg Curl

Action   Sit in the unit and place the strap over the upper thighs. With legs extended, place the back of the feet over the padded rollers (a). Flex the knees until you reach a 90° to 100° angle (b). Slowly return to the starting position.

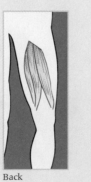

Muscles Developed
Hamstrings

Back

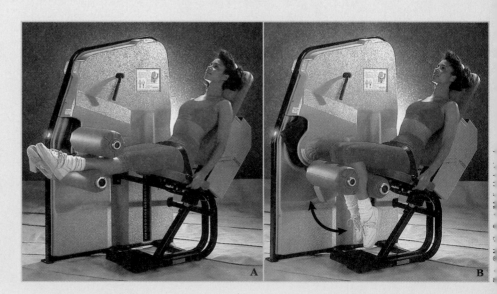

Exercise 32
Bent-Arm Pullover

Machine   Sit back into the chair and grasp the bar behind your head (a). Pull the bar over your head all the way down to your abdomen (b) and slowly return to the original position.

Free Weights   Lie on your back on an exercise bench with the head over the edge of the bench. Hold a barbell over your chest with the hands less than shoulder-width apart (a). Keeping the elbows shoulder-width apart, lower the weight over your head until your shoulders are completely extended (b). Slowly return the weight to the starting position.

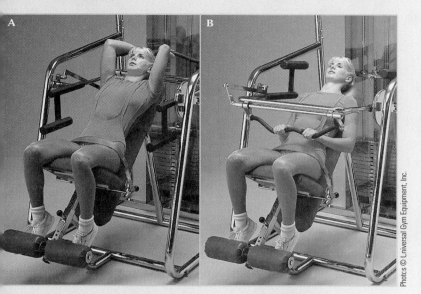

A   B

Photos © Universal Gym Equipment, Inc.

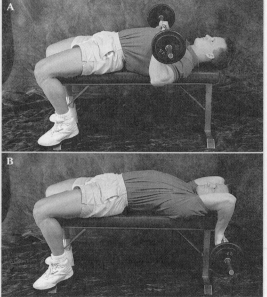

A

B

Photos by Eric Risberg

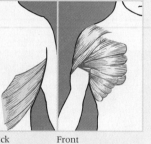

Muscles Developed
Latissimus dorsi, pectoral muscles, deltoid, and serratus anterior

Back   Front

Exercise 33
Triceps Extension

Action   Using a palms-down grip, grasp the bar slightly closer than shoulder-width and start with the elbows almost completely bent (a). Extend the arms fully (b), then return to starting position.

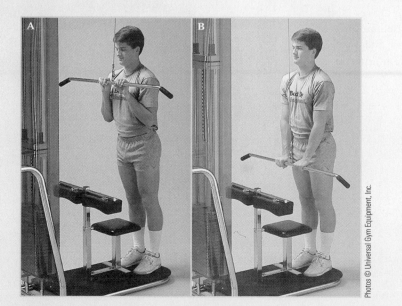

A   B

Photos © Universal Gym Equipment, Inc.

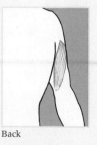

Back

Muscles Developed
Triceps

Exercise 34
Dip

Action   Start with the elbows flexed (a), then extend the arms fully (b), and return slowly to the initial position.

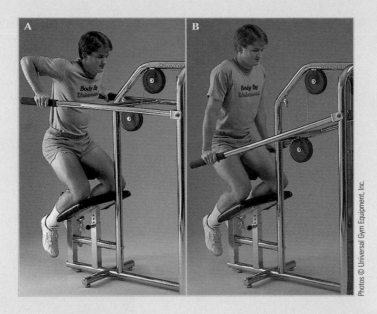

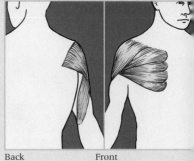

Back   Front

Muscles Developed
Triceps, deltoid, and pectoralis major

Photos © Universal Gym Equipment, Inc.

Exercise 35
Back Extension

Action   Place your feet under the ankle rollers and the hips over the padded seat. Start with the trunk in a flexed position and the arms crossed over the chest (a). Slowly extend the trunk to a horizontal position (b), hold the extension for 2 to 5 seconds, then slowly flex (lower) the trunk to the original position.

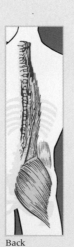

Muscles Developed
Erector spinae, gluteus maximus, and quadratus lumborum (lower back)

Back

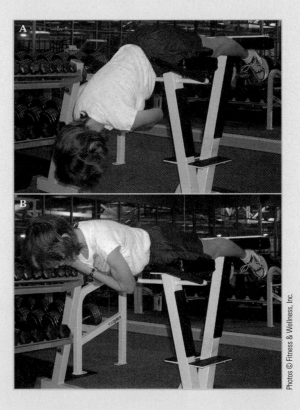

Photos © Fitness & Wellness, Inc.

Lab 7A

MUSCULAR STRENGTH AND ENDURANCE ASSESSMENT

Name: _____   Date: _____   Grade: _____

Instructor: _____   Course: _____   Section: _____

Necessary Lab Equipment

A Lafayette hand grip dynamometer model 78010 is recommended for the Hand Grip Test. A metronome, gymnasium bleachers, and a stopwatch are needed for the Muscular Endurance Test. A metronome is also needed for the Muscular Strength and Endurance Test.

Objective

To determine muscular strength and/or endurance and the respective fitness classification.

Lab Preparation

Wear exercise clothing and avoid strenuous strength training 48 hours prior to this lab.

I. Hand Grip Strength Test

The instructions for the Hand Grip Strength Test are provided in Figure 7.2, page 202. Perform the test according to the instructions and look up your results in Table 7.1, page 202.

Hand used: ☐ Right   ☐ Left

Reading: _____ lbs.

Fitness category (see Figure 7.2, page 202): _____

II. Muscular Endurance Test

Conduct this test using the guidelines provided in Figure 7.3 and Table 7.2, pages 203–204. Record your repetitions, fitness category, and points in the spaces provided below.

Exercise	Metronome Cadence	Repetitions	Fitness Category	Points
Bench jumps	none			
Modified dips — men only	56 bpm			
Modified push-ups — women only	56 bpm			
Bent-leg curl-ups	40 bpm			
Abdominal crunches	60 bpm			

Total Points: _____

Overall muscular endurance fitness category (see Figure 7.3, page 203–204): _____

III. Muscular Strength and Endurance Test

Perform the Muscular Strength and Endurance Test according to the procedure outlined in Figure 7.4, page 205. Record the results, fitness category, and points in the appropriate blanks provided below.

Body weight: _____ lbs.

Lift	Percent of Body Weight (pounds) Men	Women	Resistance	Repetitions
Lat pull-down	.70	.45		
Leg extension	.65	.50		
Bench press	.75	.45		
Bent-leg curl-up or abdominal crunch	NA*	NA*		
Leg curl	.32	.25		
Arm curl	.35	.18		

*Not applicable—no resistance required. Use test described in Figure 7.3, pages 203–204.

IV. Muscular Strength and Endurance Goals

Indicate the muscular strength/endurance category that you would like to achieve by the end of the term: _____

Briefly state your feelings about your current strength level and indicate how you are planning to achieve your strength objective:

_____

_____

_____

_____

_____

_____

_____

_____

_____

_____

_____

_____

_____

_____

Lab 7B

STRENGTH-TRAINING PROGRAM

Name: _____

Date: _____

Grade: _____

Instructor: _____

Course: _____

Section: _____

Necessary Lab Equipment

Free weights, strength-training machines, or no equipment if the "Strength-Training Exercises without Weights" program is selected.

Objective

To develop your personal strength-training exercise program.

Lab Preparation

Wear exercise clothing and prepare to participate in a sample strength-training exercise session. All of the strength-training exercises are illustrated on pages 221–234.

I. Stage of Change for Muscular Strength or Endurance

Using Figure 2.4 (page 41) and Table 2.3 (page 41), identify your current stage of change for participation in a muscular strength or muscular endurance program:

_____

II. Instructions

Select one of the two strength-training exercise programs. Perform all of the recommended exercises and, with the exception of the abdominal curl-up exercises, determine the resistance required to do approximately 10 repetitions maximum. For "Strength-Training Exercises without Weights," simply indicate the total number of repetitions performed. For the abdominal crunches or curl-up exercises, perform or build up to about 20 repetitions.

1. **Strength-Training Exercises without Weights**

Exercise	Repetitions
Step-up	
Rowing torso	
Push-up	
Abdominal curl-up or abdominal crunch	
Leg curl	
Modified dip	
Pull-up or arm curl	
Heel raise	
Leg abduction and adduction	
Reverse crunch	
Pelvic tilt	
Lateral bridge	
Prone bridge	

2. Strength-Training Exercises with Weights

Exercise	Repetitions	Resistance
Bench press, shoulder press, or chest press (select and circle one)		
Leg press or squat (select one)		
Abdominal curl-up or abdominal crunch (select one)		N/A
Rowing torso		
Arm curl or upright rowing (select one)		
Leg curl or seated leg curl (select one)		
Seated back		
Heel raise		
Lat pull-down or bent-arm pullover (select one)		
Rotary torso		
Triceps extension or dip (select one)		
Leg extension		
Back extension		

III. Your Personalized Strength-Training Program

Once you have performed activity 1 or 2 above (or both), and depending on your personal preference (strength versus endurance), design your strength-training program selecting a minimum of eight exercises. Indicate the number of sets, repetitions, and approximate resistance that you will use. Also state the days of the week, time, and facility that will be used for this program.

Strength-training days: M ☐ T ☐ W ☐ Th ☐ F ☐ Sa ☐ Su ☐   Time of day: _____   Facility: _____

Exercise	Sets / Reps / Resistance		Exercise	Sets / Reps / Resistance
1.		9.		
2.		10.		
3.		11.		
4.		12.		
5.		13.		
6.		14.		
7.		15.		
8.		16.		

Muscular Flexibility

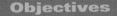

Objectives

- ◼ Explain the importance of muscular flexibility to adequate fitness and preventive health care.
- ◼ Identify the factors that affect muscular flexibility.
- ◼ Explain the health-fitness benefits of stretching.
- ◼ Become familiar with a battery of tests to assess overall body flexibility (Modified Sit-and-Reach Test, Total Body Rotation Test, Shoulder Rotation Test).
- ◼ Be able to interpret flexibility test results according to health-fitness and physical-fitness standards.
- ◼ Learn the principles that govern muscular flexibility development.
- ◼ List some exercises that may cause injury.
- ◼ Become familiar with a program for preventing and rehabilitating low-back pain.

Profile Plus CD Connections

- ◼ Create your personal flexibility profile.
- ◼ Check how well you understand the chapter's concepts.

Most fitness participants underestimate and overlook the contribution of good muscular flexibility to overall fitness and preventive health care. **Flexibility** refers to the achievable range of motion at a joint or group of joints without causing injury. Most people who exercise don't take the time to stretch, and many of those who do stretch don't stretch properly. When joints are not regularly moved through their normal range of motion, muscles and ligaments shorten in time, and flexibility decreases.

Some muscular/skeletal problems and injuries are related to a lack of flexibility. In daily life, we often have to make rapid or strenuous movements we are not accustomed to making. Abruptly forcing a tight muscle beyond its achievable range of motion may lead to injury.

A decline in flexibility can cause poor posture and subsequent aches and pains that lead to limited and painful joint movement. Inordinate tightness is uncomfortable and debilitating. Approximately 80 percent of all low-back problems in the United States stem from improper alignment of the vertebral column and pelvic girdle, a direct result of inflexible and weak muscles. This backache syndrome costs U.S. industry billions of dollars each year in lost productivity, health services, and worker compensation.

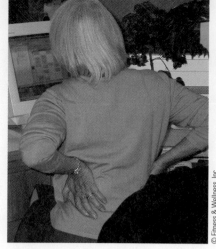

Excessive sitting and lack of physical activity lead to chronic back pain.

© Fitness & Wellness, Inc.

Benefits of Good Flexibility

Improving and maintaining good range of motion in the joints enhances the quality of life. Good flexibility promotes healthy muscles and joints. Improving elasticity of muscles and connective tissue around joints enables greater freedom of movement and the individual's ability to participate in many types of sports and recreational activities. Adequate flexibility also makes activities of daily living such as turning, lifting, and bending much easier to perform. A person must take care, however, not to overstretch joints. Too much flexibility leads to unstable and loose joints, which may increase injury rate, including joint dislocation and **subluxation**.

Taking part in a regular **stretching** program increases circulation to the muscle(s) being stretched, prevents low-back and other spinal column problems, improves and maintains good postural alignment, promotes proper and graceful body movement, improves personal appearance and self-image, and helps to develop and maintain motor skills throughout life.

Flexibility exercises have been prescribed successfully to treat **dysmenorrhea**[1] (painful menstruation), general neuromuscular tension (stress), and knots (trigger points) in muscles and fascia. Regular stretching helps decrease the aches and pains caused by psychological stress and contributes to a decrease in anxiety, blood pressure, and breathing rate.[2] Stretching also helps relieve muscle cramps encountered at rest or during participation in exercise.

Mild stretching exercises, in conjunction with calisthenics, are helpful in warm-up routines to prepare for more vigorous aerobic or strength-training exercises, and in cool-down routines following exercise to facilitate the return to a normal resting state. Fatigued muscles tend to contract to a shorter-than-average resting length, and stretching exercises help fatigued muscles reestablish their normal resting length.

Flexibility in Older Adults

Similar to muscular strength, good range of motion is critical in older life (see discussion in Chapter 9). Because of decreased flexibility, older adults lose mobility and may be unable to perform simple daily tasks such as bending forward or turning. Many older adults cannot turn their head or rotate their trunk to look over their shoulder but, rather, must step around 90° to 180° to see behind them. Adequate flexibility is also important for driving. Individuals who lose range of motion with age are unable to look over their shoulder to switch lanes or to parallel-park, increasing the risk for automobile accidents.

Physical activity and exercise can be hampered severely by lack of good range of motion. Because of the pain during activity, older people who have tight hip flexors (muscles) cannot jog or walk very far. A vicious circle ensues, because the condition usually worsens with further inactivity. Lack of flexibility also may be a cause of falls and subsequent injury in older adults. A simple stretching program can alleviate or prevent this problem and help people return to an exercise program.

Factors Affecting Flexibility

Total range of motion around a joint is highly specific and varies from one joint to another (hip, trunk, shoulder), as well as from one individual to the next. Muscular flexibility relates primarily to genetic factors and to physical activity. Joint structure (shape of the bones), joint cartilage, ligaments, tendons, muscles, skin, tissue injury, and adipose tissue (fat)—all influence range of motion about a joint. Body temperature, age, and gender also affect flexibility.

The range of motion about a given joint depends mostly on the structure of that joint. Greater range of motion, however, can be attained through plastic and elastic elongation. **Plastic elongation** is the permanent lengthening of soft tissue. Even though joint capsules, ligaments, and tendons are basically nonelastic, they can undergo plastic elongation. This permanent lengthening, accompanied by increased range of motion, is best attained through slow-sustained stretching exercises.

Elastic elongation is the temporary lengthening of soft tissue. Muscle tissue has elastic properties and responds to stretching exercises by undergoing elastic or temporary lengthening. Elastic elongation increases extensibility, or ability to stretch the muscles.

Changes in muscle temperature can increase or decrease flexibility by as much as 20 percent. Individuals who warm up properly have better flexibility than people who do not. Cool temperatures have the opposite effect, impeding range of motion. Because of the effects of temperature on muscular flexibility, many people prefer to do their stretching exercises after the aerobic phase of their workout. Aerobic activities raise body temperature, facilitating plastic elongation.

Another factor that influences flexibility is the amount of adipose (fat) tissue in and around joints and muscle tissue. Excess adipose tissue will increase resistance to movement, and the added bulk also hampers joint mobility because of the contact between body surfaces.

On the average, women have better flexibility than men do, and they seem to retain this advantage throughout life. Aging does decrease the extensibility of soft tissue, though, resulting in less flexibility in both sexes.

The most significant contributor to lower flexibility is sedentary living. With less physical activity, muscles lose their elasticity, and tendons and ligaments tighten and shorten. Inactivity also tends to be accompanied by an increase in adipose tissue, which further decreases the range of motion around a joint. Finally, injury to muscle tissue and tight skin from excessive scar tissue have negative effects on range of motion.

Assessment of Flexibility

Many flexibility tests developed over the years were specific to certain sports or not practical for the general population. Their application in health and fitness programs was limited. For example, the Front-to-Rear Splits Test and the Bridge-Up Test had applications in

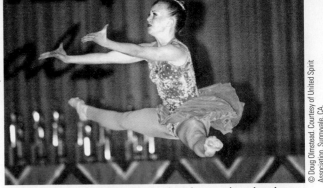

Adequate flexibility helps to develop and maintain sports skill throughout life.

© Doug Olmstead. Courtesy of United Spirit Association, Sunnyvale, CA.

sports such as gymnastics and several track-and-field events, but they did not represent actions that most people encounter in daily life.

Profile Plus
How flexible are you? Create your personal flexibility profile on your CD-ROM.

Because of the lack of practical flexibility tests, most health and fitness centers rely strictly on the Sit-and-Reach Test as an indicator of overall flexibility. This test measures flexibility of the hamstring muscles (back of the thigh) and, to a lesser extent, the lower back muscles.

Flexibility is joint-specific. This means that a lot of flexibility in one joint does not necessarily indicate that other joints are just as flexible. Therefore, the Total Body Rotation Test and the Shoulder Rotation Test—indicators of ability to perform everyday movements such as reaching, bending, and turning—are included to determine your flexibility profile.

The Sit-and-Reach Test has been modified from the traditional test to take length of arms and legs into consideration in determining the score (see Figure 8.1). In the original Sit-and-Reach Test, the 15-inch mark of the yardstick used to measure flexibility was always set at the edge of the box where the feet are placed. This does not take into consideration an individual with long arms and/or short legs or one with short arms and/or long legs.[3] All other factors being equal, an individual with longer arms or shorter legs, or both, receives a better rating because of the structural advantage.

The procedures and norms for the flexibility tests are described in Figures 8.1 through 8.3 and Tables 8.1 through 8.3. The flexibility test results in

Flexibility Refers to the achievable range of motion at a joint or group of joints without causing injury.

Subluxation Partial dislocation of a joint.

Stretching Moving the joints beyond the accustomed range of motion.

Dysmenorrhea Painful menstruation.

Plastic elongation Permanent lengthening of soft tissue.

Elastic elongation Temporary lengthening of soft tissue.

FIGURE 8.1 Procedure for the Modified Sit-and-Reach Test.

To perform this test, you will need the Acuflex I* Sit-and-Reach Flexibility Tester, or you may simply place a yardstick on top of a box approximately 12" high.

1. Warm up properly before the first trial.
2. Remove your shoes for the test. Sit on the floor with the hips, back, and head against a wall, the legs fully extended, and the bottom of the feet against the Acuflex I or sit-and-reach box.
3. Place the hands one on top of the other and reach forward as far as possible without letting the head and back come off the wall (the shoulders may be rounded as much as possible, but neither the head nor the back should come off the wall at this time). The technician then can slide the reach indicator on the Acuflex I (or yardstick) along the top of the box until the end of the indicator touches the participant's fingers. The indicator

then must be held firmly in place throughout the rest of the test.

4. Now your head and back can come off the wall. Gradually reach forward three times, the third time stretching forward as far as possible on the indicator (or yardstick) and holding the final position for at least 2 seconds. Be sure that during the test you keep the backs of the knees flat against the floor.
5. Record the final number of inches reached to the nearest 1/2".

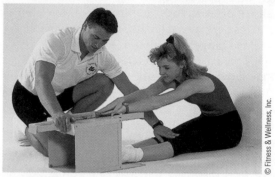

Modified Sit-and-Reach Test.

You are allowed two trials, and an average of the two scores is used as the final test score. The respective percentile ranks and fitness categories for this test are given in Tables 8.1 and 8.4.

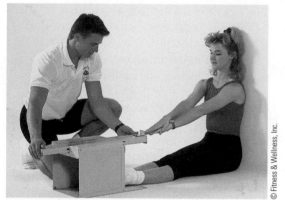

Determining the starting position for the Modified Sit-and-Reach Test.

* The Acuflex I Flexibility Tester for the Modified Sit-and-Reach Test can be obtained from Figure Finder Collection, Novel Products, P. O. Box 408, Rockton, IL 61072-0480. Phone: 800-323-5143, Fax 815-624-4866.

TABLE 8.1 Percentile Ranks for the Modified Sit-and-Reach Test

Age Category—Men

Percentile Rank	≤18 in.	≤18 cm	19–35 in.	19–35 cm	36–49 in.	36–49 cm	≥50 in.	≥50 cm
99	20.8	52.8	20.1	51.1	18.9	48.0	16.2	41.1
95	19.6	49.8	18.9	48.0	18.2	46.2	15.8	40.1
90	18.2	46.2	17.2	43.7	16.1	40.9	15.0	38.1
80	17.8	45.2	17.0	43.2	14.6	37.1	13.3	33.8
70	16.0	40.6	15.8	40.1	13.9	35.3	12.3	31.2
60	15.2	38.6	15.0	38.1	13.4	34.0	11.5	29.2
50	14.5	36.8	14.4	36.6	12.6	32.0	10.2	25.9
40	14.0	35.6	13.5	34.3	11.6	29.5	9.7	24.6
30	13.4	34.0	13.0	33.0	10.8	27.4	9.3	23.6
20	11.8	30.0	11.6	29.5	9.9	25.1	8.8	22.4
10	9.5	24.1	9.2	23.4	8.3	21.1	7.8	19.8
05	8.4	21.3	7.9	20.1	7.0	17.8	7.2	18.3
01	7.2	18.3	7.0	17.8	5.1	13.0	4.0	10.2

Age Category—Women

Percentile Rank	≤18 in.	≤18 cm	19–35 in.	19–35 cm	36–49 in.	36–49 cm	≥50 in.	≥50 cm
99	22.6	57.4	21.0	53.3	19.8	50.3	17.2	43.7
95	19.5	49.5	19.3	49.0	19.2	48.8	15.7	39.9
90	18.7	47.5	17.9	45.5	17.4	44.2	15.0	38.1
80	17.8	45.2	16.7	42.4	16.2	41.1	14.2	36.1
70	16.5	41.9	16.2	41.1	15.2	38.6	13.6	34.5
60	16.0	40.6	15.8	40.1	14.5	36.8	12.3	31.2
50	15.2	38.6	14.8	37.6	13.5	34.3	11.1	28.2
40	14.5	36.8	14.5	36.8	12.8	32.5	10.1	25.7
30	13.7	34.8	13.7	34.8	12.2	31.0	9.2	23.4
20	12.6	32.0	12.6	32.0	11.0	27.9	8.3	21.1
10	11.4	29.0	10.1	25.7	9.7	24.6	7.5	19.0
05	9.4	23.9	8.1	20.6	8.5	21.6	3.7	9.4
01	6.5	16.5	2.6	6.6	2.0	5.1	1.5	3.8

High physical fitness standard   Health fitness standard

FIGURE 8.2 Procedure for the Total Body Rotation Test.

An Acuflex II* Total Body Rotation Flexibility Tester or a measuring scale with a sliding panel is needed to administer this test. The Acuflex II or scale is placed on the wall at shoulder height and should be adjustable to accommodate individual differences in height. If you need to build your own scale, use two measuring tapes and glue them above and below the sliding panel centered at the 15" mark. Each tape should be at least 30" long. If no sliding panel is available, simply tape the measuring tapes onto a wall oriented in opposite directions as shown below. A line also must be drawn on the floor and centered with the 15" mark.

1. Warm up properly before beginning this test.
2. Stand with one side toward the wall, an arm's length away from the wall, with the feet straight ahead, slightly separated, and the toes touching the center line drawn on the floor. Hold out the arm away from the wall horizontally from the body, making a fist with the hand. The Acuflex II measuring scale, or tapes should be shoulder height at this time.
3. Rotate the trunk, the extended arm going backward (always maintaining a horizontal plane) and making contact with the panel, gradually sliding it forward as far as possible. If no panel is available, slide the fist alongside the tapes as far as possible. Hold the final position at least 2 seconds. Position the hand with the little finger side forward during the entire sliding movement. **Proper hand position is crucial. Many people attempt to open the hand, or push with extended fingers, or slide the panel with the knuckles—none of which is acceptable.** During the test the knees can be bent slightly, but **the feet cannot be moved or rotated**—they must point forward. The body must be kept as straight (vertical) as possible.

4. Conduct the test on either the right or the left side of the body. Perform two trials on the selected side. Record the farthest point reached, measured to the nearest half inch and held for at least 2 seconds. Use the average of the two trials as the final test score. Refer to Tables 8.2 and 8.4 to determine the percentile rank and flexibility fitness category for this test.

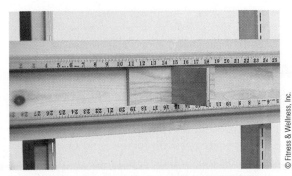

Acuflex II measuring device for the Total Body Rotation Test.

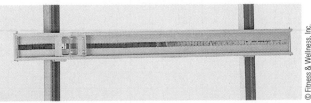

Homemade measuring device for the Total Body Rotation Test.

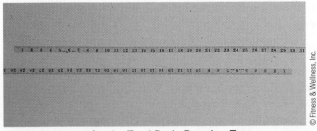

Measuring tapes for the Total Body Rotation Test.

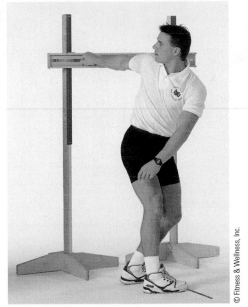

Total Body Rotation Test.

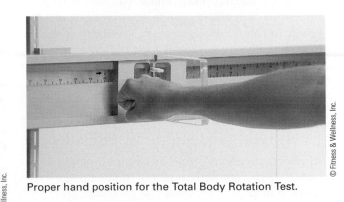

Proper hand position for the Total Body Rotation Test.

---

* The Acuflex II Flexibility Tester for the Total Body Rotation Test can be obtained from Figure Finder Collection, Novel Products, P.O. Box 408, Rockton, IL 61072-0408. Phone: 800-323-5143, Fax 815-624-4866.

TABLE 8.2 Percentile Ranks for the Total Body Rotation Test

		Left Rotation								Right Rotation							
		≤18		19–35		36–49		≥50		≤18		19–35		36–49		≥50	
	Percentile Rank	in.	cm	in.	cm	in.	cm	in.	cm	in.	cm	in.	cm	in.	cm	in.	cm
Men	99	29.1	73.9	28.0	71.1	26.6	67.6	21.0	53.3	28.2	71.6	27.8	70.6	25.2	64.0	22.2	56.4
	95	26.6	67.6	24.8	63.0	24.5	62.2	20.0	50.8	25.5	64.8	25.6	65.0	23.8	60.5	20.7	52.6
	90	25.0	63.5	23.6	59.9	23.0	58.4	17.7	45.0	24.3	61.7	24.1	61.2	22.5	57.1	19.3	49.0
	80	22.0	55.9	22.0	55.9	21.2	53.8	15.5	39.4	22.7	57.7	22.3	56.6	21.0	53.3	16.3	41.4
	70	20.9	53.1	20.3	51.6	20.4	51.8	14.7	37.3	21.3	54.1	20.7	52.6	18.7	47.5	15.7	39.9
	60	19.9	50.5	19.3	49.0	18.7	47.5	13.9	35.3	19.8	50.3	19.0	48.3	17.3	43.9	14.7	37.3
	50	18.6	47.2	18.0	45.7	16.7	42.4	12.7	32.3	19.0	48.3	17.2	43.7	16.3	41.4	12.3	31.2
	40	17.0	43.2	16.8	42.7	15.3	38.9	11.7	29.7	17.3	43.9	16.3	41.4	14.7	37.3	11.5	29.2
	30	14.9	37.8	15.0	38.1	14.8	37.6	10.3	26.2	15.1	38.4	15.0	38.1	13.3	33.8	10.7	27.2
	20	13.8	35.1	13.3	33.8	13.7	34.8	9.5	24.1	12.9	32.8	13.3	33.8	11.2	28.4	8.7	22.1
	10	10.8	27.4	10.5	26.7	10.8	27.4	4.3	10.9	10.8	27.4	11.3	28.7	8.0	20.3	2.7	6.9
	05	8.5	21.6	8.9	22.6	8.8	22.4	0.3	0.8	8.1	20.6	8.3	21.1	5.5	14.0	0.3	0.8
	01	3.4	8.6	1.7	4.3	5.1	13.0	0.0	0.0	6.6	16.8	2.9	7.4	2.0	5.1	0.0	0.0
Women	99	29.3	74.4	28.6	72.6	27.1	68.8	23.0	58.4	29.6	75.2	29.4	74.7	27.1	68.8	21.7	55.1
	95	26.8	68.1	24.8	63.0	25.3	64.3	21.4	54.4	27.6	70.1	25.3	64.3	25.9	65.8	19.7	50.0
	90	25.5	64.8	23.0	58.4	23.4	59.4	20.5	52.1	25.8	65.5	23.0	58.4	21.3	54.1	19.0	48.3
	80	23.8	60.5	21.5	54.6	20.2	51.3	19.1	48.5	23.7	60.2	20.8	52.8	19.6	49.8	17.9	45.5
	70	21.8	55.4	20.5	52.1	18.6	47.2	17.3	43.9	22.0	55.9	19.3	49.0	17.3	43.9	16.8	42.7
	60	20.5	52.1	19.3	49.0	17.7	45.0	16.0	40.6	20.8	52.8	18.0	45.7	16.5	41.9	15.6	39.6
	50	19.5	49.5	18.0	45.7	16.4	41.7	14.8	37.6	19.5	49.5	17.3	43.9	14.6	37.1	14.0	35.6
	40	18.5	47.0	17.2	43.7	14.8	37.6	13.7	34.8	18.3	46.5	16.0	40.6	13.1	33.3	12.8	32.5
	30	17.1	43.4	15.7	39.9	13.6	34.5	10.0	25.4	16.3	41.4	15.2	38.6	11.7	29.7	8.5	21.6
	20	16.0	40.6	15.2	38.6	11.6	29.5	6.3	16.0	14.5	36.8	14.0	35.6	9.8	24.9	3.9	9.9
	10	12.8	32.5	13.6	34.5	8.5	21.6	3.0	7.6	12.4	31.5	11.1	28.2	6.1	15.5	2.2	5.6
	05	11.1	28.2	7.3	18.5	6.8	17.3	0.7	1.8	10.2	25.9	8.8	22.4	4.0	10.2	1.1	2.8
	01	8.9	22.6	5.3	13.5	4.3	10.9	0.0	0.0	8.9	22.6	3.2	8.1	2.8	7.1	0.0	0.0

▓ High physical fitness standard   ░ Health fitness standard

these three tables are provided in both inches and centimeters (cm). Be sure to use the proper column to read your percentile score based on your test results. For the flexibility profile, you should take all three tests. You will be able to assess your flexibility profile in Lab 8A. Because of the specificity of flexibility, pinpointing an "ideal" level of flexibility is difficult. Nevertheless, flexibility is important to health and independent living, so assessment will give an indication of level of flexibility.

Interpreting Flexibility Test Results

After obtaining your scores and fitness ratings for each test, you can determine the fitness category for each flexibility test using the guidelines given in Table 8.4. You also should look up the number of points assigned for each fitness category in this table. The overall flexibility fitness category is obtained by totaling the number of points from all three tests and using the ratings given in Table 8.5.

Evaluating Body Posture

Posture tests are used to detect deviations from normal body alignment and prescribe corrective exercises or procedures to improve alignment. These analyses are best conducted early in life, because certain postural deviations are more difficult to correct in older people. If deviations are allowed to go uncorrected, they usually become more serious as the person grows older. Consequently, corrective exercises or other medical procedures should be used to stop or slow postural degeneration.

A leading cause of chronic low-back problems is faulty posture together with weak and inelastic muscles. Thus, evaluation is crucial to prevent and rehabilitate low-back pain. The results of these tests can be used to prescribe corrective exercises.

Adequate body mechanics also help alleviate chronic low-back pain. Proper body mechanics means using correct positions in all the activities of

FIGURE 8.3 Procedure for the Shoulder Rotation Test.

This test can be done using the Acuflex III* Flexibility Tester, which consists of a shoulder caliper and a measuring device for shoulder rotation. If this equipment is unavailable, you can construct your own device quite easily. The caliper can be built with three regular yardsticks. Nail and glue two of the yardsticks at one end at a 90° angle, and use the third one as the sliding end of the caliper. Construct the rotation device by placing a 60" measuring tape on an aluminum or wood stick, starting at about 6" or 7" from the end of the stick.

1. Warm up before the test.
2. Using the shoulder caliper, measure the biacromial width to the nearest ¼" (use the top scale on the Acuflex III). Measure biacromial width between the lateral edges of the acromion processes of the shoulders.
3. Place the Acuflex III or homemade device behind the back and use a reverse grip (thumbs out) to hold on to the device. Place the index finger of the right hand next to the zero point of the scale or tape (lower scale on the Acuflex III) and hold it firmly in place throughout the test. Place the left hand on the other end of the measuring device wherever comfortable.

4. Standing straight up and extending both arms to full length, with elbows locked, slowly bring the measuring device over the head until it reaches about forehead level. For subsequent trials, depending on the resistance encountered when rotating the shoulders, move the left grip in ½" to 1" at a time, and repeat the task until you no longer can rotate the shoulders without undue strain or starting to bend the elbows. Always keep the right-hand grip against the zero point of the scale. Measure the last successful trial to the nearest ½". Take this measurement at the inner edge of the left hand on the side of the little finger.
5. Determine the final score for this test by subtracting the biacromial width from the best score (shortest distance) between both hands on the rotation test. For example, if the best score is 35" and the biacromial width is 15", the final score is 20" (35 − 15 = 20). Using Tables 8.3 and 8.4, determine the percentile rank and flexibility fitness category for this test.

*The Acuflex III Flexibility Tester for the Shoulder Rotation Test can be obtained from Figure Finder Collection, Novel Products, Inc., P. O. Box 408, Rockton, IL 61072-0408. Phone: (800) 323-5143, Fax 815-624-4866.

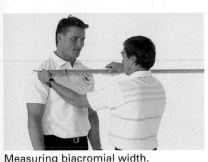
Measuring biacromial width.

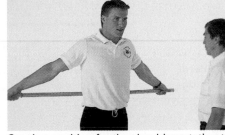
Starting position for the shoulder rotation test (note the reverse grip used for this test).

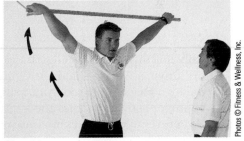
Shoulder rotation test.

Photos © Fitness & Wellness, Inc.

TABLE 8.3 Percentile Ranks for the Shoulder Rotation Test

Percentile Rank	Age Category—Men								Percentile Rank	Age Category—Women							
	≤18		19–35		36–49		≥50			≤18		19–35		36–49		≥50	
	in.	cm	in.	cm	in.	cm	in.	cm		in.	cm	in.	cm	in.	cm	in.	cm
99	2.2	5.6	−1.0	−2.5	18.1	46.0	21.5	54.6	99	2.6	6.6	−2.4	−6.1	11.5	29.2	13.1	33.3
95	15.2	38.6	10.4	26.4	20.4	51.8	27.0	68.6	95	8.0	20.3	6.2	15.7	15.4	39.1	16.5	41.9
90	18.5	47.0	15.5	39.4	20.8	52.8	27.9	70.9	90	10.7	27.2	9.7	24.6	16.8	42.7	20.9	53.1
80	20.7	52.6	18.4	46.7	23.3	59.2	28.5	72.4	80	14.5	36.8	14.5	36.8	19.2	48.8	22.5	57.1
70	23.0	58.4	20.5	52.1	24.7	62.7	29.4	74.7	70	16.1	40.9	17.2	43.7	21.5	54.6	24.3	61.7
60	24.2	61.5	22.9	58.2	26.6	67.6	29.9	75.9	60	19.2	48.8	18.7	47.5	23.1	58.7	25.1	63.8
50	25.4	64.5	24.4	62.0	28.0	71.1	30.5	77.5	50	21.0	53.3	20.0	50.8	23.5	59.7	26.2	66.5
40	26.3	66.8	25.7	65.3	30.0	76.2	31.0	78.7	40	22.2	56.4	21.4	54.4	24.4	62.0	28.1	71.4
30	28.2	71.6	27.3	69.3	31.9	81.0	31.7	80.5	30	23.2	58.9	24.0	61.0	25.9	65.8	29.9	75.9
20	30.0	76.2	30.1	76.5	33.3	84.6	33.1	84.1	20	25.0	63.5	25.9	65.8	29.8	75.7	31.5	80.0
10	33.5	85.1	31.8	80.8	36.1	91.7	37.2	94.5	10	27.2	69.1	29.1	73.9	31.1	79.0	33.1	84.1
05	34.7	88.1	33.5	85.1	37.8	96.0	38.7	98.3	05	28.0	71.1	31.3	79.5	33.4	84.8	34.1	86.6
01	40.8	103.6	42.6	108.2	43.0	109.2	44.1	112.0	01	32.5	82.5	37.1	94.2	34.9	88.6	35.4	89.9

▒ High physical fitness standard   ░ Health fitness standard

TABLE 8.4 Flexibility Fitness Categories According to Percentile Ranks

Percentile Rank	Fitness Category	Points
≥90	Excellent	5
70–80	Good	4
50–60	Average	3
30–40	Fair	2
≤20	Poor	1

TABLE 8.5 Overall Flexibility Fitness Categories

Total Points	Flexibility Category
≥13	Excellent
10–12	Good
7–9	Average
4–6	Fair
≤3	Poor

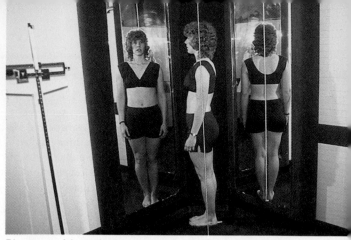

Photographic technique used for posture evaluation.

TABLE 8.6 Posture Evaluation Standards

Total Points	Category
≥45	Excellent
40–44	Good
30–39	Average
20–29	Fair
≤19	Poor

daily life, including sleeping, sitting, standing, walking, driving, working, and exercising. Because of the high incidence of low-back pain, illustrations of proper body mechanics and a series of corrective and preventive exercises are shown in Figure 8.7 on pages 253–254.

Most people are unaware of how faulty their posture is until they see themselves in a photograph. This can be quite a shock and is often enough to motivate them to institute change.

Besides engaging in the recommended exercises to elicit changes in postural alignment, individuals need to be continually aware of the corrections they are trying to make. As their posture improves, people frequently become motivated to change other aspects, such as improving muscular strength and flexibility and decreasing body fat.

Proper body alignment has been difficult to evaluate because most experts still don't know exactly what constitutes good posture. To objectively analyze a person's posture, an observer either must be adequately trained or must have some guidelines to identify abnormalities and assign ratings according to the amount of deviation from "normal" posture.

A posture rating chart, such as that in Lab 8B, provides simple guidelines for evaluating posture. Assuming that the drawings in the left column illustrate proper alignment and the drawings in the right column are extreme deviations from normal, an observer is able to rate each body segment on a scale from 1 to 5.

Postural analysis can be done with more precision with the aid of a plumb line, two mirrors, and a Polaroid camera. The mirrors are placed at an 80 to 85 percent angle, and the plumb line is centered in front of the mirrors. Another line is drawn down the center of the mirror on the right. The person should stand with the left side to the plumb line. The plumb line is used as a reference to divide the body into front and back halves (try to center the line with the hip joint and the shoulder). The line on the back (right) mirror should divide the body into right and left halves. A picture then is taken (like the photo above) that can be compared to the rating chart given in Lab 8B.

The photographic procedure allows for a better comparison of the different body segment alignments and a more objective analysis. If no mirrors and camera are available, the participant should stand with his or her side to the line, then repeat with the back to the line, while the evaluator does the assessment.

A final posture score is determined according to the sum of the ratings obtained for each body segment. Table 8.6 contains the various categories as determined by the final posture score.

Principles of Muscular Flexibility Prescription

Even though genetics play a crucial role in body flexibility, the range of joint mobility can be increased and maintained through a regular stretching program. Because range of motion is highly specific to each body part (ankle, trunk, shoulder), a comprehensive stretching program should include all body parts and follow the basic guidelines for flexibility development.

The overload and specificity of training principles (discussed in conjunction with strength development in Chapter 7) also apply to the development of muscular flexibility. To increase the total range of motion of a joint, the specific muscles surrounding that joint have to be stretched progressively beyond their accustomed length. The principles of mode, intensity, repetitions, and frequency of exercise can also be applied to flexibility programs.

Mode of Training

Three modes of stretching exercises can increase flexibility:

1. Ballistic stretching.
2. Slow-sustained stretching.
3. Proprioceptive neuromuscular facilitation (PNF) stretching.

Although research has indicated that all three types of stretching are effective in improving flexibility, each technique has certain advantages.

BALLISTIC STRETCHING

Ballistic (or **dynamic**) **stretching** exercises are done with jerky, rapid, and bouncy movements that provide the necessary force to lengthen the muscles. This type of stretching helps to develop flexibility, but the ballistic actions may cause muscle soreness and injury from small tears to the soft tissue.

Precautions must be taken not to overstretch ligaments, because they will undergo plastic or permanent elongation. If the stretching force cannot be controlled—as often occurs in fast, jerky movements—ligaments can easily be overstretched. This, in turn, leads to excessively loose joints, increasing the risk for injuries. Slow, gentle, and **controlled ballistic stretching** (instead of jerky, rapid, and bouncy movements), however, is effective in developing flexibility, and most individuals can perform it safely.

SLOW-SUSTAINED STRETCHING

With the **slow-sustained stretching** technique, muscles are lengthened gradually through a joint's complete range of motion and the final position is held for a few seconds. A slow-sustained stretch causes the muscles to relax and thereby achieve greater length. This type of stretch causes little pain and has a low risk for injury. Slow-sustained stretching exercises are the most frequently used and recommended in flexibility-development programs.

PROPRIOCEPTIVE NEUROMUSCULAR FACILITATION (PNF)

Proprioceptive neuromuscular facilitation (PNF) stretching is based on a "contract-and-relax" method and requires the assistance of another person. The procedure is as follows:

1. The person assisting with the exercise provides initial force by pushing slowly in the direction of the desired stretch. This first stretch does not cover the entire range of motion.
2. The person being stretched then applies force in the opposite direction of the stretch, against the assistant, who tries to hold the initial degree of stretch as close as possible. This results in an isometric contraction at the angle of the stretch.
3. After 4 or 5 seconds of isometric contraction, the person being stretched relaxes the target muscle completely. The assistant then increases the degree of stretch slowly to a greater angle.
4. The isometric contraction is repeated for another 4 or 5 seconds, after which the muscle is relaxed again. The assistant then can increase the degree of stretch, slowly, one more time.

Steps 1 through 4 are repeated two to five times, until the exerciser feels mild discomfort. On the last trial, the final stretched position should be held for several seconds.

Theoretically, with the PNF technique, the isometric contraction helps relax the muscle being stretched, which results in lengthening the muscle. Some fitness leaders believe PNF is more effective than slow-sustained stretching. Another benefit of PNF is an increase in strength of the muscle(s) being stretched. Research has shown approximately 17 and 35 percent increases in absolute strength and muscular endurance, respectively, in the hamstring muscle group after 12 weeks of PNF stretching.[4] The

---

Ballistic (dynamic) stretching Exercises done with jerky, rapid, bouncy movements, or slow, short, and sustained movements.

Controlled ballistic stretching Exercises done with slow, short, and sustained movements.

Slow-sustained stretching Exercises in which the muscles are lengthened gradually through a joint's complete range of motion.

Proprioceptive neuromuscular facilitation (PNF) Mode of stretching that uses reflexes and neuromuscular principles to relax the muscles that are being stretched.

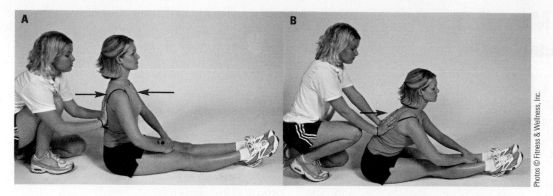

Proprioceptive neuromuscular facilitation (PNF) stretching technique: (A) isometric phase, (B) stretching phase.

results were consistent in both men and women and are attributed to the isometric contractions performed during PNF. Disadvantages of PNF are (1) more pain, (2) the need for a second person to assist, and (3) the need for more time to conduct each session.

Intensity

The **intensity**, or degree of stretch, when doing flexibility exercises should be only to a point of mild discomfort. Pain does not have to be part of the stretching routine. Excessive pain is an indication that the load is too high and may cause injury.

All stretching should be done to slightly below the pain threshold. As participants reach this point, they should try to relax the muscle being stretched as much as possible. After completing the stretch, the body part is brought back gradually to the starting point.

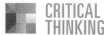

CRITICAL THINKING

Carefully consider the relevance of stretching exercises to your personal fitness program. How much importance do you place on these exercises? Have some conditions improved through your stretching program, or have certain specific exercises contributed to your health and well-being?

Repetitions

The time required for an exercise session for flexibility development is based on the number of **repetitions** and the length of time each repetition is held in the final stretched position. As a general recommendation, each exercise should be done four or five times, holding the final position each time for 10 to 30 seconds.

As flexibility increases, a person can gradually increase the time each repetition is held, to a maximum of 1 minute. Individuals who are susceptible to flexibility injuries should limit each stretch to 20 seconds. Pilates exercises are recommended for these individuals, as they increase joint stability (also see Chapter 7, page 214).

FIGURE 8.4 Guidelines for flexibility development.

Mode:	Static or dynamic (slow ballistic or proprioceptive neuromuscular facilitation) stretching to include every major joint of the body
Intensity:	Stretch to the point of mild discomfort
Repetitions:	Repeat each exercise at least 4 times and hold the final stretched position for 10 to 30 seconds
Frequency:	2–3 days per week

Based on American College of Sports Medicine, "Position Stand: The Recommended Quantity and Quality of Exercise for Developing and Maintaining Cardiorespiratory and Muscular Fitness, and Flexibility in Healthy Adults," *Medical Science Sports Exercise* 30 (1998): 975–991.

Frequency of Exercise

Flexibility exercises should be conducted five or six times a week in the early stages of the program. After 6 to 8 weeks of almost daily stretching, flexibility can be maintained with only two or three sessions per week, doing about three repetitions of 10 to 30 seconds each. Figure 8.4 summarizes the flexibility development guidelines.

When to Stretch?

Many people do not differentiate a warm-up from stretching. Warming up means starting a workout slowly with walking, cycling, or slow jogging, followed by gentle stretching (not through the entire range of motion). Stretching implies movement of joints through their full range of motion and holding the final degree of stretch according to recommended guidelines.

A warm-up that progressively increases muscle temperature and mimics movement that will occur during training enhances performance. For some activities, gentle stretching is recommended in conjunction with warm-up routines. Before steady activities (walking, jogging, cycling), a warm-up of 3 to 5 minutes is recommended. Up to 10 minutes is the recommendation before stop-and-go activities (racquet sports, basketball, soccer) and athletic participation in general (football, gymnastics). Activities that require abrupt changes in direction are more likely to cause muscle strains if they are performed without proper warm-up that includes mild stretching.

Sports-specific/pre-exercise stretching can improve performance in sports that require greater-than-average range of motion, such as gymnastics, dance, swimming, and figure skating. Some evidence, however, suggests that intense stretching during warm-up can lead to a temporary short-term (up to 60 minutes) decrease in strength. Thus, extensive stretching conducted prior to participation in athletic events that rely on strength and power for peak performance is not recommended.[5]

In terms of preventing injuries, the best time to stretch is controversial. In limited studies on athletic populations, the evidence is unclear as to whether stretching before or after exercise is more beneficial in preventing injury. Additional research is necessary to clarify this issue.

In general, a good time to stretch is after aerobic workouts. Higher body temperature in itself helps to increase the joint range of motion. Muscles also are fatigued following exercise, and a fatigued muscle tends to shorten, which can lead to soreness and spasms. Stretching exercises help fatigued muscles reestablish their normal resting length and prevent unnecessary pain.

Flexibility Exercises

To improve body flexibility, each major muscle group should be subjected to at least one stretching exercise. A complete set of exercises for developing muscular flexibility is presented on pages 257–258.

You may not be able to hold a final stretched position with some of these exercises (such as lateral head tilts and arm circles), but you still should perform the exercise through the joint's full range of motion. Depending on the number and length of repetitions, a complete workout will last between 15 and 30 minutes.

Contraindicated Exercises

Most strength and flexibility exercises are relatively safe to perform, but even safe exercises can be hazardous if they are performed incorrectly. Some exercises may be safe to perform occasionally but, when executed repeatedly, may cause trauma and

injury. Preexisting muscle or joint conditions (old sprains or injuries) can further increase the risk of harm during certain exercises. As you develop your exercise program, you are encouraged to follow the exercise descriptions and guidelines given in this book.

A few exercises, however, are not recommended because of the potential high risk for injury. These exercises are sometimes performed in videotaped workouts and some fitness classes. **Contraindicated exercises** may cause harm because of the excessive strain placed on muscles and joints, in particular the spine, lower back, knees, neck, or shoulders.

Illustrations of contraindicated exercises are presented in Figure 8.5. Safe alternative exercises are listed below each contraindicated exercise and are illustrated in the exercises for strength (pages 221–234) and flexibility (pages 257–258). In isolated instances, a qualified physical therapist may select one or a few of the contraindicated exercises to treat a specific injury or disability in a carefully supervised setting. Unless you are specifically instructed to use one of these exercises, it is best that you select safe exercises from this book.

Preventing and Rehabilitating Low-Back Pain

Few people make it through life without having low-back pain at some point. An estimated 60 to 80 percent of the population has been afflicted by back pain or injury. Estimates indicate that more than 75 million Americans suffer from chronic back pain each year.

Back pain is considered chronic if it persists longer than 3 months. It has been determined that backache syndrome is preventable about 80 percent of the time, and is caused by (a) physical inactivity, (b) poor postural habits and body mechanics, (c) excessive body weight, and/or (d) psychological stress. Data also indicate that back injuries are more common among smokers.

More than 95 percent of all back pain is related to muscle/tendon injury, and only 1 to 5 percent is related to intervertebral disk damage.[6] Usually, back pain is the result of repeated micro-injuries that occur over an extended time (sometimes years) until a certain movement, activity, or excessive overload causes a significant injury to the tissues.[7]

Intensity (for flexibility exercises) Degree of stretch when doing flexibility exercises.

Repetitions Number of times a given resistance is performed.

Contraindicated exercises Exercises that are not recommended because they may cause injury to a person.

FIGURE 8.5 Contraindicated exercises.

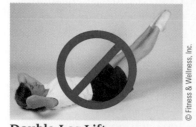

Double-Leg Lift

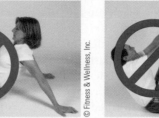

Upright Double-Leg Lifts

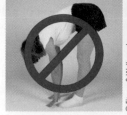

V-Sits

All three of these exercises cause excessive strain on the spine and may harm disks.

Alternatives: Strength Exercises 4 and 17, pages 222 and 226

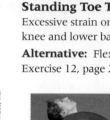

Standing Toe Touch

Excessive strain on the knee and lower back.

Alternative: Flexibility Exercise 12, page 258

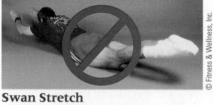

Swan Stretch

Excessive strain on the spine; may harm intervertebral disks.

Alternative: Flexibility Exercise 20, page 259

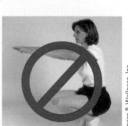

Cradle

Excessive strain on the spine, knees, and shoulders.

Alternatives: Flexibility Exercises 20, 8, and 6, pages 259, 258, and 257

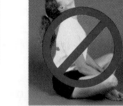

Full Squat

Excessive strain on the knees.

Alternatives: Flexibility Exercise 8, page 258; Strength Exercises 1, 16, 26, pages 221, 226, and 230

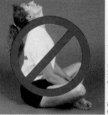

Head Rolls

May injure neck disks.

Alternative: Flexibility Exercise 1, page 257

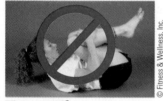

Knee to Chest

(with hands over the shin) Excessive strain on the knee.

Alternative: Flexibility Exercises 15 and 16, page 259

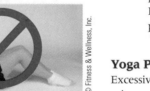

Sit-Ups with Hands Behind the Head

Excessive strain on the neck.

Alternatives: Strength Exercises 4 and 17, pages 222 and 226

Yoga Plow

Excessive strain on the spine, neck, and shoulders.

Alternatives: Flexibility Exercises 12, 15, 16, 17, and 19, pages 258 and 259

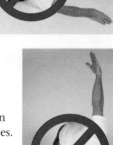
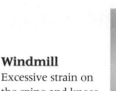
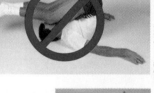
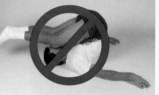

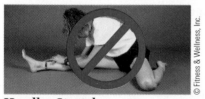

Hurdler Stretch

Excessive strain on the bent knee.

Alternatives: Flexibility Exercises 8 and 12, page 258

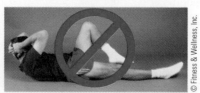

The Hero

Excessive strain on the knees.

Alternatives: Flexibility Exercises 8 and 14, pages 258 and 259

Windmill

Excessive strain on the spine and knees.

Alternatives: Flexibility Exercises 12 and 21, pages 258 and 260

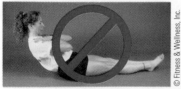

Straight-Leg Sit-Ups

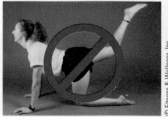

Alternating Bent-Leg Sit-Ups

These exercises strain the lower back.

Alternatives: Strength Exercises 4 and 17, pages 222 and 226

Donkey Kicks

Excessive strain on the back, shoulders, and neck.

Alternatives: Flexibility Exercises 20, 14, and 1, pages 259 and 257

FIGURE 8.6 Incorrect (left) and correct (right) pelvic alignment.

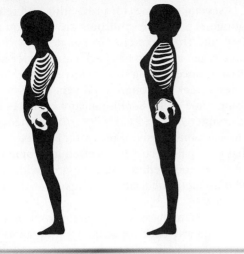

People tend to think of back pain as a problem with the skeleton. In fact, the spine's curvature, alignment, and movement are controlled by surrounding muscles. Lack of physical activity is the most common reason for chronic low-back pain. In particular, a major contributor to back pain is excessive sitting, which causes back muscles to shorten, stiffen, and become weaker.

Deterioration or weakening of the abdominal and gluteal muscles, along with tightening of the lower back (erector spinae) muscles, brings about an unnatural forward tilt of the pelvis (Figure 8.6). This tilt puts extra pressure on the spinal vertebrae, causing pain in the lower back. Accumulation of fat around the midsection of the body contributes to the forward tilt of the pelvis, which further aggravates the condition.

Low-back pain frequently is associated with faulty posture and improper body mechanics, or body positions in all of life's daily activities, including sleeping, sitting, standing, walking, driving, working, and exercising. Incorrect posture and poor mechanics, such as prolonged static postures, repetitive bending and pushing, twisting a loaded spine, and prolonged sitting with little movement (more than an hour) increase strain on the lower back and many other bones, joints, muscles, and ligaments. Figure 8.7 provides a summary of proper body mechanics that promote back health.

In the majority of back injuries, pain is present only with movement and physical activity. If the pain is severe and persists even at rest, the first step is to consult a physician, who can rule out any disc damage and may prescribe proper bed rest using several pillows under the knees for leg support

(see Figure 8.7). This position helps release muscle spasms by stretching the muscles involved. In addition, a physician may prescribe a muscle relaxant or anti-inflammatory medication (or both) and some type of physical therapy.

In most cases of low-back pain, even with severe pain, people feel better within days or weeks without treatment from health care professionals.[8] To relieve symptoms, you may use over-the-counter pain relievers and hot or cold packs. You should also stay active to avoid further weakening of the back muscles. Low-impact activities such as walking, swimming, water aerobics, and cycling are recommended. Once you are pain-free in the resting state, you need to start correcting the muscular imbalance by stretching the tight muscles and strengthening the weak ones. Stretching exercises always are performed first.

If there is no indication of disease or injury (such as leg numbness or pain), a herniated disk, or fractures, spinal manipulation by a chiropractor or other health care professional can provide pain relief. Spinal manipulation as a treatment modality for low-back pain has been endorsed by the federal Agency for Health Care Policy and Research. The guidelines suggest that spinal manipulation may help to alleviate discomfort and pain during the first few weeks of an acute episode of low-back pain. Generally, benefits are seen in fewer than 10 treatments. People who have had chronic pain for more than 6 months should avoid spinal manipulation

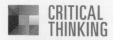
until they have been thoroughly examined by a physician.

Back pain can be reduced greatly through aerobic exercise, muscular flexibility exercise, and muscular strength and endurance training that includes specific exercises to strengthen the spine-stabilizing muscles. Exercise requires effort by the patient, and it may create discomfort initially, but exercise promotes circulation, healing, muscle size, and muscle strength and endurance. Many patients abstain from aggressive physical therapy because they are unwilling to commit the time required for the program.

Aerobic exercise is beneficial because it helps decrease body fat and psychological stress. During an episode of back pain, however, people often avoid activity and cope by getting more rest. Rest is recommended if the pain is associated with a herniated disc, but if your physician rules out a serious problem, exercise is a better choice of treatment. Exercise helps restore physical function, and individuals who start and maintain an aerobic exercise program have back pain less frequently. Individuals who exercise are also less likely to require surgery or other invasive treatments.

In terms of flexibility, regular stretching exercises that help the hip and trunk go through a functional range of motion, as opposed to increasing the range of motion, are recommended. That is, for proper back care, stretching exercises should not be performed to the extreme range of motion. Individuals with a greater spinal range of motion also have a higher incidence of back injury. Spinal stability, instead of mobility, is desirable for back health.[9]

A strengthening program for a healthy back should be conducted around the endurance threshold—10 to 12 repetitions to near fatigue. Muscular endurance of the muscles that support the spine is more important than absolute strength because these muscles perform their work during the course of an entire day.

Several exercises for preventing and rehabilitating the backache syndrome are given on pages 259–260. These exercises can be done twice or more daily when a person has back pain. Under normal circumstances, doing these exercises three or four times a week is enough to prevent the syndrome. Using some of the additional core exercises listed in Chapter 7 (page 213) will further enhance your low-back management program. Data have shown that back pain recurs more often in people who rely solely on medication, compared with people who use both medication and exercise therapy to recover.[10]

Lab 8C allows you to develop your own flexibility and low-back conditioning programs. The recommendation calls for isometric contractions of 2 to 20 seconds during each repetition for some of the exercises listed for back health (see Lab 8C) to further increase spinal stability and muscular strength endurance. The length of the hold depends on your current fitness level and the difficulty of each exercise. For most exercises, you may start with a 2- to 10-second hold. Over the course of several weeks, you can increase the length of the hold from 10 to 30 seconds.

Psychological stress may also lead to back pain.[11] Excessive stress causes muscles to contract. In the case of the lower back, frequent tightening of the muscles can throw the back out of alignment and constrict blood vessels that supply oxygen and nutrients to the back. Chronic stress also increases the release of hormones that have been linked to muscle and tendon injuries. Furthermore, people under stress tend to forget proper body mechanics, placing themselves at unnecessary risk for injury. If you are undergoing excessive stress and back pain at the same time, proper stress management (see Chapter 10) should be a part of your comprehensive back-care program.

FIGURE 8.7 Your back and how to care for it.

Whatever the cause of low-back pain, part of its treatment is the correction of faulty posture. But good posture is not simply a matter of "standing tall." It refers to correct use of the body at all times. In fact, for the body to function in the best of health it must be so used that no strain is put upon the muscles, joints, bones, and ligaments. To prevent low-back pain, avoiding strain must become a way of life, practiced while lying, sitting, standing, walking, working, and exercising. When body position is correct, internal organs have enough room to function normally and blood circulates more freely.

With the help of this guide, you can begin to correct the positions and movements that bring on or aggravate backache. Particular attention should be paid to the positions recommended for resting, since it is possible to strain the muscles of the back and neck even while lying in bed. By learning to live with good posture, under all circumstances, you will gradually develop the proper carriage and stronger muscles needed to protect and support your hard-working back.

How to Stay on Your Feet Without Tiring Your Back

To prevent strain and pain in everyday activities, it is restful to change from one task to another before fatigue sets in. Housewives can lie down between chores; others should check body position frequently, drawing in the abdomen, flattening the back, bending the knees slightly.

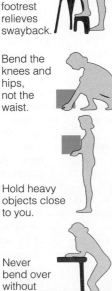

Not this way

Use of a footrest relieves swayback.

Not this way

Bend the knees and hips, not the waist.

Not this way

Hold heavy objects close to you.

Not this way

Never bend over without bending the knees.

Check Your Carriage Here

In correct, fully erect posture, a line dropped from the ear will go through the tip of the shoulder, middle of hip, back of kneecap, and front of anklebone.

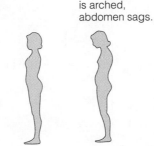

Incorrect
Lower back is arched or hollow.

Incorrect
Upper back is stooped, lower back is arched, abdomen sags.

Incorrect
Note how, in strained position, pelvis tilts forward, chin is out, and ribs are down, crowding internal organs.

Correct
In correct position, chin is in, head up, back flattened, pelvis held straight.

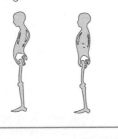

To find the correct standing position: Stand one foot away from wall. Now sit against wall, bending knees slightly. Tighten abdominal and buttock muscles. This will tilt the pelvis back and flatten the lower spine. Holding this position, inch up the wall to standing position, by straightening the legs. Now walk around the room, maintaining the same posture. Place back against wall again to see if you have held it.

How to Sit Correctly

A back's best friend is a straight, hard chair. If you can't get the chair you prefer, learn to sit properly on whatever chair you get. *To correct sitting position from forward slump:* Throw head well back, then bend it forward to pull in the chin. This will straighten the back. Now tighten abdominal muscles to raise the chest. Check position frequently.

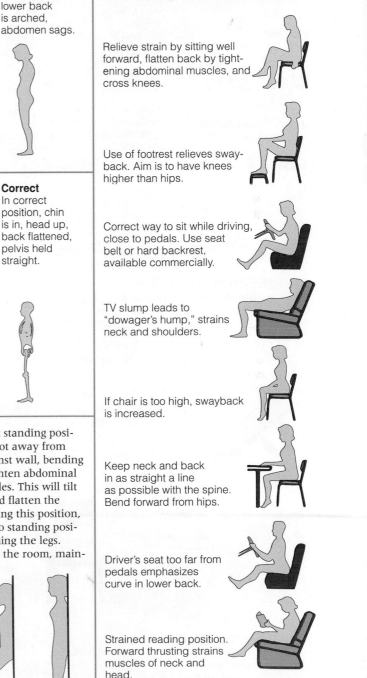

Relieve strain by sitting well forward, flatten back by tightening abdominal muscles, and cross knees.

Use of footrest relieves swayback. Aim is to have knees higher than hips.

Correct way to sit while driving, close to pedals. Use seat belt or hard backrest, available commercially.

TV slump leads to "dowager's hump," strains neck and shoulders.

If chair is too high, swayback is increased.

Keep neck and back in as straight a line as possible with the spine. Bend forward from hips.

Driver's seat too far from pedals emphasizes curve in lower back.

Strained reading position. Forward thrusting strains muscles of neck and head.

Continued

FIGURE 8.7 (Continued)

How to Put Your Back to Bed

For proper bed posture, a firm mattress is essential. Bedboards, sold commercially, or devised at home, may be used with soft mattresses. Bedboards, preferably, should be made of 3/4-inch plywood. Faulty sleeping positions intensify swayback and result not only in backache but in numbness, tingling, and pain in arms and legs.

Incorrect:
Lying flat on back makes swayback worse.

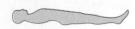

Use of high pillow strains neck, arms, shoulders.

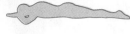

Sleeping face down exaggerates swayback, strains neck and shoulders.

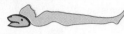

Bending one hip and knee does not relieve swayback.

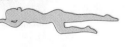

Correct:
Lying on side with knees bent effectively flattens the back. Flat pillow may be used to support neck, especially when shoulders are broad.

Sleeping on back is restful and correct when knees are properly supported.

Raise the foot of the mattress eight inches to discourage sleeping on the abdomen.

Proper arrangement of pillows for resting or reading in bed.

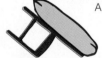

A straight-back chair used behind a pillow makes a serviceable backrest.

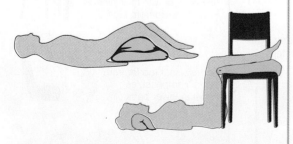

When Doing Nothing, Do it Right

- Rest is the first rule for the tired, painful back. The following positions relieve pain by taking all pressure and weight off the back and legs.
- Note pillows under knees to relieve strain on spine.
- For complete relief and relaxing effect, these positions should be maintained from 5 to 25 minutes.

Exercise Without Getting Out of Bed

Exercises to be performed while lying in bed are aimed not so much at strengthening muscles as at teaching correct positioning. But muscles used correctly become stronger and in time are able to support the body with the least amount of effort.

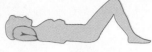

Do all exercises in this position. Legs should not be straightened.

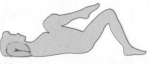

Bring knee up to chest. Lower slowly but do not straighten leg. Relax. Repeat with each leg 10 times.

Bring both knees slowly up to chest (place your hands on the lower thigh behind the knees). Tighten muscles of abdomen, press back flat against bed. Hold knees to chest 20 seconds, then lower slowly. Relax. Repeat 5 times. This exercise gently stretches the shortened muscles of the lower back, while strengthening abdominal muscles.

Rules to Live By—From Now On

1. Never bend from the waist only; bend the hips and knees.
2. Never lift a heavy object higher than your waist.
3. Always turn and face the object you wish to lift.
4. Avoid carrying unbalanced loads; hold heavy objects close to your body.
5. Never carry anything heavier than you can manage with ease.
6. Never lift or move heavy furniture. Wait for someone to do it who knows the principles of leverage.
7. Avoid sudden movements, sudden "overloading" of muscles. Learn to move deliberately, swinging the legs from the hips.
8. Learn to keep the head in line with the spine, when standing, sitting, lying in bed.
9. Put soft chairs and deep couches on your "don't sit" list. During prolonged sitting, cross your legs to rest your back.
10. Your doctor is the only one who can determine when low-back pain is due to faulty posture and he is the best judge of when you may do general exercises for physical fitness. When you do, omit any exercise that arches or overstrains the lower back: backward bends, or forward bends, touching the toes with the knees straight.
11. Wear shoes with moderate heels, all about the same height. Avoid changing from high to low heels.
12. Put a footrail under the desk and a footrest under the crib.
13. Diaper the baby sitting next to him or her on the bed.
14. Don't stoop and stretch to hang the wash; raise the clothesbasket and lower the washline.
15. Beg or buy a rocking chair. Rocking rests the back by changing the muscle groups used.
16. Train yourself vigorously to use your abdominal muscles to flatten your lower abdomen. In time, this muscle contraction will become habitual, making you the envied possessor of a youthful body-profile!
17. Don't strain to open windows or doors.
18. For good posture, concentrate on strengthening "nature's corset"—the abdominal and buttock muscles. The pelvic roll exercise is especially recommended to correct the postural relation between the pelvis and the spine.

file
s
ate how
you
rstand
oncepts
ented in
chapter
the
ess Your
vledge"
"Practice
es"
ns
ur
OM.

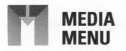

ASSESS YOUR KNOWLEDGE

1. Muscular flexibility is defined as
   a. the capacity of joints and muscles to work in a synchronized manner.
   b. the ability of a joint to move freely through its full range of motion.
   c. the capability of muscles to stretch beyond their normal resting length without injury to the muscles.
   d. the capacity of muscles to return to their proper length following the application of a stretching force.
   e. the limitations placed on muscles as the joints move through their normal planes.

2. Good flexibility
   a. promotes healthy muscles and joints.
   b. decreases the risk of injury.
   c. improves posture.
   d. decreases the risk of chronic back pain.
   e. All are correct choices.

3. Plastic elongation is a term used in reference to
   a. permanent lengthening of soft tissue.
   b. increased flexibility achieved through dynamic stretching.
   c. temporary elongation of muscles.
   d. the ability of a muscle to achieve a complete degree of stretch.
   e. lengthening of a muscle against resistance.

4. The most significant contributors to loss of flexibility are
   a. sedentary living and lack of physical activity.
   b. weight and power training.
   c. age and injury.
   d. muscular strength and endurance.
   e. excessive body fat and low lean tissue.

5. Which of the following is *not* a mode of stretching?
   a. proprioceptive neuromuscular facilitation
   b. elastic elongation
   c. ballistic stretching
   d. slow-sustained stretching
   e. All are modes of stretching.

6. PNF can help increase
   a. muscular strength.
   b. muscular flexibility.
   c. muscular endurance.
   d. range of motion.
   e. All are correct choices.

7. When performing stretching exercises, the degree of stretch should be
   a. through the entire arc of movement.
   b. to about 80 percent of capacity.
   c. to the point of mild discomfort.
   d. applied until the muscle(s) start shaking.
   e. progressively increased until the desired stretch is attained.

8. When stretching, the final stretch should be held for
   a. 1 to 10 seconds.
   b. 10 to 30 seconds.
   c. 30 to 90 seconds.
   d. 1 to 3 minutes.
   e. as long as the person is able to sustain the stretch.

9. Low-back pain is primarily associated with
   a. physical inactivity.
   b. faulty posture.
   c. excessive body weight.
   d. improper body mechanics.
   e. All are correct choices.

10. The following exercise helps stretch the lower back and hamstring muscles:
    a. adductor stretch
    b. sit-and-reach stretch
    c. back extension stretch
    d. single-knee-to-chest stretch
    e. quad stretch

Correct answers can be found at the back of the book.

MEDIA MENU

PROFILE PLUS CD CONNECTIONS

■ Create your personal flexibility profile.

■ Check how well you understand the chapter's concepts.

INTERNET CONNECTIONS

■ Stretching and Flexibility: Everything You Never Wanted to Know. This very comprehensive and academic site describes the physiology of muscles, types of flexibility, types of stretching, and factors limiting flexibility. It includes how to stretch and specific exercises, as well as references.

http://www.cmcrossroads.com/bradapp/docs/rec/stretching/

■ Specific stretching exercises, with diagrams. This site is sponsored by Shape Up, America, and is easy to understand.

http://www.shapeup.org/publications/fitting.fitness.in/noframes/stretches.htm

■ Yoga and other stretching exercises. This site features information on the techniques of yoga, pilates, and other forms of stretching exercises.

http://www.yoga.com

■ Stretching to Increase Flexibility. In addition to a comprehensive description of the health benefits of regular stretching, this site features a series of exercises tailored to one of three levels of fitness levels based on the frequency that you perform stretching exercises.

http://k2.kirtland.cc.mi.us/~balbachl/flex.htm

Notes

1. American College of Obstetricians and Gynecologists, *Guidelines for Exercise During Pregnancy*, 1994.

2. "Stretch Yourself Younger," *Consumer Reports on Health* 11 (August 1999): 6–7.

3. W. W. K. Hoeger and D. R. Hopkins, "A Comparison Between the Sit and Reach and the Modified Sit and Reach in the Measurement of Flexibility in Women," *Research Quarterly for Exercise and Sport* 63 (1992): 191–195.

   W. W. K. Hoeger, D. R. Hopkins, S. Button, and T. A. Palmer, "Comparing the Sit and Reach with the Modified Sit and Reach in Measuring Flexibility in Adolescents," *Pediatric Exercise Science* 2 (1990): 156–162.

   D. R. Hopkins and W. W. K. Hoeger, "A Comparison of the Sit and Reach and the Modified Sit and Reach in the Measurement of Flexibility for Males," *Journal of Applied Sports Science Research* 6 (1992): 7–10.

4. J. Kokkonen and S. Lauritzen, "Isotonic Strength and Endurance Gains Through PNF Stretching," *Medicine and Science in Sports and Exercise* 27 (1995): S22, 127.

5. S. B. Thacker, J. Gilchrist, D. F. Stroup, and C. D. Kimsey. Jr., "The Impact of Stretching on Sports Injury Risk: A Systematic Review of the Literature," *Medicine and Science in Sports and Exercise* 36 (2004): 371–378.

6. D. B. J. Andersson, L. J. Fine, and B. A. Silverstein, "Musculoskeletal Disorders," Occupational Health: Recognizing and Preventing Work-Related Disease, edited by B. S. Levy and D. H. Wegman (Boston: Little, Brown and Company, 1995).

7. M. R. Bracko, "Can We Prevent Back Injuries?" *ACSM's Health & Fitness Journal* 8, no. 4 (2004): 5–11.

8. R. Deyo, "Chiropractic Care for Back Pain: The Physician's Perspective," *HealthNews* 4 (September 10, 1998).

9. See note 7.

10. J. A. Hides, G. A. Jull, and C. A. Richardson, "Long-Term Effects of Specific Stabilizing Exercises for First-Episode Low Back Pain," *Spine* 26 (2001): E243–248.

11. A. Brownstein, "Chronic Back Pain Can Be Beaten," *Bottom Line/Health* 13 (October 1999): 3–4.

Suggested Readings

Alter, M. J. *The Science of Stretching*. Champaign, IL: Human Kinetic Press, 1996.

Alter, M. J. *Sports Stretch*. Champaign, IL: Human Kinetics, 2004.

Anderson, B. *Stretching*. Bolinas, CA: Shelter Publications, 1999.

Bracko, M. R. "Can We Prevent Back Injuries?" *ACSM's Health & Fitness Journal* 8, no. 4 (2004): 5–11.

Hoeger, W. W. K. *The Assessment of Muscular Flexibility: Test Protocols and National Flexibility Norms for the Modified Sit-and-Reach Test, Total Body Rotation Test, and Shoulder Rotation Test*. Rockton, IL: Figure Finder Collection Novel Products, Inc., 2004.

Liemohn, W. and G. Pariser. "Core Strength: Implications for Fitness and Low Back Pain." *ACSM's Health and Fitness Journal* 6, no. 5 (2002): 10–16.

McAtee, R. E. and J. Charland. *Facilitated Stretching*. Champaign, IL: Human Kinetics, 1999.

Flexibility Exercises

Exercise 1
Lateral Head Tilt

Action Slowly and gently tilt the head laterally. Repeat several times to each side.

Areas Stretched
Neck flexors and extensors; ligaments of the cervical spine

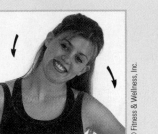

Exercise 2
Arm Circles

Action Gently circle your arms all the way around. Conduct the exercise in both directions.

Areas Stretched
Shoulder muscles and ligaments

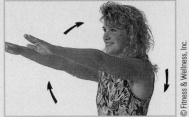

Exercise 3
Side Stretch

Action Stand straight up, feet separated to shoulder-width, and place your hands on your waist. Now move the upper body to one side and hold the final stretch for a few seconds. Repeat on the other side.

Areas Stretched
Muscles and ligaments in the pelvic region

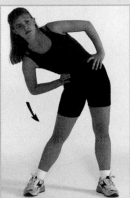

Exercise 4
Body Rotation

Action Place your arms slightly away from your body and rotate the trunk as far as possible, holding the final position for several seconds. Conduct the exercise for both the right and left sides of the body. You also can perform this exercise by standing about 2 feet away from the wall (back toward the wall) and then rotating the trunk, placing the hands against the wall.

Areas Stretched
Hip, abdominal, chest, back, neck, and shoulder muscles; hip and spinal ligaments

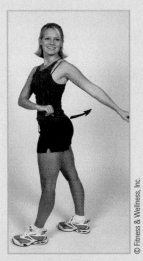

Exercise 5
Chest Stretch

Action Place your hands on the shoulders of your partner, who will in turn push you down by your shoulders. Hold the final position for a few seconds.

Areas Stretched
Chest (pectoral) muscles and shoulder ligaments

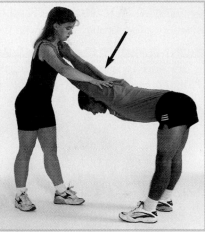

Exercise 6
Shoulder Hyperextension Stretch

Action Have a partner grasp your arms from behind by the wrists and slowly push them upward. Hold the final position for a few seconds.

Areas Stretched
Deltoid and pectoral muscles; ligaments of the shoulder joint

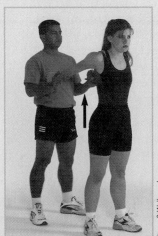

Exercise 7
Shoulder Rotation Stretch

Action With the aid of surgical tubing or an aluminum or wood stick, place the tubing or stick behind your back and grasp the two ends using a reverse (thumbs-out) grip. Slowly bring the tubing or stick over your head, keeping the elbows straight. Repeat several times (bring the hands closer together for additional stretch).

Areas Stretched
Deltoid, latissimus dorsi, and pectoral muscles; shoulder ligaments

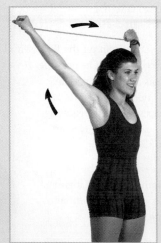

Exercise 8
Quad Stretch

Action   Lie on your side and move one foot back by flexing the knee. Grasp the front of the ankle and pull the ankle toward the gluteal region. Hold for several seconds. Repeat with the other leg.

Areas Stretched   Quadriceps muscle, hip flexors; knee and ankle ligaments

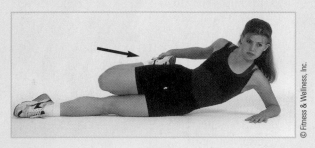

Exercise 9
Heel Cord Stretch

Action   Stand against the wall or at the edge of a step and stretch the heel downward, alternating legs. Hold the stretched position for a few seconds.

Areas Stretched Heel cord (Achilles tendon), gastrocnemius and soleus muscles

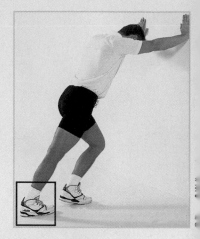

Exercise 10
Adductor Stretch

Action   Stand with your feet about twice shoulder-width apart and place your hands slightly above the knees. Flex one knee and slowly go down as far as possible, holding the final position for a few seconds. Repeat with the other leg.

Areas Stretched   Hip adductor muscles

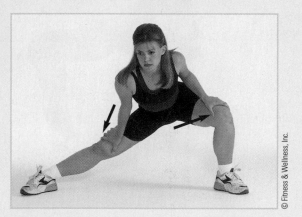

Exercise 11
Sitting Adductor Stretch

Action   Sit on the floor and bring your feet in close to you, allowing the soles of the feet to touch each other. Now place your forearms (or elbows) on the inner part of the thighs and push the legs downward, holding the final stretch for several seconds.

Areas Stretched Hip adductor muscles

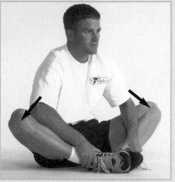

Exercise 13
Triceps Stretch

Action   Place the right hand behind your neck. Grasp the right arm above the elbow with the left hand. Gently pull the elbow backward. Repeat the exercise with the opposite arm.

Areas Stretched Back of upper arm (triceps muscle); shoulder joint

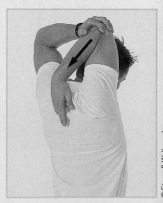

Exercise 12
Sit-and-Reach Stretch

Action   Sit on the floor with legs together and gradually reach forward as far as possible. Hold the final position for a few seconds. This exercise also may be performed with the legs separated, reaching to each side as well as to the middle.

Areas Stretched Hamstrings and lower back muscles; lumbar spine ligaments

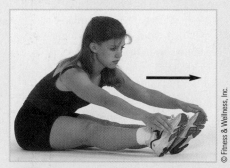

NOTE: Exercises 14 through 21 and 23 are also flexibility exercises and can be added to your stretching program.

Exercises for the Prevention and Rehabilitation of Low-Back Pain

Exercise 14
Hip Flexors Stretch

Action Kneel down on an exercise mat or a soft surface, or place a towel under your knees. Raise the left knee off the floor and place the left foot about 3 feet in front of you. Place your left hand over your left knee and the right hand over the back of the right hip. Keeping the lower back flat, slowly move forward and downward as you apply gentle pressure over the right hip. Repeat the exercise with the opposite leg forward.

Areas Stretched Flexor muscles in front of the hip joint

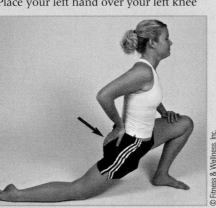

Exercise 15
Single-Knee-to-Chest Stretch

Action Lie down flat on the floor. Bend one leg at approximately 100° and gradually pull the opposite leg toward your chest. Hold the final stretch for a few seconds. Switch legs and repeat the exercise.

Areas Stretched Lower back and hamstring muscles; lumbar spine ligaments

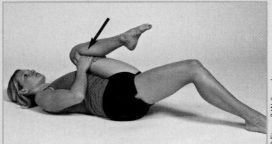

Exercise 16
Double-Knee-to-Chest Stretch

Action Lie flat on the floor and then curl up slowly into a fetal position. Hold for a few seconds.

Areas Stretched Upper and lower back and hamstring muscles; spinal ligaments

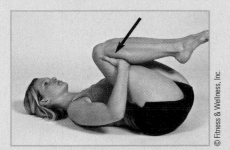

Exercise 17
Upper- and Lower-Back Stretch

Action Sit on the floor and bring your feet in close to you, allowing the soles of the feet to touch each other. Holding on to your feet, bring your head and upper chest gently toward your feet.

Areas Stretched Upper and lower back muscles and ligaments

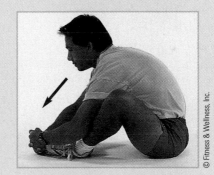

Exercise 18
Sit-and-Reach Stretch

(see Exercise 12, in this chapter, on page 258)

Exercise 19
Gluteal Stretch

Action Sit on the floor, bend your right leg, and place your right ankle slightly above the left knee. Grasp the left thigh with both hands and gently pull the leg toward your chest. Repeat the exercise with the opposite leg.

Areas Stretched Buttock area (gluteal muscles)

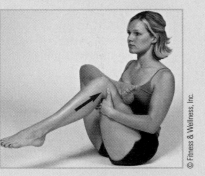

Exercise 20
Back Extension Stretch

Action Lie face down on the floor with the elbows by the chest, forearms on the floor, and the hands beneath the chin. Gently raise the trunk by extending the elbows until you reach an approximate 90° angle at the elbow joint. Be sure the forearms remain in contact with the floor at all times. DO NOT extend the back beyond this point. Hyperextension of the lower back may lead to or aggravate an existing back problem. Hold the stretched position for about 10 seconds.

Areas Stretched Abdominal region

Additional Benefits Restore lower back curvature

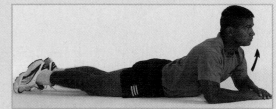

Exercise 21
Trunk Rotation and Lower Back Stretch

Action   Sit on the floor and bend the right leg, placing the right foot on the outside of the left knee. Place the left elbow on the right knee and push against it. At the same time, try to rotate the trunk to the right (clockwise). Hold the final position for a few seconds. Repeat the exercise with the other side.

Areas Stretched
Lateral side of the hip and thigh; trunk and lower back

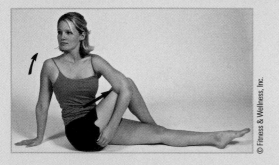

Exercise 24
Abdominal Crunch or Abdominal Curl-Up
(see Exercise 4 in Chapter 7, page 222)

It is important that you do not stabilize your feet when performing either of these exercises, because doing so decreases the work of the abdominal muscles. Also, remember not to "swing up" but, rather, to curl up as you perform these exercises.

Exercise 26
Supine Bridge

Action   Lie face up on the floor with the knees bent at about 120°. Do a pelvic tilt (Exercise 12, page 225) and maintain the pelvic tilt while you raise the hips off the floor until the upper body and upper legs are in a straight line. Hold this position for several seconds.

Areas Strengthened
Gluteal and abdominal flexor muscles

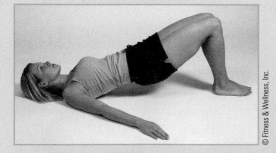

Exercise 22
Pelvic Tilt
(see Exercise 12 in Chapter 7, page 225)

Note:
This is perhaps the most important exercise for the care of the lower back. It should be included as a part of your daily exercise routine and should be performed several times throughout the day when pain in the lower back is present as a result of muscle imbalance.

Exercise 25
Reverse Crunch
(see Exercise 11 in Chapter 7, page 224)

Exercise 27
Pelvic Clock

Action   Lie face up on the floor with the knees bent at about 120°. Fully extend the hips as in the supine bridge (Exercise 26). Now progressively rotate the hips in a clockwise manner (2 o'clock, 4 o'clock, 6 o'clock, 8 o'clock, 10 o'clock, and 12 o'clock), holding each position in an isometric contraction for about 1 second. Repeat the exercise counterclockwise.

Areas Strengthened
Gluteal, abdominal, and hip flexor muscles

Exercise 28
Lateral Bridge
(see Exercise 13 in Chapter 7, page 225)

Exercise 23
The Cat

Action   Kneel on the floor and place your hands in front of you (on the floor) about shoulder-width apart. Relax your trunk and lower back (a). Now arch the spine and pull in your abdomen as far as you can and hold this position for a few seconds (b). Repeat the exercise 4–5 times.

Areas Stretched
Low back muscles and ligaments

Areas Strengthened
Abdominal and gluteal muscles

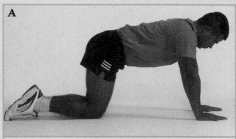

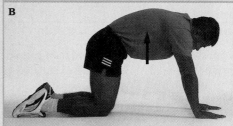

Exercise 29
Prone Bridge
(see Exercise 14 in Chapter 7, page 225)

Exercise 30
Leg Press
(see Exercise 16 in Chapter 7, page 226)

Exercise 31
Seated Back
(see Exercise 21 in Chapter 7, page 228)

Exercise 32
Lat Pull-Down
(see Exercise 23 in Chapter 7, page 229)

Exercise 33
Back Extension
(see Exercise 35 in Chapter 7, page 234)

Lab 8A

 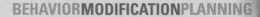

MUSCULAR FLEXIBILITY ASSESSMENT

Name: _____ Date: _____ Grade: _____

Instructor: _____ Course: _____ Section: _____

Necessary Lab Equipment

Acuflex I, Acuflex II, and Acuflex III Flexibility Testers*
or homemade flexibility testing equipment as described
in Figures 8.1, 8.2, and 8.3.

Objective

To assess muscular flexibility and the respective fitness
categories.

Lab Preparation

The procedures for the flexibility tests* administered in
this lab are explained in this Chapter (Figures 8.1, 8.2,
and 8.3, pages 242–245. It is important that you warm up
properly before you perform any of these tests. Do gentle
stretching exercises specific to the tests that will be
administered. Wear loose exercise clothing for this lab.
Be sure to circle either inches or cm, depending on which
system you use.

Profile Plus

I. Modified Sit-and-Reach Test (page 242)

Trials: 1. _____ inches _____ cm 2. _____ inches _____ cm (circle either inches or cm)

Average score: _____ inches _____ cm Percentile rank: _____ Points: _____

(Table 8.4, page 246)

Fitness category: _____

II. Total Body Rotation Test (pages 243–244)

Right Side   Left Side   (circle one)

Trials: 1. _____ inches _____ cm 2. _____ inches _____ cm (circle either inches or cm)

Average score: _____ inches _____ cm Percentile rank: _____ Points: _____

(Table 8.4, page 246)

Fitness category: _____

III. Shoulder Rotation Test (page 245)

Biacromial width: _____ inches _____ cm   Rotation score: _____ inches _____ cm

Final score = Rotation score − biacromial width

Final score = _____ − _____ = _____ inches / cm (circle one)   Percentile rank: _____

Fitness category: _____   Points: _____

(Table 8.4, page 246)

* The Acuflex I, II, and III Flexibility Testers can be obtained from Figure Finder Collection, Novel Products, Inc., P. O. Box 408, Rockton, IL 61072-0408,
Phone (800) 323-5143, Fax 815-624-4866.

IV. Overall Flexibility Rating

Test	Points
Modified sit-and-reach:	
Total body rotation (right, left — circle one):	
Shoulder rotation:	
Total Points:	

Overall flexibility category (see Table 8.5, page 246):

V. Flexibility Goals

1. Indicate the flexibility category that you would like to achieve by the end of the term:

2. Describe your feelings about your current body flexibility and any potential implications that your current flexibility levels may have on your health and wellness. Also, briefly state how you plan to achieve your flexibility objective by the end of the term.

Lab 8B

POSTURE EVALUATION

Name: _____ Date: _____ Grade: _____

Instructor: _____ Course: _____ Section: _____

Necessary Lab Equipment
A plumb line, two large mirrors set at about an 85° angle, and a Polaroid camera (the mirrors and the camera are optional—see "Evaluating Body Posture" (pages 244 and 246).

Objective
To determine current body alignment.

Lab Preparation
To conduct the posture analysis, men should wear shorts only and women, shorts and a tank top. Shoes should also be removed for this test.

Lab Assignment
The class should be divided in groups of four students each. The group should carefully study the posture form given in this lab, then proceed to fill out the form for each member according to the instructions given under "Evaluating Body Posture" (pages 244 and 246). If no mirrors and camera are available, three members of the group are to rate the fourth person's posture while he/she first stands with the side of the body and then with the back to the plumb line. A final score is obtained by totaling the points given for each body segment and looking up the posture rating according to the total score found in the table provided below.

Results

Total points: _____

Category: _____

Posture Evaluation Standards	
Total Points	**Category**
≥45	Excellent
40–44	Good
30–39	Average
20–29	Fair
≤19	Poor

Posture Improvement

Indicate how you feel about your posture, identify areas to correct, and specify the steps you can take to make those improvements.

_____
_____
_____
_____
_____
_____
_____
_____
_____

	Good — 5	Fair — 3	Poor — 1	Score
HEAD Left Right	head erect, gravity passes directly through center	head twisted or turned to one side slightly	head twisted or turned to one side markedly	
SHOULDERS Left Right	shoulders level horizontally	one shoulder slightly higher	one shoulder markedly higher	
SPINE Left Right	spine straight	spine slightly curved	spine markedly curved laterally	
HIPS Left Right	hips level horizontally	one hip slightly higher	one hip markedly higher	
KNEES and ANKLES	feet pointed straight ahead, legs vertical	feet pointed out, legs deviating outward at the knee	feet pointed out markedly, legs deviate markedly	
NECK and UPPER BACK	neck erect, head in line with shoulders, rounded upper back	neck slightly forward, chin out, slightly more rounded upper back	neck markedly forward, chin markedly out, markedly rounded upper back	
TRUNK	trunk erect	trunk inclined to rear slightly	trunk inclined to rear markedly	
ABDOMEN	abdomen flat	abdomen protruding	abdomen protruding and sagging	
LOWER BACK	lower back normally curved	lower back slightly hollow	lower back markedly hollow	
LEGS	legs straight	knees slightly hyper-extended	knees markedly hyperextended	
			Total Score	

Adapted from *The New York Physical Fitness Test: A Manual for Teachers of Physical Education,* New York State Education Department (Division of HPER), 1958.

Lab 8C

FLEXIBILITY DEVELOPMENT AND LOW-BACK CONDITIONING PROGRAMS

Name:		Date:		Grade:	
Instructor:		Course:		Section:	

Necessary Lab Equipment

Minor implements such as a chair, a table, an elastic band (surgical tubing or a wood or aluminum stick), and a stool or steps.

Objective

To develop a flexibility exercise program and a conditioning program for the prevention and rehabilitation of low-back pain.

Lab Preparation

Wear exercise clothing and prepare to participate in a sample stretching exercise session. All of the flexibility and low-back conditioning exercises are illustrated on pages 257–258.

I. Stage of Change for Flexibility Training

Using Figure 2.4 (page 41) and Table 2.3 (page 41), identify your current stage of change for participation in a muscular stretching program:

II. Instruction

Perform all of the recommended flexibility exercises given on pages 257–258. Use a combination of slow-sustained and proprioceptive neuromuscular facilitation stretching techniques. Indicate the technique(s) used for each exercise and, where applicable, the number of repetitions performed and the length of time that the final degree of stretch was held.

Stretching Exercises

Exercise	Stretching Technique	Repetitions	Length of Final Stretch
Lateral head tilt			NA*
Arm circles			NA
Side stretch			
Body rotation			
Chest stretch			
Shoulder hyperextension stretch			
Shoulder rotation stretch			NA
Quad stretch			
Heel cord stretch			
Adductor stretch			
Sitting adductor stretch			
Sit-and-reach stretch			
Triceps stretch			

*Not Applicable

Stretching Schedule (Indicate days, time, and place where you will stretch):

Flexibility-training days: M ☐ T ☐ W ☐ Th ☐ F ☐ Sa ☐ Su ☐   Time of day: ☐   Place: ☐

Low-Back Conditioning Program

Perform all of the recommended exercises for the prevention and rehabilitation of low-back pain given on pages 259–260. Indicate the number of repetitions performed for each exercise.

Flexibility Exercises	Repetitions		Strength/Endurance Exercises	Repetitions	Seconds Held
Hip flexors stretch	☐		Pelvic tilt	☐	☐
Single-knee-to-chest stretch	☐		The cat	☐	☐
Double-knee-to-chest stretch	☐		Abdominal crunch or abdominal curl-up	☐	
Upper- and lower-back stretch	☐		Reverse crunch	☐	
Sit-and-reach stretch	☐		Supine bridge	☐	☐
Gluteal stretch	☐		Pelvic clock	☐	☐
Back extension stretch	☐		Lateral bridge	☐	☐
Trunk rotation and lower back stretch	☐		Prone bridge	☐	☐
			Leg press	☐	
			Seated back	☐	
			Lat pull-down	☐	
			Back extension	☐	☐

Proper Body Mechanics

Perform the following tasks using the proper body mechanics given in Figure 8.7 (pages 253–254). Check off each item as you perform the task:

☐ Standing (carriage) position   ☐ Resting position for tired and painful back

☐ Sitting position   ☐ Lifting an object

☐ Bed posture

"Rules to Live By — From Now On"

Read the 18 "Rules to Live By—From Now On" given in Figure 8.7 (pages 253–254) and indicate below those rules that you need to work on to improve posture and body mechanics and prevent low-back pain.

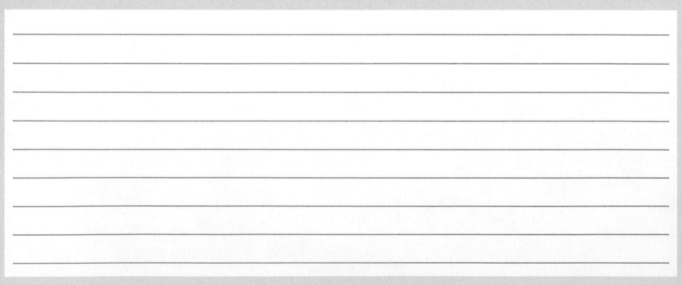

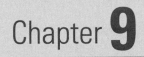

Chapter **9**

Skill Fitness and Fitness Programming

© John Kelly/The Image Bank/Getty Images

Objectives

- Enumerate the benefits of good skill-related fitness.
- Identify and define the six components of skill-related fitness.
- Describe performance tests to assess skill-related fitness.
- Dispel common misconceptions related to physical fitness and wellness.
- Become aware of safety considerations for exercise participation.
- Describe some common injuries and how to prevent and treat them.
- Explain the relationship between fitness and aging.
- Define and explain the concepts of interval training, overtraining, and periodization.

Profile Plus CD Connections

- Evaluate your skill-related fitness levels.
- Check how well you understand the chapter's concepts.

Skill-related fitness is important for successful motor performance in athletic events and in lifetime sports and activities such as basketball, racquetball, golf, hiking, soccer, and water skiing. Good skill-related fitness also enhances overall quality of life by helping people cope more effectively in emergency situations.

Outstanding gymnasts, for example, must achieve good skill-related fitness in all six components. A significant amount of *agility* is necessary to perform a double back somersault with a full twist—a skill during which the athlete must simultaneously rotate around one axis and twist around a different one. They must have good *balance*. Static balance is essential for maintaining a handstand or a scale. Dynamic balance is needed to perform many of the gymnastics routines (such as those on the balance beam, parallel bars, and pommel horse). *Coordination* is important to successfully integrate multiple skills, each with its own degree of difficulty, into one routine. *Power* and *speed* are needed to propel the body into the air, such as when tumbling or vaulting. Quick *reaction* time is necessary to determine when to end rotation upon a visual clue, such as spotting the floor on a dismount.

The principle of specificity of training applies to skill-related components just as it does to health-related fitness components. The development of agility, balance, coordination, and reaction time is highly task-specific. That is, to develop a certain task or skill, the individual must practice that same task many times. There seems to be very little crossover learning effect.

For instance, properly practicing a handstand (balance) will lead eventually to performing the skill successfully, but complete mastery of this skill does not ensure that the person will have immediate success when attempting to perform other static-balance positions in gymnastics. In contrast, power and speed may improve with a specific strength-training program or frequent repetition of the specific task to be improved, or both.

The rate of learning in skill-related fitness varies from person to person, mainly because these components seem to be determined to a large extent by genetics. Individuals with good skill-related fitness tend to do better and learn faster when performing a wide variety of skills, but few individuals enjoy complete success in all skill-related components. Although skill-related fitness can be enhanced with practice, improvements in reaction time and speed are limited and seem to be related to genetic endowment.

Benefits of Skill-Related Fitness

Although we do not know how much skill-related fitness is desirable, everyone should attempt to develop and maintain a better-than-average level.

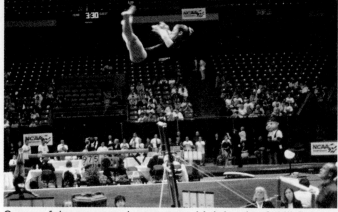
Successful gymnasts demonstrate high levels of skill-fitness.

As pointed out earlier, this type of fitness is crucial for athletes, and it also enables fitness participants to lead a better and happier life. Improving skill-related fitness affords an individual more enjoyment and success in lifetime sports (for example, tennis, racquetball, basketball) and also can help a person cope more effectively in emergency situations. Some of the benefits are as follows.

1. Good reaction time, balance, coordination, and/or agility can help you avoid a fall or break a fall and thereby minimize injury.
2. The ability to generate maximum force in a short time (power) may be crucial to ameliorate injury or even preserve life if you ever have to lift a heavy object that has fallen on another person or even on yourself.
3. In our society, where the average lifespan continues to expand, maintaining speed can be especially important for elderly people. Many of these individuals and, for that matter, many unfit/overweight young people no longer have the speed they need to cross an intersection safely before the light changes or run for help if someone else needs assistance.

Regular participation in a health-related fitness program can heighten performance of skill-related components. For example, significantly overweight people do not have good agility or speed. Because participating in aerobic and strength-training programs helps take off body fat, an overweight individual who loses weight through such an exercise program can improve agility and speed. A sound flexibility program decreases resistance to motion about body joints, which may increase agility, balance, and overall coordination. Improvements in strength definitely help develop power. People who have good

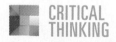

CRITICAL THINKING

If you are interested in health fitness, should you participate in skill-fitness activities? Explain the pros and cons of participating in skill-fitness activities. Should you participate in skill-fitness activities to get fit, or should you get fit to participate in skill-fitness activities?

skill-related fitness usually participate in lifetime sports and games, which in turn helps develop and/or maintain health-related fitness.

Performance Tests for Skill-Related Fitness

Several performance tests will assess the various components of skill-related fitness. Results of the performance tests, expressed in percentile ranks, are given in Table 9.1 (men) and Table 9.2 (women) on page 273. Fitness categories for skill-fitness components are established according to percentile rankings only. These rankings fall into categories that are similar to those given for muscular strength and endurance and for flexibility (see Table 9.3 on page 273).

Agility

Agility is the ability to quickly and efficiently change body position and direction. Agility is important in sports such as basketball, soccer, and racquetball, in which the participant must change direction rapidly and also maintain proper body control.

SEMO AGILITY TEST[1]

Objective
To measure general body agility

Procedure
The free-throw area of a basketball court or any other smooth area 12 feet by 19 feet with adequate running space around it can be used for this test. Four plastic cones or similar objects are needed, with one placed at each corner of the free-throw lane, as shown in Figure 9.1.

Start on the outside of the free-throw lane at point A, with your back to the free-throw line. When given the "go" command, sidestep from A to B (do not make crossover steps), backpedal from B to D, sprint forward from D to A, again backpedal from A to C, sprint forward from C to B, and sidestep from B to the finish line at A.

During the test, always go outside each corner cone. A stopwatch is started at the "go" command and stopped when you cross the finish line. Take a practice trial, and then use the best of two trials as the final test score. Record the time to the nearest tenth of a second.

Balance

The ability to maintain the body in proper equilibrium, **balance** is vital in activities such as gymnastics, diving, ice skating, skiing, and even football and wrestling, in which the athlete attempts to upset the opponent's equilibrium.

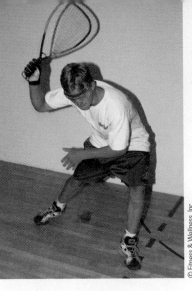

Good racquetball players have excellent agility.

© Fitness & Wellness, Inc.

FIGURE 9.1 Graphic depiction of the SEMO test for agility.

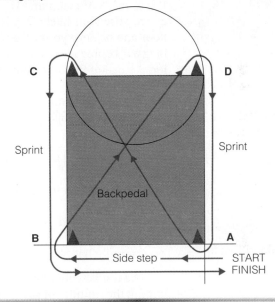

ONE-FOOT STAND TEST
(preferred foot, without shoes)

Objective
To measure the static balance of the participant

Procedure
A flat, smooth floor, not carpeted, is used for this test. Remove your shoes and socks and stand on

Skill-related fitness Fitness components important for success in skillful activities and athletic events; encompasses agility, balance, coordination, power, reaction time, and speed.

Agility Ability to change body position and direction quickly and efficiently.

Balance Ability to maintain the body in proper equilibrium.

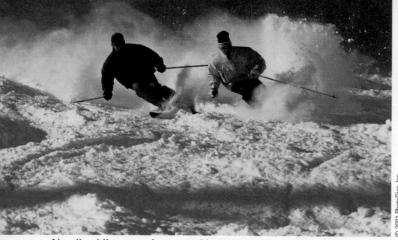

Nordic skiing requires good balance.

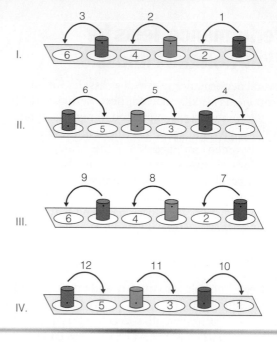

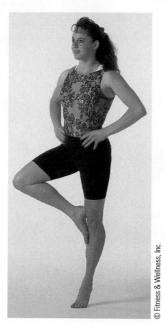

One-Foot Stand Test for balance.

your preferred foot, placing the other foot on the inside of the supporting knee, and the hands on the sides of the hips. When the "go" command is given, raise your heel off the floor and balance yourself as long as possible without moving the ball of the foot from its initial position.

The test is terminated when any of the following conditions occurs:

1. The supporting foot moves (shuffles).
2. The raised heel touches the floor.
3. The hands are moved from the hips.
4. A minute has elapsed.

The test is scored by recording the number of seconds that the testee maintains balance on the selected foot, starting with the "go" command. After a practice trial, use the best of two trials as the final performance score. Record the time to the nearest tenth of a second.

Coordination

Coordination integrates the nervous system and the muscular system to produce correct, graceful, and harmonious body movements. This component is important in a wide variety of motor activities such as golf, baseball, karate, soccer, and racquetball, in which hand–eye and/or foot–eye movements, or both, must be integrated.

SODA POP TEST

Objective
To assess overall motor/muscular control and movement time.

Procedure
Administrator: Homemade equipment is necessary to perform this test. Draw a straight line lengthwise through the center of a piece of cardboard approximately 32 inches long by 5 inches wide. Draw six marks exactly 5 inches away from each other on this line (draw the first mark about 2½ inches from the edge of the cardboard). Using a compass, draw six circles, each 3¼ inches in diameter (a radius of 1 centimeter larger than a can of soda pop), which must be centered on the six marks along the line. See Figure 9.2.

For the purpose of this test, each circle is assigned a number starting with 1 for the first circle on the right of the test taker and ending with 6 for the last circle on the left. The cardboard, three unopened (full) cans of soda pop, a table, a chair, and a stopwatch are needed to perform the test.

Place the cardboard on a table and have the person sit in front of it with the center of the cardboard bisecting the body. Use the preferred hand for this test. If this is the right hand, place the three cans of soda pop on the cardboard in the following manner: can one centered in circle 1 (farthest to the right), can two in circle 3, and can three in circle 5.

Participant: To start the test, place the right hand, with the thumb up, on can one with the elbow joint bent at about 100 percent to 120 percent. When the tester gives the signal and the stopwatch is started, turn the cans of soda pop upside

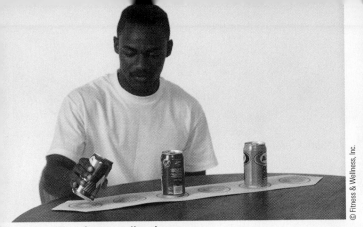

Soda Pop Test for coordination.

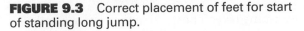

Fast starts in bob sleigh require exceptional leg power.

FIGURE 9.3 Correct placement of feet for start of standing long jump.

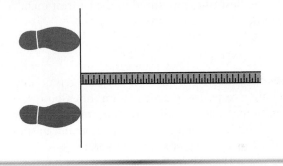

down, placing can one inside circle 2, followed by can two inside circle 4, and then can three inside circle 6. Immediately return all three cans, starting with can one, then can two, and can three, turning them right side up to their original placement. On this "return trip," grasp the cans with the hand in a thumb-down position.

The entire procedure is done twice, without stopping, and is counted as one trial. Two "trips" down and up are required to complete one trial. The watch is stopped when the last can of soda pop is returned to its original position, following the second trip back. The preferred hand (in this case, the right hand) is used throughout the entire task, and the objective of the test is to perform the task as fast as possible, making sure the cans are always placed within each circle.

If the person misses a circle at any time during the test (that is, if a can is placed on a line or outside a circle), the trial must be repeated from the start.

If using the left hand, the participant follows the same procedure, except the cans are placed starting from the left, with can one in circle 6, can two in circle 4, and can three in circle 2. The procedure is initiated by turning can one upside down onto circle 5, can two onto circle 3, and so on.

Prior to initiating the test, two practice trials are allowed. Two test trials then are administered, and the best time, recorded to the nearest tenth of a second, is used as the test score. If the person has a mistrial (misses a circle), the test is repeated until two consecutive successful trials are accomplished.

Power

Power is defined as the ability to produce maximum force in the shortest time. The two components of power are speed and force (strength). An effective combination of these two components allows a person to produce explosive movements such as in jumping, putting the shot, and spiking/throwing/ hitting a ball.

Power is necessary to perform many activities of daily living that require strength and speed, such as climbing stairs, lifting objects, preventing falls, or hurrying to catch a bus. Power is also beneficial in sports such as soccer, tennis, softball, golf, and volleyball.

STANDING LONG JUMP TEST[2]

Objective
To measure leg power

Procedure
Administrator: Draw a takeoff line on the floor, and place a 10-foot-long tape measure perpendicular to this line. Have the participant stand with the feet several inches apart, centered on the tape measure, and toes just behind the takeoff line (see Figure 9.3).

Participant: Prior to the jump, swing your arms backward and bend your knees. Perform the jump by extending your knees and swinging your arms forward at the same time.

The distance is recorded from the takeoff line to the heel or other body part that touches the floor

Coordination The integration of the nervous and the muscular systems to produce correct, graceful, and harmonious body movements.

Power The ability to produce maximum force in the shortest time.

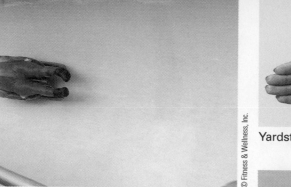

Luge athletes exhibit excellent reaction time and coordination.

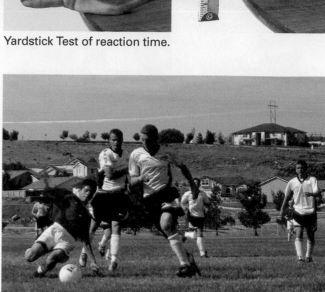

Yardstick Test of reaction time.

Speed is essential in the sport of soccer.

nearest the takeoff line. Three trials are allowed, and the best trial, measured to the nearest inch, becomes the final test score.

Reaction Time

Reaction time is defined as the time required to initiate a response to a given stimulus. Good reaction time is important for starts in track and swimming, when playing tennis at the net, and in sports such as ping pong, boxing, and karate.

YARDSTICK TEST
(preferred hand)

Objective

To measure hand reaction time in response to a visual stimulus

Procedure

Administrator: For this test you will need a regular yardstick with a shaded "concentration zone" marked on the first 2 inches of the stick (see photo). Administer the test with the participant sitting in a chair adjacent to a table and the preferred forearm and hand resting on the table.

Participant: Hold the tips of the thumb and fingers in a "ready-to-pinch" position, about 1 inch apart and 3 inches beyond the edge of the table, with the upper edges of the thumb and index finger parallel to the floor. With the person administering the test holding the yardstick near the upper end and the zero point of the stick even with the upper edge of your thumb and index finger (the administrator may steady the middle of the stick with the other hand), look at the "concentration zone" and react by catching the stick when it is dropped. Do not look at the administrator's hand or move your hand up or down while trying to catch the stick.

Twelve trials make up the test, each preceded by the preparatory command "ready." The administrator makes a random 1- to 3-second count between the "ready" command and each drop of the stick. Each trial is scored to the nearest half inch, read just above the upper edge of the thumb. Three

practice trials are given before the actual test to be sure the person understands the procedure. The three lowest and the three highest scores are discarded, and the average of the middle six is used as the final test score. The testing area should be as free from distractions as possible.

Speed

Speed is the ability to rapidly propel the body or a part of the body from one point to another. Examples of activities that require good speed for success are soccer, basketball, sprints in track, and stealing a base in baseball. In everyday life, speed can be important in a wide variety of emergency situations.

50-YARD DASH[3]

Objective

To measure speed

Procedure

Two participants take their positions behind the starting line. The starter raises one arm and asks, "Are you ready?" and then gives the command "go" while swinging the raised arm downward as a signal for the timer (or timers) at the finish line to start the stopwatch (or stopwatches).

The score is the time that elapses between the starting signal and the moment the participant crosses the finish line, recorded to the nearest tenth of a second.

TABLE 9.1 Percentile Ranks and Fitness Category for Skill-Related Fitness Components—Men

	Agility*	Balance*	Coordination*	Power**	Reaction Time*	Speed**
99	9.5	59.8	5.8	9'10"	3.5	5.4
95	10.3	46.9	7.5	8'5"	4.2	5.9
90	10.6	41.1	7.7	8'2"	4.5	6.0
80	11.1	24.9	8.5	7'10"	4.9	6.3
70	11.5	15.4	8.9	7'7"	5.3	6.4
60	11.7	12.0	9.3	7'5"	5.5	6.5
50	11.9	9.2	9.6	7'2"	5.8	6.6
40	12.1	7.3	9.9	7'0"	6.1	6.8
30	12.4	5.8	10.2	6'8"	6.5	7.0
20	12.9	4.3	10.7	6'4"	6.7	7.1
10	13.7	3.1	11.3	5'10"	7.2	7.5
5	14.0	2.6	11.8	5'3"	7.4	7.9

*Norms developed at Boise State University, Department of Kinesiology.

**From *AAHPERD Youth Fitness: Test Manual.* 1976.

TABLE 9.2 Percentile Ranks and Fitness Category for Skill-Related Fitness Components—Women

	Agility*	Balance*	Coordination*	Power**	Reaction Time*	Speed**
99	11.1	59.9	7.5	7'6"	3.3	6.4
95	12.0	39.1	8.0	6'9"	4.5	6.8
90	12.2	25.8	8.2	6'6"	4.7	7.0
80	12.5	16.7	8.6	6'2"	5.1	7.3
70	12.9	11.9	9.0	5'11"	5.3	7.5
60	13.2	9.8	9.2	5'9"	5.9	7.6
50	13.4	7.6	9.5	5'5"	6.1	7.9
40	13.9	6.2	9.6	5'3"	6.4	8.0
30	14.2	5.0	9.9	5'0"	6.7	8.2
20	14.8	4.2	10.3	4'9"	7.2	8.5
10	15.5	2.9	10.7	4'4"	7.8	9.0
5	16.2	1.8	11.2	4'1"	8.4	9.5

*Norms developed at Boise State University, Department of Kinesiology.

**From *AAHPERD Youth Fitness: Test Manual.* 1976.

Interpreting Test Results

Look up your score for each test in Table 9.1 or 9.2, then use Table 9.3 to see your level of fitness in that skill.

Specific Exercise Considerations

In addition to the exercise-related issues already discussed in this book, many other concerns require clarification or are somewhat controversial. Let's examine some of these issues.

1. Does aerobic exercise make a person immune to heart and blood vessel disease?

Although aerobically fit individuals as a whole have a lower incidence of cardiovascular disease, a regular aerobic exercise program by itself does not offer an absolute guarantee against cardiovascular disease. Overall management of the risk factors is the best way to minimize the risk for cardiovascular disease. Many factors, including a genetic predisposition, can increase the person's risk. In any case, experts believe that a regular aerobic exercise program will delay the onset of cardiovascular problems and also will improve the chances of surviving a heart attack.

Even moderate increases in aerobic fitness significantly lower the incidence of premature deaths from cardiovascular diseases. Data from the research study on death rates by physical fitness groups (illustrated in Chapter 1) indicate that the decrease in cardiovascular mortality is greatest between the

TABLE 9.3 Skill-Fitness Categories

Percentile Rank	Fitness Category
≥81	Excellent
61–80	Good
41–60	Average
21–40	Fair
≤20	Poor

unfit and the moderately fit groups. A further decrease in cardiovascular mortality is observed between the moderately fit and the highly fit groups, although the difference is not as pronounced as that between the unfit and the moderately fit groups.

2. How much aerobic exercise is required to decrease the risk for cardiovascular disease?

Even though research has not yet indicated the exact amount of aerobic exercise required to lower the risk for cardiovascular disease, some general recommendations have been set forth. In their study, Dr. Ralph Paffenbarger and his co-researchers showed that expending 2,000 calories per week as a result of physical activity yielded the lowest risk for cardiovascular disease among a group of almost 17,000 Harvard alumni.[4] The expenditure of 2,000

Reaction time The time required to initiate a response to a given stimulus.

Speed The ability to propel the body or a part of the body rapidly from one point to another.

calories per week represents about 300 calories per daily exercise session.

3. Do people get a "physical high" during aerobic exercise?

During vigorous exercise, **endorphins** are released from the pituitary gland in the brain. Endorphins can create feelings of euphoria and natural well-being. Higher levels of endorphins often result from aerobic endurance activities and may remain elevated for as long as 30 to 60 minutes following exercise. Many experts believe these higher levels explain the physical high that some people get during and after prolonged exercise.

Endorphin levels have also been shown to increase during pregnancy and childbirth. Endorphins act as painkillers. The higher levels could explain a woman's greater tolerance for the pain and discomfort of natural childbirth and her pleasant feelings shortly after the baby's birth. Several reports have indicated that well-conditioned women have shorter and easier labor. These women may attain higher endorphin levels during delivery, making childbirth less traumatic than it is for untrained women.

4. Can people with asthma exercise?

Asthma, a condition that causes difficulty in breathing, is characterized by coughing, wheezing, and shortness of breath induced by narrowing of the airway passages because of contraction (bronchospasm) of the airway muscles, swelling of the mucous membrane, and excessive secretion of mucus. In a few people, asthma can be triggered by exercise itself, particularly in cool and dry environments. This type of condition is referred to as *exercise-induced asthma* (EIA).

People with asthma need to obtain proper medication from a physician prior to initiating an exercise program. A regular program is best, because random exercise bouts are more likely to trigger asthma attacks. In the initial stages of exercise, an intermittent program (with frequent rest periods during the exercise session) is recommended. Gradual warm-up and cool-down are also essential to reduce the risk of an acute attack. Furthermore, exercising in warm and humid conditions (such as swimming) is better because it helps to moisten the airways and thus minimizes the asthmatic response. For land-based activities (such as walking or aerobics), drinking water before, during, and after exercise helps to keep the airways moist, decreasing the risk of an attack. During the winter months, wearing an exercise mask is recommended to increase warmth and humidity of inhaled air. People with asthma should not exercise alone and should always carry their medication with them during workouts.

5. What types of activities are recommended for people with arthritis?

Individuals who have arthritis should participate in a combined stretching, aerobic, and strength-

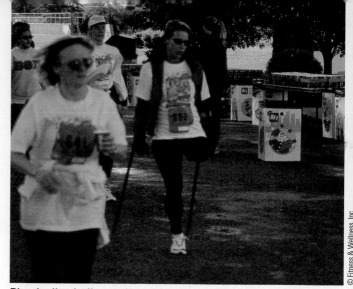

Physically challenged people can participate in and derive health and fitness benefits from a high-intensity exercise program.

© Fitness & Wellness, Inc.

training program. Mild stretching should be performed prior to aerobic exercise to relax tight muscles. A regular flexibility program following aerobic exercise is encouraged to help maintain good joint mobility. During the aerobic portion of the exercise program, people with arthritis should avoid high-impact activities, because they may cause greater trauma to arthritic joints. Low-impact activities such as swimming, water aerobics, or cycling are recommended. A complete strength-training program is also recommended, with special emphasis on exercises that will help support the affected joint(s). As with any other program, individuals with arthritis should start with low intensity or resistance and build up gradually to a higher fitness level.

6. What precautions should diabetics take with respect to exercise?

According to the Centers for Disease Control and Prevention, there were more than 18 million reported diabetics in the United States in 2004 and more than 1 million new cases are diagnosed each year. At the current rate, one in three children born in the United States will develop the disease. There are two types of diabetes:

■ type 1, or insulin-dependent diabetes (IDDM)
■ type 2, or non–insulin-dependent diabetes (NIDDM).

In type 1, found primarily in young people, the pancreas produces little or no insulin. With type 2, the pancreas may not produce enough insulin or the cells become insulin-resistant, thereby keeping glucose from entering the cell. Type 2 accounts for more than 90 percent of all diabetes cases, and it occurs mainly in overweight people. (A more thorough discussion of the types of diabetes is given in Chapter 11.)

If you have diabetes, consult your physician before you start exercising. You may not be able to start until the diabetes is under control. Never exercise alone, and always wear a bracelet that identifies your condition. If you take insulin, the amount and timing of each dose may have to be regulated with your physician. If you inject insulin, do so over a muscle that won't be exercised, then wait an hour before exercising. For type 1 diabetics, it is recommended that you ingest 15 to 30 grams of carbohydrates during each 30 minutes of intense exercise and follow it with a carbohydrate snack after exercise.

Both types of diabetes improve with exercise, although the results are more notable in patients with type 2 diabetes. Exercise usually lowers blood sugar and helps the body use food more effectively. The degree to which blood glucose level can be controlled in overweight type 2 diabetics seems to be directly related to how long and how hard a person exercises. Normal or near-normal blood glucose levels can be achieved through a proper exercise program.

As with any fitness program, the exercise must be done regularly to be effective against diabetes. The benefits of a single exercise bout on blood glucose are highest between 12 and 24 hours following exercise. These benefits are completely lost within 72 hours after exercise. Thus, regular participation is crucial to derive ongoing benefits. In terms of fitness, all diabetic patients can achieve higher fitness levels, including reductions in weight, blood pressure, and total cholesterol and triglycerides.

According to the ACSM, patients with type 2 diabetes should adhere to the following guidelines to make their exercise program safe and derive the most benefit:[5]

- Expend a minimum of 1,000 calories per week through your exercise program.
- Exercise at a low-to-moderate intensity (40 to 70 percent of HRR). Start your program with 10 to 15 minutes per session, on at least 3 nonconsecutive days, but preferably exercise 5 days per week. Gradually increase the time you exercise to 30 minutes until you achieve your goal of at least 1,000 calories weekly. Diabetic individuals with a weight problem should build up daily physical activity to 60 minutes per session.
- Choose an activity that you enjoy doing and stay with it. As you select your activity, be aware of your condition. For example, if you have lost sensation in your feet, swimming or stationary cycling is better than walking or jogging to minimize the risk for injury.
- Check blood glucose levels before and after exercise. If you are on insulin or diabetes medication, monitor blood glucose regularly and

TABLE 9.4 Contraindications to Exercise During Pregnancy

Stop exercise and seek medical advice if you experience any of the following symptoms:

- Unusual pain or discomfort, especially in the chest or abdominal area
- Cramping, primarily in the pelvic or lower back areas
- Muscle weakness, excessive fatigue, or shortness of breath
- Abnormally high heart rate or a pounding (palpitations) heart rate
- Decreased fetal movement
- Insufficient weight gain
- Amniotic fluid leakage
- Nausea, dizziness, or headaches
- Persistent uterine contractions
- Vaginal bleeding or rupture of the membranes
- Swelling of ankles, calves, hands, or face

check it at least twice within 30 minutes of starting exercise.
- Schedule your exercise 1 to 3 hours after a meal, and avoid exercise when your insulin is peaking.
- Be ready to treat low blood sugar with a fast-acting source of sugar, such as juice, raisins, or other source recommended by your doctor.
- Discontinue exercise immediately if you feel that a reaction is about to occur. Check your blood glucose level and treat the condition as needed.
- When you exercise outdoors, always do so with someone who knows what to do in a diabetes-related emergency.

In addition, strength training twice per week, using 8 to 10 exercises with a minimum of one set of 10 to 15 repetitions to near fatigue, is recommended for individuals with diabetes. A complete description of strength-training programs is provided in Chapter 7.

7. Is exercise safe during pregnancy?

Exercise is beneficial during pregnancy. According to the American College of Obstetricians and Gynecologists (ACOG), in the absence of contraindications, healthy pregnant women are encouraged to participate in regular moderate-intensity physical activities to continue to derive health benefits during pregnancy.[6] Pregnant women, however, should consult with their respective physicians to ensure that there are no contraindications to exercise during pregnancy (see Table 9.4).

Endorphins Morphine-like substances released from the pituitary gland (in the brain) during prolonged aerobic exercise; thought to induce feelings of euphoria and natural well-being.

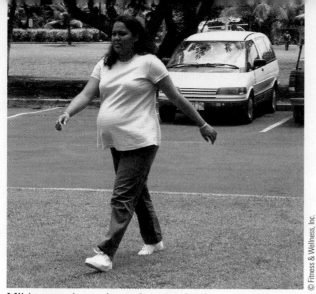

Mild-to-moderate intensity exercise is recommended throughout pregnancy.

As a general rule, healthy pregnant women can also accumulate 30 minutes of moderate-intensity physical activity on most, if not all, days of the week. Physical activity strengthens the body and helps prepare for the challenges of labor and childbirth.

The average labor and delivery lasts 10–12 hours. In most cases, labor and delivery are highly intense, with repeated muscular contractions interspersed with short rest periods. Proper conditioning will better prepare the body for childbirth. Moderate exercise during pregnancy also helps to prevent back pain and excessive weight gain, and it speeds up recovery following childbirth.

The most common recommendations for exercise during pregnancy for healthy pregnant women with no additional risk factors are as follows:

- Do not start a new or more rigorous exercise program without proper medical clearance.
- Accumulate 30 minutes of moderate-intensity physical activities on most days of the week.
- Instead of using heart rate to monitor intensity, exercise at an intensity level between "fairly light" and "somewhat hard," using the Rate of Perceived Exertion (RPE) scale in Chapter 6 (see page 175).
- Gradually switch from weight-bearing and high-impact activities such as jogging and aerobics, to nonweight-bearing/lower-impact activities such as walking, stationary cycling, swimming, and water aerobics. The latter activities minimize the risk of injury and may allow exercise to continue throughout pregnancy.
- Avoid exercising at an altitude above 6,000 feet (1,800 meters); and scuba diving may compromise availability of oxygen to the fetus.
- Women who are accustomed to strenuous exercise may continue in the early stages of pregnancy but should gradually decrease the amount, intensity,

and exercise mode as pregnancy advances (most healthy pregnant women, however, slow down during the first few weeks of pregnancy until morning sickness and fatigue subside).

- Pay attention to the body's signals of discomfort and distress, and never exercise to exhaustion. When fatigued, slow down or take a day off. Do not stop exercising altogether unless you experience any of the contraindications for exercise listed in Table 9.4.
- To prevent fetal injury, avoid activities that involve potential contact, loss of balance, or cause even mild trauma to the abdomen. Examples of these activities are basketball, soccer, volleyball, Nordic or water skiing, ice skating, road cycling, horseback riding, and motorcycle riding.
- Do not exercise for weight-loss purposes during pregnancy.
- Get proper nourishment (pregnancy requires between 150 and 300 extra calories per day), and eat a small snack or drink some juice 20 to 30 minutes prior to exercise.
- Prevent dehydration by drinking a cup of fluids 20 to 30 minutes before exercise, and drink 1 cup of liquid every 15 to 20 minutes during exercise.
- During the first 3 months in particular, do not exercise in the heat. Wear clothing that allows for proper dissipation of heat. A body temperature above 102.6°F (39.2°C) can harm the fetus.
- After the first trimester, avoid exercises that require lying on the back. This position can block blood flow to the uterus and the baby.
- Perform stretching exercises gently because hormonal changes during pregnancy increase the laxity of muscles and connective tissue. Although these changes facilitate delivery, they also make women more susceptible to injuries during exercise.

8. Does exercise help relieve dysmenorrhea?

Even though exercise has not been shown to either cure or aggravate **dysmenorrhea**, it has been shown to relieve menstrual cramps because it improves circulation to the uterus. Less severe menstrual cramps also could be related to higher levels of endorphins produced during prolonged physical activity, which may counteract pain. Particularly, stretching exercises of the muscles in the pelvic region seem to reduce and prevent painful menstruation that is not the result of disease.[7]

9. Does participation in exercise hinder menstruation?

In some instances, highly trained athletes develop **amenorrhea** during training and competition. This condition is seen most often in extremely lean women who also engage in sports that require strenuous physical effort over a sustained time. It is by no means irreversible. At present, we do not know whether the condition is caused by physical or emotional stress related to high-intensity training, excessively low body fat, or other factors.

Although, on the average, women have a lower physical capacity during menstruation, medical surveys at the Olympic games have shown that women have broken Olympic and world records at all stages of the menstrual cycle. Menstruation should not keep a woman from exercising, and it will not necessarily have a negative impact on performance.

10. Does exercise offset the detrimental effects of cigarette smoking?

Physical exercise often motivates a person to stop smoking, but it does not offset any ill effects of smoking. Smoking greatly decreases the ability of the blood to transport oxygen to working muscles.

Oxygen is carried in the circulatory system by hemoglobin, the iron-containing pigment of the red blood cells. Carbon monoxide, a byproduct of cigarette smoke, has 210 to 250 times greater affinity for hemoglobin over oxygen. Consequently, carbon monoxide combines much faster with hemoglobin, decreasing the oxygen-carrying capacity of the blood.

Chronic smoking also increases airway resistance, requiring the respiratory muscles to work much harder and consume more oxygen just to ventilate a given amount of air. If a person quits smoking, exercise does help increase the functional capacity of the pulmonary system.

A regular exercise program seems to be a powerful incentive to quit smoking. A random survey of 1,250 runners conducted at the 6.2-mile Peachtree Road Race in Atlanta provided impressive results. The survey indicated that, of the men and women who smoked cigarettes when they started running, 81 percent and 75 percent, respectively, had quit before the date of the race.

11. How long should a person wait after a meal before exercising strenuously?

The length of time to wait before exercising after a meal depends on the amount of food eaten. On the average, after a regular meal, you should wait about 2 hours before participating in strenuous physical activity. A walk or some other light physical activity is fine following a meal, though. If anything, it helps burn extra calories and may help the body metabolize fats more efficiently.

12. What type of clothing should I wear when I exercise?

The type of clothing you wear during exercise is important. In general, clothing should fit comfortably and allow free movement of the various body parts. Select clothing according to air temperature, humidity, and exercise intensity. Avoid nylon and rubberized materials and tight clothes that interfere with the cooling mechanism of the human body or obstruct normal blood flow. Choose fabrics made of polypropylene, Capilene, Thermax, or any synthetic

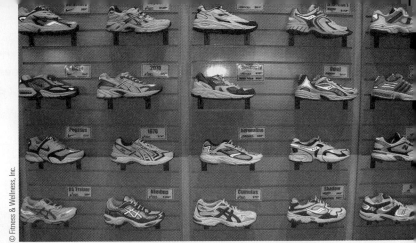

© Fitness & Wellness, Inc.

Activity-specific shoes are recommended to prevent lower-extremity injuries.

that draws (wicks) moisture away from the skin, enhancing evaporation and cooling of the body. It's also important to consider your exercise intensity, because the harder you exercise, the more heat your body produces.

When exercising in the heat, avoid the hottest time of the day—between 11:00 A.M. and 5:00 P.M. Surfaces such as asphalt, concrete, and artificial turf absorb heat, which then radiates to the body. Therefore, these surfaces are not recommended. (Also see the discussion about heat and humidity in Question 14, pages 278–279.)

Only a minimal amount of clothing is necessary during exercise in the heat, to allow for maximal evaporation. Clothing should be lightweight, light-colored, loose-fitting, airy, and absorbent. Examples of commercially available products that can be used during exercise in the heat are Asic's Perma Plus, Cool-max, and Nike's Dri-F.I.T. Double-layer acrylic socks are more absorbent than cotton and help to prevent blistering and chafing of the feet. A straw-type hat can be worn to protect the eyes and head from the sun. (Clothing for exercise in the cold is discussed in Question 16, page 280.)

A good pair of shoes is vital to prevent injuries to lower limbs. Shoes manufactured specifically for your choice of activity are a must (see Figure 9.4). When selecting proper footwear, you should consider body type, tendency toward pronation (rotating foot outward) or supination (rotating foot inward), and exercise surfaces. Shoes should have good stability, motion control, and comfortable fit. Purchase shoes in the middle of the day when your feet have expanded and might be one-half size larger. For increased breathability, choose shoes with nylon or mesh uppers. Generally, salespeople at reputable

Dysmenorrhea Painful menstruation.

Amenorrhea Cessation of regular menstrual flow.

FIGURE 9.4 What to look for in a good pair of shoes.

Choosing the Right Shoe

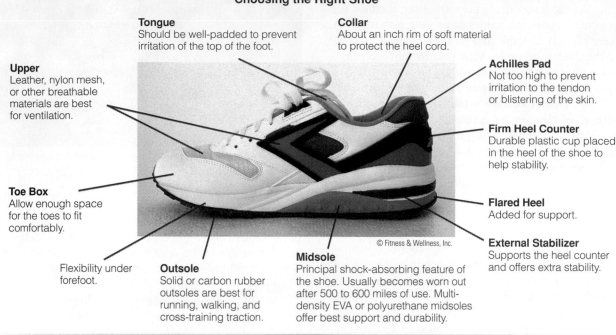

Tongue
Should be well-padded to prevent irritation of the top of the foot.

Collar
About an inch rim of soft material to protect the heel cord.

Upper
Leather, nylon mesh, or other breathable materials are best for ventilation.

Achilles Pad
Not too high to prevent irritation to the tendon or blistering of the skin.

Firm Heel Counter
Durable plastic cup placed in the heel of the shoe to help stability.

Toe Box
Allow enough space for the toes to fit comfortably.

Flared Heel
Added for support.

External Stabilizer
Supports the heel counter and offers extra stability.

© Fitness & Wellness, Inc.

Flexibility under forefoot.

Outsole
Solid or carbon rubber outsoles are best for running, walking, and cross-training traction.

Midsole
Principal shock-absorbing feature of the shoe. Usually becomes worn out after 500 to 600 miles of use. Multi-density EVA or polyurethane midsoles offer best support and durability.

---

athletic shoe stores are knowledgeable and can help you select a good shoe that fits your needs. After 300 to 500 miles or 6 months, examine your shoes and obtain a new pair if they are worn out. Old shoes are frequently responsible for injuries to the lower limbs.

13. What time of the day is best for exercise?

You can do intense exercise almost any time of the day, with the exception of about 2 hours following a heavy meal or the mid-day and early afternoon hours on hot, humid days. Moderate exercise seems to be beneficial shortly after a meal, because exercise enhances the **thermogenic response**. A walk shortly after a meal burns more calories than a walk several hours after a meal.

Many people enjoy exercising early in the morning because it gives them a boost to start the day. People who exercise in the morning also seem to stick with it more than others, because the chances of putting off the exercise session for other reasons are minimized. Some prefer the lunch hour for weight-control reasons. By exercising at noon, they do not eat as big a lunch, which helps keep down the daily caloric intake. Highly stressed people seem to like the evening hours because of the relaxing effects of exercise.

14. Why is exercising in hot and humid conditions unsafe?

When a person exercises, only 30 to 40 percent of the energy the body produces is used for mechanical work or movement. The rest of the energy (60 to 70 percent) is converted into heat. If this heat cannot be dissipated properly because the weather is too hot or the relative humidity is too high, body temperature increases and, in extreme cases, it can result in death.

The specific heat of body tissue (the heat required to raise the temperature of the body by 1 degree C) is .38 calories per pound of body weight (.38 cal/lb). This indicates that if no body heat is dissipated, a 150-pound person has to burn only 57 calories (150 × .38) to increase total body temperature by 1 degree C. If this person were to conduct an exercise session requiring 300 calories (e.g., running about 3 miles) without any heat dissipation, the inner body temperature would increase by 5.3° C, which is the equivalent of going from 98.6° F to 108.1° F.

This example illustrates clearly the need for caution when exercising in hot or humid weather. If the relative humidity is too high, body heat cannot be lost through evaporation because the atmosphere already is saturated with water vapor. In one instance, a football casualty occurred when the temperature was only 64 degrees F—but the relative humidity was 100 percent. People must be cautious when air temperature is above 90° F and the relative humidity is above 60 percent.

The American College of Sports Medicine recommends avoiding strenuous physical activity when the readings of a wet-bulb globe thermometer exceed

SYMPTOMS OF HEAT ILLNESS

If any of these symptoms occur, stop physical activity, get out of the sun, and start drinking fluids.

- ■ Decreased perspiration
- ■ Cramping
- ■ Weakness
- ■ Flushed skin
- ■ Throbbing head
- ■ Nausea/vomiting
- ■ Diarrhea
- ■ Numbness in the extremities
- ■ Blurred vision
- ■ Unsteadiness
- ■ Disorientation
- ■ Incoherency

82.4° F. With this type of thermometer, the wet bulb is cooled by evaporation, and on dry days it shows a lower temperature than the regular (dry) thermometer. On humid days, the cooling effect is less because of less evaporation; hence, the difference between the wet and dry readings is not as great.

Following are descriptions of, and first-aid measures for, the three major signs of heat illness:

- ■ **Heat cramps**. Symptoms include cramps, spasms, and muscle twitching in the legs, arms, and abdomen. To relieve heat cramps, stop exercising, get out of the heat, massage the painful area, stretch slowly, and drink plenty of fluids (water, fruit drinks, or electrolyte beverages).
- ■ **Heat exhaustion**. Symptoms include fainting; dizziness; profuse sweating; cold, clammy skin; weakness; headache; and a rapid, weak pulse. If you incur any of these symptoms, stop and find a cool place to rest. If conscious, drink cool water. Do not give water to an unconscious person. Loosen or remove clothing, and rub your body with a cool, wet towel or apply ice packs. Place yourself in a supine position with the legs elevated 8 to 12 inches. If you are not fully recovered in 30 minutes, seek immediate medical attention.
- ■ **Heat stroke**. Symptoms include serious disorientation; warm, dry skin; no sweating; rapid, full pulse; vomiting; diarrhea; unconsciousness; and high body temperature. As the body temperature climbs, unexplained anxiety sets in. When the body temperature reaches 104° F to 105° F, the individual may feel a cold sensation in the trunk of the body, goosebumps, nausea, throbbing in the temples, and numbness in the extremities. Most people become incoherent after this stage. When body temperature reaches 105° F to 107° F, disorientation, loss of fine-motor control, and

muscular weakness set in. If the temperature exceeds 106° F, serious neurologic injury and death may be imminent.

Heat stroke requires immediate emergency medical attention. Request help and get out of the sun and into a cool, humidity-controlled environment. While you are waiting to be taken to the hospital emergency room, you should be placed in a semi-seated position and your body should be sprayed with cool water and rubbed with cool towels. If possible, cold packs should be placed in areas that receive an abundant blood supply, such as the head, neck, armpits, and groin. Fluids should not be given if you are unconscious. In any case of heat-related illness, if the person refuses water, vomits, or starts to lose consciousness, call for an ambulance immediately. Proper initial treatment of heat stroke is critical.

15. What should a person do to replace fluids lost during prolonged aerobic exercise?

The main objective of fluid replacement during prolonged aerobic exercise is to maintain the blood volume so circulation and sweating can continue at normal levels. Adequate water replacement is the most important factor in preventing heat disorders. Drinking about 6 to 8 ounces of cool water every 15 to 20 minutes during exercise is ideal to prevent dehydration. Cold fluids seem to be absorbed more rapidly from the stomach.

Other relevant points are the following:

- ■ Drinking commercially prepared sports drinks is recommended when exercise will be strenuous and carried out for more than an hour. For exercise lasting less than an hour, water is just as effective in replacing lost fluid. The sports drinks you select may be based on your personal preference. Try different drinks at 6 to 8 percent glucose concentration to see which drink you tolerate best and suits your tastes as well.
- ■ Commercial fluid-replacement solutions (such as Powerade® and Gatorade®) contain about 6 to 8 percent glucose, which seems to be optimal for fluid absorption and performance. Sugar does not become available to the muscles until about 30 minutes after a glucose solution is consumed.
- ■ Drinks high in fructose or with a glucose concentration above 8 percent are not recommended

Thermogenic response Amount of energy required to digest food.

Heat cramps Muscle spasms caused by heat-induced changes in electrolyte balance in muscle cells.

Heat exhaustion Heat-related fatigue.

Heat stroke Emergency situation resulting from the body being subjected to high atmospheric temperatures.

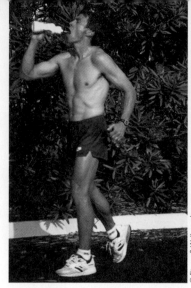

Fluid and carbohydrate replacement are essential when exercising in the heat or for a prolonged period.

© Fitness & Wellness, Inc.

because they slow down water absorption when exercising in the heat.

■ Most sodas (both cola, non-cola) contain between 10 and 12 percent glucose, which is too high for proper rehydration during exercise in the heat.

16. What precautions must a person take when exercising in the cold?

When exercising in the cold, the two factors to consider are frostbite and **hypothermia**. In contrast to hot and humid conditions, cold weather usually does not threaten health because clothing can be selected for heat conservation, and exercise itself increases the production of body heat.

Most people actually overdress for exercise in the cold. Because exercise increases body temperature, a moderate workout on a cold day makes a person feel that the temperature is 20 to 30 degrees warmer than it actually is. Overdressing for exercise can make the clothes damp from excessive perspiration. The risk for hypothermia increases when a person is wet or after exercise stops—when the person is not moving around sufficiently to increase (or maintain) body heat.

Initial warning signs of hypothermia include shivering, loss of coordination, and difficulty speaking. With a continued drop in body temperature, shivering stops, the muscles weaken and stiffen, and the person has feelings of elation or intoxication and eventually loses consciousness. To prevent hypothermia, use common sense, dress properly, and be aware of environmental conditions.

The popular belief that exercising in cold temperatures (32° F and lower) freezes the lungs is false, because the air is warmed properly in the air passages before it reaches the lungs. Cold is not what poses a threat; wind velocity is what increases the chill factor most.

For example, exercising at a temperature of 25° F with adequate clothing is not too cold to exercise, but if the wind is blowing at 25 miles per hour, the chill factor lowers the actual temperature to 15° F. This effect is even worse if a person is wet and exhausted. When the weather is windy, the individual should exercise (jog or cycle) against the wind on the way out and with the wind upon returning.

Even though the lungs are under no risk when you exercise in the cold, your face, head, hands, and feet should be protected, because they are subject to frostbite. Watch for signs of frostbite—numbness and discoloration. In cold temperatures, as much as half of the body's heat can be lost through an unprotected head and neck. A wool or synthetic cap, hood, or hat will help to hold in body heat. Mittens are better than gloves, because they keep the fingers together so the surface area from which to lose heat is less. Inner linings of synthetic material to wick moisture away from the skin are recommended. Avoid cotton next to the skin, because once cotton gets wet—whether from perspiration, rain, or snow—it loses its insulating properties.

Wearing several layers of lightweight clothing is preferable to wearing one single, thick layer because warm air is trapped between layers of clothes, enabling greater heat conservation. As body temperature increases, you can remove layers as necessary.

The first layer of clothes should wick moisture away from the skin. Polypropylene, Capilene, and Thermax are recommended materials. Next, a layer of wool, dacron, or polyester fleece insulates well even when wet. Lycra tights or sweatpants help protect the legs. The outer layer should be waterproof, wind-resistant, and breathable. A synthetic material such as Gortex is best, so moisture can still escape from the body. A ski mask or face mask helps protect the face. In extremely cold conditions, exposed skin, such as the nose, cheeks, and around the eyes, can be insulated with petroleum jelly.

For lengthy or long-distance workouts (cross-country skiing or long runs), take a small backpack to carry the clothing that is removed. You also can carry extra warm and dry clothes in case you stop exercising away from shelter. If you remain outdoors following exercise, added clothing and continuous body movement are essential to maintain body temperature and avoid hypothermia.

17. Should I exercise when I have a cold or the flu?

The most important consideration in deciding to exercise when you have a cold or flu is to use common sense and pay attention to your symptoms. Typically, you may continue to exercise if your symptoms are limited to a runny nose, sneezing, or a scratchy throat, but if your symptoms include fever, muscle ache, vomiting, diarrhea, or a hacking cough, you should avoid exercise. Following an illness, be sure to ease back gradually into your program. Do not attempt to return at the same intensity and duration that you were used to prior to your illness.

Exercise-Related Injuries

To enjoy and maintain physical fitness, preventing injury during a conditioning program is essential. Exercise-related injuries, nonetheless, are common in individuals who participate in exercise programs. Surveys indicate that more than half of all new participants incur injuries during the first 6 months after beginning the conditioning program.

Causes of Injuries

The four most common causes of injuries are:

1. High-impact activities
2. Rapid conditioning programs (doing too much too quickly)
3. Improper shoes or training surfaces
4. Anatomical predisposition (body propensity)

By far the most common causes of injuries are high-impact activities and a significant increase in quantity, intensity, and duration of activities. The body requires time to adapt to more intense activities. Most of these injuries can be prevented through a more gradual and correct conditioning (low-impact) program.

Proper shoes for specific activities are essential. Shoes should be replaced when they show a lot of wear and tear. Softer training surfaces, such as grass and dirt, produce less trauma than asphalt and concrete.

Because few people have perfect body alignment, injuries associated with overtraining may occur eventually. In case of injury, proper treatment can avert a lengthy recovery process. A summary of common exercise-related injuries and how to manage them follows.

Acute Sports Injuries

The best treatment always has been prevention. If an activity causes unusual discomfort or chronic irritation, you need to treat the cause by decreasing the intensity, switching activities, substituting equipment, or upgrading clothing (such as buying proper-fitting shoes).

In cases of acute injury, the standard treatment is rest, cold application, compression or splinting (or both), and elevation of the affected body part. This is commonly referred to as "**RICE**":

R = rest
I = ice (cold) application
C = compression
E = elevation

Cold should be applied three to five times a day for 15 minutes at a time during the first 24 to 36 hours, by submerging the injured area in cold water, using an ice bag, or applying ice massage to the affected part. An elastic bandage or wrap can be used for compression. Elevating the body part decreases blood flow (and therefore swelling) in that body part.

The purpose of these treatment modalities is to minimize swelling in the area, which hastens recovery time. After the first 36 to 48 hours, heat can be used if the injury shows no further swelling or inflammation. If you have doubts as to the nature or seriousness of the injury (such as suspected fracture), you should seek a medical evaluation.

Obvious deformities (exhibited by fractures, dislocations, or partial dislocations, as examples) call for splinting, cold application with an ice bag, and medical attention. Do not try to reset any of these conditions by yourself, because you could further damage muscles, ligaments, and nerves. Treatment of these injuries always should be in the hands of specialized medical personnel. A quick reference guide for the signs or symptoms and treatment of exercise-related problems is provided in Table 9.5.

Muscle Soreness and Stiffness

Individuals who begin an exercise program or participate after a long layoff from exercise often develop muscle soreness and stiffness. The acute soreness that sets in the first few hours after exercise is thought to be related to a lack of blood (oxygen) flow and general fatigue of the exercised muscles.

Delayed muscle soreness that appears several hours after exercise (usually about 12 hours later) and lasts 2 to 4 days may be related to actual tiny tears in muscle tissue, muscle spasms that increase fluid retention (stimulating the pain nerve endings), and overstretching or tearing of connective tissue in and around muscles and joints.

Mild stretching before and adequate stretching after exercise help to prevent soreness and stiffness. Gradually progressing into an exercise program is important, too. A person should not attempt to do too much too quickly. To relieve pain, mild stretching, low-intensity exercise to stimulate blood flow, and a warm bath might help.

Hypothermia A breakdown in the body's ability to generate heat; a drop in body temperature below 95° F.

RICE An acronym used to describe the standard treatment procedure for acute sports injuries: Rest, Ice (cold application), Compression, and Elevation.

TABLE 9.5 Reference Guide for Exercise-Related Problems

Injury	Signs/Symptoms	Treatment*
Bruise (contusion)	Pain, swelling, discoloration	Cold application, compression, rest
Dislocation / Fracture	Pain, swelling, deformity	Splinting, cold application, seek medical attention
Heat cramp	Cramps, spasms, and muscle twitching in the legs, arms, and abdomen	Stop activity, get out of the heat, stretch, massage the painful area, drink plenty of fluids
Heat exhaustion	Fainting, profuse sweating, cold/clammy skin, weak/rapid pulse, weakness, headache	Stop activity, rest in a cool place, loosen clothing, rub body with cool/wet towel, drink plenty of fluids, stay out of heat for 2–3 days
Heat stroke	Hot/dry skin, no sweating, serious disorientation, rapid/full pulse, vomiting, diarrhea, unconsciousness, high body temperature	**Seek immediate medical attention**, request help and get out of the sun, bathe in cold water/spray with cold water/rub body with cold towels, drink plenty of cold fluids
Joint sprain	Pain, tenderness, swelling, loss of use, discoloration	Cold application, compression, elevation, rest, heat after 36 to 48 hours (if no further swelling)
Muscle cramp	Pain, spasm	Stretch muscle(s), use mild exercises for involved area
Muscle soreness and stiffness	Tenderness, pain	Mild stretching, low-intensity exercise, warm bath
Muscle strain	Pain, tenderness, swelling, loss of use	Cold application, compression, elevation, rest, heat after 36 to 48 hours (if no further swelling)
Shin splints	Pain, tenderness	Cold application prior to and following any physical activity, rest, heat (if no activity is carried out)
Side stitch	Pain on the side of the abdomen below the rib cage	Decrease level of physical activity or stop altogether, gradually increase level of fitness
Tendonitis	Pain, tenderness, loss of use	Rest, cold application, heat after 48 hours

* Cold should be applied three to four times a day for 15 minutes. Heat can be applied three times a day for 15 to 20 minutes.

Exercise Intolerance

When starting an exercise program, participants should stay within the safe limits. The best method to determine whether you are exercising too strenuously is to check your heart rate and make sure it does not exceed the limits of your target zone. Exercising above this target zone may not be safe for unconditioned or high-risk individuals. You do not have to exercise beyond your target zone to gain the desired cardiorespiratory benefits.

Several physical signs will tell you when you are exceeding your functional limitations—that is, experiencing **exercise intolerance**. Signs of intolerance include rapid or irregular heart rate, difficult breathing, nausea, vomiting, lightheadedness, headache, dizziness, unusually flushed or pale skin, extreme weakness, lack of energy, shakiness, sore muscles, cramps, and tightness in the chest. Learn to listen to your body. If you notice any of these symptoms, seek medical attention before continuing your exercise program.

Recovery heart rate is another indicator of overexertion. To a certain extent, recovery heart rate is related to fitness level. The higher your cardiorespiratory fitness level, the faster your heart rate will decrease following exercise. As a rule, heart rate should be below 120 beats per minute 5 minutes into recovery. If your heart rate is above 120, you most likely have overexerted yourself or possibly could have some other cardiac abnormality. If you lower the intensity or duration of exercise, or both, and you still have a fast heart rate 5 minutes into recovery, you should consult your physician.

Side Stitch

Side stitch can develop in the early stages of participation in exercise. It occurs primarily in unconditioned beginners and in trained individuals when they exercise at higher intensities than usual. As one's physical condition improves, this condition tends to disappear unless training is intensified.

The exact cause is unknown. Some experts suggest that it could relate to a lack of blood flow to the respiratory muscles during strenuous physical exertion. Some people encounter side stitch during downhill running. If you experience side stitch during exercise, slow down. If it persists, stop altogether. Lying down on your back and gently bringing both knees to the chest and holding that position for 30 to 60 seconds also helps.

Some people get side stitch if they eat or drink juice shortly before exercise. Drinking only water 1–2 hours prior to exercise sometimes prevents side stitch. Other individuals have problems with commercially available sports drinks during high-intensity exercise. Unless carbohydrate replacement is crucial to complete an event (such as a marathon or a triathlon), drink cool water for fluid replacement or try a different carbohydrate solution.

Shin Splints

Shin splints, one of the most common injuries to the lower limbs, usually results from one or more of the following: (a) lack of proper and gradual conditioning, (b) doing physical activities on hard surfaces (wooden floors, hard tracks, cement, or asphalt), (c) fallen arches, (d) chronic overuse, (e) muscle fatigue, (f) faulty posture, (g) improper shoes, or (h) participating in weight-bearing activities when excessively overweight.

To manage shin splints:

1. Remove or reduce the cause (exercise on softer surfaces, wear better shoes or arch supports, or completely stop exercise until the shin splints heal);
2. Do stretching exercises before and after physical activity;
3. Use ice massage for 10 to 20 minutes before and after exercise;
4. Apply active heat (whirlpool and hot baths) for 15 minutes, two to three times a day; or
5. Use supportive taping during physical activity (a qualified athletic trainer can teach you the proper taping technique).

Muscle Cramps

Muscle cramps are caused by the body's depletion of essential electrolytes or a breakdown in the coordination between opposing muscle groups. If you have a muscle cramp, you should first attempt to stretch the muscles involved. In the case of the calf muscle, for example, pull your toes up toward the knees. After stretching the muscle, rub it down gently, and, finally, do some mild exercises requiring the use of that muscle.

In pregnant and lactating women, muscle cramps often are related to a lack of calcium. If women get cramps during these times, calcium supplements usually relieve the problem. Tight clothing also can cause cramps by decreasing blood flow to active muscle tissue.

Leisure-Time Physical Activity

Recognizing that individuals have notable differences, the average person in developed countries has about 3.5 hours of "free" or leisure time daily. In our current automated society, most of this time is spent in sedentary living. People would be better off doing some physical activities based on personal interests. Motivational factors include health, aesthetics, weight control, competition and challenge, fun, social interaction, mental arousal, relaxation, and stress management.

Frequently, leisure-time physical activity does not include exercise performed during a regular exercise program. It consists of activities such as walking, hiking, gardening, yardwork, occupational work and chores, and moderate sports such as tennis, table tennis, badminton, golf, or croquet.

Every small increase in daily physical activity contributes to better health and wellness. Small increases in physical activity have a large impact in decreasing early risks for disease and premature death. Therefore, a new, concerted effort must be made to spend leisure time in activities that will promote the expenditure of energy, provide a break from daily tasks, and contribute to health-related fitness.

Exercise and Aging

For the first time in U.S. history, the elderly constitute the fastest-growing segment of the population. The number of Americans ages 65 and older has increased from 3.1 million in 1900 (4.1 percent of the population) to more than 34 million (12.8 percent) in 1996. By the year 2030, more than 70 million people, or 22 percent of the U.S. population, are expected to be older than age 65.

The main objective of fitness programs for older adults should be to help them improve their functional status and contribute to healthy aging. This implies the ability to maintain independent living status and to avoid disability. Older adults are encouraged to participate in programs that will help develop cardiorespiratory endurance, muscular strength and endurance, muscular flexibility, agility, balance, and motor coordination.

Exercise intolerance   Inability to function during exercise because of excessive fatigue or extreme feelings of discomfort.

Side stitch   A sharp pain in the side of the abdomen.

Shin splints   Injury to the lower leg characterized by pain and irritation in the shin region of the leg.

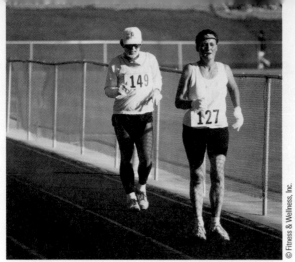

Older adults who exercise enjoy better health, increase their quality of life, and live longer than physically inactive adults.

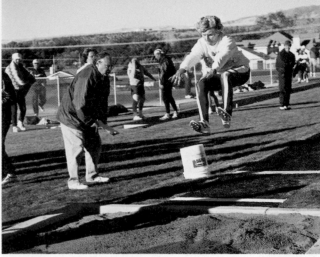

A high level of physical fitness can be maintained throughout the life span.

Physical Training in Older Adults

Regular participation in physical activity provides both physical and psychological benefits to older adults.[8] Cardiorespiratory endurance training helps to increase functional capacity, decrease the risk for disease, improve health status, and increase life expectancy. Strength training decreases the rate at which strength and muscle mass are lost. Among the psychological benefits are preserved cognitive function, reduced symptoms and behaviors related to depression, and improved self-confidence and self-esteem.

The trainability of older men and women alike and the effectiveness of physical activity in enhancing health have been demonstrated in prior research. Older adults who increase their physical activity experience significant changes in cardiorespiratory endurance, strength, and flexibility. The extent of the changes depends on their initial fitness level and the types of activities they select for their training (walking, cycling, strength training, and so on).

Improvements in maximal oxygen uptake in older adults are similar to those of younger people, although older people seem to require a longer training period to achieve these changes. Declines in maximal oxygen uptake average about 1 percent per year between age 25 and 75.[9] A slower rate of decline is seen in people who maintain a lifetime aerobic exercise program.

Results of research on the effects of aging on the cardiorespiratory system of male exercisers versus non-exercisers showed that the maximal oxygen

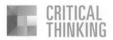

CRITICAL THINKING

You have been exercising regularly and you are enjoying many exercise-related benefits. Other friends and members of your family, however, do not exercise and think that something is wrong with you because of your love for physical activity. How do you respond so that they will be supportive and maybe even start an exercise program of their own?

TABLE 9.6 Effects of Physical Activity and Inactivity on Older Men

	Exercisers	Non-exercisers
Age (yrs)	68.0	69.8
Weight (lbs)	160.3	186.3
Resting heart rate (bpm)	55.8	66.0
Maximal heart rate (bpm)	157.0	146.0
Heart rate reserve* (bpm)	101.2	80.0
Blood pressure (mm Hg)	120/78	150/90
Maximal oxygen uptake (ml/kg/min)	38.6	20.3

*Heart rate reserve = maximal heart rate − resting heart rate.

Data from F. W. Kash, J. L. Boyer, S. P. Van Camp, L. S. Verity, and J. P. Wallace, "The Effect of Physical Activity on Aerobic Power in Older Men (A Longitudinal Study)," *The Physician and Sports Medicine* 18, no. 4 (1990): 73–83.

uptake of regular exercisers was almost twice that of the non-exercisers (see Table 9.6).[10] The study revealed a decline in maximal oxygen uptake between ages 50 and 68 of only 13 percent in the active group, compared to 41 percent in the inactive group. These changes indicate that about one-third of the loss in maximal oxygen uptake results from aging and two-thirds of the loss comes from inactivity. Blood pressure, heart rate, and body weight also were remarkably better in the exercising group. Furthermore, aerobic training seems to decrease high blood pressure in the older patients at the same rate as in young hypertensive people.[11]

In terms of aging, muscle strength declines by 10 to 20 percent between ages 20 and 50, but between ages 50 and 70, it drops by another 25 to

30 percent. Through strength training, frail adults in their 80s or 90s can double or triple their strength in just a few months. The amount of muscle hypertrophy achieved, however, decreases with age. Strength gains close to 200 percent have been found in previously inactive adults over age 90.[12] In fact, research has shown that regular strength training improves balance, gait, speed, **functional independence**, morale, depression symptoms, and energy intake.[13] (The health-related components of strength and flexibility fitness are addressed in Chapters 7 and 8, respectively.)

Although muscle flexibility drops by about 5 percent per decade of life, 10 minutes of stretching every other day can prevent most of this loss as a person ages.[14] Improved flexibility also enhances mobility skills.[15] The latter promotes independence because it helps older adults successfully perform activities of daily living.

In terms of body composition, inactive adults continue to gain body fat after age 60 despite their tendency toward lower body weight. The increase in body fat is most likely related to a decrease in basal metabolic rate and physical activity along with increased caloric intake above that required to maintain daily energy requirements.[16]

Older adults who wish to initiate or continue an exercise program are strongly encouraged to have a complete medical exam, including a stress electrocardiogram test (see Chapter 11). Recommended activities for older adults include calisthenics, walking, jogging, swimming, cycling, and water aerobics.

Older people should avoid isometric and very high intensity weight-training exercises (see Chapter 7). Activities that require all-out effort or require participants to hold their breath tend to lessen blood flow to the heart, cause a significant increase in blood pressure, and increase the load placed on the heart. Older adults should participate in activities that require continuous and rhythmic muscular activity (about 40 to 60 percent of HRR). These activities do not cause large increases in blood pressure or overload the heart.

Preparing for Participation in Sports*

To enhance your participation in sports, keep in mind that in most cases it is better to get fit before playing sports instead of playing sports to get fit. A good pre-season training program will help make the season more enjoyable and prevent exercise-related injuries.

Properly conditioned individuals can safely participate in sports and enjoy the activities to their fullest with few or no limitations. Unfortunately, sport injuries are often the result of poor fitness and a lack of sport-specific conditioning. Many injuries occur when fatigue sets in following overexertion by unconditioned individuals.

Base Fitness Conditioning

Pre-activity screening that includes a health history (see page 25) and/or a medical evaluation appropriate to your sport selection is recommended. Once cleared for exercise, start by building a base of general athletic fitness that includes the four health-related fitness components: cardiorespiratory fitness, muscular strength and endurance, flexibility, and recommended body composition. The base fitness conditioning program should last a minimum of 6 weeks.

As explained in Chapter 6, for cardiorespiratory fitness select an activity that you enjoy (such as walking, jogging, cycling, step aerobics, cross-country skiing, stair climbing, endurance games) and train three to five times per week at a minimum of 20 minutes of continuous activity per session. Exercise in the moderate- to high-intensity zones for adequate conditioning. You should feel as though you are training "somewhat hard" to "hard" at these intensity levels.

Strength (resistance) training helps maintain and increase muscular strength and endurance. Following the guidelines provided in Chapter 7, select 8 to 10 exercises that involve the major muscle groups of the body and train two or three times per week on nonconsecutive days. Select a resistance (weight) that allows you to do 8 to 12 repetitions to near fatigue. That is, the resistance will be heavy enough so that when you perform a set of an exercise, you will not be able to do more than 12 repetitions at that weight. Begin your program slowly and perform between one and three sets of each exercise. Recommended exercises include the bench press, lat pulldown, leg press, leg curl, triceps extension, arm curl, rowing torso, heel raise, abdominal crunch, and back extension.

Flexibility is important in sports participation to enhance the range of motion in the joints. Using the guidelines from Chapter 8, schedule flexibility training two or three days per week. Perform each stretching exercise four times, and hold each stretch for 10 to 30 seconds. Examples of stretching exercises include the side body stretch, body rotation, chest

*Adapted from W. W. K. Hoeger and J. R. Moore, "Preparing for Outdoor Winter Sports," *ACSM Fit Society Page*, Fall 2002 (www.acsm.org).

Functional independence Ability to carry out activities of daily living without assistance from other individuals.

stretch, shoulder stretch, sit-and-reach stretch, adductor stretch, quad stretch, heel cord stretch, and knee-to-chest stretch.

In terms of body composition, excess body fat hinders sports performance and increases the risk for injuries. Depending on the nature of the activity, fitness goals for body composition range from 12 percent to 20 percent body fat for men and 17 percent to 25 percent for most women.

Sport-Specific Conditioning

Once the general fitness base is achieved, continue with the program but make adjustments to add sport-specific training. This training should match the sport's requirements for aerobic/anaerobic capabilities, muscular strength and endurance, and range of motion.

During the sport-specific training, about half of your aerobic/anaerobic training should involve the same muscles used during your sport. Ideally, allocate 4 weeks of sport-specific training before you start participating in the sport. Then continue the sport-specific training on a more limited basis throughout the season. Depending on the nature of the sport (aerobic versus anaerobic—discussed next), once the season starts, sports participation itself can take the place of some or all of your aerobic workouts.

The next step is to look at the demands of the sport. For example, soccer, bicycle racing, cross-country skiing, and snowshoeing are aerobic activities, whereas basketball, racquetball, alpine skiing, snowboarding, and ice hockey are stop-and-go sports that require a combination of aerobic and anaerobic activity. Consequently, aerobic training may be appropriate for cross-country skiing, but it will do little to prepare your muscles for the high-intensity requirements of combined aerobic and anaerobic sports.

Interval training, performed twice per week, is added to the program at this time. The intervals consist of a 1:3 work-to-rest ratio. This means you'll work at a fairly high intensity for, say, 15 seconds, and then spend 45 seconds on low-intensity recovery. Be sure to keep moving during the recovery phase. Perform four or five intervals at first, then gradually progress to 10 intervals. As your fitness improves, progressively lengthen the high-intensity proportion of the intervals to 1 minute and use a 1:2 work-to-rest ratio—wherein you work at high intensity for 1 minute and then at low intensity for 2 minutes.

For aerobic sports, interval training once a week also improves performance. These intervals,

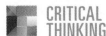

CRITICAL THINKING

Sports participation is a good predictor of adherence to exercise later in life. What experiences have you had with youth sports? Were these experiences positive, and what effect do they have on your current physical activity patterns?

however, can be done on a 3-minute to 3-minute work-to-rest ratio. A 5- to 10-minute work interval followed by 1 to 2 minutes of recovery can also be done, but the intensity of these longer intervals should not be as high, and only three to five intervals are recommended. Your interval-training workouts are not performed in addition to the regular aerobic workouts but, instead, take the place of one of these workouts.

Consider sport-specific strength requirements as well. Look at the primary muscles used in your sport, and make sure your choice of exercises works those muscles. Try to perform your strength training through a range of motion similar to that used in your sport. Aerobic/anaerobic sports require greater strength; during the season, three sets of 8 to 12 repetitions to near fatigue are recommended two or three times per week. For aerobic endurance sports, the recommendation is a minimum of one set of 8 to 12 repetitions to near fatigue performed once or twice per week during the season.

For some winter sports, such as alpine skiing and snowboarding, gravity supplies most of the propulsion and the body acts more as a shock absorber. Muscles in the hips, knees, and trunk are used to control the forces on the body and equipment. Multi-joint exercises, such as the leg press, squats, and lunges, are suggested for these activities.

Before the season starts, make sure your equipment is in proper working condition. For example, alpine skiers' bindings should be cleaned and adjusted properly so they will release as needed. This is one of the most important things you can do to help prevent knee injuries. A good pair of bindings is cheaper than knee surgery.

The first few times you participate in the sport of your choice, go easy, practice technique, and do not continue once fatigued. Gradually increase the length and intensity of your workouts. Consider taking a lesson to have someone watch your technique and help correct flaws early in the season. Even Olympic athletes have coaches watching them. Proper conditioning allows for a more enjoyable and healthier season.

Overtraining

Rest is important in any fitness conditioning program. Although the term **overtraining** is most frequently associated with athletic performance, it applies just as well to fitness participants. We all know that hard work improves fitness and performance. Hard training without adequate recovery, however, breaks down the body and leads to loss of fitness.

Physiological improvements in fitness and conditioning programs occur during the rest periods following training. As a rule, a hard day of training

- Decreased fitness
- Decreased sports performance
- Increased fatigue
- Loss of concentration
- Staleness and burnout
- Loss of competitive drive
- Increased resting and exercise heart rate
- Decreased appetite
- Loss of body weight
- Altered sleep patterns
- Decreased sex drive
- Generalized body aches and pains
- Increased susceptibility to illness and injury
- Mood disturbances
- Depression

must be followed by a rest day or a day of light training. Equally, a few weeks of increased training **volume** are to be followed by a few days of light recovery work. During these recovery periods, body systems strengthen and compensate for the training load, leading to a higher level of fitness. If proper recovery is not built into the training routine, overtraining occurs. Decreased performance, staleness, and injury are frequently seen with overtraining. Thus, to obtain optimal results, training regimens are altered during different phases of the year.

Periodization

Periodization is a training approach that uses a systematic variation in intensity and volume to enhance fitness and performance. This model was designed around the premises that the body becomes stronger as a result of training, but if similar workouts are constantly repeated, the body tires and enters a state of staleness and fatigue.

Periodization is used most frequently for athletic conditioning. Because peak fitness cannot be maintained during an entire season, most athletes seeking peak performance use a periodized training approach. Studies have documented that greater improvements in fitness are achieved by using a variety of training loads. Using the same program and attempting to increase volume and intensity over a prolonged time will be manifested in overtraining.

The periodization training system involves three cycles:

1. macrocycles
2. mesocycles
3. microcycles

These cycles vary in length depending on the requirements of the sport. Typically, the overall training period (season or year) is referred to as a macrocycle. For athletes who need to peak twice a year, such as cross-country and track runners, two macrocycles can be developed within the year.

Macrocycles are divided into smaller weekly or monthly training phases known as mesocycles. A typical season, for example, is divided into the following mesocycles: base fitness conditioning (off-season), pre-season or sport-specific conditioning, competition, peak performance, and transition (active recovery from sport-specific training and competition). In turn, mesocycles are divided into smaller weekly or daily microcycles. During microcycles, training follows the general objective of the mesocycle, but the workouts are altered to avoid boredom and fatigue.

The concept behind periodizing can be used in both aerobic and anaerobic sports. In the case of a long-distance runner, for instance, training can start with a general strength-conditioning program and cardiorespiratory endurance cross-training (jogging, cycling, swimming) during the off-season. In pre-season, the volume of strength training is decreased and the total weekly running mileage, at moderate intensities, is progressively increased. During the competitive season, the athlete maintains a limited strength-training program but now increases the intensity of the runs while decreasing the total weekly mileage. During the peaking phase, volume (miles) of training is reduced even further while the intensity is maintained at a high level. At the end of the season, a short transition period of 2 to 4 weeks, involving low- to moderate-intensity activities other than running and lifting weights, is recommended.

Periodization is frequently used for muscular strength development, progressively cycling through the various components (hypertrophy, strength, and power) of strength training. A sample sequence— one macrocycle—of periodized training is provided in Table 9.7. The program starts with high volume and low intensity. During subsequent mesocycles

Interval training A training program where high intensity speed intervals are followed by short recovery intervals.

Overtraining An emotional, behavioral, and physical condition marked by increased fatigue, decreased performance, persistent muscle soreness, mood disturbances, and feelings of "staleness" or "burnout" as a result of excessive physical training.

Volume (of training) The total amount of training performed in a given work period (day, week, month, or season).

Periodization A training approach that divides the season into three cycles (macrocycles, mesocycles, and microcycles) using a systematic variation in intensity and volume of training to enhance fitness and performance.

TABLE 9.7 Periodization Program for Strength

	One Macrocycle			
	Mesocycle 1*	**Mesocycle 2***	**Mesocycle 3***	**Mesocycle 4***
	Hypertrophy	**Strength & Hypertrophy**	**Strength & Power**	**Peak Performance**
Sets per exercise	3–5	3–5	3–5	1–3
Repetitions	8–12	6–9	1–5	1–3
Intensity (resistance)	Low	Moderate	High	Very High
Volume	High	Moderate	Low	Very Low
Weeks (microcycles)	6–8	4–6	3–5	1–2

*Each mesocycle is followed by several days of light training.

(divided among the objectives of hypertrophy, strength, and power), the volume is decreased and the intensity (resistance) increases. Following each mesocycle, up to seven days of very light training are recommended. This brief resting period allows the body to fully recuperate, preventing overtraining and risk for injury. Other models of periodization exist, but the previous example is the most commonly used training model.

Altering or cycling workouts has become popular in recent years among fitness participants. Research indicates that periodization is not limited to athletes but has been used successfully by fitness enthusiasts who are preparing for a special event such a 10K run, a triathlon, a bike race, or who are simply aiming for higher fitness. Altering training is also recommended for people who progressed nicely in the initial weeks of a program but now feel "stale" and "stagnant." Studies indicate that even among general fitness participants, systematically altering volume and intensity of training is most effective for progression in long-term fitness. Because training phases continually change during a macrocycle, periodization breaks staleness and the monotony of repeated workouts.

For the non-athlete, a periodization program does not have to account for every detail of the sport. You can periodize workouts by altering mesocycles every 2 to 8 weeks. You can use different exercises, change the number of sets and repetitions, vary the speed of the repetitions, alter recovery time between sets, and even cross-train.

Periodization is not for everyone. People who are starting an exercise program, who enjoy a set routine, or who are satisfied with their fitness routine and fitness level do not need to periodize. For new participants, the goal is to start and adhere to exercise long enough to adopt the exercise behavior.

Personal Fitness Programming: An Example

Now that you understand the principles of fitness assessment and exercise prescription given in Chapters 6 through 8 and this chapter, you can review this program to cross-check and improve the design of your own fitness program.

Mary is 20 years old. She participated in organized sports on and off throughout high school. During the last 2 years, however, she has only minimally participated in physical activity. She was not taught the principles for exercise prescription and has not participated in regular exercise to improve and maintain the various health-related components of fitness.

Mary became interested in fitness and contemplated signing up for a fitness and wellness course. As she was preparing her class schedule for the semester, she noted a "Lifetime Fitness and Wellness" course. In registering for the course, Mary anticipated some type of structured aerobic exercise. She knew that good fitness was important to health and weight management, but she didn't quite know how to plan and implement a program.

Once the new course started, she and her classmates received the "Stages of Change Questionnaire." Mary learned that she was in the Contemplation stage for cardiorespiratory endurance, the Precontemplation stage for muscular strength and endurance, the Maintenance stage for flexibility, and the Preparation stage for body composition (see Transtheoretical Model in Chapter 2, pages 34–36). Various fitness

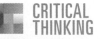

CRITICAL THINKING

In your own experience with personal fitness programs throughout the years, what factors have motivated you and helped you the most to stay with the program? What factors have kept you from being physically active and what can you do to change these factors?

assessments determined that her cardiorespiratory endurance level was fair, her muscular strength and endurance was poor, her flexibility was good, and her percent body fat was 25 percent (Moderate classification).

Cardiorespiratory Endurance

At the beginning of the semester, the instructor informed the students that the course required self-monitored participation in activities outside the regularly scheduled class hours. Thus, Mary entered the Preparation stage for cardiorespiratory endurance. She knew she would be starting exercise in the next couple of weeks.

While in this Preparation stage, Mary chose three processes of change to help her implement her program (see Table 2.1, page 37). She thought she could adopt an aerobic exercise program (Positive Outlook process of change) and set a realistic goal to reach the "Good" category for cardiorespiratory endurance by the end of the semester (Goal Setting). By staying in this course, she committed to go through with exercise (Commitment). She prepared a 12-week Personalized Cardiorespiratory Exercise Prescription (see Figure 9.5), wrote down her goal, signed the prescription (now a contract), and shared the program with her instructor and roommates.

As her exercise modalities, Mary selected walking/jogging and aerobics. Initially she walked/jogged twice a week and did aerobics once a week. By the 10th week of the program, she was jogging three times per week and participating in aerobics twice a week. She also selected Self-monitoring, Self-reevaluation, and Countering as techniques of change (see Table 2.2, page 40). Using the exercise log in Figure 6.10 (pages 185–186) and the computerized exercise log (Figure 9.6), she monitored her exercise program. At the end of 6 weeks, she scheduled a follow-up cardiorespiratory assessment test (Self-reevaluation process of change), and she's replaced her evening television hour with aerobic training (Countering).

Mary also decided to increase her daily physical activity. She chose to walk 10 minutes to and from school, take the stairs instead of elevators whenever possible, and add 5-minute walks every hour during study time. On Saturdays, she cleaned her apartment and went to a school-sponsored dance at night. On Sundays, she opted to walk to and from church and took a 30-minute leisurely walk after the dinner meal. Mary now was fully in the Action stage of change for cardiorespiratory endurance.

Muscular Strength and Endurance

After Mary had started her fitness and wellness course, she wasn't yet convinced that she wanted to strength-train. Still, she contemplated strength training because a small part of her grade depended on it. When she read the information on the importance of lean body mass in regulating basal metabolic rate and weight maintenance (the Consciousness-raising process of change), she thought that perhaps it would be good to add strength training to her program. She was also contemplating the long-term consequences of loss of lean body mass, its effect on her personal appearance, and the potential for decreased independence and quality of life (Emotional Arousal process of change).

Mary visited with her course instructor for additional guidance. Following this meeting, Mary committed herself to strength-train. While yet in the Preparation stage, she outlined a 10-week periodized training program (see Figure 9.7) and opted to aim for the "Good" strength category by the end of the program.

Because this was the first time Mary had lifted weights, the course instructor introduced Mary to two other students who were already lifting (Helping Relationships process of change). She also monitored her program with the form provided in Figure 7.7 on pages 219–220. Mary promised herself a movie and dinner out if she completed the first 5 weeks of strength training, and a new blouse if she made it through 10 weeks (Rewards process and technique for change).

Muscular Flexibility

Good flexibility was not a problem for Mary because she regularly stretched 15 to 30 minutes while watching the evening news on television. She had developed this habit the last 2 years of high school to maintain flexibility as a member of the dance-drill team (Environment Control process of change —as a team member she needed good flexibility).

Because Mary had been stretching regularly for more than 3 years, she was in the Maintenance stage for flexibility. The flexibility fitness tests revealed that she had good flexibility. These results allowed her to pursue her stretching program because she thought she would be excellent for this fitness component (Self-evaluation process of change).

To gain greater improvements in flexibility, Mary chose slow-sustained stretching and proprioceptive neuromuscular facilitation (PNF). She would need help to carry out the PNF technique. She spoke to one of her lifting classmates, and together they decided to allocate 20 minutes at the end of strength training to stretching (Helping Relationships process of change) and they chose the sequence of exercises presented in Lab 8C, pages 265–266 (Consciousness-raising and Goal Setting).

FIGURE 9.5 Sample computerized cardiorespiratory exercise prescription.

Personalized Cardiorespiratory Exercise Prescription
Fitness & Wellness Series
Wadsworth Group / Thomson Learning

Profile Plus

Mary Johnson   September 1, 2005
Maximal heart rate: 200 bpm   Resting heart rate: 76 bpm
Present cardiorespiratory fitness level: Fair   Age: 20

The following is your personal program for cardiorespiratory fitness development and maintenance. If you have been exercising regularly and you are in the average or good category, you may start at week five. If you are in the excellent category, you can start at week ten.

Week	Time (min.)	Frequency (per week)	Training Intensity (beats per minute)	Pulse (10 sec. count)
1	15	3	126 - 138	21 - 23 beats
2	15	4	126 - 138	21 - 23 beats
3	20	4	126 - 138	21 - 23 beats
4	20	5	126 - 138	21 - 23 beats
5	20	4	138 - 150	23 - 25 beats
6	20	5	138 - 150	23 - 25 beats
7	30	4	138 - 150	23 - 25 beats
8	30	5	138 - 150	23 - 25 beats
9	30	4	150 - 181	25 - 30 beats
10	30	5	150 - 181	25 - 30 beats
11	30-40	5	150 - 181	25 - 30 beats
12	30-40	5-6	150 - 181	25 - 30 beats

You may participate in any combination of activities which are aerobic and continuous in nature such as walking, jogging, swimming, cross country skiing, aerobelt exercise, rope skipping, cycling, aerobic dancing, racquetball, stair climbing, stationary running or cycling, etc. As long as the heart rate reaches the desired rate, and it stays at that level for the period of time indicated, the cardiorespiratory system will improve.

Following the twelve week program, in order to maintain your fitness level, you should exercise between 150 and 181 bpm for about 30 minutes, a minimum of three times per week on nonconsecutive days. When you exercise, allow about 5 minutes for a gradual warm-up period and another 5 for gradual cool-down. Also, when you check your exercise heart rate, only count your pulse for 10 seconds (start counting with 0) and then refer to the above 10 second pulse count. You may also multiply by 6 to obtain your rate in beats per minute.

Good cardiorespiratory fitness will greatly contribute toward the enhancement and maintenance of good health. It is especially important in the prevention of cardiovascular disease. We encourage you to be persistent in your exercise program and to participate regularly.

Training days: ✔ M ✔ T ___ W ___ Th ✔ F ✔ S ___ S   Training time: 7:00 am

Signature: _Mary Johnson_   Goal: Good Date: 9/01/05

<u>Profile Plus</u>

Exercise Log
Fitness & Wellness Series
Wadsworth Group / Thomson Learning

Mary Johnson

Date	Exercise	Body Weight (lbs)	Heart Rate (bpm)	Duration (min)	Distance (miles)	Calories Burned
09/01/2005	Walking (4.5 mph)	140.0	138	15	1.00	95
09/03/2005	Aerobics/Moderate	140.0	144	20		182
09/05/2005	Walking (4.5 mph)	141.0	138	15	1.00	95
09/06/2005	Dance/Moderate	141.0	100	60		254
09/07/2005	Walking (4.5 mph)	140.0	132	30	2.00	189
09/08/2005	Jogging (11 min/mile)	140.0	138	15	1.25	147
09/10/2005	Aerobics/Moderate	140.0	138	20		182
09/11/2005	Jogging (11 min/mile)	139.0	138	15	1.25	146
09/12/2005	Jogging (11 min/mile)	139.0	134	15	1.25	146
09/13/2005	Dance/Moderate	140.0	96	75		315
09/14/2005	Walking (4.5 mph)	139.0	126	30	2.50	188
09/15/2005	Jogging (11 min/mile)	139.0	134	20	2.00	195
09/16/2005	Strength Training	138.0	96	30		207
09/17/2005	Step-Aerobics	139.0	138	30		292
09/18/2005	Jogging (11 min/mile)	138.0	138	20	2.00	193
09/19/2005	Jogging (11 min/mile)	138.0	138	20	2.00	193
	Strength Training	138.0	96	30		207
09/20/2005	Dance/Moderate	138.0	90	30		124
09/21/2005	Walking (4.5 mph)	138.0	126	30	2.50	186
09/22/2005	Jogging (11 min/mile)	137.0	136	20	2.00	192
09/23/2005	Step-Aerobics	138.0	138	30		290
	Strength Training	138.0	96	40		276
09/24/2005	Jogging (8.5 min/mile)	138.0	144	20	2.50	248
09/25/2005	Step-Aerobics	137.0	136	20		192
09/26/2005	Strength Training	137.0	92	40		274
	Jogging (8.5 min/mile)	137.0	140	20	2.50	247
09/27/2005	Dance/Moderate	136.0	94	90		367
09/28/2005	Walking (4.5 mph)	136.0	120	30	2.50	184

Totals

				13 hr 50 min	28.25	5806

Average per exercise session
		138.5	124	30	1.88	207

Number of exercise sessions: 28

Average per day exercised
				33		232

Number of days exercised: 25

Distance summary
Total miles run: 16.8
Total miles walked: 11.5

FIGURE 9.7 Sample starting muscular strength and endurance periodization program.

	Learning Lifting Technique	Muscular Strength	Muscular Endurance	Muscular Strength
Sets per exercise	1–2	2	2	3
Repetitions	10	12	18–20	8–12 (RM)
Intensity (resistance)	Very low	Moderate	Low	High
Volume	Low	Moderate	Moderate	High
Sessions per week	2	2	2	3
Weeks	2	3	2	3

Selected exercises: Bench press, leg press, leg curl, lat pull-down, rowing torso, rotary torso, seated back, and abdominal crunch.

Training days: ☐ M ☑ T ☐ W ☐ Th ☐ F ☑ S ☐ S   Training time: **3:00 pm**

Signature: **Mary Johnson**   Goal: **Average**   Date: **9-10-05**

Body Composition

One of the motivational factors to enroll in a fitness course was Mary's desire to learn how to better manage her weight. She had gained a few pounds since entering college. To prevent further weight gain, she thought it was time to learn sound principles for weight management (Behavior Analysis process of change). She was in the Preparation stage of change because she was planning to start a diet and exercise program but wasn't sure how to get it done. All Mary needed was a little Consciousness-raising to get her into the Action stage.

With the knowledge she had now gained, Mary planned her program. At 25 percent body fat and 140 pounds, she decided to aim for 23 percent body fat so she would be in the "Good" category for body composition (Goal Setting). This meant she would have to lose about 4 pounds (see Lab 4B, page 119).

Being moderately active, Mary's daily estimated energy requirement was about 1,890 calories (140 × 13.5—see Table 5.2, page 137). Mary also figured out that she was expending an additional 450 calories per day through her newly adopted exercise program and increased level of daily physical activity. Thus, her total daily energy intake would be around 2,340 calories (1,890 + 450).

To lose weight, Mary could decrease her caloric intake by 700 calories per day (body weight × 5—see Lab 5A, page 149), yielding a target daily intake of 1,640 calories. By decreasing the intake by 700 daily calories daily, Mary should achieve her target

weight in about 20 days (4 pounds of fat × 3,500 calories per pound of fat ÷ 700 fewer calories per day = 20 days). Mary picked the 1,500 calorie diet and allowed herself one additional serving of fruit and two servings of vegetables to meet her estimated 1,640 daily calorie needs.

The processes of change that will help Mary in the Action stage for weight management are Goal Setting, Countering (exercising instead of watching television), Monitoring, Environment Control, and Rewards. To monitor her daily caloric intake, Mary uses the 1,500-calorie diet plan in Lab 5B, and once a week she cross-checks her intake with the nutrient analysis in Profile Plus 2006 (the software that accompanies this book). To further exert control over her environment, she gave away all of her junk food. She determined that she would not eat out while on the diet, and she bought only low-to-moderate fat/complex carbohydrate foods during the 3 weeks. As her reward, she achieved her target body weight of 136 pounds.

You Can Do It

Once the proper exercise, nutrition, and behavior modification guidelines are understood, implementing a fitness lifestyle program is not as difficult as people think. With adequate preparation and a personal behavioral analysis, you are now ready to design, implement, evaluate, and adhere to a lifetime fitness program that can enhance your functional capacity and zest for life.

According to the concepts provided thus far in this book, three case studies are given in Lab 9B for you to evaluate how well you have learned and are able to apply the principles of exercise prescription.

You also have an opportunity to update your current stage of change and fitness category for each health-related component of physical fitness.

ASSESS YOUR KNOWLEDGE

1. Which of the following is *not* a skill-related fitness component?
   a. agility
   b. speed
   c. power
   d. strength
   e. balance

2. The ability to quickly and efficiently change body position and direction is known as
   a. agility.
   b. coordination.
   c. speed.
   d. reaction time.
   e. mobility.

3. The two components of power are
   a. strength and endurance.
   b. speed and force.
   c. speed and endurance.
   d. strength and force.
   e. strength and speed.
   f. endurance and force.

4. Diabetics should
   a. not exercise alone.
   b. wear a bracelet that identifies their condition.
   c. exercise at a low-to-moderate intensity.
   d. check blood glucose levels before and after exercise.
   e. All four guidelines above.

5. Exercise intensity during pregnancy should be decreased by about _____ percent from the pre-pregnancy program.
   a. 5
   b. 10
   c. 20
   d. 25
   e. 50

6. During exercise in the heat, drinking about a cup of cool water every _____ minutes seems to be ideal to prevent dehydration.
   a. 5
   b. 15 to 20
   c. 30
   d. 30 to 45
   e. 60

7. One of the most common causes of activity-related injuries is
   a. high impact activities.
   b. low level of fitness.
   c. exercising without stretching.
   d. improper warm-up.
   e. All choices result in about an equal number of injuries.

8. Improvements in maximal oxygen uptake in older adults (as compared to younger adults) as a result of cardiorespiratory endurance training are
   a. lower.
   b. higher.
   c. difficult to determine.
   d. nonexistent.
   e. similar.

9. To participate in sports, it is recommended that you have
   a. basic fitness and sport-specific conditioning.
   b. at least a "Good" rating on skill-fitness.
   c. good to excellent agility.
   d. basic speed.
   e. All of the above are recommended.

10. Periodization is a training approach that
    a. uses a systematic variation in intensity and volume.
    b. enhances fitness and performance.
    c. is commonly used by athletes.
    d. helps to prevent staleness and overtraining.
    e. All are correct choices.

Correct answers can be found at the back of the book.

MEDIA MENU

PROFILE PLUS CD CONNECTIONS

■ Evaluate your skill-related fitness levels.

■ Check how well you understand the chapter's concepts.

INTERNET CONNECTIONS

■ American Council of Exercise. This site features "Fit Facts," covering sports and outdoor activities, youth

fitness, and exercise information for people with health challenges.
   http://www.acefitness.com

■ Fitness Jumpsite. This site features information on nutrition, weight management, fitness equipment, and healthy lifestyles. A comprehensive search engine is also available.
   http://www.primusweb.com/fitnesspartner

■ President's Council on Physical Fitness and Sports. This site features fitness basics, workout plans, and exercise principles.
http://www.hoptechno.com/book11.htm

■ Fitness online. This site features information on fitness goals and programs, fitness adventures, injury prevention, nutrition, and mental fitness.
http://www.fitnessonline.com/

Notes

1. R. F. Kirby, "A Simple Test of Agility," *Coach and Athlete,* June 1971: 30–31.

2. American Alliance for Health, Physical Education, Recreation and Dance (AAHPERD). *Youth Fitness: Test Manual.* Reston, VA: AAHPERD, 1976.

3. AAHPERD, note 2.

4. R. S. Paffenbarger, Jr., R. T. Hyde, A. L. Wing, and C. H. Steinmetz, "A Natural History of Athleticism and Cardiovascular Health," *Journal of the American Medical Association* 252 (1984): 491–495.

5. American College of Sports Medicine, "Position Stand: Exercise and Type 2 Diabetes," *Medicine and Science in Sports and Exercise* 32 (2000): 1345–1360.

6. University of California at Berkeley, *The Wellness Guide to Lifelong Fitness* (New York: Random House, 1993): 198.

7. American College of Obstetricians and Gynecologists," Exercise During Pregnancy and the Postpartum Period" (ACOG Committee Opinion No. 267), *International Journal of Gynecology and Obstetrics* 77 (2002): 79–81.

8. American College of Sports Medicine, "Position Stand: Exercise and Physical Activity for Older Adults," *Medicine and Science in Sports and Exercise* 30 (1998): 992–1008.

9. R. J. Shephard, "Exercise and Aging: Extending Independence in Older Adult," *Geriatrics* 48 (1993): 61–64.

10. F. W. Kash, J. L. Boyer, S. P. Van Camp, L. S. Verity, and J. P. Wallace, "The Effect of Physical Activity on Aerobic Power in Older Men (A Longitudinal Study)," *Physician and Sports Medicine* 18, no. 4 (1990): 73–83.

11. J. Hagberg, S. Blair, A. Ehsani, N. Gordon, N. Kaplan, C. Tipton, and E. Zambraski, "Position Stand: Physical Activity, Physical Fitness, and Hypertension," *Medicine and Science in Sports and Exercise* 25 (1993): i–x.

12. W. S. Evans, "Exercise, Nutrition and Aging," *Journal of Nutrition* 122 (1992): 796–801.

13. E. J. Marcinick, J. Potts, G. Schlabach, S. Will, P. Dawson, and B. F. Hurley, "Effects of Strength Training on Lactate Threshold and Endurance Performance," *Medicine and Science in Sports and Exercise* 23 (1991): 739–743.

14. The Editors, "Exercise for the Ages," *Consumer Reports on Health* (Yonkers, NY: July, 1996).

15. J. M. Walker, D. Sue, N. Miles-Elkousy, G. Ford, and H. Trevelyan, "Active Mobility of the Extremities in Older Subjects," *Physical Therapy* 64 (1994): 919–923.

16. S. B. Roberts, et al., "What are the Dietary Needs of Adults?" *International Journal of Obesity* 16 (1992): 969–976.

Suggested Readings

American College of Obstetricians and Gynecologists. "Exercise During Pregnancy and the Postpartum Period (ACOG Committee Opinion No. 267). *International Journal of Gynecology and Obstetrics* 77 (2002): 79–81.

Prentice, W., and D. D. Arnheim. *Arnheim's Principles of Athletic Training.* Boston: McGraw–Hill, 2003.

Coleman, E. *Eating for Endurance.* Palo Alto, CA: Bull Publishing, 2003.

Pfeiffer, R. P, and B. C. Mangus. *Concepts of Athletic Training.* Boston: Jones and Bartlett, 2005.

Unruh, N., S. Unruh, and E. Scantling. "Heat Can Kill: Guidelines to Prevent Heat Illness in Athletics and Physical Education." *Journal of Physical Education, Recreation & Dance* 73 no. 6 (2002): 36–38.

Lab 9A

ASSESSMENT OF SKILL-RELATED COMPONENTS OF FITNESS

Name: _____ Date: _____ Grade: _____

Instructor: _____ Course: _____ Section: _____

Necessary Lab Equipment

Agility: Free-throw area of a basketball court (or any smooth area 12 by 19 feet with sufficient running space around it), four plastic cones, and a stopwatch.

Balance: Any flat, smooth floor (not carpeted) and a stopwatch.

Coordination: A 32 inch–long by 5 inch–wide piece of cardboard with six circles drawn on it as explained in Figure 9.2, page 270, three full cans of soda pop (12 oz), and a stopwatch.

Power: A flat, smooth surface, and a 10-foot tape measure (or two standard cloth measuring tapes, each 60 inches long).

Reaction Time: A standard yardstick with a shaded "concentration zone" drawn on the first 2 inches of the stick.

Speed: A school track or premeasured 50-yard straightaway.

Objective

To assess the fitness level for each skill-related fitness component.

Lab Preparation

Wear exercise clothing, including running shoes. Do not exercise strenuously several hours prior to this lab.

Instructions

Perform all six tests for the fitness-related components as outlined in Chapter 9. Report the results below and answer the questions given at the end of this lab.

ProfilePlus

Skill-Related Fitness:	Test Results		
Agility	Trials:	1. ___ . ___	2. ___ . ___
Balance	Trials:	1. ___ . ___	2. ___ . ___
Coordination	Trials:	1. ___ . ___	2. ___ . ___
Power	Trials:	1. ___	2. ___	3. ___
Reaction Time	Trials:	1. ___ . ___	2. ___ . ___	3. ___ . ___
	4. ___ . ___	5. ___ . ___	6. ___ . ___	7. ___ . ___
	8. ___ . ___	9. ___ . ___	10. ___ . ___	11. ___ . ___
	12. ___ . ___		Average (6 middle scores) = ___ . ___
Speed	Trial:	1. ___ . ___

See Tables 9.1, 9.2, and 9.3, pages 273. Skill-Related Fitness Categories

Fitness Component/Test	Percentile Rank	Category
Agility: SEMO test		
Balance: One-foot stand		
Coordination: Soda pop test		
Power: Standing long jump		
Reaction Time: Yardstick test		
Speed: 50-yard dash		

Interpretation of Test Results

1. What conclusions can you draw from your test results?

_____

_____

_____

_____

_____

2. Briefly state how you could improve your test results and what activities you could engage in to obtain the desired results.

_____

_____

_____

_____

_____

3. Did you ever participate in organized sports, or have you found success in a particular game or sport? ☐ Yes ☐ No

   3a. If your answer is yes, list the sports, games, or events in which you enjoy(ed) success.

_____

_____

   3b. Is there a relationship between your answers to question 3a and your test results in this lab?

_____

_____

_____

Lab 9B

HEALTH-RELATED FITNESS CASE STUDIES

Name: _____ Date: _____ Grade: _____

Instructor: _____ Course: _____ Section: _____

Necessary Lab Equipment

None.

Objective

To provide an opportunity to apply exercise prescriptions concepts and to determine progress in your personal fitness goals.

I. Indicate the procedure that you would follow to clear a 66-year-old woman who wishes to initiate an exercise program. Be specific in your recommendations.

_____

_____

_____

_____

_____

_____

_____

_____

II. Design a periodized strength-training program for a 22-year-old sprint athlete who wishes to reach peak performance in 18 weeks. Include in your program the exercises (lifts), sets, and number of repetitions maximum that are to be used with each mesocycle (use additional paper as necessary).

III. Using the information that you have thus far learned in this course, design a 16-week exercise prescription for a previously inactive 60-year-old male with a resting heart rate of 76 beats per minute. Other than some minor knee problems, the individual has been cleared for cardiorespiratory exercise by a physician. Use a weekly progressive approach as outlined in Lab 6D (pages 195–196) and Figure 9.5 (page 290) that includes intensity, duration, frequency, and mode(s) of exercise.

IV. Indicate your stage of change and fitness category for the health-related components of fitness.

Fitness Component	Initial Rating		Current Rating	
	Stage of Change	Fitness Category	Stage of Change	Fitness Category
Cardiorespiratory endurance				
Muscular strength and endurance				
Muscular flexibility				
Body composition				

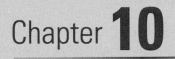

Chapter 10

Stress Management

Objectives

- Define stress, stressor, eustress, and distress.
- Explain the role of stress in maintaining health and optimal performance.
- Identify the major sources of stress in life.
- Define the two major behavior patterns.
- Explain the factors that increase vulnerability to stress and how to cope with stress.
- Describe some time-management skills.
- Explain the role of physical exercise in reducing stress.
- Describe and learn to use various stress-management techniques.

Profile Plus CD Connections

- Learn how you're affected by stress.
- Find out how vulnerable you are to stress.
- Check how well you understand the chapter's concepts.

Living in today's world is nearly impossible without encountering **stress**. In an unpredictable world that changes with every new day, most people find that stress has become the norm rather than the exception. Further, stress undermines our ability to stay well.[1] Estimates indicate that the annual cost of stress and stress-related diseases in the United States exceeds $100 billion, a direct result of health-care costs, lost productivity, and absenteeism. Many medical and stress researchers believe that "stress should carry a health warning" as well.[2]

The good news is that stress can be self-controlled. Too often, people have accepted stress as a normal part of daily life and, even though everyone has to deal with it, few seem to understand it or know how to cope effectively. It is difficult to live fully without "runs, hits, and errors." Actually, stress should not be avoided entirely. A certain amount of stress is necessary for optimum health, performance, and well-being.

Just what is stress? Dr. Hans Selye, one of the foremost authorities on stress, defined it as "the nonspecific response of the human organism to any demand that is placed upon it."[3] "Nonspecific" indicates that the body reacts in a similar fashion regardless of the nature of the event. In simpler terms, stress is the body's mental, emotional, and physiological response to any situation that is new, threatening, frightening, or exciting.

The body's response to stress has been the same ever since humans were first put on the earth. Stress prepares the organism to react to the stress-causing event, also called the **stressor**. The problem, though, is the way in which we react to stress. Many people thrive under stress; others, under similar circumstances, are unable to handle it. An individual's reaction to a stress-causing agent determines whether that stress is positive or negative.

Dr. Selye defined the ways in which we react to stress as either eustress or distress. In both cases, the nonspecific response is almost the same. In the case of **eustress**, on the one hand, health and performance continue to improve even as stress increases. On the other hand, **distress** refers to the unpleasant or harmful stress under which health and performance begin to deteriorate. The relationship between stress and performance is illustrated in Figure 10.1.

Stress is a fact of modern life, and every person does need an optimal level of stress that is most conducive to adequate health and performance. When stress levels reach mental, emotional, and

FIGURE 10.1 Relationship between stress and health and performance.

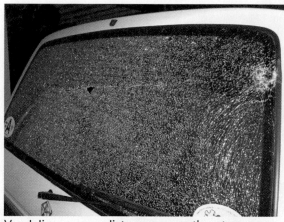

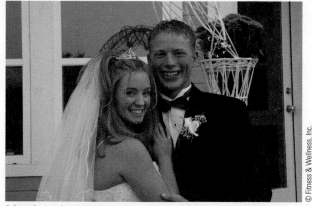
Vandalism causes distress or negative stress.

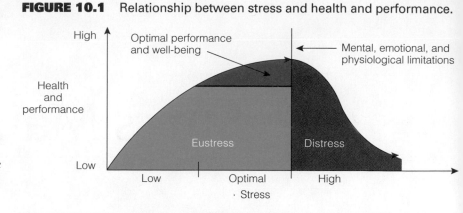
Marriage is an example of positive stress, also known as eustress.

physiological limits, however, stress becomes distress and the person no longer functions effectively.

Chronic distress raises the risk for many health disorders—including coronary heart disease, hypertension, eating disorders, ulcers, diabetes, asthma, depression, migraine headaches, sleep disorders, and chronic fatigue—and may even play a role in

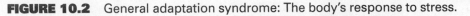

FIGURE 10.2   General adaptation syndrome: The body's response to stress.

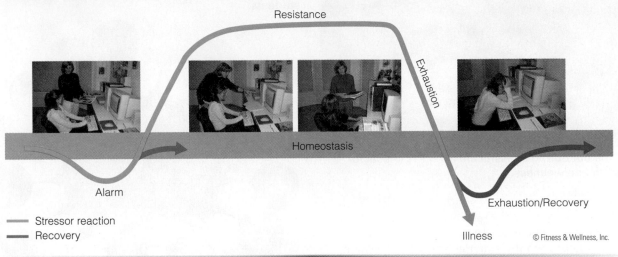

Resistance

Exhaustion

Homeostasis

Alarm

Exhaustion/Recovery

Illness   © Fitness & Wellness, Inc.

▬ Stressor reaction
▬ Recovery

the development of certain types of cancers.[4] Recognizing this and overcoming the problem quickly and efficiently are crucial in maintaining emotional and physiological stability.

Adapting to Stress

The body continually strives to maintain a constant internal environment. This state of physiological balance, known as **homeostasis**, allows the body to function as effectively as possible. When a stressor triggers a nonspecific response, homeostasis is disrupted. This reaction to stressors is best explained by Dr. Selye as the **general adaptation syndrome (GAS)**, composed of three stages—alarm reaction, resistance, and exhaustion/recovery.

Alarm Reaction

The alarm reaction is the immediate response to a stressor (whether positive or negative). During the alarm reaction, the body evokes an instant physiological reaction that mobilizes internal systems and processes to minimize the threat to homeostasis (see also "Coping with Stress" on page 307). If the stressor subsides, the body recovers and returns to homeostasis.

Resistance

If the stressor persists, the body calls upon its limited reserves to build up its resistance as it strives to maintain homeostasis. For a short while, the body

copes effectively and meets the challenge of the stressor until it can be overcome (see Figure 10.2).

Exhaustion/Recovery

If stress becomes chronic and intolerable, the body spends its limited reserves and loses its ability to cope. It enters the exhaustion/recovery stage. During this stage the body functions at a diminished capacity while it recovers from stress. In due time, following an "adequate" recovery period (which varies greatly), the body recuperates and is able to return to homeostasis. If chronic stress persists during the exhaustion stage, however, the immune function is compromised, which can damage body systems and lead to disease.

An example of the stress response through the general adaptation syndrome can be illustrated in college test performance. As you prepare to take an

Stress   The mental, emotional, and physiological response of the body to any situation that is new, threatening, frightening, or exciting.

Stressor   Stress-causing event.

Eustress   Positive stress: Health and performance continue to improve, even as stress increases.

Distress   Negative stress: Unpleasant or harmful stress under which health and performance begin to deteriorate.

Homeostasis   A natural state of equilibrium; the body attempts to maintain this equilibrium by constantly reacting to external forces that attempt to disrupt this fine balance.

General adaptation syndrome (GAS)   A theoretical model that explains the body's adaptation to sustained stress which includes three stages: Alarm reaction, resistance, and exhaustion/recovery.

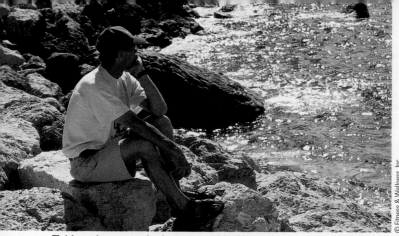

Taking time out during stressful life events is critical for good health and wellness.

exam, you experience an initial alarm reaction. If you understand the material, study for the exam, and do well (eustress), the body recovers and stress is dissipated. If, however, you are not adequately prepared and fail the exam, you trigger the resistance stage. You are now concerned about your grade, and you remain in the resistance stage until the next exam. If you prepare and do well, the body recovers. But if you fail once again and can no longer bring up your grade, exhaustion sets in and physical and emotional breakdowns may occur. Exhaustion may be further aggravated if you are struggling in other courses as well.

The exhaustion stage is often manifested by athletes and the most ardent fitness participants. Staleness is usually a manifestation of overtraining. Peak performance can be sustained for only about 2 to 3 weeks at a time. Any attempts to continue intense training after peaking leads to exhaustion, diminished fitness, and the mental and physical problems associated with overtraining (see Chapter 9, pages 286–287). Thus, athletes and some fitness participants also need an active recovery phase after attaining peak fitness.

Sources of Stress

Several instruments have been developed to assess sources of stress in life. The most practical of these is the **Life Experiences Survey**, presented in Lab 10A, in which you identify the life changes within the last 12 months that may have an impact on your physical and psychological well-being.

Profile Plus

Feeling under pressure? Discover how stress affects you with the activities on your CD-ROM.

The Life Experiences Survey is divided into two sections. Section 1, to be completed by all respondents, contains a list of 47 life events plus three blank spaces for other events experienced but not listed in the survey. Section 2 contains an additional 10 questions designed for students only (students should fill out both sections).

FIGURE 10.3 Stressors in the lives of college students.

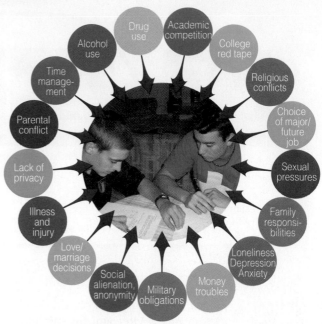

Adapted from W.W.K. Hoeger, L.W. Turner, and B.Q. Hafen. *Wellness: Guidelines for a Healthy Lifestyle.* Wadsworth/Thomson Learning, 2002.

Common stressors in the lives of college students are depicted in Figure 10.3.

The survey requires the testee to rate the extent to which his or her life events had a positive or negative impact on his or her life at the time these events occurred. The ratings are on a 7-point scale. A rating of −3 indicates an extremely undesirable impact. A rating of zero (0) suggests neither a positive nor a negative impact, called **neustress**. A rating of +3 indicates an extremely desirable impact.

After the person evaluates his or her life events, the negative and the positive points are totaled separately. Both scores are expressed as positive numbers (for example, positive ratings of 2, 1, 3, and 3 = 9 points positive score; negative ratings of −3, −2, −2, −1, and −2 = 10 points negative score). A final "total life change" score can be obtained by adding the positive score and the negative score together as positive numbers (total life change score: 9 + 10 = 19 points).

Because negative and positive changes alike can produce nonspecific responses, the total life change score is a good indicator of total life stress. Most

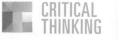 **CRITICAL THINKING**

Technological advances provide many benefits to our lives. What positive and negative effects do these advances have upon your daily living activities, and what impact are they having on your stress level?

BEHAVIOR MODIFICATION PLANNING

CHANGING A TYPE A PERSONALITY

- Make a contract with yourself to slow down and take it easy. Put it in writing. Post it in a conspicuous spot, then stick to the terms you set up. Be specific. Abstracts ("I'm going to be less uptight") don't work.
- Work on only one or two things at a time. Wait until you change one habit before you tackle the next one.
- Eat more slowly and eat only when you are relaxed and sitting down.
- If you smoke, quit.
- Cut down on your caffeine intake, because it increases the tendency to become irritated and agitated.
- Take regular breaks throughout the day, even as brief as 5 or 10 minutes, when you totally change what you're doing. Get up, stretch, get a drink of cool water, walk around for a few minutes.
- Work on fighting your impatience. If you're standing in line at the grocery store, study the interesting things people have in their carts instead of getting upset.
- Work on controlling hostility. Keep a written log. When do you flare up? What causes it? How do you feel at the time? What preceded it? Look for patterns and figure out what sets you off. Then do something about it. Either avoid the situations that cause you hostility or practice reacting to them in different ways.
- Plan some activities just for the fun of it. Load a picnic basket in the car and drive to the country with a friend. After a stressful physics class, stop at a theater and see a good comedy.
- Choose a role model, someone you know and admire who does not have a Type A personality. Observe the person carefully, then try out some techniques the person demonstrates.

- Simplify your life so you can learn to relax a little bit. Figure out which activities or commitments you can eliminate right now, then get rid of them.
- If morning is a problem time for you and you get too hurried, set your alarm clock half an hour earlier.
- Take time out during even the most hectic day to do something truly relaxing. Because you won't be used to it, you may have to work at it at first. Begin by listing things you'd really enjoy that would calm you. Include some things that take only a few minutes: Watch a sunset, lie out on the lawn at night and look at the stars, call an old friend and catch up on news, take a nap, sauté a pan of mushrooms and savor them slowly.
- If you're under a deadline, take short breaks. Stop and talk to someone for 5 minutes, take a short walk, or lie down with a cool cloth over your eyes for 10 minutes.
- Pay attention to what your own body clock is saying. You've probably noticed that every 90 minutes or so, you lose the ability to concentrate, get a little sleepy, and have a tendency to daydream. Instead of fighting the urge, put down your work and let your mind wander for a few minutes. Use the time to imagine and let your creativity run wild.
- Learn to treasure unplanned surprises: a friend dropping by unannounced, a hummingbird outside your window, a child's tightly clutched bouquet of wildflowers.
- Savor your relationships. Think about the people in your life. Relax with them and give yourself to them. Give up trying to control others and resist the urge to end relationships that don't always go as you'd like them to.

From W. W. K. Hoeger, L. W. Turner, and B. Q. Hafen, *Wellness: Guidelines for a Healthy Lifestyle* (3d ed.) (Belmont, CA: Wadsworth/Thomson Learning, 2002).

research in this area, however, suggests that the negative change score is a better predictor of potential physical and psychological illness than the total change score. More research is necessary to establish the role of total change and the role of the ratio of positive to negative stress.

Behavior Patterns

Common life events are not the only source of stress in life. All too often, individuals bring on stress as a result of their behavior patterns. The two main behavior patterns, Type A and Type B, are based on several observable characteristics.

Several attempts have been made to develop an objective scale to identify Type A individuals properly, but these questionnaires are not as valid and reliable as researchers would like them to be. Consequently, the main assessment tool to determine behavioral type is still the **structured interview**,

Life Experiences Survey A questionnaire used to assess sources of stress in life.

Neustress Neutral stress; stress that is neither harmful nor helpful.

Structured interview Assessment tool used to determine behavioral patterns that define Type A and B personalities.

during which a person is asked to reply to several questions that describe Type A and Type B behavior patterns. The interviewer notes the responses to the questions as well as the individual's mental, emotional, and physical behaviors as he or she replies to each question.

Based on the answers and the associated behaviors, the interviewer rates the person along a continuum ranging from Type A to Type B. Along this continuum, behavioral patterns are classified into five categories: A-1, A-2, X (a mix of Type A and Type B), B-3, and B-4. The Type A-1 exhibits all of the Type A characteristics, and the B-4 shows a relative absence of Type A behaviors. The Type A-2 does not exhibit a complete Type A pattern, and the Type B-3 exhibits only a few Type A characteristics.

Type A behavior characterizes a primarily hard-driving, overambitious, aggressive, at times hostile and overly competitive person. Type A individuals often set their own goals, are self-motivated, try to accomplish many tasks at the same time, are excessively achievement-oriented, and have a high degree of time urgency.

In contrast, **Type B** behavior is characteristic of calm, casual, relaxed, easygoing individuals. Type B people take one thing at a time, do not feel pressured or hurried, and seldom set their own deadlines.

Over the years, experts have indicated that individuals classified as Type A are under too much stress and have a significantly higher incidence of coronary heart disease. Based on these findings, Type A individuals have been counseled to lower their stress level by modifying their Type A behaviors.

Many of the Type A characteristics are learned behaviors. Consequently, if people can identify the sources of stress and make changes in their behavioral responses, they can move along the continuum and respond more like Type B's. The debate, however, has centered on which Type A behaviors should be changed, because not all of them are undesirable.

Even though personality questionnaires are not as valid and reliable as the structured interview in identifying Type A individuals, Drs. Meyer Friedman and Ray Rosenman, two San Francisco scientists, constructed a Type A personality assessment form, adapted from the structured interview method, to give people a general idea of Type A behavioral patterns. This assessment form is found in Lab 10A. You can use it to understand your own behavioral patterns better. If you obtain a high rating, you probably are Type A.

We also know that many individuals perform well under pressure. They typically are classified as Type A but do not demonstrate any of the detrimental effects of stress. Drs. Robert and Marilyn Kriegel came up with the term and concept of Type C to characterize people with these behaviors.[5]

BEHAVIOR MODIFICATION PLANNING

TIPS TO MANAGE ANGER

- Commit to change and gain control over the behavior.
- Remind yourself that chronic anger leads to illness and disease and may eventually kill you.
- Recognize when feelings of anger are developing and ask yourself the following questions:
  - Is the matter really that important?
  - Is the anger justified?
  - Can I change the situation without getting angry?
  - Is it worth risking my health over it?
  - How will I feel about the situation in a few hours?
- Tell yourself, "Stop, my health is worth it" every time you start to feel anger.
- Prepare for a positive response: Ask for an explanation or clarification of the situation, walk away and evaluate the situation, exercise, or use appropriate stress management techniques (breathing, meditation, imagery) before you become angry and hostile.
- Manage anger at once; do not let it build up.
- Never attack anyone verbally or physically.
- Keep a journal and ponder the situations that cause you to be angry.
- Seek professional help if you are unable to overcome anger by yourself: You are worth it.

Type C individuals are just as highly stressed as Type A's but do not seem to be at higher risk for disease than Type B's. The keys to successful Type C performance are *commitment, confidence,* and *control.* Type C people are highly committed to what they are doing, have a great deal of confidence in their ability to do their work, and are in constant control of their actions. In addition, they enjoy their work and maintain themselves in top physical condition to be able to meet the mental and physical demands of their work.

Type A behavior by itself is no longer viewed as a major risk factor for coronary heart disease, but Type A individuals who commonly express anger and hostility are at higher risk. Therefore, many behavioral modification counselors now work on changing the latter behaviors to prevent disease. The questionnaire provided at the end of Lab 10A can help you determine whether you have a hostile personality.

Anger increases heart rate and blood pressure and leads to constriction of blood vessels. Over time, these changes are thought to cause damage to the arteries and eventually lead to a heart attack. Several studies indicate that chronically angry people have up to a threefold increased risk for CHD and are seven times more likely to suffer a fatal heart attack by age 50.

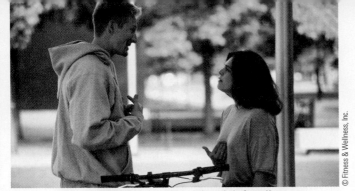
Anger and hostility can increase the risk for disease.

Many experts also believe that emotional stress is far more likely than physical stress to trigger a heart attack. People who are impatient and readily annoyed when they have to wait for someone or something—an employee, a traffic light, a table in a restaurant—are especially vulnerable.

Research is also focusing on individuals who have anxiety, depression, and feelings of helplessness when they encounter setbacks and failures in life. People who lose control of their lives or who give up on their dreams in life, knowing that they could and should be doing better, probably are more likely to have heart attacks than hard-driving people who enjoy their work.

Vulnerability to Stress

Researchers have identified a number of factors that can affect the way in which people handle stress.

Profile Plus
How vulnerable to stress are you? Find out with the activity on your CD-ROM.

How people deal with these factors can actually increase or decrease vulnerability to stress. The questionnaire provided in Lab 10B lists these factors so you can determine your vulnerability rating. Many of the items on this questionnaire are related to health, social support, self-worth, and nurturance (sense of being needed). All of these factors are crucial to a person's physical, social, mental, and emotional well-being and are essential to cope effectively with stressful life events. The more integrated people are in society, the less vulnerable they are to stress and illness.

Positive correlations have been found between social support and health outcomes. People can draw upon social support to weather crises. Knowing that someone else cares, that people are there to lean on, that support is out there, is valuable for survival (or growth) in times of need.

The health benefits of physical fitness have already been discussed extensively. The questionnaire in Lab 10B will help you identify specific areas in which you can make improvements to help you cope more efficiently.

As you complete Lab 10B, you will notice that many of the items describe situations and behaviors

that are within your own control. To make yourself less vulnerable to stress, you will want to improve the behaviors that make you more vulnerable to stress. You should start by modifying the behaviors that are easiest to change before undertaking some of the most difficult ones.

Time Management

According to Benjamin Franklin, "Time is the stuff life is made of." The present hurry-up style of American life is not conducive to wellness. The hassles involved in getting through a routine day often lead to stress-related illnesses. People who do not manage their time properly will quickly experience chronic stress, fatigue, despair, discouragement, and illness.

Surveys indicate that most Americans think time moves too fast for them, and more than half of those surveyed think they have to get everything done. The younger the respondents, the more they struggle with lack of time. Almost half wish they had more time for exercise and recreation, hobbies, and family.

Healthy and successful people are good time managers, able to maintain a pace of life within their comfort zone. In a survey of 1954 Harvard graduates from the school of business, only 27 percent had reached the goals they established in college. Every one had rated himself a superior time manager, and only 8 percent of the remaining graduates perceived themselves as superior time managers. The successful graduates attributed their success to smart work, not necessarily hard work.

Five Steps to Time Management

Trying to achieve one or more goals in a limited time can create a tremendous amount of stress. Many people don't seem to have enough hours in the day to accomplish their tasks. The greatest demands on our time, nonetheless, frequently are self-imposed. We try to do too much, too fast, too soon.

Some time killers, such as eating, sleeping, and recreation, are necessary for health and wellness, but in excess they'll lead to stress in life. You can

Type A Behavior pattern characteristic of a hard-driving, overambitious, aggressive, at times hostile, and overly competitive person.

Type B Behavior pattern characteristic of a calm, casual, relaxed, and easy-going individual.

Type C Behavior pattern of individuals who are just as highly stressed as the Type A but do not seem to be at higher risk for disease than the Type B.

BEHAVIOR MODIFICATION PLANNING

COMMON TIME KILLERS

- Watching television
- Listening to radio/music
- Sleeping
- Eating
- Daydreaming
- Shopping
- Socializing/parties
- Recreation
- Talking on the telephone
- Worrying
- Procrastinating
- Drop-in visitors
- Confusion (unclear goals)
- Indecision (what to do next)
- Interruptions
- Perfectionism (every detail must be done)

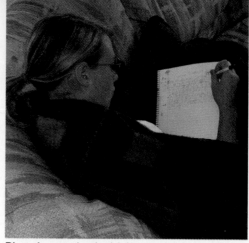

© Fitness & Wellness, Inc.

Planning and prioritizing activities will simplify your days.

follow five basic steps to make better use of your time (also see Lab 10C):

1. Find the time killers. Many people do not know how they spend each part of the day. Keep a 4- to 7-day log and record your activities at half-hour intervals. Record the activities as you go through your typical day so you will remember all of them. At the end of each day, decide when you wasted time. You may be shocked by the amount of time you spent on the phone, on the Internet, sleeping (more than 8 hours per night), or watching television.

2. Set long-range and short-range goals. Setting goals requires some in-depth thinking and helps put your life and daily tasks in perspective: What do I want out of life? Where do I want to be 10 years from now? Next year? Next week? Tomorrow? You can use Lab 10C to list these goals.

3. Identify your immediate goals and prioritize them for today and this week (Use Lab 10C—make as many copies as necessary). Each day sit down and determine what you need to accomplish that day and that week. Rank your "today" and "this week" tasks in four categories: (a) top-priority, (b) medium-priority, (c) low-priority, and (d) trash.

   Top-priority tasks are the most important. If you were to reap most of your productivity from 30 percent of your activities, which would they be? Medium-priority activities are those that must be done but can wait a day or two. Low-priority activities are those to be done only upon completing all top- and middle-priority activities. Trash activities are not worth your time (for example, cruising the hallways, channel-surfing).

4. Use a daily planner to help you organize and simplify your day. In this way, you can access your priority list, appointments, notes, references,

names, places, phone numbers, and addresses conveniently from your coat pocket or purse. Many people think that planning daily and weekly activities is a waste of time. A few minutes to schedule your time each day, however, may pay off in hours saved.

As you plan your day, be realistic and find your comfort zone. Determine the best way to organize your day. Which is the most productive time for work? study? errands? Are you a morning person, or are you getting most of your work done when people are quitting for the day? Pick your best hours for top-priority activities. Be sure to schedule enough time for exercise and relaxation. Recreation is not necessarily wasted time. You need to take care of your physical and emotional well-being. Otherwise your life will be seriously imbalanced.

5. Conduct nightly audits. Take 10 minutes each night to figure out how well you accomplished your goals that day. Successful time managers evaluate themselves daily. This simple task will help you see the entire picture. Cross off the goals you accomplished, and carry over to the next day those you did not get done. You also may realize that some goals can be moved down to low-priority or be trashed.

Time-Management Skills

In addition to the five major steps, the following can help you make better use of your time:

- *Delegate.* If possible, delegate activities that someone else can do for you. Having another person type your paper while you prepare for an exam might be well worth the expense and your time.
- *Say "no."* Learn to say no to activities that keep you from getting your top priorities done. You can do only so much in a single day. Nobody has enough time to do everything he or she would

like to get done. Don't overload either. Many people are afraid to say no because they feel guilty if they do. Think ahead, and consider the consequences. Are you doing this to please others? What will it do to your well-being? Can you handle one more task? At some point, you have to balance your activities and look at life and time realistically.

■ *Protect against boredom.* Doing nothing can be a source of stress. People need to feel that they are contributing and that they are productive members of society. It is also good for self-esteem and self-worth. Set realistic goals and work toward them each day.

■ *Plan ahead for disruptions.* Even a careful plan of action can be disrupted. An unexpected phone call or visitor can ruin your schedule. Planning your response ahead will help you deal with these saboteurs.

■ *Get it done.* Select only one task at a time, concentrate on it, and see it through. Many people do a little here, do a little there, then do something else. In the end, nothing gets done. An exception to working on just one task at a time is when you are doing a difficult task. Rather than "killing yourself," interchange with another activity that is not as hard.

■ *Eliminate distractions.* If you have trouble adhering to a set plan, remove distractions and trash activities from your eyesight. Television, radio, magazines, open doors, or studying in a park might distract you and become time killers.

■ *Set aside "overtimes."* Regularly schedule as overtime the time you didn't think you would need to complete unfinished projects. Most people underschedule rather than overschedule time. The result is (usually late-night) burnout! If you schedule overtimes and get your tasks done, enjoy some leisure time, get ahead on another project, or work on some of your trash activities.

■ *Plan time for you.* Set aside special time for yourself daily. Life is not meant to be all work. Use your time to walk, read, or listen to your favorite music.

■ *Reward yourself.* As with any other healthy behavior, positive change or a job well done deserves a reward. We often overlook the value of rewards, even if they are self-given. People practice behaviors that are rewarded and discontinue those that are not.

One more activity that you should perform weekly is to go through the list of strategies in Lab 10C to determine if you are becoming a good time manager. Provide a yes or no answer to each statement. If you are able to answer yes to most questions, congratulations. You are becoming a good time manager.

BEHAVIOR MODIFICATION PLANNING

COMMON SYMPTOMS OF STRESS

■ Headaches
■ Muscular aches (mainly in neck, shoulders, and back)
■ Grinding teeth
■ Nervous tick, finger tapping, toe tapping
■ Increased sweating
■ Increase in or loss of appetite
■ Insomnia
■ Nightmares
■ Fatigue
■ Dry mouth
■ Stuttering
■ High blood pressure
■ Tightness or pain in the chest
■ Impotence
■ Hives

■ Dizziness
■ Depression
■ Irritation
■ Anger
■ Hostility
■ Fear, panic, anxiety
■ Stomach pain, flutters
■ Nausea
■ Cold, clammy hands
■ Poor concentration
■ Pacing
■ Restlessness
■ Rapid heart rate
■ Low-grade infection
■ Loss of sex drive
■ Rash or acne

Coping with Stress

The ways in which people perceive and cope with stress seem to be more important in the development of disease than the amount and type of stress itself. If individuals perceive stress as a definite problem in their lives or if it interferes with their optimal level of health and performance, they can call upon several excellent stress-management techniques to help them cope more effectively.

First, of course, the person must recognize that a problem exists. Many people either do not want to believe they are under too much stress or they fail to recognize some of the typical symptoms of distress. Noting some of the stress-related symptoms (see "Common Symptoms of Stress") will help a person respond more objectively and initiate an adequate coping response.

When people have stress-related symptoms, they should first try to identify and remove the stressor or stress-causing agent. This is not as simple as it may seem, because in some situations eliminating the stressor is not possible, or a person may not even know the exact causal agent. If the cause is unknown, keeping a log of the time and days when the symptoms occur, as well as the events preceding and following the onset of symptoms, may be helpful.

For instance, a couple noted that every afternoon around 6 o'clock, the wife became nauseated and had abdominal pain. After seeking professional help, both were instructed to keep a log of daily events. It soon became clear that the symptoms did not appear on weekends but always started just before the husband came home from work during the week. Following some personal interviews with the couple, it was determined that the wife felt a lack of attention from her husband and responded subconsciously by becoming ill to the point at which she required personal care and affection from her husband. Once the stressor was identified, they initiated appropriate behavior changes to correct the situation.

In many instances, however, the stressor cannot be removed. Examples of these situations are the death of a close family member, the first year on the job, an intolerable boss, or a change in work responsibility. Nevertheless, stress can be managed through relaxation techniques.

The body responds to stress by activating the **fight-or-flight** mechanism, which prepares a person to take action by stimulating the body's vital defense systems. This stimulation originates in the hypothalamus and the pituitary gland in the brain. The hypothalamus activates the sympathetic nervous system, and the pituitary activates the release of catecholamines (hormones) from the adrenal glands.

These hormonal changes increase heart rate, blood pressure, blood flow to active muscles and the brain, glucose levels, oxygen consumption, and strength—all necessary for the body to fight or flee. For the body to relax, one of these actions must take place. If the person is unable to take action, however, the muscles tense up and tighten (see Figure 10.4). This increased tension and tightening can be dissipated effectively through some coping techniques, described in the following pages.

Physical Activity

The benefits of physical activity in reducing the physiological and psychological responses to stress are well-established.[6] Exercise is one of the simplest tools to control stress. The value of exercise in reducing stress is related to several factors, the main one being a decrease in muscular tension. For example, a person can be distressed because he or she has had a miserable 8 hours of work with an intolerable boss. To make matters worse, it is late and, on the way home, the car in front is going much slower than the speed limit. The fight-or-flight mechanism—already activated during the stressful day—begins again: catecholamines rise, heart rate and blood pressure shoot up, breathing quickens and deepens, muscles tense up, and all systems say "go." No action can be initiated or stress dissipated, though, because the person cannot just hit the boss or the car in front.

A real remedy would be to take action by "hitting" the swimming pool, the tennis ball, the weights, or the jogging trail. Engaging in physical

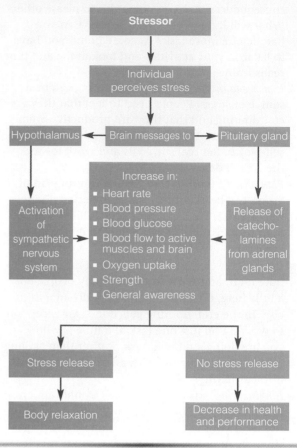

FIGURE 10.4 Physiological response to stress: fight-or-flight mechanism.

activity reduces the muscular tension and metabolizes the increased catecholamines (which were triggered by the fight-or-flight mechanism and brought about the physiological changes). Although exercise does not solve problems at work or take care of slow drivers, it certainly can help a person cope with stress and can prevent stress from becoming a chronic problem.

The early evening hours are a popular time to exercise for a lot of highly stressed executives. On the way home from work, they stop at the health club or the fitness center. Exercising at this time helps them to dissipate the stress accumulated during the day. The evening exercise helps to get rid of the stress and also provides an opportunity to enjoy the evening more. At home, the family will appreciate Dad or Mom coming home more relaxed, leaving work problems behind and being able to dedicate all energy to family activities.

Many people can relate to exercise as a means of managing stress by remembering how good they felt the last time they concluded a strenuous exercise session after a long, difficult day at the office. A

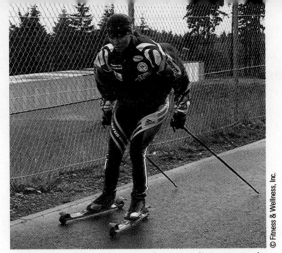

Physical activity: an excellent tool to control stress.

fatigued muscle is a relaxed muscle. For this reason, people often say that the best part of exercise is the shower afterward.

Research has also shown that physical exercise requiring continuous and rhythmic muscular activity, such as aerobic exercise, stimulates alpha-wave activity in the brain. These are the same wave patterns seen commonly during meditation and relaxation.

Further, during vigorous aerobic exercise lasting 30 minutes or longer, morphine-like substances called **endorphins** are thought to be released from the pituitary gland in the brain. These substances act as painkillers and also seem to induce the soothing, calming effect often associated with aerobic exercise.

Another way by which exercise helps lower stress is to deliberately divert stress to various body systems. Dr. Selye explains in his book *Stress without Distress* that, when one specific task becomes difficult, a change in activity can be as good or better than rest itself.[7] For example, if a person is having trouble with a task and does not seem to be getting anywhere, jogging or swimming for a while is better than sitting around and getting frustrated. In this way, the mental strain is diverted to the working muscles and one system helps the other to relax.

Other psychologists indicate that when muscular tension is removed from the emotional strain, the emotional strain disappears. In many cases, the change of activity suddenly clears the mind and helps put the pieces together.

Researchers have found that physical exercise gives people a psychological boost because exercise does all the following:

- Lessens feelings of anxiety, depression, frustration, aggression, anger, and hostility.
- Alleviates insomnia.
- Provides an opportunity to meet social needs and develop new friendships.
- Allows the person to share common interests and problems.
- Develops discipline.
- Provides the opportunity to do something enjoyable and constructive that will lead to better health and total well-being.

Beyond the short-term benefits of exercise in lessening stress, a regular aerobic exercise program actually strengthens the cardiovascular system itself. Because the cardiovascular system seems to be affected seriously by stress, a stronger system should be able to cope more effectively. For instance, good cardiorespiratory endurance has been shown to lower the resting heart rate and blood pressure. Because both heart rate and blood pressure rise in stressful situations, initiating the stress response at a lower baseline will counteract some of the negative effects of stress. Cardiorespiratory-fit individuals can cope more effectively and are less affected by the stresses of daily living.

Relaxation Techniques

Although benefits are reaped immediately after engaging in any of the several relaxation techniques, several months of regular practice may be necessary for total mastery. The relaxation exercises that follow should not be considered cure-alls. If these exercises do not prove to be effective, more specialized textbooks and professional help are called for. (Some symptoms may not be caused by stress but instead may be related to a medical disorder.)

BIOFEEDBACK

Clinical application of **biofeedback** has been used to treat various medical disorders for many years. Besides its successful application in managing stress, it is commonly used to treat medical disorders such as essential hypertension, asthma, disturbances in heart rhythm and rate, cardiac neurosis, eczematous dermatitis, fecal incontinence, insomnia, and stuttering. Biofeedback as a treatment modality has been defined as a technique in which a person learns to influence physiological responses that are not typically under voluntary control or responses that

Fight or flight Physiological response of the body to stress that prepares the individual to take action by stimulating the body's vital defense systems.

Endorphins Morphine-like substances released from the pituitary gland in the brain during prolonged aerobic exercise. They are thought to induce feelings of euphoria and natural well-being.

Biofeedback A stress-management technique in which a person learns to influence physiological responses that are not typically under voluntary control or responses that typically are regulated but for which regulation has broken down as a result of injury, trauma, or illness.

normally are regulated but regulation has broken down as a result of injury, trauma, or illness.

In simpler terms, biofeedback is the interaction with the interior self. This interaction allows a person to learn the relationship between the mind and the biological response. The person actually can "feel" how thought processes influence biological responses (such as heart rate, blood pressure, body temperature, and muscle tension) and how biological responses in turn influence the thought process.

As an illustration of this process, consider the association between a strange noise in the middle of a dark, quiet night and the heart rate response. At first the heart rate shoots up because of the stress the unknown noise induces. The individual may even feel the heart palpitating in the chest and, while still uncertain about the noise, attempts to avoid panic to prevent an even faster heart rate. Upon realizing that all is well, the person can take control and influence the heart rate to come down. The mind, now calm, is able to exert almost complete control over the biological response.

Complex electronic instruments are required to conduct biofeedback. The process itself entails a three-stage, closed-loop feedback system:

1. A biological response to a stressor is detected and amplified.
2. The response is processed.
3. Results of the response are fed back to the individual immediately.

The person uses this new input and attempts to change the physiological response voluntarily. This attempt, in turn, is detected, amplified, and processed. The results then are fed back to the person. The process continues with the intent of teaching the person to reliably influence the physiological response for the better (see Figure 10.5). The most common methods used to measure physiological responses are monitoring the heart rate, finger temperature, and blood pressure; electromyograms; and electroencephalograms. The goal of biofeedback training is to transfer the experiences learned in the laboratory to everyday living.

Although biofeedback has significant applications in treating various medical disorders, including stress, it requires adequately trained personnel and, in many cases, costly equipment. Therefore, several alternative methods that yield similar results are frequently substituted for biofeedback. For example, research has shown that exercise and progressive muscle relaxation, used successfully in stress management, seem to be just as effective as biofeedback in treating essential hypertension.

PROGRESSIVE MUSCLE RELAXATION

Progressive muscle relaxation, developed by Dr. Edmund Jacobsen in the 1930s, enables individuals

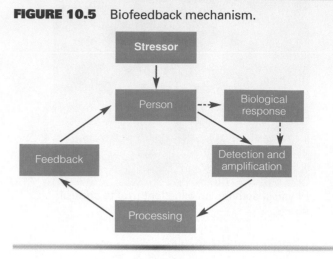

FIGURE 10.5 Biofeedback mechanism.

to relearn the sensation of deep relaxation. The technique involves progressively contracting and relaxing muscle groups throughout the body. Because chronic stress leads to high levels of muscular tension, acute awareness of how progressively tightening and relaxing the muscles feels can release the tension in the muscles and teach the body to relax at will.

Feeling the tension during the exercises also helps the person to be more alert to signs of distress, because this tension is similar to that experienced in stressful situations. In everyday life, these feelings then can cue the person to do relaxation exercises.

Relaxation exercises should be done in a quiet, warm, well-ventilated room. The recommended exercises and the duration of the routine vary from one person to the next. Most important is that the individual pay attention to the sensation that he or she feels each time the muscles are tensed and relaxed.

The exercises should encompass all muscle groups of the body. Following is an example of a sequence of progressive muscle relaxation exercises. The instructions for these exercises can be read to the person, memorized, or tape-recorded. At least 20 minutes should be set aside to complete the entire sequence. Doing the exercises any faster will defeat their purpose. Ideally, the sequence should be done twice a day.

The individual performing the exercises stretches out comfortably on the floor, face up, with a pillow under the knees, and assumes a passive attitude, allowing the body to relax as much as possible. Each muscle group is to be contracted in sequence, taking care to avoid any strain. Muscles should be tightened to only about 70 percent of the total possible tension to avoid cramping or injury to the muscle itself.

To produce the relaxation effects, the person must pay attention to the sensation of tensing up and relaxing. The person holds each contraction

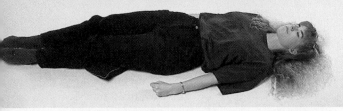

Practicing progressive muscle relaxation on a regular basis helps reduce stress.

about 5 seconds and then allows the muscles to go totally limp. The person should take enough time to contract and relax each muscle group before going on to the next.

An example of a complete progressive muscle relaxation sequence is as follows:

1. Point your feet, curling the toes downward. Study the tension in the arches and the top of the feet. Hold, continue to note the tension, then relax. Repeat once.
2. Flex the feet upward toward the face and note the tension in your feet and calves. Hold and relax. Repeat once.
3. Push your heels down against the floor as if burying them in the sand. Hold and note the tension at the back of the thigh. Relax. Repeat once.
4. Contract the right thigh by straightening the leg, gently raising the leg off the floor. Hold and study the tension. Relax. Repeat with the left leg. Hold and relax. Repeat each leg.
5. Tense the buttocks by raising your hips ever so slightly off the floor. Hold and note the tension. Relax. Repeat once.
6. Contract the abdominal muscles. Hold them tight and note the tension. Relax. Repeat once.
7. Suck in your stomach. Try to make it reach your spine. Flatten your lower back to the floor. Hold and feel the tension in the stomach and lower back. Relax. Repeat once.
8. Take a deep breath and hold it, then exhale. Repeat. Note your breathing becoming slower and more relaxed.
9. Place your arms at the sides of your body and clench both fists. Hold, study the tension, and relax. Repeat.
10. Flex the elbow by bringing both hands to the shoulders. Hold tight and study the tension in the biceps. Relax. Repeat.
11. Place your arms flat on the floor, palms up, and push the forearms hard against the floor. Note the tension on the triceps. Hold, and relax. Repeat.
12. Shrug your shoulders, raising them as high as possible. Hold and note the tension. Relax. Repeat.
13. Gently push your head backward. Note the tension in the back of the neck. Hold, and relax. Repeat.

14. Gently bring the head against the chest, push forward, hold, and note the tension in the neck. Relax. Repeat.
15. Press your tongue toward the roof of your mouth. Hold, study the tension, and relax. Repeat.
16. Press your teeth together. Hold, and study the tension. Relax. Repeat.
17. Close your eyes tightly. Hold them closed and note the tension. Relax, leaving your eyes closed. Do this one more time.
18. Wrinkle your forehead and note the tension. Hold and relax. Repeat.

When time is a factor during the daily routine and an individual is not able to go through the entire sequence, he or she may do only the exercises specific to the area that feels most tense. Performing a partial sequence is better than not doing the exercises at all. Completing the entire sequence, of course, yields the best results.

Progressive muscle relaxation A stress management technique that involves progressive contraction and relaxation of muscle groups throughout the body.

Breathing exercises A stress management technique wherein the individual concentrates on "breathing away" the tension and inhaling fresh air to the entire body.

BEHAVIOR MODIFICATION PLANNING

CHARACTERISTICS OF GOOD STRESS MANAGERS

Good stress managers

- are physically active, eat a healthy diet, and get adequate rest every day.
- believe they have control over events in their life (have an internal locus of control, see pages 33–34).
- understand their own feelings and accept their limitations.
- recognize, anticipate, monitor, and regulate stressors within their capabilities.
- control emotional and physical responses when distressed.
- use appropriate stress management techniques when confronted with stressors.
- recognize warning signs and symptoms of excessive stress.
- schedule daily time to unwind, relax, and evaluate the day's activities.
- control stress when called upon to perform.
- enjoy life despite occasional disappointments and frustrations.
- look success and failure squarely in the face and keep moving along a predetermined course.
- move ahead with optimism and energy and do not spend time and talent worrying about failure.
- learn from previous mistakes and use them as building blocks to prevent similar setbacks in the future.
- give of themselves freely to others.
- have a deep meaning in life.

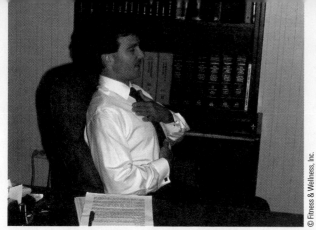
Breathing exercises help dissipate stress.

BREATHING TECHNIQUES FOR RELAXATION

Breathing exercises also can be an antidote to stress. These exercises have been used for centuries in Asia and India to improve mental, physical, and emotional stamina. In breathing exercises, the person concentrates on "breathing away" the tension and inhaling a large amount of air with each breath. Breathing exercises can be learned in only a few minutes and require considerably less time than the progressive muscle relaxation exercises.

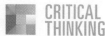

CRITICAL THINKING

List the three most common stressors you face as a college student. What techniques have you used to manage these situations, and in what way have they helped you cope?

As with any other relaxation technique, these exercises should be done in a quiet, pleasant, well-ventilated room. Any of the three examples of breathing exercises presented here will help relieve tension induced by stress.

1. *Deep breathing.* Lie with your back flat against the floor, and place a pillow under your knees. Separate the feet slightly, with the toes pointing outward. (The exercise also may be done while sitting up in a chair or standing straight up.) Place one hand on your abdomen and the other hand on your chest.

   Slowly breathe in and out so the hand on your abdomen rises when you inhale and falls as you exhale. The hand on the chest should not move much at all. Repeat the exercise about 10 times. Next, scan your body for tension and compare your present tension with the tension you felt at the beginning of the exercise. Repeat the entire process once or twice.

2. *Sighing.* Using the abdominal breathing technique, breathe in through your nose to a specific count (e.g., 4, 5, or 6). Now exhale through pursed lips to double the intake count (e.g., 8, 10, or 12). Repeat the exercise 8 to 10 times whenever you feel tense.

3. *Complete natural breathing.* Sit in an upright position, or stand straight up. Breathing through your nose, gradually fill your lungs from the bottom up. Hold your breath for several seconds. Now exhale slowly, allowing your chest and abdomen to relax completely. Repeat the exercise 8 to 10 times.

Visual Imagery

Visual or mental **imagery** has been used as a healing technique for centuries in various cultures around the world. In Western medicine, the practice of imagery is relatively new and not widely accepted among health-care professionals. Research is now being done to study the effects of imagery on the treatment of conditions such as cancer, hypertension, asthma, chronic pain, and obesity.

Visual imagery involves the creation of relaxing visual images and scenes in times of stress to elicit body and mind relaxation. Imagery works by offsetting the stressor with the visualization of relaxing scenes such as a sunny beach, a beautiful meadow, a quiet mountaintop, or some other peaceful setting. Imagery can also be used in conjunction with breathing exercises, meditation, or yoga.

As with other stress management techniques, imagery should be performed in a quiet and comfortable environment. You can either sit or lie down for the exercise. If you lie down, use a soft surface and place a pillow under your knees. Be sure that your clothes are loose and that you are as comfortable as you can be.

To start the exercise, close your eyes and take a few breaths using one of the breathing techniques previously described. You can then proceed to visualize one of your favorite scenes in nature. You may place yourself right into the scene and visualize yourself moving about and experiencing nature to its fullest. Enjoy the people, the animals, the colors, the sounds, the smells, and even the temperature in your scene. After 10 to 20 minutes of visualization, open your eyes and compare the tension in your body and mind at this point with how you felt prior to the exercise. You can repeat this exercise as often as you deem necessary when you are feeling tension or stress.

You may not always be able to find a quiet, comfortable setting in which to sit or lie down for 10 to 20 minutes. If you think imagery works for you, however, you can perform this technique while standing or sitting in an active setting. If you are able, close your eyes and disregard your surroundings for a moment and visualize one of your favorite scenes. Once you feel you have regained some control over the stressor, open your eyes and continue with your assigned tasks.

Autogenic Training

Autogenic training is a form of self-suggestion in which people place themselves in an autohypnotic

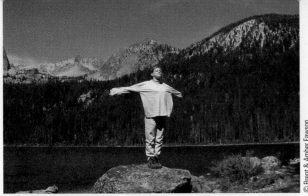

Visual imagery of beautiful and relaxing scenes helps attenuate the stress response.

state by repeating and concentrating on feelings of heaviness and warmth in the extremities. This technique was developed by Johannes Schultz, a German psychiatrist, who noted that hypnotized individuals developed sensations of warmth and heaviness in the limbs and torso. The sensation of warmth is caused by dilation of blood vessels, which increases blood flow to the limbs. Muscular relaxation produces the feeling of heaviness.

In this technique, the person lies down or sits in a comfortable position, eyes closed, and concentrates progressively on six fundamental stages and says (or thinks) the following:

1. Heaviness
   My right (left) arm is heavy.
   Both arms are heavy.
   My right (left) leg is heavy.
   Both legs are heavy.
   My arms and legs are heavy.
2. Warmth
   My right (left) arm is warm.
   Both arms are warm.
   My right (left) leg is warm.
   Both legs are warm.
   My arms and legs are warm.
3. Heart
   My heartbeat is calm and regular. (Repeat four or five times.)
4. Respiration
   My body breathes itself. (Repeat four or five times.)
5. Abdomen
   My abdomen is warm. (Repeat four or five times.)
6. Forehead
   My forehead is cool. (Repeat four or five times.)

The autogenic training technique is more difficult to master than any of those mentioned previously. The person should not move too fast through the entire exercise, because this actually may interfere with learning and relaxation. Each stage must be mastered before proceeding to the next.

Meditation

Meditation is a mental exercise that can bring about psychological and physical benefits. Regular meditation has been shown to decrease blood pressure, stress, anger, anxiety, fear, negative feelings, chronic pain, and increase activity in the brain's left frontal region—an area associated with positive emotions.[8] The objective of meditation is to gain control over one's attention by clearing the mind and blocking out the stressor(s) responsible for the higher tension.

This technique can be learned rather quickly, but first-time users often drop out before reaping benefits because they feel intimidated, confused, bored, or frustrated. In such cases, a group setting is best to get started. Many colleges, community programs, health clubs, and hospitals offer classes.

Initially, the person who is learning to meditate should choose a room that is comfortable, quiet, and free of all disturbances (including telephones). After learning the technique, the person will be able to meditate just about anywhere. A time block of approximately 10 to 15 minutes is adequate to start, but as you become more comfortable with meditation, you can lengthen the time to 30 minutes or longer. To use meditation effectively, it is best to meditate daily, as only once or twice a week may not provide noticeable benefits.

Of the several forms of meditation, the following routine is recommended to get started.

1. Sit in a chair in an upright position with the hands resting either in your lap or on the arms of the chair. Close your eyes and focus on your breathing. Allow your body to relax as much as possible. Do not try to consciously relax, because trying means work. Rather, assume a passive attitude and concentrate on your breathing.
2. Allow the body to breathe regularly, at its own rhythm, and repeat in your mind the word "one" every time you inhale, and the word "two" every time you exhale. Paying attention to these two words keeps distressing thoughts from entering into your mind.

Imagery Mental visualization of relaxing images and scenes to induce body relaxation in times of stress or as an aid in the treatment of certain medical conditions such as cancer, hypertension, asthma, chronic pain, and obesity.

Autogenic training A stress management technique using a form of self-suggestion, wherein an individual is able to place himself or herself in an autohypnotic state by repeating and concentrating on feelings of heaviness and warmth in the extremities.

Meditation A stress management technique used to gain control over one's attention by clearing the mind and blocking out the stressor(s) responsible for the increased tension.

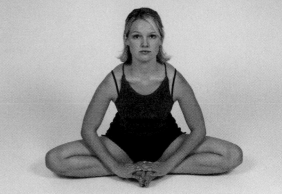

Yoga exercises help induce the relaxation response.

3. Continue to breathe in this way about 15 minutes. Because the objective of meditation is to bring about a hypometabolic state leading to body relaxation, do not use an alarm clock to remind you that the 15 minutes have expired. The alarm will only trigger your stress response again, defeating the purpose of the exercise. Opening your eyes once in a while to keep track of the time is fine, but do not rush or anticipate the end of the session. This time has been set aside for meditation, and you need to relax, take your time, and enjoy the exercise.

Yoga

Yoga is an excellent stress-coping technique. It is a school of thought in the Hindu religion that seeks to help the individual attain a higher level of spirituality and peace of mind. Although its philosophical roots can be considered spiritual, yoga is based on principles of self-care.

Yoga practitioners adhere to a specific code of ethics and a system of mental and physical exercises that promote control of the mind and the body. In Western countries, many people are familiar mainly with the exercise portion of yoga. This system of exercises (postures or asanas) can be used as a relaxation technique for stress management. The exercises include a combination of postures, diaphragmatic breathing, muscle relaxation, and meditation that help buffer the biological effects of stress.

Western interest in yoga exercises gradually developed over the last century, particularly since the 1970s. The practice of yoga exercises helps align the musculoskeletal system and increases muscular flexibility, muscular strength and endurance, and balance.[9] People pursue yoga exercises to help dispel stress by raising self-esteem, clearing the mind, slowing respiration, promoting neuromuscular relaxation, and increasing body awareness. In addition, the exercises help relieve back pain and control involuntary body functions like heart rate, blood pressure, oxygen consumption, and metabolic rate. Yoga is also used in many hospital-based programs for cardiac patients to help manage stress and decrease blood pressure.

In addition, yoga exercises have been used to help treat chemical dependency, insomnia, and prevent injury. New research on patients with coronary heart disease who practiced yoga (among other lifestyle changes) has shown that it slows down or even reverses atherosclerosis. These patients were compared with others who did not use yoga as one of the lifestyle changes.[10]

There are many different styles of yoga, and more than 60 styles are presently taught in the United States. Classes vary according to their emphasis. Some styles of yoga are athletic, and others are passive in nature.

The most popular variety in the Western world is hatha yoga, which incorporates a series of static-stretching postures, performed in specific sequences ("asanas") that help induce the relaxation response. The postures are held for several seconds while participants concentrate on breathing patterns, meditation, and body awareness.

Most yoga classes are now variations of **hatha yoga**, and many of the typical stretches used in flexibility exercises today have been adapted from hatha yoga. Examples include:

1. *integral yoga* and *viny yoga*, which focus on gentle/static stretches
2. *iyengar yoga*, which promotes muscular strength and endurance
3. *yogalates*, incorporating Pilates exercises to increase muscular strength
4. *power yoga* or *yogarobics*, a high-energy form that links many postures together in a dance-like routine to promote cardiorespiratory fitness.

As with flexibility exercises, the stretches in hatha yoga should not be performed to the point of discomfort. Instructors should not push participants beyond their physical limitations. Similar to other stress-management techniques, yoga exercises are best performed in a quiet place for about 15 to 60 minutes per session. Many yoga participants like to perform the exercises daily.

To appreciate yoga exercises, a person has to experience them. This section, nonetheless, serves only as an introduction. Although yoga exercises can be practiced with the instruction of a book or video, most participants take classes. Many of the postures are difficult and complex, and few individuals can master the entire sequence in the first few weeks.

Individuals who are interested in yoga exercises should initially pursue it under qualified instruction. Many universities offer yoga courses, and you can also check the phone book for a listing of yoga instructors or classes. Yoga courses are offered at many health clubs and recreation centers. Because instructors and yoga styles vary, you may want to sit in on a class before enrolling. The most important thing is to look for an instructor whose views on wellness parallel your own. There are no national certification standards for instructors. If you are new to yoga, you are encouraged to compare a couple of instructors before you select a class.

Which Technique Is Best?

Each person reacts to stress differently. Therefore, the best coping strategy depends mostly on the individual. Which technique is used does not really matter, as long as it works. An individual may want to experiment with several or all of them to find out which works best. A combination of two or more is best for many people.

All of the coping strategies discussed here help to block out stressors and promote mental and physical relaxation by diverting attention to a different, nonthreatening action. Some of the techniques are easier to learn and may take less time per session. As a part of your class experience, you may participate in a stress-management session (see Lab 10D). Regardless of which technique you select, the time spent doing stress-management exercises (several times a day, as needed) is well worth the effort when stress becomes a significant problem in life.

People need to learn to relax and take time out for themselves. Stress is not what makes people ill; it's the way they react to the stress-causing agent. Individuals who learn to be diligent and start taking control of themselves find that they can enjoy a better, happier, and healthier life.

Yoga A school of thought in the Hindu religion that seeks to help the individual attain a higher level of spirituality and peace of mind.

Hatha yoga A form of yoga that incorporates specific sequences of static-stretching postures to help induce the relaxation response.

file
s
uate how
you
erstand
concepts
ented in
chapter
g the
sess Your
wledge"
"Practice
zes"
ons
our
ROM.

ASSESS YOUR KNOWLEDGE

1. Positive stress is also referred to as
   a. eustress.
   b. poststress.
   c. functional stress.
   d. distress.
   e. physiostress.

2. Which of the following is not a stage of the general adaptation syndrome?
   a. alarm reaction
   b. resistance
   c. compliance
   d. exhaustion/recovery
   e. All are stages of the general adaptation syndrome.

3. The behavior pattern of highly stressed individuals who do not seem to be at higher risk for disease is known as Type
   a. A.
   b. B.
   c. C.
   d. X.
   e. Z.

4. Effective time managers
   a. delegate.
   b. learn to say "no."
   c. protect from boredom.
   d. set aside "overtimes."
   e. All of the above.

5. Hormonal changes that occur during a stress response
   a. decrease heart rate.
   b. sap the body's strength.
   c. diminish blood flow to the muscles.
   d. induce relaxation.
   e. increase blood pressure.

6. Exercise decreases stress levels by
   a. deliberately diverting stress to various body systems.
   b. metabolizing excess catecholamines.
   c. diminishing muscular tension.
   d. stimulating alpha-wave activity in the brain.
   e. All of the above.

7. Biofeedback is
   a. the interaction with the interior self.
   b. the biological response to stress.
   c. the nonspecific response to a stress-causing agent.
   d. used to identify biological factors that cause stress.
   e. most readily achieved while in a state of self-hypnosis.

8. The technique whereby a person breathes in through the nose to a specific count and then exhales through pursed lips to double the intake count is known as
   a. sighing.
   b. deep breathing.
   c. meditation.
   d. autonomic ventilation.
   e. release management.

9. During autogenic training, a person
   a. contracts each muscle to about 70 percent of capacity.
   b. concentrates on feelings of warmth and heaviness.
   c. visualizes relaxing scenes to induce body relaxation.
   d. learns to reliably influence physiological responses.
   e. notes the positive and negative impact of frequent stressors on various body systems.

10. Yoga exercises have been used successfully to
    a. stimulate ventilation.
    b. increase metabolism during stress.
    c. slow down atherosclerosis.
    d. decrease body awareness.
    e. accomplish all of the above.

Correct answers can be found at the back of the book.

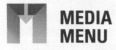

MEDIA MENU

PROFILE PLUS CD CONNECTIONS

■ Learn how you're affected by stress.

■ Find out how vulnerable you are to stress.

■ Check how well you understand the chapter's concepts.

INTERNET CONNECTIONS

■ Stress Management: A Review of Principles. Presented by Wesley E. Sime, PhD, MPH, professor of Health and Human Performance at the University of Nebraska, Lincoln. This online series of lectures on stress management education features information on the psychobiology of stress and relaxation as well as pathophysiology of stress.

   http://www.unl.edu/stress/mgmt

■ Stress: Who Has Time For It? A visually appealing site that describes the symptoms of stress and how to manage your daily stress.

   http://www.familydoctor.org/handouts/278.html

■ Workplace Stress. This site, sponsored by the American Institute of Stress, provides research-based practical information on occupational stress and its effect on health.

   http://www.stress.org/job.htm

■ Mind Tools. This site covers a variety of topics on stress management, including recognizing stress, exercise, time management, self-hypnosis, meditation, breathing exercises, coping mechanisms, and more. The site also features a free comprehensive personal self-assessment with questions pertaining to work and home stressors, physical and behavioral signs and symptoms, as well as personal coping skills and resources.

   http://www.mindtools.com/smpage.html

Notes

1. R. Booth et al., "The State of the Science: The Best Evidence for the Involvement of Thoughts and Feelings in Physical Health," *Advances in Mind–Body Medicine* 17, no. 1 (2001): 2.

2. K. Senior, "Should Stress Carry a Health Warning? *Lancet* 357 (2001): 126.

3. H. Selye, *Stress without Distress* (New York: Signet, 1974).

4. E. Gullete et al., "Effects of Mental Stress on Myocardial Ischemia during Daily Life," *Journal of the American Medical Association* 277 (1997): 1521–1525.

   C. A. Lengacher et al., "Psychoneuroimmunology and Immune System Link for Stress, Depression, Health Behaviors, and Breast Cancer," *Alternative Health Practitioner* 4 (1998): 95–108.

5. R. J. Kriegel and M. H. Kriegel, *The C Zone: Peak Performance Under Stress* (Garden City, NY: Anchor Press/Doubleday, 1985).

6. Lengacher, see note 4.

   J. Moses et al., "The Effects of Exercise Training on Mental Well-Being in the Normal Population: A Controlled Trial," *Journal of Psychosomatic Research* 33 (1989): 47–61.

   C. Shang, "Emerging Paradigms in Mind-Body Medicine," *Journal of Complementary and Alternative Medicine* 7 (2001): 83–91.

7. See note 1.

8. S. Bodian, "Meditate Your Way to Much Better Health," *Bottom Line/Health* 18 (June 2004): 11–13.

9. D. Mueller, "Yoga Therapy," *ACSM's Health & Fitness Journal* 6 (2002): 18–24.

10. S. C. Manchanda et al., "Retardation of Coronary Atherosclerosis with Yoga Lifestyle Intervention," *Journal of the Association of Physicians of India* 48 (2000): 687–694.

Suggested Readings

Girdano, D. A., D. E. Dusek, and G. S. Everly. *Controlling Stress and Tension*. San Francisco: Benjamin Cummings, 2005.

Greenberg, J. S. *Comprehensive Stress Management*. New York: McGraw-Hill/Primis Custom Publishing, 2002.

Schafer, W. *Stress Management for Wellness*. Belmont, CA: Wadsworth/Thomson Learning, 2000.

Schwartz, M. S. and F. Andrasik. *Biofeedback: A Practitioner's Guide*. New York: Guilford Press, 2004.

Selye, H. *The Stress of Life*. New York: McGraw–Hill, 1978.

Smith, J. S. *Stress Management: A Comprehensive Handbook of Techniques and Strategies*. New York: Springer, 2002.

Lab 10A

LIFE EXPERIENCES SURVEY AND TYPE A PERSONALITY ASSESSMENT

Name: _____   Date: _____   Grade: _____

Instructor: _____   Course: _____   Section: _____

Necessary Lab Equipment
None required.

Profile Plus

Objective
To determine stressful life experiences within the last 12 months that may affect your physical and psychological well-being and your Type A personality rating.

I. Life Experiences Survey

Introduction

The Life Experiences Survey contains a list of events that sometimes bring about change in the lives of those who experience them and that necessitate social readjustment. Please check events that you have experienced in the past 12 months. Be sure all checkmarks are directly across from the items to which they correspond (check only those that apply). For each item checked, please indicate the type and extent of impact the event had on your life at the time the event occurred. A rating of -3 would indicate an extremely negative impact. A rating of 0 suggests no impact either positive or negative. A rating of $+3$ would indicate an extremely positive impact.

Section 1

1. Marriage -3 -2 -1 0 $+1$ $+2$ $+3$
2. Detention in jail or comparable institution -3 -2 -1 0 $+1$ $+2$ $+3$
3. Death of spouse -3 -2 -1 0 $+1$ $+2$ $+3$
4. Major change in sleeping habits (much more or much less sleep) -3 -2 -1 0 $+1$ $+2$ $+3$
5. Death of close family member:
   a. mother -3 -2 -1 0 $+1$ $+2$ $+3$
   b. father -3 -2 -1 0 $+1$ $+2$ $+3$
   c. brother -3 -2 -1 0 $+1$ $+2$ $+3$
   d. sister -3 -2 -1 0 $+1$ $+2$ $+3$
   e. grandmother -3 -2 -1 0 $+1$ $+2$ $+3$
   f. grandfather -3 -2 -1 0 $+1$ $+2$ $+3$
   g. other (specify) -3 -2 -1 0 $+1$ $+2$ $+3$
6. Major change in eating habits (much more or much less food intake) -3 -2 -1 0 $+1$ $+2$ $+3$
7. Foreclosure on mortgage or loan -3 -2 -1 0 $+1$ $+2$ $+3$
8. Death of close friend -3 -2 -1 0 $+1$ $+2$ $+3$
9. Outstanding personal achievement -3 -2 -1 0 $+1$ $+2$ $+3$
10. Minor law violations (traffic tickets, disturbing the peace, etc.) -3 -2 -1 0 $+1$ $+2$ $+3$
11. Male: Wife/girlfriend's pregnancy -3 -2 -1 0 $+1$ $+2$ $+3$
12. Female: Pregnancy -3 -2 -1 0 $+1$ $+2$ $+3$
13. Changed work situation (different work responsibility, major change in working conditions or working hours, etc.) -3 -2 -1 0 $+1$ $+2$ $+3$
14. New job -3 -2 -1 0 $+1$ $+2$ $+3$

Continued

From Sarason, I.G., et al., "Assessing the Impact of Life Changes: Development of the Life Experiences Survey," _Journal of Consulting and Clinical Psychology_ 46 (1978): 932–946. Copyright 1978 by the American Psychological Association. Reprinted by permission.

15. Serious illness or injury of close family member:

    a. father   −3 −2 −1 0 +1 +2 +3

    b. mother   −3 −2 −1 0 +1 +2 +3

    c. sister   −3 −2 −1 0 +1 +2 +3

    d. brother   −3 −2 −1 0 +1 +2 +3

    e. grandfather   −3 −2 −1 0 +1 +2 +3

    f. grandmother   −3 −2 −1 0 +1 +2 +3

    g. spouse   −3 −2 −1 0 +1 +2 +3

    h. other (specify)   −3 −2 −1 0 +1 +2 +3

16. Sexual difficulties   −3 −2 −1 0 +1 +2 +3

17. Trouble with employer (in danger of losing job or of being suspended or demoted, etc.)   −3 −2 −1 0 +1 +2 +3

18. Trouble with in-laws   −3 −2 −1 0 +1 +2 +3

19. Major change in financial status (a lot better off or a lot worse off)   −3 −2 −1 0 +1 +2 +3

20. Major change in closeness of family members (increased or decreased closeness)   −3 −2 −1 0 +1 +2 +3

21. Gaining a new family member (through birth, adoption, family member moving in, etc.)   −3 −2 −1 0 +1 +2 +3

22. Change of residence   −3 −2 −1 0 +1 +2 +3

23. Marital separation from mate (due to conflict)   −3 −2 −1 0 +1 +2 +3

24. Major change in church activities (increased or decreased attendance)   −3 −2 −1 0 +1 +2 +3

25. Marital reconciliation with mate   −3 −2 −1 0 +1 +2 +3

26. Major change in number of arguments with spouse (a lot more or a lot less arguments)   −3 −2 −1 0 +1 +2 +3

27. Married male: Change in wife's work outside the home (beginning work, ceasing work, changing to a new job, etc.)   −3 −2 −1 0 +1 +2 +3

28. Married female: Change in husband's work (loss of job, beginning new job, retirement, etc.)   −3 −2 −1 0 +1 +2 +3

29. Major change in usual type and/or amount of recreation   −3 −2 −1 0 +1 +2 +3

30. Borrowing more than $10,000 (buying home, business etc.)   −3 −2 −1 0 +1 +2 +3

31. Borrowing less than $10,000 (buying car or TV, getting school loan, etc.)   −3 −2 −1 0 +1 +2 +3

32. Being fired from job   −3 −2 −1 0 +1 +2 +3

33. Male: Wife/girlfriend having abortion   −3 −2 −1 0 +1 +2 +3

34. Female: Having abortion   −3 −2 −1 0 +1 +2 +3

35. Major personal illness or injury   −3 −2 −1 0 +1 +2 +3

36. Major change in social activities (participation in parties, movies, visiting, etc.)   −3 −2 −1 0 +1 +2 +3

37. Major change in living conditions of family (building new home or remodeling, deterioration of home or neighborhood, etc.)   −3 −2 −1 0 +1 +2 +3

38. Divorce   −3 −2 −1 0 +1 +2 +3

39. Serious injury or illness of close friend   −3 −2 −1 0 +1 +2 +3

40. Retirement from work   −3 −2 −1 0 +1 +2 +3

41. Son or daughter leaving home (because of marriage, college, etc.)   −3 −2 −1 0 +1 +2 +3

42. End of formal schooling   −3 −2 −1 0 +1 +2 +3

43. Separation from spouse (because of work, travel, etc.)   −3 −2 −1 0 +1 +2 +3

44. Engagement   −3 −2 −1 0 +1 +2 +3

45. Breaking up with boyfriend/girlfriend ⬚−3 ⬚−2 ⬚−1 ⬚0 ⬚+1 ⬚+2 ⬚+3

46. Leaving home for the first time ⬚−3 ⬚−2 ⬚−1 ⬚0 ⬚+1 ⬚+2 ⬚+3

47. Reconciliation with boyfriend/girlfriend ⬚−3 ⬚−2 ⬚−1 ⬚0 ⬚+1 ⬚+2 ⬚+3

48. Others_____ ⬚−3 ⬚−2 ⬚−1 ⬚0 ⬚+1 ⬚+2 ⬚+3

49. _____ ⬚−3 ⬚−2 ⬚−1 ⬚0 ⬚+1 ⬚+2 ⬚+3

50. _____ ⬚−3 ⬚−2 ⬚−1 ⬚0 ⬚+1 ⬚+2 ⬚+3

Section 2

51. Beginning a new school experience at a higher academic level (college, graduate school, professional school, etc.) ⬚−3 ⬚−2 ⬚−1 ⬚0 ⬚+1 ⬚+2 ⬚+3

52. Changing to a new school at the same academic level (undergraduate, graduate, etc.) ⬚−3 ⬚−2 ⬚−1 ⬚0 ⬚+1 ⬚+2 ⬚+3

53. Academic probation ⬚−3 ⬚−2 ⬚−1 ⬚0 ⬚+1 ⬚+2 ⬚+3

54. Being dismissed from dormitory or other residence ⬚−3 ⬚−2 ⬚−1 ⬚0 ⬚+1 ⬚+2 ⬚+3

55. Failing an important exam ⬚−3 ⬚−2 ⬚−1 ⬚0 ⬚+1 ⬚+2 ⬚+3

56. Changing a major ⬚−3 ⬚−2 ⬚−1 ⬚0 ⬚+1 ⬚+2 ⬚+3

57. Failing a course ⬚−3 ⬚−2 ⬚−1 ⬚0 ⬚+1 ⬚+2 ⬚+3

58. Dropping a course ⬚−3 ⬚−2 ⬚−1 ⬚0 ⬚+1 ⬚+2 ⬚+3

59. Joining a fraternity/sorority ⬚−3 ⬚−2 ⬚−1 ⬚0 ⬚+1 ⬚+2 ⬚+3

60. Financial problems concerning school (in danger of not having sufficient money to continue) ⬚−3 ⬚−2 ⬚−1 ⬚0 ⬚+1 ⬚+2 ⬚+3

How to Score

After determining the life events that have taken place, sum the negative and the positive points separately (e.g., positive ratings: 3, 2, 1, 2 = 8 points positive score; negative ratings: −1, −3, −1, −3, −2, −3 = 13 negative points score). A final "total life change" score is obtained by adding the positive and negative scores together as positive numbers (e.g., total life change score: 8 + 13 = 21 points). The various stress ratings for the Life Experiences Survey are given below. Your negative score is the best indicator of stress (distress or negative stress) in your life.

Score Interpretation*

Stress Category	Negative Score		Total Score	
	Men	Women	Men	Women
Poor	≥13	≥15	≥27	≥27
Fair	7–12	8–14	17–26	18–26
Average	6	7	16	17
Good	1–5	1–6	5–15	6–16
Excellent	0	0	1–4	1–5

Life Experiences Survey Results

	Points	Stress Category
Negative score:	⬚	⬚
Positive score:	⬚	⬚
Total life change score:	⬚	⬚

*Adapted from I. G. Sarason et al. "Assessing the Impact of Life Changes: Development of the Life Experiences Survey." *Journal of Consulting and Clinical Psychology* 46 (1978): 932–946.

II. Type A Behavior

Instructions

Please answer "yes" or "no" for each of the items listed below. For questions 7, 15, and 16, give yourself one point for each "yes" answer. For the rest of the questions, give yourself one point for each "no" answer.

Yes	No	
☐	☐	1. Do you feel your job carries heavy responsibility?
☐	☐	2. Would you describe yourself as a hard-driving, ambitious type of person?
☐	☐	3. Do you usually try to get things done as quickly as possible?
☐	☐	4. Would family members and close friends describe you as hard-driving and ambitious?
☐	☐	5. Have people close to you ever asked you to slow down in your work?
☐	☐	6. Do you think you drive harder to accomplish things than most of your associates do?
☐	☐	7. When you play games with people your own age, do you play just for the fun of it?
☐	☐	8. If there's competition in your job, do you enjoy this?
☐	☐	9. When you are driving and there is a car in your lane going much too slowly for you, do you mutter and complain? Would anyone riding with you know you are annoyed?
☐	☐	10. If you make an appointment with someone, are you there on time in almost all cases?
☐	☐	11. If you are kept waiting, do you resent it?
☐	☐	12. If you see someone doing a job rather slowly and you know you could do it faster and better yourself, does it make you restless to watch him or her?
☐	☐	13. Would you be tempted to step in and do it yourself?
☐	☐	14. Do you eat rapidly? Walk rapidly?
☐	☐	15. After you've finished eating, do you like to sit around the table and chat?
☐	☐	16. When you go out to a restaurant and find eight or ten people waiting ahead of you for a table, will you wait?
☐	☐	17. Do you really resent having to wait in line at the bank or post office?
☐	☐	18. Do you always feel anxious to get going and finish whatever you have to do?
☐	☐	19. Do you have the feeling that time is passing too rapidly for you to accomplish all the things you'd like to get done in one day?
☐	☐	20. Do you often feel a sense of time urgency or time pressure?
☐	☐	21. Do you hurry in doing most things?

Form revised from *The Structured Interview from the Forum on Type A Behavior,* National Heart/Lung/Blood Institute, Ray M. Rosenman, MD, 1981. This form is reprinted from R. W. Patton et. al., *Implementing Health/Fitness Programs* (Champaign, IL: Human Kinetics Publisher, 1986).

How to Score

Results	Points	
Questions 7, 15, 16:	☐	(1 point for each "yes" answer)
All other questions:	☐	(1 point for each "no" answer)
Total score:	☐	

Your level of Type A: ☐

Score Interpretation

Rating	Points
High	0–7
Medium	8–13
Low	14–21

III. Hostile Personality Assessment

Hostility could harm your heart. Experts now conclude that feelings of hostility increase your risk of heart disease. Dr. Redford Williams, of Duke University Medical Center, designed a questionnaire to help you determine whether you have a hostile personality. Circle the answer that most closely fits how you would respond to the given situation:

1. **A teenager drives by my yard blasting the car stereo:**
   A. I begin to understand why teenagers can't hear.
   B. I can feel my blood pressure starting to rise.

2. **A boyfriend/girlfriend calls at the last minute "too tired to go out tonight." I'm stuck with two $15 tickets:**
   A. I find someone else to go with.
   B. I tell my friend how inconsiderate he/she is.

3. **Waiting in the express checkout line at the super- market where a sign says "No More Than 10 Items Please":**
   A. I pick up a magazine and pass the time.
   B. I glance to see if anyone has more than 10 items.

4. **Most homeless people in large cities:**
   A. Are down and out because they lack ambition.
   B. Are victims of illness or some other misfortune.

5. **At times when I've been very angry with someone:**
   A. I was able to stop short of hitting him/her.
   B. I have, on occasion, hit or shoved him/her.

6. **When I am stuck in a traffic jam:**
   A. I am usually not particularly upset.
   B. I quickly start to feel irritated and annoyed.

7. **When there's a really important job to be done:**
   A. I prefer to do it myself.
   B. I am apt to call on my friends to help.

8. **The cars ahead of me start to slow and stop as they approach a curve:**
   A. I assume there is a construction site ahead.
   B. I assume someone ahead had a fender-bender.

9. **An elevator stops too long above where I'm waiting:**
   A. I soon start to feel irritated and annoyed.
   B. I start planning the rest of my day.

10. **When a friend or co-worker disagrees with me:**
    A. I try to explain my position more clearly.
    B. I am apt to get into an argument with him or her.

11. **At times when I was really angry in the past:**
    A. I have never thrown things or slammed a door.
    B. I've sometimes thrown things or slammed a door.

12. **Someone bumps into me in a store:**
    A. I pass it off as an accident.
    B. I feel irritated at their clumsiness.

13. **When my spouse (significant other) is fixing a meal:**
    A. I keep an eye out to make sure nothing burns.
    B. I talk about my day or read the paper.

14. **Someone is hogging the conversation at a party:**
    A. I look for an opportunity to put him/her down.
    B. I soon move to another group.

15. **In most arguments:**
    A. I am the angrier one.
    B. The other person is angrier than I am.

How to Score

Score one point for each of these answers: 1. B, 2. B, 3. B, 4. A, 5. B, 6. B, 7. A, 8. B, 9. A, 10. B, 11. B, 12. B, 13. A, 14. A, 15. A. If you scored 4 or more points you may be hostile. Questions 1, 6, 9, 12, and 15 reflect anger. Questions 2, 5, 10, 11, 14, reflect aggression. Questions 3, 4, 7, 8, 13 reflect cynicism. If you scored 2 points in any category, you should work on that area of your personality.

Hostility score [ ]   Anger score [ ]   Aggression score [ ]   Cynicism score [ ]

IV. In your own words, summarize the results of all three assessment tools and express your feelings about how stress and your personality affect you in daily life.

Lab 10B

STRESS VULNERABILITY QUESTIONNAIRE

Name: _____ Date: _____ Grade: _____

Instructor: _____ Course: _____ Section: _____

Necessary Lab Equipment

None required.

Objective

To determine your stress vulnerability rating and identify areas where you can reduce your vulnerability to stress.

Instructions

Carefully read each statement and circle the number that best describes your feelings or behavior. Please be completely honest with your answers.

I. Stress Vulnerability Questionnaire

Item	Strongly Agree	Mildly Agree	Mildly Disagree	Strongly Disagree
1. I try to incorporate as much physical activity as possible in my daily schedule.	1	2	3	4
2. I exercise aerobically for 20 minutes or more at least three times per week.	1	2	3	4
3. I regularly sleep 7 to 8 hours per night.	1	2	3	4
4. I take my time eating at least one hot, balanced meal a day.	1	2	3	4
5. I drink fewer than two cups of coffee (or equivalent) per day.	1	2	3	4
6. I am at recommended body weight.	1	2	3	4
7. I enjoy good health.	1	2	3	4
8. I do not use tobacco in any form.	1	2	3	4
9. I limit my alcohol intake to no more than one drink per day.	1	2	3	4
10. I do not use hard drugs (chemical dependency).	1	2	3	4
11. There is someone I love, trust, and can rely on for help if I have a problem or need to make an essential decision.	1	2	3	4
12. There is love in my family.	1	2	3	4
13. I routinely give and receive affection.	1	2	3	4
14. I have close personal relationships with other people that provide me with a sense of emotional security.	1	2	3	4
15. There are people close by whom I can turn to for guidance in time of stress.	1	2	3	4
16. I can speak openly about feelings, emotions, and problems with people I trust.	1	2	3	4
17. Other people rely on me for help.	1	2	3	4
18. I am able to keep my feelings of anger and hostility under control.	1	2	3	4
19. I have a network of friends who enjoy the same social activities that I do.	1	2	3	4
20. I take time to do something fun at least once a week.	1	2	3	4
21. My religious beliefs provide guidance and strength in my life.	1	2	3	4
22. I often provide service to others.	1	2	3	4
23. I enjoy my job (or major or school).	1	2	3	4
24. I am a competent worker.	1	2	3	4
25. I get along well with co-workers (or students).	1	2	3	4
26. My income is sufficient for my needs.	1	2	3	4
27. I manage time adequately.	1	2	3	4

Continued

Item	Strongly Agree	Mildly Agree	Mildly Disagree	Strongly Disagree
28. I have learned to say "no" to additional commitments when I already am pressed for time.	1	2	3	4
29. I take daily quiet time for myself.	1	2	3	4
30. I practice stress management as needed.	1	2	3	4

Total Points:

Test Interpretation

Rating	Points
Excellent (great stress resistance)	0–30 points
Good (little vulnerability to stress)	31–40 points
Average (somewhat vulnerable to stress)	41–50 points
Fair (vulnerable to stress)	51–60 points
Poor (very vulnerable to stress)	≥ 61 points

This questionnaire helps you identify areas where improvements can be made to help you cope with stress more effectively. As you take this test, you will notice that most of the items describe situations and behaviors that are within your control. To make yourself less vulnerable to stress, improve the behaviors that make you more vulnerable to stress. Start by modifying behaviors that are easiest to change before undertaking the most difficult ones.

II. In the space provided below, list, in order of priority, behaviors that you would like to change to help you decrease your vulnerability to stress. Also, briefly outline how you intend to accomplish these changes.

Lab 10C

GOALS AND TIME MANAGEMENT SKILLS

Name: _____ Date: _____ Grade: _____

Instructor: _____ Course: _____ Section: _____

Necessary Lab Equipment

None required.

Objective

To help you develop time management skills.

Instructions

If you think you don't have enough hours during the day to get everything done, this lab is for you. Be sure to read the Time Management section and fill out all the forms provided with this lab.

I. Long- and Short-Term Goals

In the spaces provided below, list your goals as indicated. You may want to keep this form and review it in years to come.

1. List three goals you wish to accomplish in this life:

_____
_____
_____

2. List three goals you wish to see accomplished 10 years from now:

_____
_____
_____

3. List three goals you wish to accomplish this year:

_____
_____
_____

4. List three goals you wish to accomplish this month:

_____
_____
_____

5. List three goals you wish to accomplish this week:

_____
_____
_____

Signature: _____ Date: _____

II. Finding Time Killers

Keep a 4- to 7-day log and record at half-hour intervals the activities you do (make additional copies of this form as needed). Record the activities as you go through your typical day, so you will remember them all. At the end of each day, decide when you wasted time. Using a highlighter, identify the time killers on this form and plan necessary changes for the next day.

6:00	
6:30	
7:00	
7:30	
8:00	
8:30	
9:00	
9:30	
10:00	
10:30	
11:00	
11:30	
12:00	
12:30	
1:00	
1:30	
2:00	
2:30	
3:00	
3:30	
4:00	
4:30	
5:00	
5:30	
6:00	
6:30	
7:00	
7:30	
8:00	
8:30	
9:00	
9:30	
10:00	
10:30	
11:00	
11:30	
12:00	

III. Daily and Weekly Goals and Priorities

Take 10 minutes each morning to write down the goals or tasks you wish to accomplish that day. Rank them as top, medium, low, or "trash" priorities. (Make as many copies of this form as needed.) At the end of the day, evaluate how well you accomplished your tasks for the day. Cross off the goals you accomplished and carry over to the next day those you did not get done.

Date: ___ / ___ / ___   Day of the Week: _____

Top-Priority Goals

1. _____
2. _____
3. _____
4. _____

Medium-Priority Goals

1. _____
2. _____
3. _____
4. _____

Low-Priority Goals

1. _____
2. _____
3. _____
4. _____

Trash (do only after all other goals have been accomplished)

1. _____
2. _____
3. _____
4. _____

Take a few minutes each Sunday night to write down the goals or tasks you wish to accomplish that week. As with your daily goals, rank them as top, medium, low, or "trash" priorities. (Make as many copies of this form as needed.) At the end of the week, evaluate how well you accomplished your goals. Cross off the goals you accomplished and carry over to the next week those you did not get done.

Week: ___ / ___ / ___ to ___ / ___ / ___

Top-Priority Goals

1. _____
2. _____
3. _____
4. _____

Medium-Priority Goals

1. _____
2. _____
3. _____
4. _____

Low-Priority Goals

1. _____
2. _____
3. _____
4. _____

Trash (do only after all other goals have been accomplished)

1. _____
2. _____
3. _____
4. _____

IV. Time Management Evaluation

On a weekly basis, go through the list of strategies below and provide a "yes" or "no" answer to each statement. If you are able to answer "yes" to most questions, congratulations, you are becoming a good time manager.

Strategy Date:															
1. I evaluate my time killers periodically.															
2. I have written down my long-range goals.															
3. I have written down my short-range goals.															
4. I use a daily planner.															
5. I conduct nightly audits.															
6. I conduct weekly audits.															
7. I delegate activities that others can do.															
8. I have learned to say "no" to additional tasks when I am already in "overload."															
9. I plan activities to avoid boredom.															
10. I plan ahead for distractions.															
11. I work on one task at a time, until it's done.															
12. I have removed distractions from my work.															
13. I set aside "overtimes."															
14. I set aside special time for myself daily.															
15. I reward myself for a job well done.															

Lab 10D

STRESS MANAGEMENT

Name: _____ Date: _____ Grade: _____

Instructor: _____ Course: _____ Section: _____

Necessary Lab Equipment
None required.

Objective
To participate in a stress management session.

I. Stage of Change for Stress Management

Using Figure 2.4 (page 41) and Table 2.3 (page 41), identify your current stage of change for a stress management program:

_____

II. Stress Management

Instructions: The class should be divided into groups of about five students per group. Each group should select and go through a minimum of two of the following stress management techniques outlined in Chapter 10:

1. Progressive Muscle Relaxation
2. Breathing Techniques for Relaxation
3. Visual Imagery
4. Autogenic Training
5. Meditation
6. Yoga

A group leader is chosen who will lead the exercise according to the instructions provided for each relaxation technique in Chapter 10. Be sure this experience is conducted in a comfortable room that is as free of noise as possible. If trained personnel or a tape-recording for progressive muscle relaxation exercises is available, the entire class may participate in this experience at once. Institutions that have biofeedback equipment may use it in this laboratory as well. After completing this lab, answer the four questions given below.

1. Indicate the two relaxation techniques used in your lab:

   A. _____ B. _____

2. In your own words, relate your feelings as you were going through exercises A and B above:

   Exercise A: _____
   _____

   Exercise B: _____
   _____

3. Indicate how you felt mentally, emotionally, and physically after participating in this experience:

   _____
   _____

4. Are there situations in your daily life in which you think you would benefit from practicing the selected stress-management exercises?

   _____
   _____

III. Self-Assessment Stress Evaluation

1. Do you currently perceive stress to be a problem in your life? ☐ Yes ☐ No

2. Do you experience any of the typical stress symptoms listed in the box on page 307? If so, which ones?

3. Indicate any specific events in your life that trigger a stress response.

   _____

   _____

   _____

   _____

4. Write specific objectives to either avoid or help you manage the various stress-inducing events listed above, including one or more stress-management techniques.

   _____

   _____

   _____

   _____

5. Do you have any behavior patterns you would like to modify? List those you would like to change.

   _____

   _____

   _____

   _____

6. List specific techniques of change you will use to change undesirable behaviors (see Table 2.2, page 40).

   _____

   _____

   _____

   _____

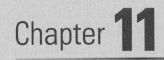

Chapter 11

Preventing Cardiovascular Disease

Objectives

- Define cardiovascular disease and coronary heart disease.
- Explain the importance of a healthy lifestyle in preventing cardiovascular disease.
- Enumerate the major risk factors that lead to the development of coronary heart disease, including physical inactivity, an abnormal cholesterol profile, hypertension, homocysteine, c-reactive protein, diabetes, and smoking.
- Assess your own risk for developing coronary heart disease.
- Outline a comprehensive program for reducing the risk for coronary heart disease and managing the overall risk for cardiovascular disease.

Profile Plus CD Connections

- Determine your risk for heart disease.
- Determine your current saturated and unsaturated fat intake.
- Check how well you understand the chapter's concepts.

The most prevalent degenerative conditions in the United States are **cardiovascular diseases**. About 20 percent of the population has some form of cardiovascular disease. Death rates are higher in men than in women (see Figure 11.1). Based on 2002 statistics, more than 35 percent of all deaths in the United States were attributable to heart and blood vessel disease.[1] According to the Centers for Disease Control and Prevention (CDC), about 60 percent of the people who die from heart disease die suddenly and unexpectedly. They had no previous symptoms of the disease. Almost half of these deaths occurred outside of the hospital, most likely because people failed to recognize early warning symptoms of a heart attack.

Some examples of cardiovascular diseases are coronary heart disease, **peripheral vascular disease**, congenital heart disease, rheumatic heart disease, atherosclerosis, strokes, high blood pressure, and congestive heart failure. According to CDC estimates, if all deaths from the major cardiovascular diseases were eliminated, life expectancy in the United States would increase by about 7 years.

The estimated cost of heart and blood vessel disease in the United States exceeded $368 billion in 2004. About 1.2 million people have new or recurrent heart attacks each year, and over 45 percent of them will die as a result. More than half of these deaths occur within 1 hour of the onset of symptoms, before the person reaches the hospital.

Although heart and blood vessel disease is still the number-one health problem in the United States, the incidence declined by 28 percent between 1960 and 2000 (see Figure 11.2), in large part because of health education. More people now are aware of the risk factors for cardiovascular disease and are changing their lifestyle to lower their potential risk for these diseases.

The heart and the coronary arteries are illustrated in Figure 11.3. The major form of cardiovascular disease is **coronary heart disease (CHD)**, in which the arteries that supply the heart muscle with oxygen and nutrients are narrowed by fatty deposits, such as cholesterol and triglycerides. Narrowing of the coronary arteries diminishes the blood supply to the heart muscle, which can precipitate a heart attack.

CHD is the single leading cause of death in the United States, accounting for about 20 percent of all deaths and approximately half of all deaths from cardiovascular disease. Approximately 80 percent of deaths from CHD in people under age 65 occurs during the first heart attack. The risk of death is also greater in the least-educated segment of the population. Each year, more than 500,000 coronary bypass operations and more than one million coronary **angioplasty** procedures are performed in the United States.

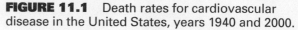

FIGURE 11.1 Death rates for cardiovascular disease in the United States, years 1940 and 2000.

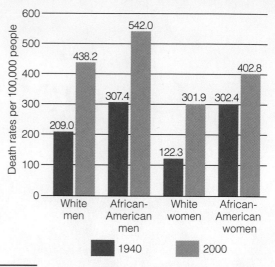

Source: American Heart Association, *Heart and Stroke Facts: 2000* (Statistical Supplement), Dallas: AHA, 1999.

FIGURE 11.2 Incidence of cardiovascular disease in the United States for selected years: 1900–2000.

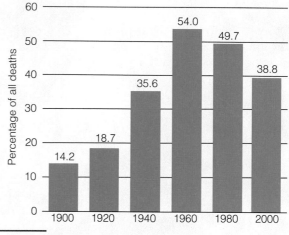

Source: Centers for Disease Control, Atlanta.

Coronary Heart Disease Risk Profile

Although genetic inheritance plays a role in CHD, the most important determinant is personal lifestyle.

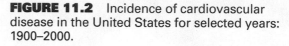

Profile Plus

Determine your risk for heart disease using the activity on your CD-ROM.

Several of the major risk factors for CHD are preventable and reversible. In this regard, CHD risk-factor analyses are administered to evaluate the impact of a person's lifestyle and genetic endowment as potential contributors to the

FIGURE 11.3 The heart and its blood vessels.

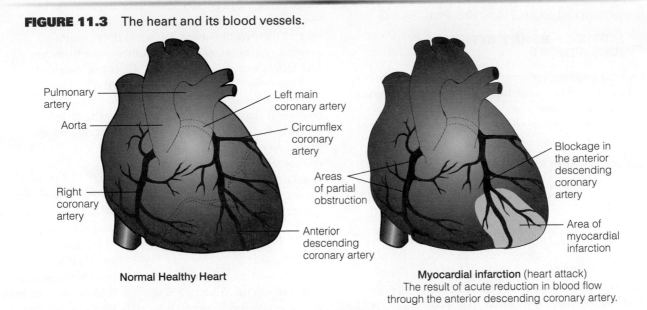

Normal Healthy Heart

Myocardial infarction (heart attack)
The result of acute reduction in blood flow
through the anterior descending coronary artery.

development of coronary disease. The specific objectives of a CHD risk factor analysis are the following:

- To screen individuals who may be at high risk for the disease.
- To educate people regarding the leading risk factors for developing CHD.
- To implement programs aimed at reducing the risks.
- To use the analysis as a starting point from which to compare changes induced by the intervention program.

Leading Risk Factors for CHD

The leading **risk factors** contributing to CHD are listed in Table 11.1. A self-assessment of risk factors for CHD is given in Lab 11A. This analysis can be done by people who have little or no medical information about their cardiovascular health, as well as those who have had a thorough medical examination. The guidelines for zero risk are outlined for each factor, making this self-analysis a valuable tool for managing CHD risk factors.

For example, a person who fills out the form learns that the ideal blood pressure is around 120/80 or lower, that risk is reduced by smoking less or quitting altogether, that HDL cholesterol should be 45 mg/dl (milligrams per deciliter) or higher for men and 55 mg/dl or higher for women, and that LDL cholesterol should be less than 100 mg/dl (if unknown, basic nutritional guidelines also are given). (The roles of HDL and LDL cholesterol, respectively,

TABLE 11.1 Weighing System for Coronary Heart Disease Risk Factors

Risk Factors	Maximal Risk Points
Abnormal cholesterol profile	12
Low HDL cholesterol	6
High LDL cholesterol	6
Inflammation	8
Physical inactivity	8
Smoking	8
Body mass index	8
Hypertension	8
Systolic blood pressure	4
Diastolic blood pressure	4
Personal history of heart disease	8
Abnormal stress electrocardiogram	8
Diabetes	6
High blood glucose	3
Known diabetes	3
Family history of heart disease	8
Elevated homocysteine	4
Age	4
Tension and stress	3
Abnormal resting electrocardiogram	3
Elevated triglycerides	2

Cardiovascular diseases The array of conditions that affect the heart and the blood vessels.

Peripheral vascular disease Narrowing of the peripheral blood vessels, excluding the cerebral and coronary arteries.

Coronary heart disease (CHD) Condition in which the arteries that supply the heart muscle with oxygen and nutrients are narrowed by fatty deposits, such as cholesterol and triglycerides.

Angioplasty A procedure in which a balloon-tipped catheter is inserted, then inflated, to widen the inner lumen of one or more arteries.

Risk factors Lifestyle and genetic variables that may lead to disease.

in protecting against and causing heart disease are discussed later in this chapter.)

To provide a meaningful score for CHD risk, a weighting system was developed to show the impact of each risk factor on developing the disease. This system is based on current research and on the work done at leading preventive medical facilities in the United States. The most significant risk factors are given the heaviest numerical weight.

For example, a poor cholesterol profile seems to be the largest predictor for developing CHD. Up to 12 risk points are assigned to individuals with very high LDL cholesterol levels and very low HDL cholesterol levels. The least heavily weighted risk factor is triglycerides, with a maximum of only 2 risk points assigned to this factor. Each risk factor also is assigned a zero-risk level—the level at which it apparently does not increase the risk for disease at all.

Based on actual test results, a person receives a score anywhere from zero to the maximum number of points for each factor. When the risk points from all of the risk factors are totaled, the final number is used to place an individual in one of five overall risk categories for potential development of CHD (see Lab 11A).

The "Very Low" CHD risk category designates the group at lowest risk for developing heart disease based on age and gender. Low CHD suggests that, even though people in this category are taking good care of their cardiovascular health, they can improve it (unless all of the risk points come from age and family history). "Moderate" CHD risk means that the person can definitely improve his or her lifestyle to lower the risk for disease, or medical treatment may be required. A score in the "High" or "Very High" CHD risk category points to a strong probability of developing heart disease within the next few years and calls for immediate implementation of a personal risk-reduction program, including professional medical, nutritional, and exercise intervention.

The leading risk factors for CHD are discussed next, along with the general recommendations for risk reduction.

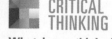

CRITICAL THINKING

What do you think about your own risk for diseases of the cardiovascular system? Is this something you need to concern yourself with at this point in your life? Why or why not?

Physical Inactivity

Physical inactivity is responsible for low levels of cardiorespiratory endurance (the ability of the heart, lungs, and blood vessels to deliver enough oxygen to the cells to meet the demands of prolonged physical activity). The level of cardiorespiratory endurance (or fitness) is given most commonly by the maximal amount of oxygen (in milliliters) that every kilogram (2.2 pounds) of body weight is able to utilize per minute of physical activity (ml/kg/min). As maximal oxygen uptake increases, so does efficiency of the cardiorespiratory system.

Even though physical inactivity has not been assigned the most risk points (8 points for a poor level of fitness, versus 12 for a poor cholesterol profile—see Table 11.1), improving cardiorespiratory endurance through daily physical activity and aerobic exercise greatly reduces the overall risk for heart disease.

Although specific recommendations can be followed to improve each risk factor, daily physical activity and a regular aerobic exercise program help to control most of the major risk factors that lead to heart disease. Physical activity and aerobic exercise will

■ Increase cardiorespiratory endurance.
■ Decrease and control blood pressure.
■ Reduce body fat.
■ Lower blood lipids (cholesterol and triglycerides).
■ Improve HDL cholesterol.
■ Help control diabetes.
■ Decrease low-grade (hidden) inflammation in the body.

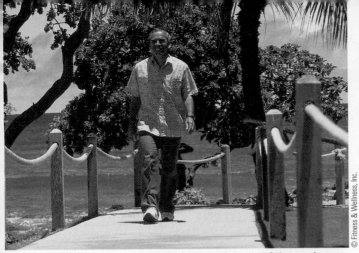

Regular physical activity helps to control most of the major risk factors that lead to heart disease.

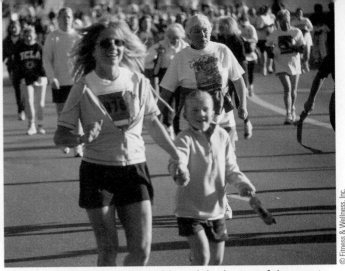

Lifetime participation in aerobic activity is one of the most important factors in preventing cardiovascular disease.

- Increase and maintain good heart function, sometimes improving certain ECG abnormalities.
- Motivate toward smoking cessation.
- Alleviate tension and stress.
- Counteract a personal history of heart disease.

Data from the research summarized in Figure 1.9, page 11, clearly show the tie between physical activity and mortality, regardless of age and other risk factors.[2] A higher level of physical fitness benefits even those who exhibit other risk factors, such as high blood pressure and serum cholesterol, cigarette smoking, and a family history of heart disease. In most cases, less-fit people in the study without these risk factors had higher death rates than highly fit people with these same risk factors.

The findings show that the higher the level of cardiorespiratory fitness, the longer the life, but the largest drop in premature death is seen between the "Unfit" and the "Moderately Fit" groups. Even small improvements in cardiorespiratory endurance greatly decrease the risk for cardiovascular mortality. Most adults who engage in a moderate exercise program can attain these fitness levels easily. A 2-mile walk in 30 to 40 minutes, five to seven days a week, is adequate to decrease risk.

Subsequent research published in the *New England Journal of Medicine* substantiated the importance of exercise in preventing CHD.[3] The benefits to previously inactive adults of starting a moderate-to-vigorous physical activity program were as important as quitting smoking, managing blood pressure, or controlling cholesterol. In relative risk for death from CHD, the increase in physical activity led to the same decrease as giving up cigarette smoking. Based on the overwhelming amount of scientific data in this area, evidence of the benefits of aerobic exercise in reducing heart disease is far too impressive to be ignored.

Even though aerobically fit individuals have a lower incidence of cardiovascular disease, regular physical activity and aerobic exercise by themselves do not guarantee a lifetime free of cardiovascular problems. Poor lifestyle habits—such as smoking, eating too many fatty/salty/sweet foods, being overweight, and having high stress levels—increase cardiovascular risk and will not be eliminated completely through an active lifestyle.

Overall management of risk factors is the best guideline to lower the risk for cardiovascular disease. Still, aerobic exercise is one of the most important factors in preventing and reducing cardiovascular problems. The basic principles for cardiorespiratory exercise are given in Chapter 6.

As more research studies are conducted, the addition of strength training is increasingly recommended for good heart function. The American Heart Association recommends strength training even for individuals who have had a heart attack or have high blood pressure, as long as they do so under a physician's advice. Strength training helps control body weight and blood sugar and lowers cholesterol and blood pressure.

Abnormal Electrocardiograms

The **electrocardiogram (ECG** or **EKG)** is a valuable measure of the heart's function. The ECG provides a record of the electrical impulses that stimulate the heart to contract (see Figure 11.4). In reading an ECG, doctors interpret five general areas: heart rate, heart rhythm, axis of the heart, enlargement or hypertrophy of the heart, and myocardial infarction.

During a standard 12-lead ECG, 10 electrodes are placed on the person's chest. From these 10 electrodes, 12 tracings, or "leads," of the electrical

Electrocardiogram (ECG or EKG) A recording of the electrical activity of the heart.

FIGURE 11.4 Normal electrocardiogram.

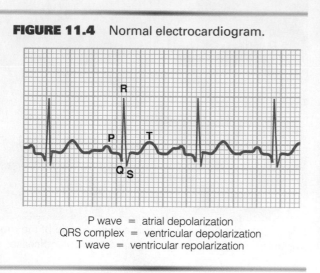

P wave = atrial depolarization
QRS complex = ventricular depolarization
T wave = ventricular repolarization

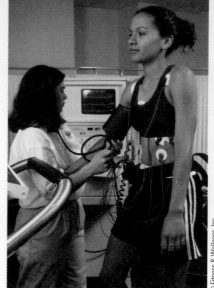

Exercise tolerance test with 12-lead electrocardiographic monitoring (an exercise stress-ECG).

© Fitness & Wellness, Inc.

FIGURE 11.5 Abnormal electrocardiogram showing a depressed S-T segment.

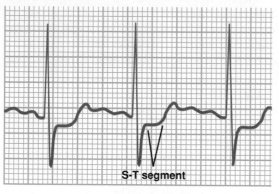

S-T segment

impulses as they travel through the heart muscle, or **myocardium,** are studied from 12 different positions. By looking at ECG tracings, doctors can identify abnormalities in heart functioning (see Figure 11.5). Based on the findings, the ECG may be interpreted as normal, equivocal, or abnormal. An ECG will not always identify problems, so a normal tracing is not an absolute guarantee. Conversely, an abnormal tracing does not necessarily signal a serious condition.

ECGs are taken at rest, during the stress of exercise, and during recovery. A **stress electrocardiogram** is also known as a "graded exercise stress test" or a "maximal exercise tolerance test." Similar to a high-speed test on a car, a stress ECG reveals the tolerance of the heart to increased physical activity. It is a much better test than a resting ECG to discover CHD.

Stress ECGs also are used to assess cardiorespiratory fitness levels, to screen individuals for preventive and cardiac rehabilitation programs, to detect abnormal blood pressure response during exercise, and to establish actual or functional maximal

heart rate for exercise prescription. The recovery ECG is another important diagnostic tool to monitor the return of the heart's activity to normal conditions.

Not every adult who wishes to start or continue an exercise program needs a stress ECG. This type of test, however, should be administered to the following:

1. Men over age 45 and women over age 55.
2. Anyone with total cholesterol level above 200 mg/dl or an HDL cholesterol below 35 mg/dl.
3. Hypertensive and diabetic patients.
4. Cigarette smokers.
5. Individuals with a family history of CHD, syncope, or sudden death before age 60.
6. People with an abnormal resting ECG.
7. All individuals with symptoms of chest discomfort, dysrhythmias (abnormal heartbeat), syncope (brief loss of consciousness), or chronotropic incompetence (heart rate that increases slowly during exercise and never reaches maximum).

At times, the stress ECG has been questioned as a reliable predictor of CHD. Nevertheless, it remains the most practical, inexpensive, noninvasive procedure available to diagnose latent (undiagnosed/unknown) CHD. The test is accurate in diagnosing CHD about 65 percent of the time. The sensitivity of the test increases along with the severity of the disease, and more accurate results are seen in people who are at high risk for cardiovascular disease, in particular men over age 45 and women over age 55.

Abnormal Cholesterol Profile

Cholesterol has received much attention because of its direct relationships to heart disease. **Blood lipids** (cholesterol and triglycerides) are carried in the bloodstream by molecules of protein known as

FIGURE 11.6 The atherosclerotic process.

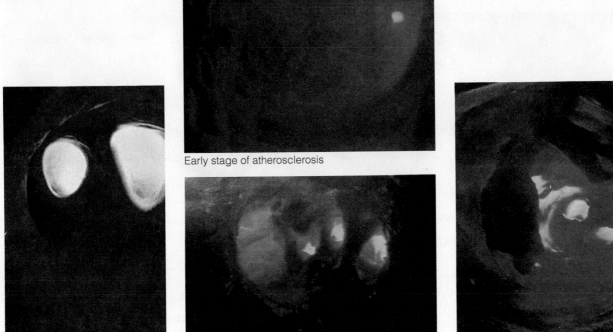

Early stage of atherosclerosis

Normal artery

Progression of the atherosclerotic plaque

Advanced stage of atherosclerosis

high-density lipoproteins (HDLs), low-density lipoproteins (LDLs), very low-density lipoproteins (VLDLs), and chylomicrons. An increased risk for CHD has been established in people with high total cholesterol, high LDL cholesterol, and low HDL cholesterol.

An abnormal cholesterol profile contributes to **atherosclerosis**, the build-up of fatty tissue in the walls of the arteries (see Figures 11.6 and 11.7). As the plaque builds up, it blocks the blood vessels that supply the myocardium with oxygen and nutrients (the coronary arteries), and these obstructions can trigger a **myocardial infarction**, or heart attack.

Unfortunately, the heart disguises its problems quite well, and typical symptoms of heart disease, such as **angina pectoris**, do not start until the arteries are about 75 percent blocked. In many cases, the first symptom is sudden death.

The most recent recommendation released in 2001 by the National Cholesterol Education Program (NCEP) is to keep total cholesterol levels below 200 mg/dl. Other health professionals recommend that total cholesterol in individuals age 30 and younger should not be higher than 180 mg/dl, and for children the level should be below 170 mg/dl. Cholesterol levels between 200 and 239 mg/dl are borderline high, and levels of 240 mg/dl and above indicate high risk for disease (see Table 11.2). The risk for heart attack increases 2 percent for every 1 percent increase in total cholesterol.[4] More

Myocardium Heart muscle.

Stress electrocardiogram An exercise test during which the workload is gradually increased until the individual reaches maximal fatigue, with blood pressure and 12-lead electrocardiographic monitoring throughout the test.

Cholesterol A waxy substance, technically a steroid alcohol, found only in animal fats and oil; used in making cell membranes, as a building block for some hormones, in the fatty sheath around nerve fibers, and in other necessary substances.

Blood lipids (fat) Cholesterol and triglycerides.

High-density lipoproteins (HDLs) Cholesterol-transporting molecules in the blood ("good" cholesterol) that help clear cholesterol from the blood.

Low-density lipoproteins (LDLs) Cholesterol-transporting molecules in the blood ("bad" cholesterol) that tend to increase blood cholesterol.

Very low-density lipoproteins (VLDLs) Triglyceride, cholesterol, and phospholipid-transporting molecules in the blood that tend to increase blood cholesterol.

Chylomicron Triglyceride-transporting molecule.

Atherosclerosis Fatty/cholesterol deposits in the walls of the arteries leading to formation of plaque.

Myocardial infarction Heart attack; damage to or death of an area of the heart muscle as a result of an obstructed artery to that area.

Angina pectoris Chest pain associated with coronary heart disease.

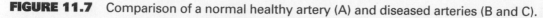

FIGURE 11.7 Comparison of a normal healthy artery (A) and diseased arteries (B and C).

The Atherosclerotic Process

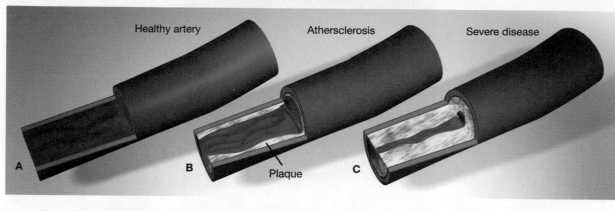

Healthy artery   Atherosclerosis   Severe disease

A   B   Plaque   C

TABLE 11.2 Cholesterol Guidelines

	Amount	Rating
Total Cholesterol	<200 mg/dl	Desirable
	200–239 mg/dl	Borderline high
	≥240 mg/dl	High risk
LDL Cholesterol	<100 mg/dl	Optimal
	100–129 mg/dl	Near or above optimal
	130–159 mg/dl	Borderline high
	160–189 mg/dl	High
	≥190 mg/dl	Very high
HDL Cholesterol	<40 mg/dl	Low (high risk)
	≥60 mg/dl	High (low risk)

From National Cholesterol Education Program.

than 50 percent, or 102,340,000 U.S. adults, have total cholesterol values of 200 mg/dl or higher. Of these, more than 41.2 million have values at or above 240 mg/dl.[5]

Many preventive medicine practitioners recommend a range between 160 and 180 mg/dl as ideal for total cholesterol. In the Framingham Heart Study (a 50-year ongoing project in the community of Framingham, Massachusetts), not a single individual with a total cholesterol level of 150 mg/dl or lower has had a heart attack. Dr. William Castelli, director of the Framingham Study, recommends a total cholesterol level of less than 150 mg/dl for possible plaque regression in people with atherosclerosis.

As important as it is, total cholesterol is not the best predictor for cardiovascular risk. Many heart attacks occur in people with only slightly elevated total cholesterol. More significant is the way in which cholesterol is carried in the bloodstream.

Cholesterol is transported primarily in the form of high-density lipoprotein (HDL) cholesterol and low-density lipoprotein (LDL) cholesterol.

In a process known as **reverse cholesterol transport**, HDLs, on the one hand, act as "scavengers," removing cholesterol from the body and preventing plaque from forming in the arteries. The strength of HDL is in the protein molecules found in its coating. When HDL comes in contact with cholesterol-filled cells, these protein molecules attach to the cells and take their cholesterol.

LDL-cholesterol, on the other hand, tends to release cholesterol, which then may penetrate the lining of the arteries and speed up the process of atherosclerosis. The NCEP guidelines given in Table 11.2 state that an LDL cholesterol value below 100 mg/dl is optimal, between 130 and 159 mg/dl is borderline-high, and 190 mg/dl and above is very high.

LDL-cholesterol particles are of two types: large or type A, and small or type B. Small particles are thought to pass through the inner lining of the coronary arteries more readily, thereby increasing the risk for a heart attack. Predominance of small particles can lead to a threefold to fivefold increase in the risk for CHD.[6] For individuals at risk for heart disease, LDL particle size should be included in the blood lipid analysis.

A genetic variation of LDL cholesterol, known as Lipoprotein-a or Lp(a), is also noteworthy because a high level of these particles promotes blood clots and earlier development of atherosclerosis. It is thought that certain substances in the arterial wall interact with Lp(a) and lead to premature formation of plaque. About 10 percent of the population has elevated levels of Lp(a). Only medications help decrease Lp(a), and drug options should be discussed with a physician.

The more HDL cholesterol (particularly the subcategory HDL$_2$), the better. HDL cholesterol, the "good cholesterol," offers some protection against heart disease. A low level of HDL cholesterol is one of the strongest predictors of CHD at all levels of total cholesterol, including levels below 200 mg/dl. Data suggest that for every 1 mg/dl increase in HDL cholesterol, the risk for CHD drops up to 3 percent in men and 5 percent in women.[7] The recommended HDL cholesterol values to minimize the risk for CHD are at least 40 mg/dl. HDL cholesterol levels above 60 mg/dl help to lower the risk for CHD.

For the most part, HDL cholesterol is determined genetically. Generally, women have higher levels than men. The female sex hormone estrogen tends to raise HDL, so premenopausal women have a much lower incidence of heart disease. African American children and adult men have higher HDL values than whites. HDL cholesterol also decreases with age.

Increasing HDL cholesterol improves the cholesterol profile and lessens the risk for CHD. Habitual aerobic exercise, weight loss, high-dose niacin, and quitting smoking help raise HDL cholesterol. Drug therapy may also promote higher HDL cholesterol levels.

Improved HDL cholesterol is clearly related to a regular aerobic exercise program (preferably high intensity, or above 6 METs, for at least 20 minutes 3 times per week—see Chapter 6). Individual responses to aerobic exercise differ, but, generally, the more you exercise, the higher your HDL cholesterol level.

Even when more LDL cholesterol is present than the cells can use, cholesterol seems not to cause a problem until it is oxidized by free radicals (see discussion on Antioxidants, Chapter 3, page 73). After cholesterol is oxidized, white blood cells invade the arterial wall, take up the cholesterol, and clog the arteries.

The antioxidant effect of vitamins C and E may provide benefits. Data suggest that a single unstable free radical (an oxygen compound produced during metabolism—see Chapter 3) can damage LDL particles, accelerating the atherosclerotic process. Vitamin C may inactivate free radicals and slow the oxidation of LDL cholesterol. Vitamin E seems to protect LDL from oxidation, preventing heart disease, but studies suggest that it does not seem to be helpful in reversing damage once it has taken place.[8]

Although the average adult in the United States consumes between 400 and 600 mg of cholesterol daily, the body actually manufactures more than that. Saturated fats raise cholesterol levels more than anything else in the diet. Saturated fats produce approximately 1,000 mg of cholesterol per day. Because of individual differences, some people can have a higher-than-normal intake of saturated fats and

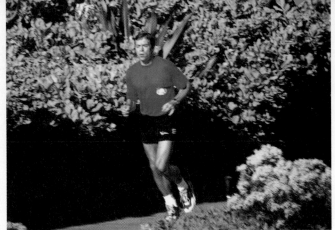

Habitual aerobic exercise helps increase HDL cholesterol ("good" cholesterol).

© Fitness & Wellness, Inc.

still maintain normal levels. Others who have a lower intake can have abnormally high levels.

Saturated fats are found mostly in meats and dairy products and seldom in foods of plant origin (see Table 11.3). Poultry and fish contain less saturated fat than beef does, but should be eaten in moderation (about 3 to 6 ounces per day—see Chapter 3). Unsaturated fats are mainly of plant origin and cannot be converted to cholesterol. Two or three omega-3-rich fish meals per week also help lower LDL cholesterol and triglycerides.

Foods that contain trans fatty acids, hydrogenated fat, or partially hydrogenated vegetable oil should be avoided. Studies indicate that these foods elevate cholesterol as much as saturated fats do. Hydrogen is frequently added to monounsaturated and polyunsaturated fats to increase shelf life and to solidify them so they are more spreadable. Hydrogenation can change the position of hydrogen atoms along the carbon chain, transforming the fat into a trans fatty acid. Margarine and spreads, commercially produced crackers and cookies, dairy products, meats, and fast foods often contain trans fatty acids. The label "partially hydrogenated" and "trans fatty acids" indicates that the product carries a health risk just as high as that of saturated fat.

LDL cholesterol that is higher than ideal can be lowered through dietary changes, by losing body fat, by taking medication, and by participating in a regular aerobic exercise program. Based on research conducted at the Aerobics Research Institute in Dallas, Texas, the data showed a higher relative risk of mortality in unfit individuals with low cholesterol than fit people with high cholesterol.[9] The lowest mortality rate, of course, is seen in fit people with low total cholesterol levels.

Reverse cholesterol transport A process in which HDL molecules attract cholesterol and carry it to the liver, where it is changed to bile and eventually excreted in the stool.

TABLE 11.3 Cholesterol and Saturated Fat Content of Selected Foods

Food	Serving Size	Cholesterol (mg)	Sat. Fat (gr)
Avocado	1/8 med.	—	3.2
Bacon	2 slices	30	2.7
Beans (all types)	any	—	—
Beef—lean, fat trimmed off	3 oz	75	6.0
Beef heart (cooked)	3 oz	150	1.6
Beef liver (cooked)	3 oz	255	1.3
Butter	1 tsp	12	0.4
Caviar	1 oz	85	—
Cheese			
American	2 oz	54	11.2
Cheddar	2 oz	60	12.0
Cottage (1% fat)	1 cup	10	0.4
Cottage (4% fat)	1 cup	31	6.0
Cream	2 oz	62	6.0
Muenster	2 oz	54	10.8
Parmesan	2 oz	38	9.3
Swiss	2 oz	52	10.0
Chicken (no skin)	3 oz	45	0.4
Chicken liver	3 oz	472	1.1
Chicken thigh, wing	3 oz	69	3.3
Egg (yolk)	1	250	1.8
Frankfurter	2	90	11.2
Fruits	any	—	—
Grains (all types)	any	—	—
Halibut, flounder	3 oz	43	0.7
Ice cream	1/2 cup	27	4.4
Lamb	3 oz	60	7.2
Lard	1 tsp	5	1.9
Lobster	3 oz	170	0.5
Margarine (all vegetable)	1 tsp	—	0.7
Mayonnaise	1 tbsp	10	2.1
Milk			
Skim	1 cup	5	0.3
Low fat (2%)	1 cup	18	2.9
Whole	1 cup	34	5.1
Nuts	1 oz	—	1.0
Oysters	3 oz	42	—
Salmon	3 oz	30	0.8
Scallops	3 oz	29	—
Sherbet	1/2 cup	7	1.2
Shrimp	3 oz	128	0.1
Trout	3 oz	45	2.1
Tuna (canned—drained)	3 oz	55	—
Turkey dark meat	3 oz	60	0.6
Turkey light meat	3 oz	50	0.4
Vegetables (except avocado)	any	—	—

BEHAVIOR MODIFICATION PLANNING

BLOOD CHEMISTRY TEST GUIDELINES

People who have never had a blood chemistry test should do so to establish a baseline for future reference. The blood test should include total cholesterol, LDL cholesterol, HDL cholesterol, triglycerides, and blood glucose.

Following an initial normal baseline test no later than age 20, for a person who adheres to the recommended dietary and exercise guidelines, a blood analysis at least every 5 years prior to age 40 should suffice. Thereafter, a blood lipid test is recommended every year, in conjunction with a regular preventive medicine physical examination.

A single baseline test is not necessarily a valid measure. Cholesterol levels vary from month to month and sometimes even from day to day. If the initial test reveals cholesterol abnormalities, the test should be repeated within a few weeks to confirm the results.

In terms of dietary modifications, a diet lower in saturated fat and cholesterol and high in fiber is recommended. Saturated fat should be replaced with monounsaturated and polyunsaturated fats because the latter tend to decrease LDL cholesterol and increase HDL cholesterol (see the discussion of "Simple Fats" in Chapter 3). Exercise is important because dietary manipulation by itself is not as effective in lowering LDL cholesterol as a combination of diet plus aerobic exercise.

To lower LDL cholesterol significantly, total daily fiber intake must be in the range of 25 to 38 grams per day (see "Fiber" in Chapter 3), total fat consumption can be in the range of 30 percent of total daily caloric intake, as long as most of the fat is unsaturated fat and the average cholesterol consumption is lower than 200 mg per day.

Among people in the United States, the average fiber intake is less than 12 grams per day. Fiber, in particular the soluble type, has been shown to lower cholesterol. Soluble fiber dissolves in water and forms a gel-like substance that encloses food particles. This property helps bind and excrete fats from the body. Soluble fibers also bind intestinal bile acids that could be recycled into additional cholesterol. Soluble fibers are found primarily in oats, fruits, barley, legumes, and psyllium.

Psyllium, a grain that is added to some multigrain breakfast cereals, also helps lower LDL cholesterol. As little as 3 daily grams of psyllium can lower LDL cholesterol by 20 percent. Commercially available fiber supplements that contain psyllium (such as Metamucil) can be used to increase soluble fiber intake. Three tablespoons daily will add about 10 grams of soluble fiber to the diet.

The incidence of heart disease is very low in populations in which daily fiber intake exceeds 30 grams per day. Further, a Harvard University Medical School study of 43,000 middle-aged men who were followed for more than 6 years showed that increasing fiber intake to 30 daily grams resulted in a 41 percent reduction in heart attacks.[10]

Research on the effects of a "typical" 30-percent-fat diet (including saturated fat) have shown that it has little or no effect in lowering cholesterol, and that CHD actually continues to progress in people who have the disease. Thus, some practitioners recommend a 10 percent or less fat-calorie diet combined with a regular aerobic exercise program while trying to lower cholesterol.

A daily 10 percent total-fat diet requires the person to limit fat intake to an absolute minimum. Some health care professionals contend that a diet like this is difficult to follow indefinitely. People with high cholesterol levels, however, may not have to follow that diet indefinitely but should adopt the 10-percent-fat diet while attempting to lower cholesterol. Thereafter, a 20- to 30-percent-fat diet may be adequate to maintain recommended cholesterol levels as long as most of the intake is from unsaturated fats (national data indicate that current fat consumption in the United States averages 34 percent of total calories—see Table 3.5, page 60).

A drawback of very low-fat diets (less than 25 percent fat) is that they tend to lower HDL cholesterol and increase triglycerides. If HDL cholesterol is already low, monounsaturated and polyunsaturated fats should be added to the diet. Examples of food items that are high in monounsaturated fats and polyunsaturated fats are olive, canola, corn, and soybean oils and nuts. The *Nutrient Analysis and Diet Planning* software of your CD-ROM can be used to determine food items that are high in monounsaturated and polyunsaturated fats (also see Figure 3.9, page 67).

The 2001 NCEP guidelines for people who are trying to decrease LDL cholesterol allow for a diet with up to 35 percent of calories from fat, including 10 percent from polyunsaturated fats and 20 percent from monounsaturated fats.[11] While attempting to lower LDL cholesterol, saturated fats should be kept to an absolute minimum. Carbohydrate intake can be in the range of 45 to 65 percent of total calories.

Soy protein is also recommended to lower total and LDL cholesterol. Soy protein increases the rate at which the liver removes LDL cholesterol from the blood, and it decreases LDL cholesterol production in the liver. Over time, a diet low in saturated fat and cholesterol that includes 25 grams of soy protein a day will lower cholesterol by an additional 5 to 7

percent, compared to the same diet without the soy protein. This benefit is seen primarily in people with total cholesterol levels above 200 mg/dl. Some people have to consume up to 60 grams a day to see an effect. Additional information on soy foods and their health benefits is given in Chapters 3 and 12.

Margarines and salad dressings that contain stanol ester, a plant-derived compound that interferes with cholesterol absorption in the intestine, are now also on the market. Over the course of several weeks, daily intake of about 3 grams of margarine or 6 tablespoons of salad dressing containing stanol ester lowers LDL cholesterol by 14 percent. Dietary guidelines to lower LDL cholesterol levels are provided in the accompanying box.

The best prescription for controlling blood lipids is the combination of a healthy diet, a sound aerobic exercise program, and weight control. If this does not work, a physician can recommend appropriate drug therapies based upon a blood test to analyze the various subcategories of lipoproteins.

The NCEP guidelines recommend that people consider drug therapy if, after 6 months on a low-cholesterol, low-saturated-fat diet, cholesterol

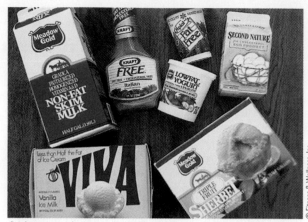

As long as the number of servings is not increased, substituting low-fat for high-fat products in the diet significantly decreases the risk for disease.

TABLE 11.4 Triglycerides Guidelines

Amount	Rating
≤125 mg/dl	Desirable
126–499 mg/dl	Borderline high
≥500 mg/dl	High risk

remains unacceptably high. An unacceptable level is an LDL cholesterol above 190 mg/dl for individuals with fewer than two risk factors and no signs of heart disease. For individuals with more than two risk factors and with a history of heart disease, LDL cholesterol above 160 mg/dl is unacceptable.

ELEVATED TRIGLYCERIDES

Triglycerides, also known as free fatty acids, make up most of the fat in our diet and most of the fat that circulates in the blood. In combination with cholesterol, triglycerides speed up formation of plaque in the arteries. Triglycerides are carried in the bloodstream primarily by very low-density lipoproteins (VLDLs) and chylomicrons.

Although they are found in poultry skin, lunch meats, and shellfish, these fatty acids are manufactured mainly in the liver from refined sugars, starches, and alcohol. High intake of alcohol and sugars (honey and fruit juices included) significantly raises triglyceride levels. To lower triglycerides, avoid pastries, candies, soft drinks, fruit juices, white bread, pasta, and alcohol. In addition, cutting down on overall fat consumption, quitting smoking, reducing weight (if overweight), and doing aerobic exercise are helpful.

The desirable blood triglyceride level is less than 150 mg/dl (see Table 11.4). For people with cardiovascular problems, this level should be below 100 mg/dl. Levels above 1,000 mg/dl pose an immediate risk for potentially fatal sudden inflammation of the pancreas.

Some people consistently have slightly elevated triglyceride levels (above 140 mg/dl) and HDL cholesterol levels below 35 mg/dl. About 80 percent of these people

CRITICAL THINKING

Are you aware of your blood lipid profile? If not, what keeps you from getting a blood chemistry test? What are the benefits of having it done now as opposed to later in life?

have a genetic condition called LDL phenotype B. Although the blood lipids may not be notably high, these people are at higher risk for atherosclerosis and CHD.

CHOLESTEROL-LOWERING MEDICATIONS

Effective medications are available to treat elevated cholesterol and triglycerides. Most notable among them are the statins group (Lipitor®, Mevacor®, Pravachol®, Lescol®, and Zocor®), which can lower cholesterol by up to 60 percent in 2 to 3 months. Statins slow down cholesterol production and increase the liver's ability to remove blood cholesterol. They also decrease triglycerides and produce a small increase in HDL levels.

In general, it is better to lower LDL cholesterol without medication, because drugs often cause undesirable side effects. Many people with heart disease, however, must take cholesterol-lowering medication, but it is best if medication is combined with lifestyle changes to augment the cholesterol-lowering effect. For example, when Zocor was taken alone over 3 months, LDL cholesterol decreased by 30 percent; but when a Mediterranean diet was adopted in combination with Zocor therapy, LDL cholesterol decreased by 41 percent.[12]

Other drugs effective in reducing LDL cholesterol are *bile acid sequestrans* that bind cholesterol found in bile acids. Cholesterol is subsequently excreted in the stools. These drugs are often used in combination with statin drugs.

High doses (1.5 to 3 grams per day) of nicotinic acid or niacin (a B vitamin) also help lower LDL cholesterol, triglycerides, and increase HDL cholesterol. A fourth group of drugs, known as *fibrates*, is used primarily to lower triglycerides.

Elevated Homocysteine

Clinical data indicating that many heart attack and stroke victims have normal cholesterol levels has led researchers to look for other risk factors that may contribute to atherosclerosis. Although it is not a blood lipid, one of these factors is a high concentration of the amino acid **homocysteine** in the blood. It is thought to enhance plaque formation and subsequent blockage of the arteries.

TABLE 11.5	Homocysteine Guidelines
Level	**Rating**
<9.0 μmol/l	Desirable
9–12 μmol/l	Mild elevation
13–15 μmol/l	Elevated
>15 μmol/l	Extreme elevation

Adapted from K. S. McCully, "What You Must Know Now About Homocysteine," *Bottom Line/Health* 18 (January 2004): 7–9.

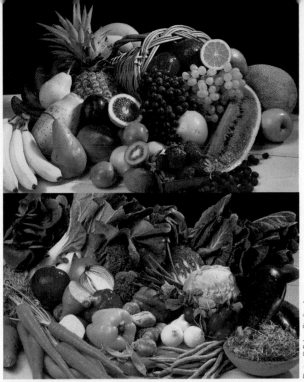

Five daily servings of fruits and vegetables can provide the necessary nutrients to keep homocysteine from causing heart disease or strokes.

The body uses homocysteine to help build proteins and carry out cellular metabolism. It is an intermediate amino acid in the interconversion of two other amino acids—methionine and cysteine. This interconversion requires the B vitamin folate (folic acid) and vitamins B_6 and B_{12}. Typically, homocysteine is metabolized rapidly, so it does not accumulate in the blood or damage the arteries.

A large number of people, however, have high blood levels of homocysteine. This might result from either a genetic inability to metabolize homocysteine or a deficiency in the vitamins required for its conversion.

Homocysteine is typically measured in micromoles per liter (μmol/l). Guidelines to interpret homocysteine levels are provided in Table 11.5. A 10-year follow-up study of people with high homocysteine levels showed that those individuals with a level above 14.25 μmol/l had almost twice the risk of stroke compared with individuals whose level was below 9.25 μmol/l.[13] Homocysteine accumulation is theorized to be toxic because it may

1. cause damage to the inner lining of the arteries (the initial step in the process of atherosclerosis),
2. stimulate the proliferation of cells that contribute to plaque formation, and
3. encourage clotting, which could completely obstruct an artery and lead to a heart attack or stroke.

Keeping homocysteine from accumulating in the blood seems to be as simple as eating the recommended daily servings of vegetables, fruits, grains, and some meat and legumes. Five servings of fruits and vegetables daily can provide sufficient levels of folate and vitamin B_6 to remove and clear homocysteine from the blood. Vitamin B_{12} is found primarily in animal flesh and animal products. Vitamin B_{12} deficiency is rarely a problem because 1 cup of milk or an egg provides the daily requirement. The body also recycles most of this vitamin; therefore, a deficiency takes years to develop. People who consume five servings of fruits and vegetables daily are unlikely to derive extra benefits from a vitamin-B-complex supplement.

Increasing evidence that folate can prevent heart attacks has led to the recommendation that people (especially women of childbearing age) consume 400 mcg per day—obtainable from five daily servings of fruits and vegetables. Unfortunately, estimates indicate that more than 80 percent of Americans do not get 400 daily mcg of folate.

Inflammation

In addition to homocysteine, scientists are looking at inflammation as a major risk factor for heart attacks. Low-grade inflammation can occur in a variety of places throughout the body. For years it has been known that inflammation plays a role in CHD and that inflammation hidden deep in the body is a common trigger of heart attacks, even when cholesterol levels are normal or low and arterial plaque is minimal.

To evaluate ongoing inflammation in the body, physicians have turned to **C-reactive protein (CRP)**, a protein whose levels in the blood increase

Triglycerides Fats formed by glycerol and three fatty acids; also called free fatty acids.

Homocysteine An amino acid that, when allowed to accumulate in the blood, may lead to plaque formation and blockage of arteries.

C-reactive protein (CRP) A protein whose blood levels increase with inflammation, at times hidden deep in the body; elevation of this protein is an indicator of potential cardiovascular events.

FIGURE 11.8 Relationship between C-reactive protein and cholesterol and risk of cardiovascular disease.

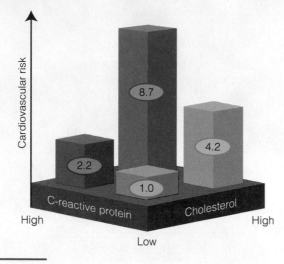

Source: Adapted from P. Libby, P. M. Ridker, and A. Maseri, "Inflammation and Atherosclerosis," *Circulation* 105 (2002): 1135–1143.

TABLE 11.6 High-Sensitivity CRP Guidelines

Amount	Rating
<1 mg/l	Low risk
1–3 mg/l	Average risk
>3 mg/l	High risk

Source: T. A. Pearson, et. al. "Markers of Inflammation and Cardiovascular Disease." *Circulation* 107 (2003): 499–511.

with inflammation. People with elevated CRP are more prone to cardiovascular events. The evidence shows that CRP blood levels elevate years before a first heart attack or stroke and that individuals with elevated CRP have twice the risk of a heart attack. The risk of a heart attack is even higher in people with both elevated CRP and cholesterol, resulting in an almost ninefold increase in risk (see Figure 11.8).

Because high CRP levels might be a better predictor of future heart attacks than high cholesterol alone, a new test known as high-sensitivity CRP (hs-CRP), which measures inflammation in the blood vessels, has been approved by the FDA. The term "high-sensitivity" was derived from the test's capability to detect small amounts of CRP in the blood.

Hs-CRP test results provide a good measure of the probability of plaque rupture within the arterial wall. There are two main types of plaque: soft and hard. Soft plaque is the most likely to rupture. Ruptured plaque releases clots into the bloodstream that can lead to a heart attack or a stroke. Other evidence has linked high CRP levels to high blood pressure and colon cancer.

Excessive intake of alcohol and high-protein diets also increase CRP. Recent evidence further indicates that high-fat, fast-food meals increase CRP levels for several hours following the meals.[14] And cooking meat and poultry at high temperatures creates damaged proteins (AGEs or advanced glycosylation end products) that trigger inflammation.

Obesity increases inflammation. With weight loss, CRP levels decrease proportional to the amount of fat lost.

An hs-CRP test is relatively inexpensive, and it is highly recommended for patients at risk for heart attack. Guidelines for hs-CRP levels are given in Table 11.6.

CRP levels decrease with statin drugs, which also lower cholesterol and reduce inflammation. Exercise, weight loss, proper nutrition, and aspirin are helpful in reducing hs-CRP. Omega-3 fatty acids (found in salmon, tuna, and mackerel fish) inhibit proteins that cause inflammation. Aspirin therapy also helps by controlling inflammation.

Diabetes

Diabetes mellitus is a condition in which blood glucose is unable to enter the cells because the pancreas totally stops producing **insulin**, or it does not produce enough to meet the body's needs, or the cells develop **insulin resistance**. The role of insulin is to "unlock" the cells and escort glucose into the cell.

Diabetes affects more than 17 million people in the United States, and about 1 million new cases are diagnosed each year. Between 1990 and 2001, the prevalence of diabetes increased by 62 percent. The National Institutes of Health estimate the cost of diabetes to be in excess of $100 billion annually.

The incidence of cardiovascular disease and death in the diabetic population is quite high. Two of three diabetics will die from cardiovascular disease. People with chronically elevated blood glucose levels may have problems metabolizing fats, which can make them more susceptible to atherosclerosis, coronary heart disease, heart attacks, high blood pressure, and strokes. Diabetics also have lower HDL cholesterol and higher triglyceride levels.

Further, chronic high blood sugar can lead to nerve damage, vision loss, kidney damage, sexual dysfunction, and decreased immune function (making the individual more susceptible to infections). Diabetics are four times more likely to become blind

TABLE 11.7 Blood Glucose Guidelines

Amount	Rating
≤126 mg/dl	Desirable
127–149 mg/dl	High
≥150 mg/dl	Very High

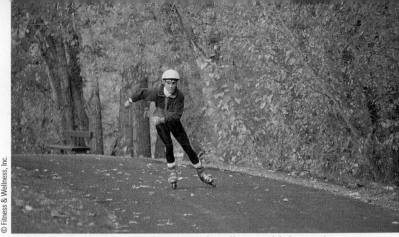

Habitual aerobic exercise increases insulin sensitivity and decreases the risk for diabetes.

and 20 times more likely to develop kidney failure. Nerve damage in the lower extremities decreases the person's awareness of injury and infection, and a small, untreated sore can result in severe infection, gangrene, and even lead to an amputation.

An 8-hour fasting blood glucose level above 126 mg/dl on two separate tests confirms a diagnosis of diabetes (see Table 11.7). A level of 127 or higher should be brought to the attention of a physician.

TYPES OF DIABETES

Diabetes is of two types: **type 1**, or insulin-dependent diabetes mellitus (IDDM), and **type 2**, or non-insulin-dependent diabetes mellitus (NIDDM). Type 1 also has been called "juvenile diabetes," because it is found mainly in young people. With type 1, the pancreas produces little or no insulin. With type 2, the pancreas either does not produce sufficient insulin or produces adequate amounts but the cells become insulin-resistant, thereby keeping glucose from entering the cell. Type 2 accounts for 90 to 95 percent of all cases of diabetes.

Although diabetes has a genetic predisposition, 60 to 80 percent of type 2 diabetes is related closely to overeating, obesity, and lack of physical activity. Type 2 diabetes, once limited primarily to overweight adults, now accounts for almost half of the new cases diagnosed in children. According to the CDC, one in three children born in the United States today will develop diabetes.

More than 80 percent of all type 2 diabetics are overweight or have a history of excessive weight. In most cases, this condition can be corrected through regular exercise, a special diet, and weight loss.

Aerobic exercise helps prevent type 2 diabetes. The protective effect is even greater in those with risk factors such as obesity, high blood pressure, and family propensity. The preventive effect is attributed to less body fat and to better sugar and fat metabolism resulting from the regular exercise program. At 3,500 calories of energy expenditure per week through exercise, the risk is cut in half versus that of a sedentary lifestyle.

Both moderate-intensity and vigorous physical activity are associated with increased insulin sensitivity and decreased risk for diabetes. The key to increase and maintain proper insulin sensitivity,

however, is regularity of the exercise program. Failure to maintain habitual physical activity voids these benefits. Thus, a simple aerobic exercise program (walking, cycling, or swimming four or five times per week) often is prescribed because it increases the body's sensitivity to insulin. Exercise guidelines for diabetic patients are discussed in detail in Chapter 9.

A diet high in complex carbohydrates (unrefined whole grains) and water-soluble fibers (found in fruits, vegetables, oats, beans, and psyllium), low in saturated fat, and low in sugar is helpful in treating diabetes. Aggressive weight loss, especially if combined with exercise, often allows diabetic patients to normalize their blood sugar level without the use of medication.

GLYCEMIC INDEX

Although complex carbohydrates are recommended in the diet, diabetics need to pay careful attention to the glycemic index (explained in Chapter 5 and detailed in Table 5.1, page 126). Refined and starchy foods (small-particle carbohydrates, which are quickly digested) rank high in the glycemic index,

Diabetes mellitus A disease in which the body doesn't produce or utilize insulin properly.

Insulin A hormone secreted by the pancreas; essential for proper metabolism of blood glucose (sugar) and maintenance of blood glucose level.

Insulin resistance Inability of the cells to respond appropriately to insulin.

Type 1 diabetes Insulin-dependent diabetes mellitus (IDDM), a condition in which the pancreas produces little or no insulin; also known as juvenile diabetes.

Type 2 diabetes Non-insulin-dependent diabetes mellitus (NIDDM), a condition in which insulin is not processed properly; also known as adult-onset diabetes.

whereas grains, fruits, and vegetables are low-glycemic foods.

Foods high in the glycemic index cause a rapid increase in blood sugar. A diet that includes many high-glycemic foods increases the risk for cardiovascular disease in people with high insulin resistance and **glucose intolerance**.[15] Combining a moderate amount of high-glycemic foods with low-glycemic foods or with some fat and protein, however, can bring down the average index.

A1C TEST

Individuals who have high blood glucose levels should consult a physician to decide on the best treatment. They also might obtain information about a new hemoglobin *A1c test* (also called Hb A1c) that measures the amount of glucose that has been in a person's blood over the last 3 months. Blood glucose can become attached to hemoglobin in the red blood cells. Once attached, it remains there for the life of the red blood cell, which is about 3 months. The higher the blood glucose, the higher is the concentration of glucose in the red blood cells. Results of this test are given in percentages.

The Hb A1c goal for diabetic patients is to keep it at less than 7 percent. At this level, or below, diabetics have a lower risk of developing diabetic-related problems of the eyes, kidneys, and nerves. Because the test tells a person how well blood glucose has been controlled over the last 3 months, a change in treatment is almost always recommended if the Hb A1c results are above 8 percent. All people with type 2 diabetes should have an Hb A1c test twice per year.

METABOLIC SYNDROME

As the cells resist the actions of insulin, the pancreas releases even more insulin in an attempt to keep blood glucose from rising. A chronic rise in insulin seems to trigger a series of abnormalities referred to as the **metabolic syndrome** or **syndrome X**. These abnormal conditions include abdominal obesity, elevated blood pressure, high blood glucose, low HDL cholesterol, high triglycerides, and an increased blood-clotting mechanism. All of these conditions increase the risk for CHD and other diabetic-related conditions (blindness, infection, nerve damage, and kidney failure). Approximately 47 million Americans are afflicted with this condition.

People with metabolic syndrome have an abnormal insulin response to carbohydrates, in particular high-glycemic foods. In contrast to the American Heart Association dietary guidelines, researchers on metabolic syndrome indicate that a low-fat, high-carbohydrate diet may not be the best for preventing CHD and could actually increase the risk for disease in people with high insulin resistance and glucose

intolerance.[16] It might be best for these people to distribute daily caloric intake so that 45 percent of the calories are derived from carbohydrates (primarily low-glycemic), 40 percent from fat, and 15 percent from protein.[17] Of the 40 percent fat calories, most of the fat should come from mono- and poly-unsaturated fats and less than 7 percent from saturated fat.

Metabolic syndrome patients also benefit from weight loss (if overweight), exercise, and smoking cessation.[18] Insulin resistance drops by about 40 percent in overweight people who lose 20 pounds. Forty-five minutes of daily aerobic exercise enhances insulin efficiency by 25 percent. Quitting smoking also decreases insulin resistance.

Hypertension

Some 60,000 miles of blood vessels run through the human body. As the heart forces the blood through these vessels, the fluid is under pressure. **Blood pressure** is measured in milliliters of mercury (mm Hg), usually expressed in two numbers. **Systolic blood pressure** is the higher number, and **diastolic blood pressure** is the lower number. Ideal blood pressure is 120/80 or lower.

STANDARDS

Statistical evidence indicates that damage to the arteries starts at blood pressures above 120/80. The risk for cardiovascular disease doubles with each increment of 20/10, starting with a blood pressure of 115/75.[19] All blood pressures above 140/90 are considered to be **hypertension** (see Table 11.8). Blood pressures ranging from 120/80 to 139/89 are referred to as prehypertension.

Based on estimates released in 2004, approximately 1 in every 3 adults are hypertensive

TABLE 11.8 Blood Pressure Guidelines (expressed in mm Hg)

Rating	Systolic	Diastolic
Normal	≤120	≤80
Prehypertension	121–139	81–89
Hypertension	≥140	≥90

Source: National Heart, Lung and Blood Institute.

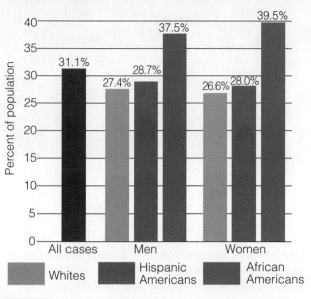

FIGURE 11.9 Incidence of high blood pressure in the United States.

Source: National Health and Nutrition Examination Study, 2004.

(Figure 11.9), up from 1 in 4 a decade earlier.[20] The incidence is higher among African Americans—in fact, it is among the highest in the world. Approximately 30 percent and 20 percent of all deaths in African-American men and women, respectively, may be caused by high blood pressure.

Even though the threshold for hypertension has been set at 140/90, many experts believe that the lower the blood pressure, the better. Even if the pressure is around 90/50, as long as that person does not have any symptoms of **hypotension**, he or she need not be concerned. Typical symptoms of hypotension are dizziness, lightheadedness, and fainting.

Blood pressure also may fluctuate during a regular day. Many factors affect blood pressure, and one single reading may not be a true indicator of the real pressure. For example, physical activity and stress increase blood pressure, and rest and relaxation decrease it. Consequently, several measurements should be taken before diagnosing high pressure.

INCIDENCE AND PATHOLOGY

Based on current estimates by the American Heart Association, 65 million Americans (age 6 and older) are hypertensive and more than 47,000 Americans die each year as a result of high blood pressure. The dramatic increase in hypertension during the last decade seems to be linked to the growing epidemic of obesity and the aging of the U.S. population. Unless appropriate, healthy, lifestyle strategies are implemented, people who do not have high blood pressure at age 55 have a 90 percent chance of developing it at some point in their lives.[21]

Hypertension has been referred to as "the silent killer." It does not hurt; it does not make you feel sick; and, unless you check it, years may go by before you even realize you have a problem. High blood pressure is a risk factor for CHD and also for congestive heart failure, strokes, kidney failure, and osteoporosis.

All inner walls of arteries are lined by a layer of smooth endothelial cells. Blood lipids cannot penetrate the healthy lining and start to build up on the walls unless the cells are damaged. High blood

pressure is thought to be a leading contributor to destruction of this lining. As blood pressure rises, so does the risk for atherosclerosis. The higher the pressure, the greater is the damage to the arterial wall, making the vessels susceptible to fat deposits, especially if serum cholesterol is also high. Blockage of the coronary vessels decreases blood supply to the heart muscle and can lead to heart attacks. When brain arteries are involved, strokes may follow.

A clear example of the connection between high blood pressure and atherosclerosis can be seen

Glucose intolerance A condition characterized by slightly elevated blood glucose levels.

Syndrome X (metabolic syndrome) An array of metabolic abnormalities that contribute to the development of atherosclerosis triggered by insulin resistance. These conditions include low HDL-cholesterol, high triglycerides, high blood pressure, and an increased blood clotting mechanism.

Blood pressure A measure of the force exerted against the walls of the vessels by the blood flowing through them.

Systolic blood pressure Pressure exerted by blood against walls of arteries during forceful contraction (systole) of the heart; higher of the two numbers in blood pressure readings.

Diastolic blood pressure Pressure exerted by blood against walls of arteries during relaxation phase (diastole) of the heart; lower of the two numbers in blood pressure readings.

Hypertension Chronically elevated blood pressure.

Hypotension Low blood pressure.

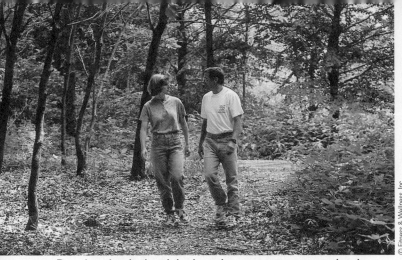

Regular physical activity is an important way to maintain healthy blood pressure.

CRITICAL THINKING

Do you know what your most recent blood pressure reading was, and did you know at the time what the numbers meant? How would you react if your doctor were to instruct you to take blood pressure medication?

by comparing blood vessels in the human body. Even when atherosclerosis is present throughout major arteries, fatty plaques rarely are seen in the pulmonary artery, which goes from the right part of the heart to the lungs. The pressure in this artery normally is below 40 mm Hg, and at such low pressure, significant deposits do not occur. This is one of the reasons people with low blood pressure have a lower incidence of cardiovascular disease.

Constantly elevated blood pressure also causes the heart to work much harder. At first the heart does well, but in time this continual strain produces an enlarged heart, followed by congestive heart failure. Furthermore, high blood pressure damages blood vessels to the kidneys and eyes, which can result in kidney failure and loss of vision.

TREATMENT

Of all hypertension, 90 percent has no definite cause. Called "essential hypertension," it is treatable. Aerobic exercise, weight reduction, a low-salt/low-fat and high-potassium/high-calcium diet, lower alcohol and caffeine intake, smoking cessation, stress management, and antihypertensive medication all have been used effectively to treat essential hypertension.

The remaining 10 percent of hypertensive cases are caused by pathological conditions, such as narrowing of the kidney arteries, glomerulonephritis (a kidney disease), tumors of the adrenal glands, and narrowing of the aortic artery. With this type of hypertension, the pathological cause has to be treated before the blood pressure problem can be corrected.

Antihypertensive medicines often are the first choice of treatment, but they produce many side effects. These include lethargy, sleepiness, sexual difficulties, higher blood cholesterol and glucose levels, lower potassium levels, and elevated uric acid levels. A physician may end up treating these side effects as much as the hypertension itself. Because of the many side effects, about half of the patients stop taking the medication within the first year of treatment.

Another factor contributing to elevated blood pressure is too much sodium in the diet (salt, or sodium chloride, contains approximately 40 percent sodium). With a high sodium intake, the body retains more water, which increases the blood volume and, in turn, drives up the pressure. High intake of potassium seems to regulate water retention and lower the pressure slightly. According to the Institute of Medicine of the National Academy of Sciences, we need to consume at least 4,700 mg of potassium per day. Most Americans get only half that amount.[22] Food items high in potassium include vegetables (especially leafy green), citrus fruit, dairy products, fish, beans, and nuts.

Although sodium is essential for normal body functions, the body can function with as little as 200 mg, or a tenth of a teaspoon daily. Even under strenuous conditions of job and sports participation that incite heavy perspiration, the amount of sodium required is seldom more than 3,000 mg per day. Yet, sodium intake in the typical U.S. diet ranges between 3,100 and 4,700 mg per day in men and 2,300 to 3,100 in women (the average daily intake is lower in women because they tend to eat fewer calories than men, not because they limit their sodium intake).

A 2004 government report now indicates that, to either prevent or postpone the onset of hypertension and to help some hypertensives control their blood pressure, we should consume even less sodium than previously recommended.[23] These new guidelines are provided in Table 11.9. The upper limit has been set at 2,300 mg per day. Among Americans and Canadians, about 95 percent of men and 75 percent of women exceed this limit.

Where does all the sodium come from? Part of the answer is given in Table 11.10. People do not realize the amount of sodium in various foods (the list in Table 11.10 does not include salt added at the table). Unfortunately, most of the sodium in our diets comes from prepared foods, in which the consumer does not have control over the ingredients.

When treating high blood pressure (unless it is extremely high), before recommending medication, many sports medicine physicians suggest a combination of aerobic exercise, weight loss, and less sodium in the diet. In most instances, this treatment brings blood pressure under control.

TABLE 11.9 Sodium and Potassium Levels of Selected Foods

Food	Serving Size	Sodium (mg)	Potassium (mg)
Asparagus	1 cup	2	330
Avocado	1/2	4	680
Banana	1 med	1	440
Beans			
Kidney (canned)	1/2 cup	436	330
Lima (cooked)	1/2 cup	2	478
Pinto (cooked)	1/2 cup	2	398
Refried (canned)	1/2 cup	16	336
Bologna	3 oz	1,107	133
Bouillon cube	1	960	4
Brussels sprouts (cooked)	1/2 cup	16	247
Cantaloupe	1/4	17	341
Carrot (raw)	1	34	225
Cheese			
American	2 oz	614	93
Cheddar	2 oz	342	56
Muenster	2 oz	356	77
Parmesan	2 oz	1,056	53
Swiss	2 oz	148	64
Chicken (light meat)	6 oz	108	700
Corn (natural)	1/2 cup	3	136
Frankfurter	1	627	136
Haddock	6 oz	300	594
Hamburger (reg)	1	500	321
Milk (whole)	1 cup	120	351
Milk (skim)	1 cup	126	406
Nuts			
Brazil	1 nut	1	120
Walnuts	1/2 cup	1	327
Orange	1 med	1	263
Peach	1 med	2	308
Peas (canned)	1/2 cup	200	82
Pizza (cheese — 14" diam.)	1/8	456	85
Potato	1 med	6	763
Salami	3 oz	1,047	170
Salmon (baked)	4 oz	75	424
Salmon (canned)	6 oz	198	756
Salt	1 tsp	2,132	0
Soups			
Chicken Noodle	1 cup	979	55
Cream of Mushroom	1 cup	955	98
Vegetable Beef	1 cup	1,046	162
Soy sauce	1 tsp	1,123	22
Spaghetti (tomato sauce and cheese)	6 oz	648	276
Spinach (cooked, fresh)	1 cup	126	838
Strawberries	1 cup	1	244
Tomato (raw)	1 med	3	444
Tuna (drained)	3 oz	38	255

TABLE 11.10 Recommended Daily Sodium Recommendations for the Prevention and Treatment of High Blood Pressure

Age	Sodium (mg/day)
19–50	1,500
51–70	1,300
>70	1,200

The relative risk for mortality ranked by blood pressure and fitness levels is similar to that of physical fitness and cholesterol. The data show that, in men and women alike, the relative risk of early mortality is lower in fit people with high systolic blood pressure (140 mm Hg or higher) than in unfit people with a healthy systolic blood pressure (120 mm Hg or lower).[24]

The link between hypertension and obesity seems to be quite strong. Blood volume increases with excess body fat, and each additional pound of fat requires an estimated extra mile of blood vessels to feed this tissue. Furthermore, blood capillaries are constricted by the adipose tissues as these vessels run through them. As a result, the heart muscle must work harder to pump the blood through a longer, constricted network of blood vessels.

The role of regular physical activity in managing blood pressure is becoming more important each day. On the average, fit individuals have a lower blood pressure than unfit people do. Aerobic exercise of moderate intensity supplemented by strength training is recommended for individuals with high blood pressure.[25]

Comprehensive reviews on the effects of aerobic exercise on blood pressure found that, in general, an individual can expect exercise-induced reductions of approximately 4 to 5 mm Hg in resting systolic blood pressure and 3 to 4 mm Hg in resting diastolic blood pressure.[26] Although these reductions do not seem large, a decrease of about 5 mm Hg in resting diastolic blood pressure has been associated with a 40 percent decrease in the risk for stroke and a 15 percent reduction in the risk for coronary heart disease.[27] Even in the absence of any decrease in resting blood pressure, hypertensive individuals who exercise have a lower risk of all-cause mortality compared to hypertensive/sedentary individuals. The research data also show that exercise, not weight loss, is the major contributor to the lower blood pressure of exercisers. If they discontinue aerobic exercise, they do not maintain these changes.

Another extensive review of research studies on the effects of at least 4 weeks of strength training on resting blood pressure yielded similar results.[28] Both

TABLE 11.11 Effects of Long-term (14–18 years) Aerobic Exercise on Resting Blood Pressure

	Initial	Final
Exercise Group		
Age	44.6	68.0
Blood Pressure	120/79	120/78
Non-exercise Group		
Age	51.6	69.7
Blood Pressure	135/85	150/90

Note: The aerobic exercise program consisted of an average four training sessions per week, each 66 minutes long, at about 76 percent of heart rate reserve.

Based on data from F. W. Kash, J. L. Boyer, S. P. Van Camp, L. S. Verity, and J. P. Wallace, "The Effect of Physical Activity on Aerobic Power in Older Men (A Longitudinal Study)," *The Physician and Sports Medicine* 18, no. 4 (1990): 73–83.

systolic and diastolic blood pressures decreased by an average of 3 mm Hg. Participants in these studies, however, were primarily individuals with normal blood pressure. Of greater significance, the results showed that strength training did not cause an increase in resting blood pressure. More research remains to be done on hypertensive subjects.

The effects of long-term participation in exercise are apparently much more remarkable. An 18-year follow-up study on exercising and non-exercising subjects showed much lower blood pressures in the active group.[29] The exercise group had an average resting blood pressure of 120/78 compared to 150/90 for the non-exercise group (see Table 11.11).

Aerobic exercise programs for hypertensive patients should be of moderate intensity. Training at 40 to 60 percent intensity (12 to 13 on the RPE scale) seems to have the same effect in lowering blood pressure as training at 70 percent. High-intensity training (above 70 percent) in hypertensive patients may not lower the blood pressure as much as moderate-intensity exercise. Even so, a person may be better off being highly fit and having high blood pressure than being unfit and having low blood pressure. The death rates for unfit individuals with low systolic blood pressure are much higher than for highly fit people with high systolic blood pressure. Strength training for hypertensive individuals should be performed with a minimum of one set of 10 to 15 repetitions that elicit a "somewhat hard" RPE rating, using 8 to 10 exercises involving multi-joint exercises, two to three times per week.

Most important is a preventive approach. Keeping blood pressure under control is easier than trying to bring it down once it is high. Regardless of your blood pressure history, high or low, you should have

GUIDELINES TO STOP HYPERTENSION

- Participate in moderate-intensity aerobic exercise program (50% intensity) for 30 to 45 minutes 5 to 7 times per week.
- Participate in a moderate-resistance strength-training program (use 12 to 15 repetitions to near-fatigue on each set) 2 times per week (seek your physician's approval and advice for this program).
- Lose weight if you are above recommended body weight.
- Eat less salt- and sodium-containing foods.
- Do not smoke cigarettes or use tobacco in any other form.
- Practice stress management.
- Do not consume more than two alcoholic beverages a day if you are a man or one if you are a woman.
- Consume more potassium-rich foods.
- Follow the Dietary Approach to Stop Hypertension (DASH Diet):
  - Seven or eight daily servings of grains, bread, cereal, or pasta.
  - Eight to ten daily servings of fruits and vegetables.
  - Two or three daily servings of nonfat/low-fat dairy products.
  - Two or less daily servings of meat, poultry, or fish (less than 3 ounces per serving).
  - Follow the Dietary Approach to Stop Hypertension (DASH) diet.

Food Group	Servings
Whole grains	7–8 per day
Fruits and vegetables	8–10 per day
Low-fat or fat-free dairy foods	2–13 per day
Meat, poultry, or fish*	2 or less per day
Beans, peas, nuts, or seeds	4–15 *per week*
Fats and oils	2–3 servings per day
Snacks and sweets	4–5 *per week*

*Less than 3 ounces per serving

it checked routinely. To keep your blood pressure as low as possible, exercise regularly, lose excess weight, eat less salt and sodium-containing foods, do not smoke, practice stress management, do not consume more than two alcoholic beverages a day if you are a man, or one if you are a woman, and consume more potassium-rich foods such as potatoes, bananas, orange juice, cantaloupe, tomatoes, and beans (see "Guidelines To Stop Hypertension"). The Dietary Approach to Stop Hypertension (DASH)—which emphasizes fruits, vegetables, grains, and dairy products—lowers systolic blood pressure by 11 points and diastolic pressure by 5.5 points.[30]

Those who are taking medication for hypertension should not stop unless the prescribing physician gives the go-ahead. If it is not treated properly, high blood pressure can kill. By combining medication with the other treatments, drug therapy eventually may be reduced or completely eliminated.

Excessive Body Fat

Body composition refers to the ratio of lean body weight to fat weight. If the body contains too much fat, the person is considered overweight or obese (see Table 4.10, page 113).

Although some experts recognize obesity as an independent risk factor for CHD, the risks attributed to obesity may actually be augmented by other risk factors that usually accompany excessive body fat. Risk factors such as high blood lipids, hypertension, and diabetes are typically seen in conjunction with obesity. All of these risk factors usually improve with increased physical activity.

Attaining recommended body composition helps to improve some of the CHD risk factors and also helps to reach a better state of health and wellness. People who have a weight problem and want to get down to recommended weight must implement the following:

1. Increase daily physical activity, and participate in aerobic and strength-training programs.
2. Follow a diet lower in fat and refined sugars and high in complex carbohydrates and fiber.
3. Reduce total caloric intake moderately while getting the necessary nutrients to sustain normal body functions.

Additional recommendations for weight reduction and weight control are discussed in Chapter 5.

Smoking

More than 47 million adults and 3.5 million adolescents in the United States smoke cigarettes. Smoking is the single largest preventable cause of illness and premature death in the United States. Smoking has been linked to cardiovascular disease, cancer, bronchitis, emphysema, and peptic ulcers. In relation to coronary disease, smoking speeds up the process of atherosclerosis and carries a threefold increase in the risk of sudden death following a myocardial infarction.

According to estimates, about 20 percent of all deaths from cardiovascular diseases are attributable to smoking. Smoking prompts the release of nicotine and another 1,200 toxic compounds into the bloodstream. Similar to hypertension, many of these substances are destructive to the inner membrane that protects the walls of the arteries. Once the lining is damaged, cholesterol and triglycerides can be deposited readily in the arterial wall. As the plaque builds up, it obstructs blood flow through the arteries.

Furthermore, smoking encourages the formation of blood clots, which can completely block an artery already narrowed by atherosclerosis. In addition, carbon monoxide, a byproduct of cigarette smoke, decreases the blood's oxygen-carrying capacity. A combination of obstructed arteries, less oxygen, and nicotine in the heart muscle heightens the risk for a serious heart problem.

Smoking also increases heart rate, raises blood pressure, and irritates the heart, which can trigger fatal cardiac **arrhythmias**. Another harmful effect is a decrease in HDL cholesterol, the "good" type that helps control blood lipids. Smoking actually presents a much greater risk of death from heart disease than from lung disease.

Pipe and cigar smoking and chewing tobacco also increase the risk for heart disease. Even if the smoker inhales no smoke, he or she absorbs toxic substances through the membranes of the mouth, and these end up in the bloodstream. Individuals who use tobacco in any of these three forms also have a much greater risk for cancer of the oral cavity.

The risks for both cardiovascular disease and cancer start to decrease the moment a person quits smoking. One year after quitting, the risk of CHD decreases by half, and within 15 years, the relative risk of dying from cardiovascular disease and cancer approaches that of a lifetime non-smoker. A more thorough discussion of the harmful effects of cigarette smoking, the benefits of quitting, and a complete program for quitting are detailed in Chapter 13.

Tension and Stress

Tension and stress have become a part of life. Everyone has to deal daily with goals, deadlines, responsibilities, pressures. Almost everything in life (whether positive or negative) can be a source of stress. The stressor itself is not what creates the health hazard but, rather, the individual's response to it.

The human body responds to stress by producing more **catecholamines**, which prepare the body for quick physical action—often called "fight or flight." These hormones increase heart rate, blood pressure, and blood glucose levels, enabling the person to take action. If the person actually fights or flees, the higher levels of catecholamines are metabolized and the body can return to a normal state. If, however, a person is under constant stress and unable to take action (as in the death of a close relative or friend, loss of a job, trouble at work, or financial insecurity), the catecholamines remain elevated in the bloodstream.

Arrhythmias Irregular heart rhythms.

Catecholamines "Fight-or-flight" hormones, including epinephrine and norepinephrine.

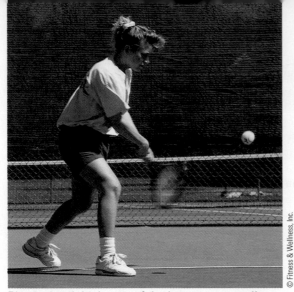

Physical activity is one of the best ways to relieve stress.

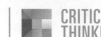

People who are not able to relax place a constant low-level strain on the cardiovascular system that could manifest itself as heart disease. In addition, when a person is in a stressful situation, the coronary arteries that feed the heart muscle constrict, reducing the oxygen supply to the heart. If the blood vessels are largely blocked by atherosclerosis, arrhythmias or even a heart attack may follow.

Individuals who are under a lot of stress and do not cope well with it need to take measures to counteract the effects of stress in their lives. One way is to identify the sources of stress and learn how to cope with them. People need to take control of themselves, examine and act upon the things that are most important in their lives, and ignore less meaningful details.

Physical activity is one of the best ways to relieve stress. When a person takes part in physical activity, the body metabolizes excess catecholamines and is able to return to a normal state. Exercise also steps up muscular activity, which contributes to muscular relaxation after completing the physical activity.

Many executives in large cities are choosing the evening hours for their physical activity programs, stopping after work at the health or fitness club. In doing this, they are able to "burn up" the excess tension accumulated during the day and enjoy the evening hours. This has proved to be one of the best stress-management techniques. More information on stress management techniques is presented in Chapter 10.

Personal and Family History

Individuals who have had cardiovascular problems are at higher risk than those who have never had a problem. People with this history should control the other risk factors as much as they can. Many of the risk factors are reversible, so this will greatly decrease the risk for future problems. The more time that passes after the cardiovascular problem occurred, the lower is the risk for recurrence.

A genetic predisposition toward heart disease has been demonstrated clearly. All other factors being equal, a person with blood relatives who now have or did have heart disease run a greater risk than someone with no such history. Premature CHD is defined as a heart attack before age 55 in a close male relative or before age 65 in a close female relative. The younger the age at which the relative incurred the cardiovascular incident, the greater is the risk for the disease.

In some cases, there is no way of knowing whether the heart problem resulted from a person's genetic predisposition or simply poor lifestyle habits. A person may have been physically inactive, been overweight, smoked, and had bad dietary habits—all of which contributed to a heart attack. Regardless, blood relatives fall in the "family history" category. Because we have no reliable way to differentiate all the factors contributing to cardiovascular disease, a person with a family history should watch all other factors closely and maintain the lowest risk level possible. In addition, the person should have a blood chemistry analysis annually to make sure the body is handling blood lipids properly.

Age

Age is a risk factor because of the higher incidence of heart disease as people get older. This tendency may be induced partly by other factors stemming from changes in lifestyle as we get older—less physical activity, poorer nutrition, obesity, and so on. Young people should not think they are exempt from heart disease, though. The process begins early in life. Autopsies conducted on American soldiers killed at age 22 and younger revealed that approximately 70 percent had early stages of atherosclerosis. Other studies found elevated blood cholesterol levels in children as young as 10 years old.

Although the aging process cannot be stopped, it certainly can be slowed. Physiological age versus chronological age is important in preventing disease. Some individuals in their 60s or older have the body of a 30-year-old. And 30-year-olds often are in such poor condition and health that they almost seem to have the body of 60-year-olds. The best ways to slow the natural aging process are to engage in risk-factor management and positive lifestyle habits.

Other Risk Factors for CHD

Additional evidence points to a few other factors that may be linked to coronary heart disease. One of these factors is gum disease. The oral bacteria that build up with dental plaque can enter the bloodstream and contribute to inflammation, formation of blood vessel plaque, blood clotting, and thus increase the risk for heart attack. Data on women who have periodontal disease indicate that these women also have higher blood levels of CRP and lower HDL cholesterol. Daily flossing, using a power brush, scraping the tongue, and irrigating the gums with water are all preventive measures that will help protect you from gum disease.

Another factor that has been linked to cardiovascular disease is loud snoring. People who snore heavily may suffer from sleep apnea, a sleep disorder in which the throat closes for a brief moment, causing breathing to stop. Individuals who snore heavily may triple their risk of a heart attack and quadruple the risk of a stroke.

Low birth weight, considered to be under 5.5 pounds, also has been linked to heart disease, hypertension, and diabetes. Individuals with low birth weight should bring this information to the attention of their personal physician and regularly monitor the risk factors for CHD.

Aspirin therapy is also recommended to prevent heart disease. For individuals at moderate risk or higher, a daily aspirin dose of about 81 mg per day (the equivalent of a baby aspirin) can prevent or dissolve clots that cause heart attack or stroke. With daily use, the incidence of nonfatal heart attack is decreased by about a third.

Cardiovascular Risk Reduction

Using Lab 11A, you can chart a program to reduce your own cardiovascular risk. Most of the risk factors are reversible and preventable. Having a family history of heart disease and/or possessing some of the other risk factors because of neglect in lifestyle does not mean you are doomed. A healthier lifestyle—free of cardiovascular problems—is something over which you have extensive control. Be persistent! Willpower and commitment are required to develop patterns that eventually will turn into healthy habits and contribute to your total well-being and longevity.

ofile
us
___
luate how
ll you
derstand
concepts
sented in
s chapter
ng the
ssess Your
owledge"
d "Practice
izzes"
ions
your
-ROM.

ASSESS YOUR KNOWLEDGE

1. Coronary heart disease
   a. is the single leading cause of death in the United States.
   b. is the leading cause of sudden cardiac deaths.
   c. is a condition in which the arteries that supply the heart muscle with oxygen and nutrients are narrowed by fatty deposits.
   d. accounts for approximately 20 percent of all cardiovascular deaths.
   e. All of the above.

2. The incidence of cardiovascular disease during the past 40 years in the United States has
   a. increased.
   b. decreased.
   c. remained constant.
   d. increased in some years and decreased in others.
   e. fluctuated according to medical technology.

3. Regular aerobic activity helps
   a. lower LDL cholesterol.
   b. lower HDL cholesterol.
   c. increase triglycerides.
   d. decrease insulin sensitivity.
   e. All of the above.

4. The risk of heart disease increases with
   a. high LDL cholesterol.
   b. low HDL cholesterol.
   c. high concentration of homocysteine.
   d. high levels of hs-CRP.
   e. All of the above factors.

5. An optimal level of LDL cholesterol is
   a. between 200 and 239 mg/dl.
   b. at about 200 mg/dl.
   c. between 150 and 200 mg/dl.
   d. between 100 and 150 mg/dl.
   e. below 100 mg/dl.

6. As a part of a CHD-prevention program, saturated fat intake should be kept below
   a. 35 percent.
   b. 30 percent.
   c. 22 percent.
   d. 15 percent.
   e. 7 percent.

7. Statin drugs
   a. increase the liver's ability to remove blood cholesterol.
   b. decrease LDL cholesterol.
   c. slow cholesterol production.
   d. help reduce inflammation.
   e. All of the above.

8. Type 1 diabetes is related closely to
   a. overeating.
   b. obesity.
   c. lack of physical activity.
   d. insulin resistance.
   e. All of the above factors.

9. Metabolic syndrome is related to
   a. low HDL cholesterol.
   b. high triglycerides.
   c. increased blood-clotting mechanism.
   d. an abnormal insulin response to carbohydrates.
   e. All of the above.

10. Comprehensive reviews on the effects of aerobic exercise on blood pressure found that, in general, an individual can expect exercise-induced reductions of approximately
    a. 3 to 5 mm Hg.
    b. 5 to 10 mm Hg.
    c. 10 to 15 mm Hg.
    d. over 15 mm Hg.
    e. There is no significant change in blood pressure with exercise.

Correct answers can be found at the back of the book.

MEDIA MENU

PROFILE PLUS CD CONNECTIONS

■ Determine your risk for heart disease.

■ Determine your current saturated and unsaturated fat intake.

■ Check how well you understand the chapter's concepts.

INTERNET CONNECTIONS

■ American Heart Association. This comprehensive site provides research, cardiac information for health professionals and the general public, as well as advocacy. The site features information on a variety of cardiovascular illnesses, healthy lifestyles, and CPR. It also offers a heart and stroke searchable encyclopedia and a ten-question "Healthy Heart Workout" quiz.

http://www.americanheart.org

■ National Cholesterol Education Program. This comprehensive site features interactive sessions on planning a low-cholesterol diet and lots more. It provides you with information to prevent heart disease as well as information for people who already have heart disease. You can also hear radio messages from the Heart Beat Radio Network. This site is highly recommended.

http://rover.nhlbi.nih.gov/chd

■ The Heart: An Online Exploration. This very informative and interesting site, developed by the Franklin Institute of Science, provides an interactive multimedia tour of the heart, statistical information, resources, and links. You can learn how to monitor your heart's health by becoming aware of your vital signs, read more about diagnostic tests, and listen to heart sounds via the site's audio and video clips.

http://www.fi.edu/biosci/heart.html

■ Check Your Healthy Heart IQ. This site is sponsored by the National Heart, Lung, and Blood Institute. Test your knowledge about heart disease and its risk factors (high blood pressure, high blood cholesterol, smoking, lack of exercise, and overweight) and learn ways to reduce your risk.

http://www.nhlbi.nih.gov/health/public/heart/other/

Notes

1. U. S. Department of Health and Human Services, Centers for Disease Control and Prevention, National Center for Health Statistics, National Vital Statistics System, *Deaths: Preliminary Data for 2002* 52, no. 13 (February 11, 2004).

2. S. N. Blair, H. W. Kohl III, R. S. Paffenbarger, Jr., D. G. Clark, K. H. Cooper, and L. W. Gibbons, "Physical Fitness and All-Cause Mortality: A Prospective Study of Healthy Men and Women," *Journal of the American Medical Association* 262 (1989): 2395–2401.

3. R. S. Paffenbarger, Jr., R. T. Hyde, A. L. Wing, I. Lee, D. L. Jung, and J. B. Kampert, "The Association of Changes in Physical-Activity Level and Other Lifestyle Characteristics with Mortality Among Men," *New England Journal of Medicine* 328 (1993): 538–545.

4. "Lipid Research Clinics Program: The Lipid Research Clinic Coronary Primary Prevention Trial Results," *Journal of the American Medical Association* 251 (1984): 351–364.

5. American Heart Association, *Heart Disease and Stroke Statistics—2004 Update* (Dallas: AHA, 2003).

6. M. Mogadam, "5 Little-Known Ways to Lower Heart Attack Risk," *Bottom Line/Health* 18 (May 2004): 5–6.

7. "HDL on the Rise," *HealthNews*, September 10, 1999.

8. "From Starring Role to Bit Part: Has the Curtain Come Down on Vitamin E?" *Environmental Nutrition* 25 no. 5 (May 2002): 1, 4.

9. See note 2.

10. E. B. Rimm, A. Ascherio, E. Giovannucci, D. Spiegelman, M. J. Stampfer, and W. C. Willett, "Vegetable,

Fruit, and Cereal Fiber Intake and Risk of Coronary Heart Disease Among Men," *Journal of the American Medical Association* 275 (1996): 447–451.

11. National Cholesterol Education Program Expert Panel, "Summary of the Third Report of the National Cholesterol Education Program (NCEP) Expert Panel on Detection, Evaluation, and Treatment of High Blood Cholesterol in Adults (Adult Treatment Panel III)," *Journal of the American Medical Association* 285 (2001): 2486–2497.

12. A. Jula et al., "Effects of Diet and Simvastatin on Serum Lipids, Insulin, and Antioxidants in Hypercholesterolemic Men," *Journal of the American Medical Association* 287 (2002): 598–605.

13. "The Homocysteine–CVD Connection," *HealthNews* (October 25, 1999).

14. "Inflammation May Be Key Cause of Heart Disease and More: Diet's Role" *Environmental Nutrition* 27 no. 7 (July 2004): 1, 4.

15. S. Liu et al., "A Prospective Study of Dietary Glycemic Load, Carbohydrate Intake, and Risk of Coronary Heart Disease in the U.S.," *American Journal of Clinical Nutrition* 71 (2000): 1455–1461.

16. E. J. Mayer et al., "Intensity and Amount of Physical Activity in Relation to Insulin Sensitivity," *Journal of the American Medical Association* 279 (1998): 669–674.

17. G. M. Reaven, T. K. Strom, and B. Fox, *Syndrome X: Overcoming the Silent Killer That Can Give You a Heart Attack* (Englewood Cliffs, NJ: Simon & Schuster, 2000).

18. G. M. Reaven, "Syndrome X: The Little Known Cause of Many Heart Attacks," *Bottom Line/Health* 14 (June 2000).

19. A. V. Chobanian, et al., "The Seventh Report of the Joint National Committee on Prevention, Detection, Evaluation, and Treatment of High Blood Pressure," *Journal of the American Medical Association* 289 (2003): 2560–2571.

20. L. E. Fields, et al., "The Burden of Adult Hypertension in the United States 1999 to 2000: A Rising Tide," *Hypertension On Line First*, August 23, 2004.

21. See note 20.

22. "Water, Sodium, Potassium: The Verdict Is In," *University of California at Berkeley Wellness Letter* (Palm Coast, FL: The Editors, May 2004).

23. See note 22.

24. See note 2.

25. L. S. Pescatello et al., "Exercise and Hypertension Position Stand," *Medicine and Science in Sports and Exercise* 36 (2004): 533–553.

26. G. Kelley, "Dynamic Resistance Exercise and Resting Blood Pressure in Adults: A Meta-analysis," *Journal of Applied Physiology* 82 (1997): 1559–1565.

G. A. Kelley and Z. Tran, "Aerobic Exercise and Normotensive Adults: A Meta-analysis," *Medicine and Science in Sports and Exercise* 27 (1995): 1371–1377.

G. Kelley and P. McClellan, "Antihypertensive Effects of Aerobic Exercise: A Brief Meta-analytic Review of Randomized Controlled Trials," *American Journal of Hypertension* 7 (1994): 115–119.

27. R. Collins et al., "Blood Pressure, Stroke, and Coronary Heart Disease; Part 2, Short-term Reductions in Blood Pressure: Overview of Randomized Drug Trials in Their Epidemiological Context," *Lancet* 335 (1990): 827–838.

28. G. A. Kelley and K. S. Kelley, "Progressive Resistance Exercise and Resting Blood Pressure: A Meta-Analysis of Randomized Controlled Trials," *Hypertension* 35 (2000): 838–843.

29. F. W. Kash, J. L. Boyer, S. P. Van Camp, L. S. Verity, and J. P. Wallace, "The Effect of Physical Activity on Aerobic Power in Older Men (A Longitudinal Study)," *Physician and Sports Medicine* 18, no. 4 (1990): 73–83.

30. S. G. Sheps, "High Blood Pressure Can Often Be Controlled without Medication," *Bottom Line/Health*, November, 1999.

Suggested Readings

American Heart Association. *2005 Heart and Stroke Facts Statistical Update*. Dallas: AHA, 2004.

American Heart Association. *Heart and Stroke Facts*. Dallas: AHA, 2004.

Cooper, K. H. "Control Your Cholesterol without Drugs." *Bottom Line/Health* 17 (August 2003): 3–4.

National Cholesterol Education Program Expert Panel. "Summary of the Third Report of the National Cholesterol Education Program (NCEP) Expert Panel on Detection, Evaluation, and Treatment of High Blood Cholesterol in Adults (Adult Treatment Panel III)." *Journal of the American Medical Association* 285 (2001): 2486–2497.

Lab 11A

SELF-EVALUATION OF CARDIOVASCULAR RISK AND BEHAVIOR MODIFICATION PROGRAM

Name: _____   Date: _____   Grade: _____

Instructor: _____   Course: _____   Section: _____

Necessary Lab Equipment

Basic lab equipment to repeat the body composition and blood pressure tests, and if possible, a blood chemistry analysis should be performed prior to this lab.

Objective

To assess your current risk for coronary heart disease (CHD) and develop a behavior modification program.

Profile Plus

I. Self-Assessment: Coronary Heart Disease Risk Factor Analysis

Instructions   The disease process for cardiovascular disease starts early in life, primarily as a result of poor lifestyle habits. Studies have shown beginning stages of atherosclerosis and elevated blood lipids in children as young as 10 years old. Consequently, the purpose of this lab is to establish a baseline CHD risk profile and to point out the "zero-risk" level for each coronary risk factor.

You may want to repeat the body composition and blood pressure tests to obtain current values for this lab experience. If time does not allow for reassessment of these parameters, use the results obtained in previous labs. In addition, if you have had a blood chemistry analysis performed recently that included total cholesterol, HDL cholesterol, triglycerides, and glucose levels, you may use the results for this lab.

			Score
1. Physical Activity	Do you participate in a regular aerobic exercise program (brisk walking, jogging, swimming, bicycling, aerobics, etc.) for more than 20 minutes:		
	Once a week or less	8	
	Two times per week	3	
	Three or more times per week	0	

2. Resting and Stress Electrocardiograms (ECG)	Add scores for both ECGs			
	ECG	Resting	Stress	
	Normal	(0)	(0)	0
	Equivocal	(1)	(4)	1–5
	Abnormal	(3)	(8)	3–11

3. HDL Cholesterol	Men	Women	
(If unknown, answer	≥45	≥55	0
Question 6)	35–44	45–54	3
	≤34	≤44	6

4. LDL Cholesterol	<130	0
(If unknown, answer	130–159	3
Question 6)	≥160	6

5. Triglycerides	≤125	0
(If unknown, answer	126–499	1
Question 6)	≥500	2

Subtotal Risk Score: _____

Subtotal Risk Score (from previous page):

6. Diet (Do not answer if Questions 3, 4 and 5 have been answered)

Does your regular diet include (high score if all apply):
One or more daily servings of red meat; 7 or more eggs/week; daily butter, cheese, whole milk, sweets and alcohol.. 10–14

Four to six servings of red meat/week; 4–6 eggs per week; 1% or 2% milk; some cheese, sweets, and alcohol.............. 4–10

Fish, poultry, red meat fewer than three times/week; fewer than 3 eggs/week; skim milk and skim milk products; moderate sweets and alcohol 0–3

7. Homocysteine

Does your daily diet include:
2 and 3 servings of fruits and vegetables respectively.................. 0
Less than 2 and 3 servings of fruits and vegetables respectively........ 4

8. Inflammation (as measured by High-Sensitivity C-Reactive Protein or hs-CRP)

<1 mg/l.. 0
1–3 mg/l 2
>3 mg/l 8

9. Diabetes/Glucose

≤120.. 0
121–128.. 1
129–136.. 1.5
137–144 2
145–149 .... 2.5
≥150 3
Diabetics add another 3 points 3

10. Blood Pressure

Add scores for both readings (e.g., 144/88 score = 4)

Systolic	Diastolic	
≤120 .... (0)	≤80............ (0)	0
121–130......... (1)	81–90 .... (1)	1–2
131–140......... (2)	91–98 .... (2)	2–4
141–150......... (3)	99–106 .... (3)	3–6
≥151 .... (4)	≥107 .... (4)	4–8

11. Body Mass Index (BMI)

≤25.0 0
25.0–29.99 2
30.0–39.99 4
≥40.0 8

12. Smoking

Lifetime non-smoker 0
Ex-smoker more than 1 year 0
Ex-smoker less than 1 year 1
Smoke 1 cigarette/day or none 1
Nonsmoker, but live or work in smoking environment 2
Pipe or cigar smoker, or chew tobacco 3
Smoke 1–9 cigarettes/day 3
Smoke 10–19 cigarettes/day 4
Smoke 20–29 cigarettes/day 5
Smoke 30–39 cigarettes/day 6
Smoke 40 or more cigarettes/day 8

Subtotal Risk Score:

Subtotal Risk Score (from previous page): [ ]

13. Tension and Stress	Are you:	
	Sometimes tense	0
	Often tense..	1
	Nearly always tense	2
	Always tense	3

14. Personal History	Have you ever had a heart attack, stroke, coronary disease, or any known heart problem:	
	During the last year	8
	1–2 years ago...	5
	2–5 years ago...	3
	More than 5 years ago...	2
	Never had heart disease	0

15. Family History	Have any of your blood relatives (parents, uncles, brothers, sisters, grandparents) had cardiovascular disease (heart attack, strokes, bypass surgery):	
	One or more before age 51	8
	One or more between 51 and 60......................................	4
	One or more after age 60	2
	None had cardiovascular disease	0

16. Age	29 or younger	0
	30–39	1
	40–49	2
	50–59	3
	≥60	4

Total Risk Score: [ ]

How to Score

Risk Category	Total Risk Score
Very Low	5 or fewer points
Low	Between 6 and 15 points
Moderate	Between 16 and 25 points
High	Between 26 and 35 points
Very High	36 or more points

II. Stage of Change for Cardiovascular Disease Prevention

Using Figure 2.4 (page 41) and Table 2.3 (page 41), identify your current stage of change for participation in a cardiovascular disease risk-reduction program:

III. In a few sentences, discuss your family and personal risk for cardiovascular disease:

IV. Discuss lifestyle changes that you have already implemented in this course, as well as additional changes that you can make to decrease your own risk of developing cardiovascular disease in the future.

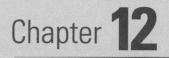

Chapter **12**

Cancer Prevention

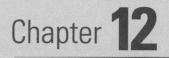

Objectives

- Define cancer and understand how it starts and spreads.
- Cite guidelines for preventing cancer.
- Delineate the major risk factors that lead to specific types of cancer.
- Assess the risk of developing certain types of cancer.

Profile Plus CD Connections

- Assess your risk for cancer.
- Check how well you understand the chapter's concepts.

361

© Carol Kohen/The Image Bank/Getty Images

FIGURE 12.1 Mutant (cancer) cells.

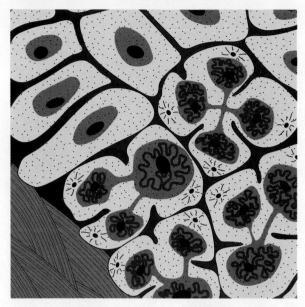

Adapted from American Cancer Society, *Youth Looks at Cancer* (New York: American Cancer Society, 1982) p. 4.

FIGURE 12.2 Erosion of chromosome telomeres in normal cells.

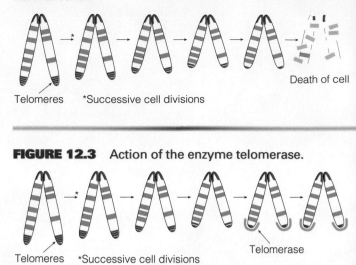

Telomeres   *Successive cell divisions   Death of cell

FIGURE 12.3 Action of the enzyme telomerase.

Telomeres   *Successive cell divisions   Telomerase

The human body has approximately 100 trillion cells. Under normal conditions, these cells reproduce themselves in an orderly way. Cell growth (cell reproduction) takes place to replace and repair old, worn-out tissue.

Cell growth is controlled by **deoxyribonucleic acid (DNA)** and **ribonucleic acid (RNA)**, found in the nucleus of each cell. When nuclei lose their ability to regulate and control cell growth, cell division is disrupted and mutant cells can develop (see Figure 12.1). Some of these cells might grow uncontrollably and abnormally, forming a mass of tissue called a tumor, which can be either **benign** or **malignant**. Benign tumors do not invade other tissues. Although they can interfere with normal bodily functions, they rarely cause death. A malignant tumor is a **cancer**. More than 100 types of cancer can develop in any tissue or organ of the human body.

The process of cancer actually begins with an alteration in DNA. Within DNA are **oncogenes** and tumor **suppressor genes**, which normally work together to repair and replace cells. Defects in these genes—caused by external factors such as radiation, chemicals, and viruses, as well as internal factors such as immune conditions, hormones, and genetic mutations—ultimately allow the cell to grow into a tumor.

A healthy cell can duplicate as many as 100 times in its lifetime. Normally, the DNA molecule is duplicated perfectly during cell division. In the few cases when the DNA molecule is not replicated exactly, specialized enzymes make repairs quickly.

Occasionally, however, cells with defective DNA keep dividing and ultimately form a small tumor. As more mutations occur, the altered cells continue to divide and can become malignant. A decade or more might pass between exposure to carcinogens or mutations and the time cancer is diagnosed.

The process of abnormal cell division is related indirectly to chromosome segments called **telomeres** (see Figure 12.2). Each time a cell divides, chromosomes lose some telomeres. After many cell divisions, chromosomes eventually run out of telomeres and the cell then invariably dies.

Scientists have discovered that human tumors make an enzyme known as **telomerase**. In cancer cells, telomerase keeps the chromosome from running out of telomeres entirely. The shortened strand of telomeres (see Figure 12.3) now allows cells to reproduce indefinitely, creating a malignant tumor.

Telomerase seems to have another function that is still under investigation: After many cell divisions, cancer cells grow old by nature, but telomerase keeps them from dying. If scientists can confirm that telomerase plays such a crucial role in the formation of tumors, research will be directed to finding a way to block the action of telomerase, thereby making cancerous cells die.

Cancer starts with the abnormal growth of one cell, which then can multiply into billions of cancerous cells. A critical turning point in the development of cancer is when a tumor reaches about one million cells. At this stage, it is referred to as **carcinoma in situ**. Such an undetected tumor may go for months or years without any significant growth. While it remains encapsulated, it does not pose a serious

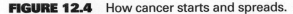

FIGURE 12.4   How cancer starts and spreads.

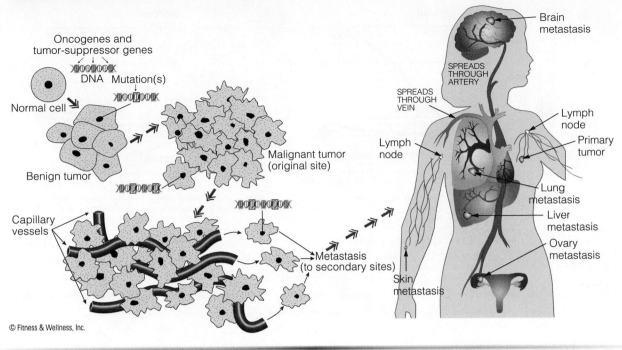

Oncogenes and tumor-suppressor genes
DNA Mutation(s)
Normal cell
Benign tumor
Malignant tumor (original site)
Capillary vessels
Metastasis (to secondary sites)

© Fitness & Wellness, Inc.

Brain metastasis
SPREADS THROUGH ARTERY
SPREADS THROUGH VEIN
Lymph node
Lymph node
Primary tumor
Lung metastasis
Liver metastasis
Ovary metastasis
Skin metastasis

threat to human health. To grow, however, the tumor requires more oxygen and nutrients.

In time, a few of the cancer cells start producing chemicals that enhance **angiogenesis**, or capillary (blood vessel) formation into the tumor. Angiogenesis is the precursor of **metastasis**. Through the new blood vessels formed by angiogenesis, cancerous cells now can break away from a malignant tumor and migrate to other parts of the body, where they can cause new cancer (Figure 12.4).

Most adults have precancerous or cancerous cells in their bodies. By middle age, our bodies contain millions of precancerous cells. The immune system and the blood turbulence destroy most cancer cells, but only one abnormal cell lodging elsewhere is enough to start a new cancer. These cells grow and multiply uncontrollably, invading and destroying normal tissue. The rate at which cancer cells grow varies from one type to another. Some types grow fast, and others take years.

Once cancer cells metastasize, treatment becomes more difficult. Although therapy can kill most cancer cells, a few cells might become resistant to treatment. These cells then can grow into a new tumor that will not respond to the same treatment.

Incidence of Cancer

According to mortality statistics for 2002 from the National Center for Health Statistics, cancer was the cause of 22.8 percent of all deaths in the United States. It is the second leading cause of death in the country and the leading cause in children between ages 1 and 14. The major contributor to the increase in incidence of cancer during the last five decades is lung cancer. Tobacco use alone is responsible for 87 percent of lung cancer and accounts for 30 percent of all deaths from cancer. Death rates for most major cancer sites are declining, except for lung cancer in women (see Figure 12.5).

Deoxyribonucleic acid (DNA) Genetic substance of which genes are made; molecule that contains cell's genetic code.

Ribonucleic acid (RNA) Genetic material that guides the formation of cell proteins.

Benign Noncancerous.

Malignant Cancerous.

Cancer Group of diseases characterized by uncontrolled growth and spread of abnormal cells.

Oncogenes Genes that initiate cell division.

Suppressor genes Genes that deactivate the process of cell division.

Telomeres A strand of molecules at both ends of a chromosome.

Telomerase An enzyme that allows cells to reproduce indefinitely.

Carcinoma in situ Encapsulated malignant tumor that has not spread.

Angiogenesis Formation of blood vessels (capillaries).

Metastasis The movement of cells from one part of the body to another.

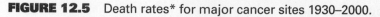

FIGURE 12.5 Death rates* for major cancer sites 1930–2000.

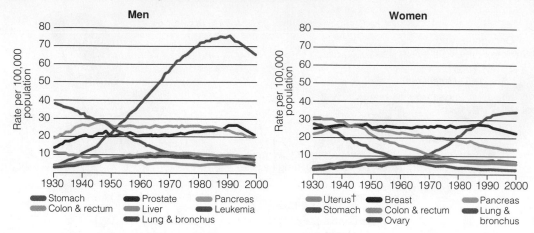

Men

Rate per 100,000 population

Stomach • Prostate • Pancreas
Colon & rectum • Liver • Leukemia
Lung & bronchus

Women

Rate per 100,000 population

Uterus† • Breast • Pancreas
Stomach • Colon & rectum • Lung & bronchus
Ovary

*Per 100,000, age-adjusted to the 1970 U. S. standard population.   †Uterus cancer deaths are for uterine cervix and uterine corpus combined.

Note: Due to changes in ICD coding, numerator information has changed over time. Rates for cancers of the liver, lung, and bronchus, and colon and rectum are affected by these coding changes.

Source: Reprinted with permission from the American Cancer Society, *Cancer Facts & Figures.* © 2004, American Cancer Society, Inc. www.cancer.org.

Cancer will develop in approximately one of every two men and one of three women in the United States, striking approximately three of every four families. About 563,700 Americans died from cancer in 2004, and approximately 1,368,030 new cases were diagnosed that same year.[1] The incidence of cancer is higher in African Americans than in any other racial or ethnic group.

Statistical estimates of the incidence of cancer and deaths by sex and site for the year 2004 are given in Figure 12.6. These estimates exclude **nonmelanoma skin cancer** and carcinoma in situ.

Like coronary heart disease, cancer is largely preventable. As much as 80 percent of all human cancer is related to lifestyle or environmental factors (including diet and obesity, tobacco use, sedentary lifestyle, excessive use of alcohol, and exposure to occupational hazards—see Figure 12.7). Most of these cancers could be prevented through positive lifestyle habits.

Research sponsored by the American Cancer Society and the National Cancer Institute showed that individuals who have a healthy lifestyle have some of the lowest cancer mortality rates ever reported in scientific studies. A group of about 10,000 members of the Church of Jesus Christ of Latter-Day Saints (commonly referred to as the Mormon church) in California was reported to have only about one-third (men) to one-half (women) the rate of cancer mortality of the general white population[2] (Figure 12.8). In this study, the investigators looked at three

general health habits in the participants: lifetime abstinence from smoking, regular physical activity, and sufficient sleep. In addition, healthy lifestyle guidelines (encouraged by the church since 1833) include abstaining from all forms of tobacco, alcohol, and drugs and adhering to a well-balanced diet based on grains, fruits, and vegetables, and moderate amounts of poultry and red meat. Lifestyle is definitely an important factor in the risk for cancer.

Equally important is that approximately 9.6 million Americans with a history of cancer were alive in 2004. Currently, 6 in 10 people diagnosed with cancer are expected to be alive 5 years after the initial diagnosis.[3]

Guidelines for Preventing Cancer

The biggest factor in fighting cancer today is health education. People need to be informed about the risk factors for cancer and the guidelines for early detection. The most effective way to protect against cancer is to change negative lifestyle habits and behaviors. Following are some guidelines for preventing cancer.

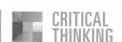

CRITICAL THINKING

Have you ever had, or d you now have, any fam members with cancer? Can you identify lifesty or environmental facto as possible contributor to the disease? If not, a you concerned about your genetic predisposi tion, and, if so, are you making lifestyle chang to decrease your risk?

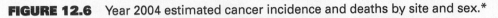

FIGURE 12.6 Year 2004 estimated cancer incidence and deaths by site and sex.*

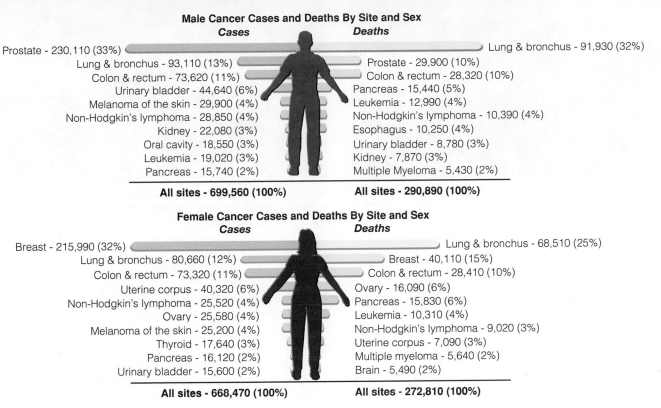

Male Cancer Cases and Deaths By Site and Sex

Cases | *Deaths*

Prostate - 230,110 (33%) — Lung & bronchus - 91,930 (32%)
Lung & bronchus - 93,110 (13%) — Prostate - 29,900 (10%)
Colon & rectum - 73,620 (11%) — Colon & rectum - 28,320 (10%)
Urinary bladder - 44,640 (6%) — Pancreas - 15,440 (5%)
Melanoma of the skin - 29,900 (4%) — Leukemia - 12,990 (4%)
Non-Hodgkin's lymphoma - 28,850 (4%) — Non-Hodgkin's lymphoma - 10,390 (4%)
Kidney - 22,080 (3%) — Esophagus - 10,250 (4%)
Oral cavity - 18,550 (3%) — Urinary bladder - 8,780 (3%)
Leukemia - 19,020 (3%) — Kidney - 7,870 (3%)
Pancreas - 15,740 (2%) — Multiple Myeloma - 5,430 (2%)

All sites - 699,560 (100%) | **All sites - 290,890 (100%)**

Female Cancer Cases and Deaths By Site and Sex

Cases | *Deaths*

Breast - 215,990 (32%) — Lung & bronchus - 68,510 (25%)
Lung & bronchus - 80,660 (12%) — Breast - 40,110 (15%)
Colon & rectum - 73,320 (11%) — Colon & rectum - 28,410 (10%)
Uterine corpus - 40,320 (6%) — Ovary - 16,090 (6%)
Non-Hodgkin's lymphoma - 25,520 (4%) — Pancreas - 15,830 (6%)
Ovary - 25,580 (4%) — Leukemia - 10,310 (4%)
Melanoma of the skin - 25,200 (4%) — Non-Hodgkin's lymphoma - 9,020 (3%)
Thyroid - 17,640 (3%) — Uterine corpus - 7,090 (3%)
Pancreas - 16,120 (2%) — Multiple myeloma - 5,640 (2%)
Urinary bladder - 15,600 (2%) — Brain - 5,490 (2%)

All sites - 668,470 (100%) | **All sites - 272,810 (100%)**

*Excludes basal and squamous cell skin cancers and in situ carcinoma except urinary bladder. Percentages may not total 100% due to rounding.

Source: From American Cancer Society, *Cancer Facts & Figures.* © 2004, American Cancer Society, Inc.

FIGURE 12.7 Estimates of the relative role of the major cancer-causing factors.

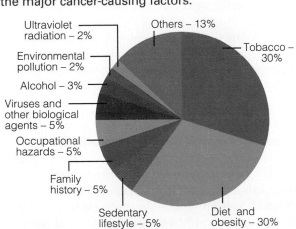

Ultraviolet radiation – 2%
Others – 13%
Tobacco – 30%
Environmental pollution – 2%
Alcohol – 3%
Viruses and other biological agents – 5%
Occupational hazards – 5%
Family history – 5%
Sedentary lifestyle – 5%
Diet and obesity – 30%

Source: Harvard Center for Cancer Prevention. *Causes of Human Cancer, Harvard Report on Cancer Prevention*, 1 (1996).

FIGURE 12.8 Effects of a healthy lifestyle on cancer mortality rate.

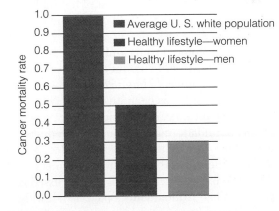

■ Average U. S. white population
■ Healthy lifestyle—women
■ Healthy lifestyle—men

Note: Healthy lifestyle factors include proper nutrition, abstinence from cigarette smoking, regular sleep (7–8 hours per night), and regular physical activity.

Source: "Health Practices and Cancer Mortality Among Active California Mormons," *Journal of the National Cancer Institute* 81 (1989): 1807–1814.

Nonmelanoma skin cancer Cancer that spreads or grows at the original site but does not metastasize to other regions of the body.

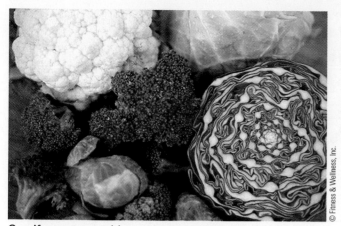

Cruciferous vegetables are recommended in a cancer-prevention diet.

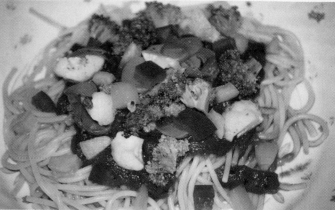

Nutrition guidelines for a cancer-prevention program include a diet low in fat and high in fiber, with ample amounts of fruits and vegetables.

Make Dietary Changes

The American Cancer Society estimates that one-third of all cancer in the United States is related to nutrition. A healthy diet, therefore, is crucial to decrease the risk for cancer. The diet should be predominately vegetarian, high in fiber, and low in fat (particularly from animal sources). **Cruciferous vegetables**, tea, soy products, calcium, and omega-3 fats are encouraged. Protein intake should be kept within the recommended nutrient guidelines. If alcohol is used, it should be used in moderation. Obesity should be avoided.

Green and dark yellow vegetables, cruciferous vegetables (cauliflower, broccoli, cabbage, Brussels sprouts, and kohlrabi), and beans (legumes) seem to protect against cancer. Folate, found naturally in dark green leafy vegetables, dried beans, and orange juice, may reduce the risk for colon and cervical cancers. Brightly colored fruits and vegetables also contain **carotenoids** and vitamin C. Lycopene, one of the many carotenoids (a phytochemical—see the following discussion), has been linked to lower risk of cancers of the prostate, colon, and cervix. Lycopene is especially abundant in cooked tomato products.

Researchers believe the antioxidant effect of vitamins and the mineral selenium help protect the body from oxygen free radicals. As discussed in Chapter 3 (under "Antioxidants," page 73), during normal metabolism most of the oxygen in the human body is converted into stable forms of carbon dioxide and water. A small amount, however, ends up in an unstable form known as "oxygen free radicals," which are thought to attack and damage the cell membrane and DNA, leading to the formation of cancers. Antioxidants are thought to absorb free radicals before they can cause damage and also interrupt the sequence of reactions once damage has begun.

PHYTOCHEMICALS

A promising horizon in preventing cancer is the discovery of **phytochemicals**. These compounds, found in abundance in fruits and vegetables, apparently prevent cancer by blocking the formation of cancerous tumors and disrupting the process at almost every step of the way. Phytochemicals exert their protective action in the following ways:

- Removing **carcinogens** from cells before they cause damage.
- Activating enzymes that detoxify cancer-causing agents.
- Keeping carcinogens from locking onto cells.
- Preventing carcinogens from binding to DNA.
- Breaking up cancer-causing precursors to benign forms.
- Disrupting the chemical combination of cell molecules that can produce carcinogens.
- Keeping small tumors from accessing capillaries (small blood vessels) to get oxygen and nutrients.

Examples of phytochemicals and their effects are found in Table 12.1. Experts in this area recommend that to obtain the best possible protection, vegetables should be consumed several times during the day (instead of in one meal) to maintain phytochemicals at effective levels throughout the day. Research indicates that phytochemical blood levels drop within 3 hours of consuming the food containing phytochemicals.[4]

FIBER

Although one recent study failed to show an association, many studies have linked low intake of fiber to increased risk for colon cancer. Fiber binds to bile acids in the intestine for excretion from the body in the stools. The interaction of bile acids with intestinal bacteria releases carcinogenic byproducts. The

TABLE 12.1 Selected Phytochemicals: Their Effects, and Sources

Phytochemical	Effect	Good Sources
Sulforaphane	Removes carcinogens from cells	Broccoli
PEITC	Keeps carcinogens from binding to DNA	Broccoli
Genistein	Prevents small tumors from accessing capillaries to get oxygen and nutrients	Soybeans
Flavonoids	Helps keep cancer-causing hormones from locking onto cells	Most fruits and vegetables
p-coumaric and chlorogenic acids	Disrupts the chemical combination of cell molecules that can produce carcinogens	Strawberries, green peppers, tomatoes, pineapple
Capsaicin	Keeps carcinogens from binding to DNA	Hot chili peppers

production of bile acid increases with higher fat content in the small intestine (created, of course, by higher fat content in the diet).

Daily consumption of 25 (women) to 38 (men) grams of fiber is recommended. Grains are high in fiber and contain vitamins and minerals—folate, selenium, and calcium—which seem to decrease the risk for colon cancer. Selenium protects against prostate cancer and, possibly, lung cancer. Calcium may protect against colon cancer by preventing the rapid growth of cells in the colon, especially in people with colon polyps.

TEA

Polyphenols (a phytochemical) are potent cancer-fighting antioxidants found in tea. Green, black, and red tea all seem to provide protection. Evidence also points to certain components in tea that can block the spread of cancers to other parts of the body.

Polyphenols are known to block the formation of **nitrosamines** and quell the activation of carcinogens. Green tea and black tea have similar amounts of polyphenols. Polyphenols are also thought to fight cancer by shutting off the formation of cancer cells, turning up the body's natural detoxification defenses and thereby suppressing progression of the disease.

Green tea seems to be especially helpful in preventing gastrointestinal cancers, including those of the stomach, small intestines, pancreas, and colon. Consumption of green tea also has been linked to a lower incidence of lung, esophageal, and estrogen-related cancers, including most breast cancers.

Research on tea-drinking habits in China showed that people who regularly drank green tea had about half the risk for chronic gastritis and stomach cancer and the risk decreased further as the number of years of drinking green tea increased.[5]

In Japan, where people drink green tea regularly but smoke twice as much as people in the United States, the incidence of lung cancer is half that of the United States. The antioxidant effect of one of the polyphenols in green tea, epigallocatechin gallate, or EGCG, is at least 25 times more effective than vitamin E and 100 times more effective than vitamin C at protecting cells and the DNA from damage believed to cause cancer, heart disease, and other diseases associated with free radicals.[6] EGCG is also twice as strong as the red wine antioxidant resveratrol in helping prevent heart disease.

A cancer-prevention diet recommends drinking two or more cups of green tea daily. Herbal teas do not provide the same benefits as regular tea.

DIETARY FAT

High fat intake may promote cancer and excessive weight. Some experts actually recommend that total fat intake be limited to less than 20 percent of total daily calories.[7] Fat intake should consist of primarily monounsaturated and omega-3 fats (found in flaxseed and many types of fish), which seem to offer protection against colorectal, pancreatic, breast, oral, esophageal, and stomach cancers. Omega-3 fats block the synthesis of prostaglandins, bodily compounds that promote growth of tumors.

PROCESSED MEAT AND PROTEIN

Salt-cured, smoked, and nitrite-cured foods have been associated with cancers of the esophagus and stomach. Processed meats should be consumed sparingly and always with orange juice or other vitamin C-rich foods, as vitamin C seems to discourage the formation of nitrosamines. These potentially cancer-causing compounds are formed when nitrites

Cruciferous vegetables Plants that produce cross-shaped leaves (cauliflower, broccoli, cabbage, Brussels sprouts, and kohlrabi); they seem to have a protective effect against cancer.

Carotenoids Pigment substances in plants that are often precursors to vitamin A. More than 600 carotenoids are found in nature, about 50 of which are precursors to vitamin A, the most potent one being beta-carotene.

Phytochemicals Compounds found in fruits and vegetables that block formation of cancerous tumors and disrupt the progress of cancer.

Carcinogens Substances that contribute to the formation of cancers.

Nitrosamines Potentially cancer-causing compounds formed when nitrites and nitrates, which are used to prevent the growth of harmful bacteria in processed meats, combine with other chemicals in the stomach.

and nitrates, which are used to prevent the growth of harmful bacteria in processed meats, combine with other chemicals in the stomach.

Further, nutritional guidelines discourage the excessive intake of protein. The daily protein intake for some people is almost twice the amount the human body needs. Too much animal protein apparently decreases blood enzymes that prevent precancerous cells from developing into tumors. According to the National Cancer Institute, eating substantial amounts of red meat may increase the risk of colorectal, pancreatic, breast, prostate, and renal cancer.

Research also suggests that grilling protein (fat or lean) at high temperatures for a long time increases the formation of carcinogenic substances on the skin or surface of the meat. Microwaving the meat for a couple of minutes before barbecuing decreases the risk, as long as the fluid released by the meat is discarded. Most of the potential carcinogens collect in this solution. Removing the skin before serving and cooking at lower heat to "medium" rather than "well done" also seem to lower the risk.

SOY

Soy protein seems to decrease the formation of carcinogens during cooking of meats. Soy foods may help because soy contains chemicals that prevent cancer. Although further research is merited, isoflavones (phytochemicals) found in soy are structurally similar to estrogen and may prevent breast cancer, prostate, lung, and colon cancers. Isoflavones, frequently referred to as "phytoestrogens" or "plant estrogens," also block angiogenesis. Presently, it is not known if the health benefits of soy are derived from isoflavones by themselves or in combination with other nutrients found in soy.

One drawback of soy was found in animal studies in which animals with tumors were given very large amounts of soy. The estrogen-like activity of soy isoflavones actually led to the growth of estrogen-dependent tumors. Experts, therefore, caution women with breast cancer or a history of this disease to limit their soy intake because it could stimulate cancer cells by closely imitating the actions of estrogen. No specific recommendations are presently available as to the amount of daily soy protein intake for cancer prevention.

Based on the traditional diets of people (including children) in China and Japan who regularly consume soy foods, there doesn't appear to be an unsafe natural level of consumption. Soy protein powder supplementation, however, may elevate soy protein intake to an unnatural (and perhaps unsafe) level.

ALCOHOL

Alcohol should be consumed in moderation, because too much alcohol raises the risk for developing

certain cancers, especially when it is combined with tobacco smoking or smokeless tobacco. In combination, these substances significantly increase the risk for cancers of the mouth, larynx, throat, esophagus, and liver. Approximately 17,000 deaths from cancer yearly are attributed to excessive use of alcohol, often in combination with smoking. The combined action of heavy alcohol and tobacco use can increase the odds of developing cancer of the oral cavity fifteenfold.

Maintaining recommended body weight is encouraged. Based on estimates, excess weight accounts for 14 percent of cancer deaths in men and 20 percent in women, respectively. Furthermore, obese

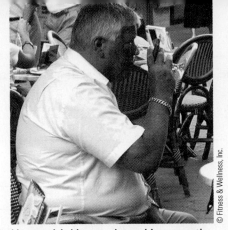
Heavy drinking and smoking greatly increase risk for oral cancer.

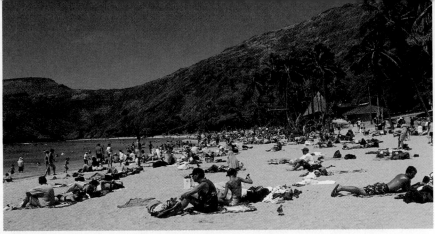
Tanning poses a risk for skin cancer from overexposure to ultraviolet rays. Tanned skin is the body's natural reaction to permanent and irreversible damage—a precursor to severe or fatal skin cancer.

men and women have an increased risk of more than 50 percent of dying from any form of cancer.[8] Obesity has been associated with cancers of the colon, rectum, breast, prostate, endometrium, and kidney.

Abstain from Tobacco

Cigarette smoking by itself is a major health hazard. If we include all related deaths, smoking is responsible for more than 435,000 unnecessary deaths in the United States each year. The World Health Organization estimates that smoking causes 5 million deaths worldwide annually. The average life expectancy for a chronic smoker is about 15 years shorter than for a non-smoker.[9]

The biggest carcinogenic exposure in the workplace is cigarette smoke. Of all cancers, at least 30 percent are tied to smoking, and 87 percent of lung cancers are linked to smoking. Use of smokeless tobacco also can lead to nicotine addiction and dependence as well as increased risk for mouth, larynx, throat, and esophageal cancers.

Avoid Excessive Exposure to Sun

Too much exposure to ultraviolet radiation (both UVB and UVA rays) is a major contributor to skin cancer. The most common sites of skin cancer are the areas exposed to the sun most often (face, neck, and back of the hands).

The three types of skin cancer are

1. Basal cell carcinoma
2. Squamous cell carcinoma
3. Malignant melanoma

Nearly 90 percent of the almost one million cases of basal cell or squamous cell skin cancers reported yearly in the United States could have been prevented by protecting the skin from the sun's rays. **Melanoma,** the most deadly type, caused

approximately 7,600 deaths in 2003. One in every six Americans will develop some type of skin cancer eventually.

Nothing is healthy about a "healthy tan." Tanning of the skin is the body's natural reaction to permanent and irreversible damage from too much exposure to the sun. Even small doses of sunlight add up to a greater risk for skin cancer and premature aging. The tan fades at the end of the summer season, but the underlying skin damage does not disappear. Ultraviolet rays are strongest when the sun is high in the sky. Therefore, you should avoid sun exposure between 10:00 A.M. and 4:00 P.M. Take the shadow test: If your shadow is shorter than you, the UV rays are at their strongest.

The stinging sunburn comes from **ultraviolet B (UVB) rays,** which also are thought to be the main cause of premature wrinkling and skin aging, roughened/leathery/sagging skin, and skin cancer. Unfortunately, the damage may not become evident until up to 20 years later. By comparison, skin that has not been overexposed to the sun remains smooth and unblemished, and, over time, shows less evidence of aging.

Sun lamps and tanning parlors provide mainly ultraviolet A (UVA) rays. Once thought to be safe, they, too, are now known to be damaging and have been linked to melanoma. As little as 15 to 30 minutes of exposure to UVA can be as dangerous as a day spent in the sun. Similar to regular sun exposure, short-term exposure to recreational tanning at a salon causes DNA alterations that can lead to skin cancer.[10]

Melanoma The most virulent, rapidly spreading form of skin cancer.

Ultraviolet B (UVB) rays Portion of sunlight that causes sunburn and encourages skin cancers.

Sunscreen lotion should be applied about 30 minutes before lengthy exposure to the sun because the skin takes that long to absorb the protective ingredients. A **sun protection factor (SPF)** of at least 15 is recommended. SPF 15 means that the skin takes 15 times longer to burn than it would with no lotion. If you ordinarily get a mild sunburn after 20 minutes of noonday sun, an SPF 15 allows you to remain in the sun about 300 minutes before burning. The higher the number, the stronger the protection. When swimming or sweating, you should reapply waterproof sunscreens more often, because all sunscreens lose strength when they are diluted.

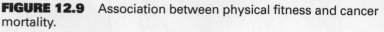

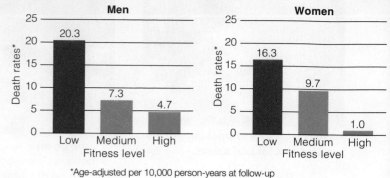

FIGURE 12.9 Association between physical fitness and cancer mortality.

*Age-adjusted per 10,000 person-years at follow-up

Source: S. N. Blair, H. W. Kohl III, R. S. Paffenbarger, Jr., D. G. Clark, K. H. Cooper, and L. W. Gibbons, "Physical Fitness and All-Cause Mortality: A Prospective Study of Healthy Men and Women," *Journal of the American Medical Association* 262 (1989): 2395–2401.

Monitor Estrogen, Radiation Exposure, and Potential Occupational Hazards

Intake of estrogen has been linked to endometrial cancer in some studies, but other evidence contradicts those findings. As to exposure to radiation—although it increases the risk for cancer, the benefits of X-rays may outweigh the risk involved, and most medical facilities use the lowest dose possible to keep the risk to a minimum. Occupational hazards—such as asbestos fibers, nickel and uranium dusts, chromium compounds, vinyl chloride, and bischlormethyl ether—increase the risk for cancer. Cigarette smoking magnifies the risk from occupational hazards.

Engage in Physical Activity

An active lifestyle has been shown to have a protective effect against cancer. Although the mechanism is not clear, physical fitness and cancer mortality in men and women may have a graded and consistent inverse relationship (see Figure 12.9). A daily 30-minute, moderate-intensity exercise program lowers the risk for colon cancer and may lower the risk for cancers of the breast and reproductive system. Research has shown that regular exercise lowers the risk for breast cancer in women by 20 to 30 percent. In addition, growing evidence suggests that the body's autoimmune system may play a role in preventing cancer and that moderate exercise improves the autoimmune system.

Early Detection

Fortunately, many cancers can be controlled or cured through early detection. The real problem comes when cancerous cells spread, because they

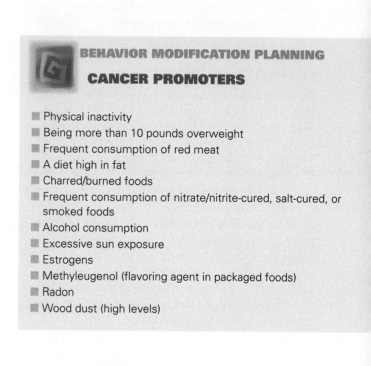

BEHAVIOR MODIFICATION PLANNING

CANCER PROMOTERS

- Physical inactivity
- Being more than 10 pounds overweight
- Frequent consumption of red meat
- A diet high in fat
- Charred/burned foods
- Frequent consumption of nitrate/nitrite-cured, salt-cured, or smoked foods
- Alcohol consumption
- Excessive sun exposure
- Estrogens
- Methyleugenol (flavoring agent in packaged foods)
- Radon
- Wood dust (high levels)

become more difficult to destroy. Therefore, effective prevention, or at least early detection, is crucial. Herein lies the importance of periodic screening. Once a month, women should practice breast self-examination (BSE) (see Figure 12.13, page 377) and men, testicular self-examination (TSE) (see Figure 12.14, page 379). Men should pick a regular day each month (for example, the first day of each month) to practice TSE, and women should perform BSE two or three days after the menstrual period is over.

Other Factors

The contributions of many of the other much-publicized factors are not as significant as those just pointed out. Intentional food additives, saccharin, processing agents, pesticides, and packaging materials currently used in the United States and other developed countries seem to have minimal consequences. High levels of tension and stress and poor coping may affect the autoimmune system negatively and render the body less effective in dealing with the various cancers. In the workplace, the biggest carcinogenic exposure is cigarette smoke.

Genetics plays a role in susceptibility in about 10 percent of all cancers. Most of the effect is seen in the early childhood years. Some cancers are a combination of genetic and environmental liability; genetics may add to the environmental risk of certain types of cancers. "Environment," however, means more than pollution and smoke. It incorporates diet, lifestyle-related events, viruses, and physical agents such as X-rays and exposure to the sun.

Warning Signals of Cancer

Everyone should become familiar with the following seven warning signals for cancer and bring them to a physician's attention if any are present:

1. Change in bowel or bladder habits.
2. Sore that does not heal.
3. Unusual bleeding or discharge.
4. Thickening or lump in the breast or elsewhere.
5. Indigestion or difficulty in swallowing.
6. Obvious change in wart or mole.
7. Nagging cough or hoarseness.

The recommendations for early detection of cancer in asymptomatic people by the American Cancer Society, outlined in Table 12.2, should be heeded in regular physical examinations as part of a cancer-prevention program. In Lab 12A, you will be able to determine how well you are doing in terms of a cancer-prevention program and also respond to a questionnaire developed by the American Medical Association to alert people to symptoms that may indicate a serious health problem. Although in most cases nothing serious will be found, any of the symptoms calls for a physician's attention as soon as possible. Scientific evidence and testing procedures for prevention and early detection of cancer do change. Studies continue to provide new information. The intent of cancer-prevention programs is to educate and guide individuals toward a lifestyle that will help prevent cancer and enable early detection of malignancy.

Treatment of cancer should always be left to specialized physicians and cancer clinics. Current treatment modalities include surgery, radiation, radioactive substances, chemotherapy, hormones, and immunotherapy.

Assessing Your Risks

The Texas Division of the American Cancer Society designed a self-testing questionnaire, shown in Figure 12.10, to help people assess their risk for cancer. These are the major risk factors for specific cancer sites and by no means represent the only ones that might be involved. Men and women alike should complete the questions for lung, colon-rectum, and skin cancer. Three additional types of cancer—breast, cervical, and endometrial—are included for women.

Check your status against the factors contained in this questionnaire, total your scores, then locate your "Total Risk" in the sections below. Record in Lab 12B your risk-level totals for each cancer site. Individual numbers for specific questions are not to be interpreted as a precise measure of relative risk, but the totals for a given site should give you a general indication of your risk.

Explanations of the risk factors for each type of cancer follows. If you are at higher risk, you are advised to discuss the results with your physician.

Common Sites of Cancer

Lung Cancer

RISK FACTORS

1. *Gender*. Men have a higher risk for developing lung cancer than women do, when type, amount, and duration of smoking are equal. Because more women are smoking cigarettes for a longer duration than previously, however, their incidence of lung and upper respiratory tract (mouth, tongue, and larynx) cancer is increasing. By type of cancer, lung cancer is now number one in mortality for women.
2. *Age*. The occurrence of lung and upper respiratory tract cancers increases with age.
3. *Smoking status*. Cigarette smokers have 20 times or even greater risk than non-smokers. The rates for ex-smokers who have not smoked for 10 years, however, approaches those for non-smokers.
4. *Type of smoking*. Pipe and cigar smokers are at higher risk for lung cancer than non-smokers. Cigarette smokers are at much higher risk than non-smokers or pipe and cigar smokers. All forms of tobacco, including chewing, markedly

Sun protection factor (SPF) Degree of protection offered by ingredients in sunscreen lotion; at least SPF 15 is recommended.

TABLE 12.2 Summary of Recommendations for Early Detection of Cancer in Asymptomatic People

Site	Recommendation
Breast	■ Yearly mammograms are recommended starting at age 40. The age at which screening should be stopped should be individualized by considering the potential risks and benefits of screening in the context of overall health status and longevity.
	■ Clinical breast exam should be part of a perodic health exam, about every three years for women in their 20s and 30s, and every year for women 40 and older.
	■ Women should know how their breasts normally feel and report any breast change promptly to their health care providers. Breast self-exam is an option for women starting in their 20s.
	■ Women at increased risk (e.g., family history, genetic tendency, past breast cancer) should talk with their doctors about the benefits and limitations of starting mammography screening earlier, having additional tests (i.e., breast ultrasound and MRI), or having more frequent exams.
Colon & Rectum	Beginning at age 50, men and women should follow one of the examination schedules below: ■ A fecal occult blood test (FOBT) or fecal immunochemical test (FIT) every year ■ A flexible sigmoidoscopy (FSIG) every five years ■ Annual FOBT or FIT and flexible sigmoidoscopy every five years* ■ A double-contrast barium enema every five years ■ A colonoscopy every 10 years * Combined testing is preferred over either annual FOBT or FIT, or FSIG every five years, alone. People who are at moderate or high risk for colorectal cancer should talk with a doctor about a different testing schedule.
Prostate	The PSA test and the digital rectal exam should be offered annually, beginning at age 50, to men who have a life expectancy of at least 10 years. Men at high risk (African-American men and men with a strong family history of one or more first-degree relatives diagnosed with prostate cancer at an early age) should begin testing at age 45. For both men at average risk and high risk, information should be provided about what is known and what is uncertain about the benefits and limitations of early detection and treatment of prostate cancer so that they can make an informed decision about testing.
Uterus	**Cervix:** Screening should begin approximately three years after a woman begins having vaginal intercourse, but no later than 21 years of age. Screening should be done every year with regular Pap tests or every two years using liquid-based tests. At or after age 30, women who have had three normal test results in a row may get screen every two to three years. Alternatively, cervical cancer screening with HPV DNA testing and conventional or liquid-based cytology could be performed every three years. However, doctors may suggest a woman get screened more often if she has certain risk factors, such as HIV infection or a weak immune system. Women 70 years and older who have had three or more consecutive normal Pap tests in the last 10 years may choose to stop cervical cancer screening. Screening after total hysterectomy (with removal of the cervix) is not necessary unless the surgery was done as a treatment for cervical cancer.
	Endometrium: The American Cancer Society recommends that at the time of menopause all women should be informed about the risks and symptoms of endometrial cancer, and strongly encouraged to report any unexpected bleeding or spotting to their physicians. Annual screening for endometrial cancer with endometrial biopsy beginning at age 35 should be offered to women with or at risk for hereditary nonpolyposis colon cancer (HNPCC).
Cancer-related Checkup	For individuals undergoing periodic health examinations, a cancer-related checkup should include health counseling and, depending on a person's age and gender, might include examinations for cancers of the thyroid, oral cavity, skin, lymph nodes, testes, and ovaries, as well as for some nonmalignant diseases.

From *Cancer Facts and Figures.* © 2004, American Cancer Society, Inc.

increase the user's risk of developing cancer of the mouth.

5. *Number of cigarettes smoked per day.* Males who smoke less than half a pack per day have lung cancer rates five times higher than nonsmokers. Males who smoke one to two packs per day have 15 times higher lung cancer rates than non-smokers. Males who smoke more than two packs per day are 20 times more likely than non-smokers to develop lung cancer.

6. *Type of cigarette.* Smokers of low-tar/nicotine cigarettes have slightly lower lung cancer rates.

7. *Duration of smoking.* The frequency of lung and upper respiratory tract cancers increase with the length of time people have smoked.

8. *Type of industrial work.* Exposure to materials used in the industries mentioned in Figure 12.10 (Question 8) have been demonstrated to be associated with lung cancer. Exposure to materials in other industries also carry a higher risk.

FIGURE 12.10 Cancer questionnaire: Assessing your risks.

Assessing Your Risks for Cancer

Read each question concerning each site and its specific risk factors. Be honest in your responses. Place the number in parentheses (risk points) in the box provided to the left of each question. For example, Question #2 on lung cancer: If you are 53 years old (age 50 to 59), then enter 5 (risk points) as your score on the left. At the end of each site, total your number of points for that site. Record the final number of points in Lab 12B, page 387.

Lung Cancer

1. Sex
   a. Male (2)
   b. Female (1)

2. Age
   a. 39 or less (1)
   b. 40–49 (2)
   c. 50–59 (5)
   d. 60+ (7)

3. Smoking status
   a. Smoker (8)
   b. Nonsmoker (1)

4. Type of smoking
   a. Current cigarettes or little cigars (10)
   b. Pipe and/or cigar, but not cigarettes (3)
   c. Ex-cigarette smoker (2)

5. Amount of cigarettes smoked per day
   a. 0 cigarettes (1)
   b. Less than 1 pack per day (5)
   c. 1 pack (9)
   d. 1–2 packs (15)
   e. 2+ packs (20)

6. Type of cigarette
   a. High tar/nicotine (10)*
   b. Medium T/N (9)
   c. Low T/N (7)
   d. Nonsmoker (1)

7. Duration of smoking
   a. Never smoked (1)
   b. Ex-smoker (3)
   c. Up to 15 years (5)
   d. 15–25 years (10)
   e. 25+ years (20)

8. Type of industrial work
   a. Mining (3)
   b. Asbestos (7)
   c. Uranium and radioactive products (5)

Total

Colon-Rectum Cancer

1. Age
   a. 39 or less (10)
   b. 40–59 (20)
   c. 60+ (50)

2. Has anyone in your immediate family ever had
   a. Colon cancer (20)
   b. One or more polyps of the colon (10)
   c. Neither (1)

3. Have you ever had
   a. Colon cancer (100)
   b. One or more polyps of the colon (40)
   c. Ulcerative colitis (20)
   d. Cancer of the breast or uterus (10)
   e. None (1)

4. Bleeding from the rectum (other than obvious hemorrhoids or piles)
   a. Yes (75)
   b. No (1)

Total

Skin Cancer

1. Frequent work or play in the sun:
   a. Yes (10)
   b. No (1)

2. Work in mines, around coal tars, or around radioactivity:
   a. Yes (10)
   b. No (1)

3. Complexion—fair and/or light skin:
   a. Yes (10)
   b. No (1)

Total

(continued)

Adapted from the Texas Division of the American Cancer Society. (*Note:* This questionnaire is not available nationwide; distribution is limited to Texas residents only.)

FIGURE 12.10 (Continued)

Breast Cancer

1. Age group
   a. 20–34 (10)
   b. 35–49 (40)
   c. 50+ (90)

2. Race group
   a. Oriental (5)
   b. African American (20)
   c. White (25)
   d. Hispanic American (10)

3. Family history
   a. Mother, sister, aunt, or grandmother with breast cancer (30)
   b. None (10)

4. Your history
   a. Previous lumps or cysts (25)
   b. No breast disease (10)
   c. Previous breast cancer (100)

5. Maternity
   a. First pregnancy before 25 (10)
   b. First pregnancy after 25 (15)
   c. No pregnancies (20)

   Total

Cervical Cancer

(Lower portion of uterus. These questions do not apply to a woman who has had a total hysterectomy.)

1. Age group
   a. Less than 25 (10)
   b. 25–39 (20)
   c. 40–54 (30)
   d. 55+ (30)

2. Race
   a. Oriental (10)
   b. Puerto Rican (20)
   c. African American (20)
   d. White (10)
   e. Hispanic American (20)

3. Number of pregnancies
   a. 0 (10)
   b. 1–3 (20)
   c. 4 and over (30)

4. Viral infections
   a. Herpes and other viral infections or ulcer formations on the vagina (10)
   b. Never (1)

5. Age at first intercourse
   a. Before 15 (40)
   b. 15–19 (30)
   c. 20–24 (20)
   d. 25 and over (10)
   e. Never (5)

6. Bleeding between periods or after intercourse
   a. Yes (40)
   b. No (1)

   Total

Endometrial Cancer

(Body of uterus. These questions do not apply to a woman who has had a total hysterectomy.)

1. Age group
   a. 39 or less (5)
   b. 40–49 (20)
   c. 50+ (60)

2. Race
   a. Oriental (10)
   b. African American (10)
   c. White (20)
   d. Hispanic American (10)

3. Births
   a. None (15)
   b. 1 to 4 (7)
   c. 5 or more (5)

4. Weight
   a. 50 or more pounds overweight (50)
   b. 20–49 pounds overweight (15)
   c. Underweight for height (10)
   d. Normal (10)

5. Diabetes (elevated blood sugar)
   a. Yes (3)
   b. No (1)

6. Estrogen hormone intake
   a. Yes, regularly (15)
   b. Yes, occasionally (12)
   c. None (10)

7. Abnormal uterine bleeding
   a. Yes (40)
   b. No (1)

8. Hypertension (high blood pressure)
   a. Yes (3)
   b. No (1)

   Total

Smokers who work in these industries have greatly increased risks. Exposure to arsenic, radon, radiation from occupational/medical/environmental sources, and air pollution increase the risk for lung cancer.

TOTAL RISK

24 or less   You have a low risk for lung cancer (low-risk category).

25–49   You may be a light smoker and have a good chance of kicking the habit (light risk).

50–74   As a moderate smoker, your risks for cancers of the lung and upper respiratory tract cancers are increased. If you stop smoking now, these risks will decrease (moderate risk).

75 or over   As a heavy cigarette smoker, your chances of getting cancer of the lung and upper respiratory tract are greatly increased. Your best bet is to stop smoking now—for the health of it. If you have a nagging cough, hoarseness, persistent pain, or a sore in the mouth or throat, see your doctor (high risk).

Colon/Rectum Cancer

RISK FACTORS

1. *Age.* Colon cancer occurs more frequently after 50 years of age.
2. *Family predisposition.* Colon cancer is more common in families that have a previous history of this disease.
3. *Personal history.* Polyps and bowel diseases are associated with colon cancer.
4. *Rectal bleeding.* Rectal bleeding may be a sign of colorectal cancer.

TOTAL RISK

29 and under   You are at low risk for colon/rectum cancer.

30–69   This is a moderate-risk category. Testing by your physician may be indicated.

70 and over   This is a high-risk category. You should see your physician for the following tests: digital rectal exam, guaiac (stool) slide test, and proctoscopic exam.

In addition to the risk factors mentioned in the questionnaire, a diet high in fat and low in fiber, inadequate consumption of fruits and vegetables, physical inactivity, a history of breast or endometrial cancer, and inflammatory bowel disease also increase the risk for colon or rectum cancer.

FIGURE 12.11 Warning signs of melanoma: ABCD rule.

A. *Asymmetry:* One half of a mole or lesion doesn't look like the other half.

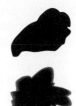

B. *Border:* A mole has an irregular, scalloped, or not clearly defined border.

C. *Color:* The color varies or is not uniform from one area of a mole or lesion to another, whether the color is tan, brown, black, white, red, or blue.

D. *Diameter:* The lesion is larger than 6 millimeters (¼ inch) or larger than a pencil eraser.

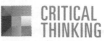

Adapted from *FDA Consumer*, May 1991.

Skin Cancer

RISK FACTORS

1. *Sun exposure.* Excessive ultraviolet light is a culprit in skin cancer. Protect yourself with a sunscreen medication.
2. *Work environment.* Working in mines, around coal tar, or around radioactive materials can cause cancer of the skin.
3. *Complexion.* Individuals with light complexions need more protection than others.

TOTAL RISK

Numerical risks for skin cancer are difficult to state. For instance, a person with a dark complexion can work longer in the sun and be less likely to develop cancer than a light-skinned person. Furthermore, a person wearing a long-sleeved shirt and a wide-brimmed hat who spends hours working in the sun has less risk than a person wearing a swimsuit who sunbathes for only a short period. The risk increases greatly with age, and family history also plays a role.

If any of these conditions apply to you, you need to protect your skin from the sun or any other toxic material. Changes in moles, warts, or skin sores are important and should be evaluated by your doctor (see Figure 12.11).

> **CRITICAL THINKING**
>
> **What significance does a "healthy tan" have in your social life? Are you a "sun worshiper," or are you concerned about skin damage, premature aging, and potential skin cancer in your future?**

SKIN SELF-EXAM

One of the easiest and quickest self-exams is a brief survey to detect possible skin cancers (see Figure 12.12). A simple skin self-exam can reduce deaths from melanoma by as much as 63 percent, saving as many as 4,500 lives in the United States each year.

■ Make a drawing of yourself. Include a full frontal view, a full back view, and close-up views of your head (both sides), the soles of your feet, the tops of your feet, and the backs of your hands.

■ After you get out of the bath or shower, examine yourself closely in a full-length mirror. On your sketch, make note of any moles, warts, or other skin marks you find anywhere on your body. Pay particular attention to areas that are exposed to the sun constantly, such as your face, the tops of your ears, and your hands.

■ Briefly describe each mark on your sketch: its size, color, texture, and so on.

■ Repeat the exam about once a month. Watch for changes in the size, texture, or color of moles, wart, or other skin mark. If you notice any difference, contact your physician. You also should contact a doctor if you have a sore that does not heal.

Breast Cancer

RISK FACTORS

1. *Age*. The risk for breast cancer increases significantly after 50 years of age.
2. *Race*. Breast cancer occurs more frequently in white women than any other group.
3. *Family history*. The risk for breast cancer is higher in women with a family history of this type of cancer. The risk is even higher if more than one family member has developed breast cancer and is further enhanced by the closeness of the relationship of family member(s) (e.g., a mother or sister with breast cancer indicates a higher risk than a cousin with breast cancer).
4. *Personal history*. A previous history of breast or ovarian cancer indicates a greater risk.
5. *Maternity*. The risk is higher in women who never have had children and in women who bear children after 30 years of age.

TOTAL RISK

Under 100	Low-risk women should practice monthly breast self-examination (BSE—see Figure 12.13) and have their breasts examined by a doctor as a part of a cancer-related check-up.
100–199	Moderate-risk women should practice monthly BSE and have their

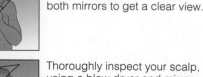

FIGURE 12.12 Self-exam for skin cancer.

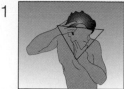

1 Examine your face, especially the nose, lips, mouth, and ears —front and back. Use one or both mirrors to get a clear view.

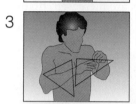

2 Thoroughly inspect your scalp, using a blow dryer and mirror to expose each section to view. Get a friend or family member to help, if you can.

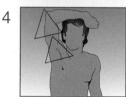

3 Check your hands carefully: palms and backs, between the fingers, and under the fingernails. Continue up the wrists to examine both front and back of your forearms.

4 Standing in front of a full-length mirror, begin at the elbows and scan all sides of your upper arms. Don't forget the underarms.

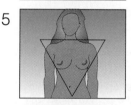

5 Next focus on the neck, chest, and torso. Women should lift breasts to view the underside.

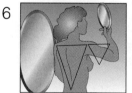

6 With your back to the full-length mirror, use the hand mirror to inspect the back of your neck, shoulders, upper back, and any part of the back of your upper arms you could not view in step 4.

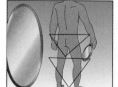

7 Still using both mirrors, scan your lower back, buttocks, and backs of both legs.

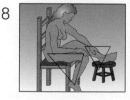

8 Sit down; prop each leg in turn on another stool or chair. Use the hand mirror to examine the genitals. Check front and sides of both legs, thigh to shin; ankles, tops of feet, between toes, and under toenails. Examine soles of feet and heels.

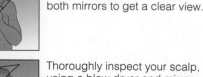

Reprinted with permission from *Family Practice Recertification* 14, no. 3 (March 1992).

FIGURE 12.13 Breast self-examination.

Looking

Stand in front of a mirror with your upper body unclothed. Look for changes in the shape and size of the breast, and for dimpling of the skin or "pulling in" of the nipples. Any changes in the breast may be made more noticeable by a change in position of the body or arms. Look for any of the above signs or for changes in shape from one breast to the other.

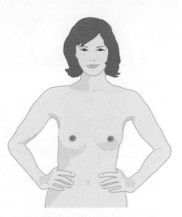

1. Stand with your arms down.

2. Raise your arms overhead.

3. Place your hands on your hips and tighten your chest and arm muscles by pressing firmly.

Feeling

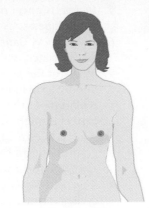

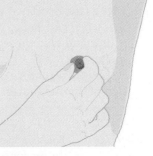

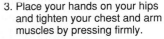

1. Lie flat on your back. Place a pillow or towel under one shoulder, and raise that arm over your head. With the opposite hand, you'll feel with the pads, not the fingertips, of the three middle fingers, for lumps or any change in the texture of the breast or skin.

2. The area you'll examine is from your collarbone to your bra line and from your breastbone to the center of your armpit. Imagine the area divided into vertical strips. Using small circular motions (the size of a dime), move your fingers up and down the strips. Apply light, medium, and deep pressure to examine each spot. Repeat this same process for your other breast.

3. Gently squeeze the nipple of each breast between your thumb and index finger. Any discharge, clear or bloody, should be reported to your doctor immediately.

Source: From *An Invitation to Health*, 11th edition, by Hales. © 2005. Reprinted with permission of Wadsworth, a division of Thomson Learning, Inc.

breasts examined by a doctor as part of a cancer-related check-up. Periodic mammograms (see below) should be included as recommended.

200 and over High-risk women should practice monthly BSE and have their breasts examined regularly by a doctor. See your doctor for the recommended examinations (including mammograms and physical exam of breasts).

Clinical breast exams by a physician are recommended every 3 years for women between ages 20 and 40 and every year for women over age 40. The American Cancer Society also recommends an annual **mammogram** for women over age 40.

The latter is still an area of debate among health-care practitioners, and personal risk factors should be considered to determine the frequency of mammograms.

Other possible risk factors for breast cancer not listed in the questionnaire are a long menstrual history (onset of menstruation prior to age 13 and ending later in life), recent use of oral contraceptives or postmenopausal estrogens, drinking two or more alcoholic beverages per day, chronic cystic disease, and ionizing radiation. A diet high in fat has also

Mammogram Low-dose X-rays of the breasts used as a screening technique for the early detection of breast cancer.

been viewed as a predisposing factor, although more recent research has questioned its link to breast cancer.

Cervical Cancer (Women)

RISK FACTORS

1. *Age*. The highest occurrence is in the 40-and-over age group. The scoring numbers in the questionnaire represent the relative rates of cancer for different age groups—that is, a 45-year-old woman has a risk three times greater than a 20-year-old.
2. *Race*. Puerto Ricans, African Americans, and Hispanic Americans have higher rates of cervical cancer.
3. *Number of pregnancies*. Women who have delivered several children have a higher occurrence.
4. *Viral infections*. Viral infections of the cervix and vagina are associated with cervical cancer.
5. *Age at first intercourse*. Women with earlier intercourse and with more sexual partners are at a higher risk.
6. *Bleeding*. Irregular vaginal bleeding may be a sign of uterine cancer.

TOTAL RISK

40–69	This is a low-risk group. Ask your doctor for a Pap test. You will be advised how often you should be tested after your first test.
70–99	In this moderate-risk group, more frequent Pap tests may be required.
100 and over	You are in a high-risk group and should have a Pap test (and pelvic exam) as advised by your doctor.

Early detection through a Pap test during a pelvic exam should be performed annually in women who are or have been sexually active or who have reached the age of 18. Following three normal tests during three consecutive years, the Pap test may be done less frequently, at the discretion of the physician.

Endometrial Cancer (Women)

RISK FACTORS

1. *Age*. Endometrial cancer is seen in older age groups. The scoring numbers by the age groups represent relative rates of endometrial cancer at different ages—for example, a 50-year-old woman has a risk 12 times higher than that of a 35-year-old woman.
2. *Race*. White women have a higher occurrence.
3. *Births*. The fewer children the woman has delivered, the greater is the risk for endometrial cancer.

4. *Weight*. Women who are overweight are at greater risk.
5. *Diabetes*. Cancer of the endometrium is associated with diabetes.
6. *Estrogen use*. Cancer of the endometrium may be associated with prolonged and continuous intake of the estrogen hormone. This occurs in only a small number of women. Hormone replacement therapy (progesterone plus estrogen) is thought to offset the increased risk related to estrogen use. You should consult your physician before starting or stopping any estrogen medication.
7. *Abnormal bleeding*. Women who do not have cyclic menstrual periods are at greater risk.
8. *Hypertension*. Cancer of the endometrium is associated with high blood pressure.

TOTAL RISK

49–59	Low risk for developing endometrial cancer.
60–99	Slightly higher risk (moderate risk). Report any abnormal bleeding immediately to your doctor. Tissue sampling at menopause is recommended.
100 or over	Much greater risk (high risk). See your doctor for tests as appropriate.

Additional risk factors that may be associated with endometrial cancer but are not included in the questionnaire are infertility, a prolonged history of failure to ovulate, and menopause occurring after age 55. Women over age 40 should have a yearly pelvic exam by a physician.

Other Cancer Sites

Following are other types of cancers whose risk factors are not defined as clearly as those in Figure 12.10. Risk factors and prevention techniques for these types of cancer have been outlined in *The Causes of Cancer*,[11] published by the American Cancer Society, as well as in a series of pamphlets titled "Facts on Cancer," also available from the American Cancer Society. These types of cancer are presented, along with the risk factors associated with each type and preventive techniques to decrease the risk. No numeric weights for the risk factors have been assigned. As you read the information, however, rate yourself on a scale from 1 to 3 (1 for low risk, 2 for moderate risk, 3 for high risk) for each cancer site, and record your results in Lab 12B.

Prostate Cancer (Men)

The prostate gland is actually a cluster of smaller glands that encircles the top section of the urethra (urinary channel) at the point where it leaves the bladder. Although the function of the prostate is not entirely clear, the muscles of these small glands help squeeze prostatic secretions into the urethra.

RISK FACTORS

1. *Advancing age*. The highest incidence of prostate cancer (75 percent of cases) is found in men over age 65. The incidence is also higher among African Americans than whites, and more married men than single men develop this type of cancer.
2. *Family history*.
3. *Race*. African Americans have the highest rate in the world.
4. *Diet*. A diet high in fat.

PREVENTION AND WARNING SIGNALS

Prostate cancer is difficult to detect and control because the causes are not known. Death rates can be lowered through early detection and awareness of the warning signals. Detection is done by a digital rectal exam of the gland and a prostate-specific antigen (PSA) blood test once a year after the age of 50. Possible warning signals include difficulties in urination (especially at night), painful urination, blood in the urine, and constant pain in the lower back or hip area.

Other factors that decrease the risk include increasing the consumption of selenium-rich foods (up to 200 micrograms per day), including consumption of tomato-rich foods and fatty fish in the diet two or three times per week, avoiding a high-fat (especially animal fat) diet, increasing daily consumption of produce and grains, taking a daily supplement of vitamin E (preferably mixed tocopherols), and maintaining recommended vitamin D intake (found in multivitamins, fortified milk, and manufactured by the body when exposed to sunlight).

Testicular Cancer (Men)

Testicular cancer accounts for only 1 percent of all male cancers, but it is the most common type of cancer seen in men between ages 25 and 35. The incidence is slightly higher in whites than in African Americans, and it is rarely seen in middle-aged and older men. The malignancy rate of testicular tumors is 96 percent, but if it is diagnosed early, this type of cancer is highly curable.

RISK FACTORS

1. *Undescended testicle* not corrected before age 6.
2. *Atrophy of the testicle* following mumps or virus infection.
3. *Family history* of testicular cancer.
4. *Recurring injury* to the testicle.

FIGURE 12.14 Testicular self-examination.

How To Examine The Testicles

You can increase your chances of early detection of testicular cancer by regularly performing a testicular self examination (TSE). The following procedure is recommended:

■ Perform the self-exam once a month. Select an easy day to remember such as the first day or first Sunday of the month.

■ Learn how your testicle feels normally so that it will be easier to identify changes. A normal testicle should feel oval, smooth, and uniformly firm, like a hard-boiled egg.

■ Perform TSE following a warm shower or bath, when the scrotum is relaxed.

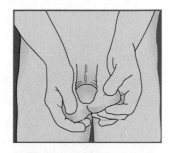

■ Gently roll each testicle between your thumb and the first three fingers until you have felt the entire surface. Pay particular attention to any lumps, change in size or texture, pain, or a dragging or heavy sensation since your last self-exam. Do not confuse the epididymis at the rear of the testicle for an abnormality.

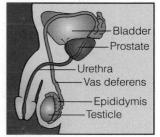

■ Bring any changes to the attention of your physician. A change does not necessarily indicate a malignancy, but only a physician is able to determine that.

5. *Abnormalities of the endocrine system* (e.g., high hormone levels of pituitary gonadotropin or androgens).
6. *Incomplete testicular development*.

PREVENTION AND WARNING SIGNALS

The incidence of testicular cancer is quite high in males born with an undescended testicle. Therefore, this condition should be corrected early in life. Parents of infant males should make sure that the child is checked by a physician to ensure that the testes have descended into the scrotum. Testicular self-examination (TSE) once a month following a warm bath or shower (when the scrotal skin is relaxed) is recommended. Guidelines for performing a TSE are given in Figure 12.14.

Some of the warning signs associated with testicular cancer are a small lump on the testicle, slight enlargement (usually painless) and change in consistency of the testis, sudden build-up of blood or fluid in the scrotum, pain in the groin and lower abdomen or discomfort accompanied by a sensation of dragging and heaviness, breast enlargement or tenderness, and enlarged lymph glands.

Early diagnosis of testicular cancer is essential, because this type of cancer spreads rapidly to other parts of the body. Because in most cases no early symptoms or pain is associated with testicular cancer, most people do not see a physician for months after discovering a lump or a slightly enlarged testis. Unfortunately, this delay allows almost 90 percent of testicular cancer to metastasize (spread) before a diagnosis is made.

Pancreatic Cancer

The pancreas is a thin gland that lies behind the stomach. This gland releases insulin and pancreatic juice. Insulin regulates blood sugar, and pancreatic juice contains enzymes that aid in digesting food.

POSSIBLE RISK FACTORS
1. *Increased incidence between ages 35 and 70,* but significantly higher around age 55.
2. *Cigarette smoking.*
3. *Chronic pancreatitis.*
4. *Cirrhosis.*
5. *Diabetes.*
6. *High-fat diet.*

PREVENTION AND WARNING SIGNALS
Detection of pancreatic cancer is difficult because (a) no symptoms are apparent in the early stages, and (b) advanced disease symptoms are similar to those of other diseases. Only a biopsy can provide a definite diagnosis, but because it is primarily a "silent" disease, the need for a biopsy is apparent only when the disease is already in an advanced stage.

Warning signals that may be related to pancreatic cancer include pain in the abdomen or lower back, jaundice, loss of weight and appetite, nausea, weakness, agitated depression, loss of energy and feeling weary, dizziness, chills, muscles spasms, double vision, and coma.

Kidney and Bladder Cancer

The kidneys are the organs that filter the urine, and the bladder stores and empties the urine. Most of these two types of cancer are caused by environmental factors. Bladder cancer occurs most frequently between the ages of 50 and 70. Of all bladder cancers, 80 percent are seen in men, and the incidence among white males is twice that of African American males.

POSSIBLE RISK FACTORS
1. *Heavy cigarette smoking.* Smoking is responsible for almost half of all deaths from bladder cancer in men and one-third of deaths from bladder cancer in women.
2. Congenital (inborn) abnormalities of either organ (these conditions are detected by a physician).
3. *Exposure to certain chemical compounds* such as aniline dyes, naphthalenes, or benzidines.
4. *History of schistosomiasis* (a parasitic bladder infection).
5. *Frequent urinary tract infections,* particularly after age 50.

PREVENTION AND WARNING SIGNALS
Avoiding cigarette smoking and occupational exposure to cancer-causing chemicals is important to decrease the risk. Bloody urine, especially in repeated occurrences, is always a warning sign and requires immediate evaluation. Bladder cancer is diagnosed through urine analysis and examination of the bladder with a cystoscope (a small tube that is inserted into the tract through the urethra).

Oral Cancer

Oral cancer includes the mouth, lips, tongue, salivary glands, pharynx, larynx, and floor of the mouth. Most of these cancers seem to be related to cigarette smoking and excessive consumption of alcohol.

RISK FACTORS
1. *Heavy use of tobacco* (cigarette, cigar, pipe, or smokeless) and/or alcohol drinking.
2. *Broken or ill-fitting dentures.*
3. *Broken tooth* that irritates the inside of the mouth.
4. *Excessive sun exposure* (lip cancer).

PREVENTION AND WARNING SIGNALS
Regular examinations and good dental hygiene help in prevention and early detection of oral cancer. Warning signals include a sore that doesn't heal or a white patch in the mouth, a lump, problems with chewing and swallowing, or a constant feeling of having "something" in the throat. A person with any of these conditions should be evaluated by a physician or a dentist. A tissue biopsy normally is conducted to diagnose the presence of cancer.

Esophageal and Stomach Cancer

The incidence of gastric cancer in the United States has dropped about 40 percent in the last 30 years. Cancer experts attribute this drastic decrease to changes in dietary habits and refrigeration. This type of cancer is more common in men, and the incidence is higher in African American males than in white males.

RISK FACTORS

1. *A diet high in starch and low in fresh fruits and vegetables.*
2. *High consumption of salt-cured, smoked, and nitrate-cured foods.*
3. *Imbalance in stomach acid.*
4. *History of pernicious anemia.*
5. *Chronic gastritis or gastric polyps.*
6. *Family history* of these types of cancer.

PREVENTION AND WARNING SIGNALS

Prevention is accomplished primarily by increasing dietary intake of complex carbohydrates and fiber and decreasing the intake of salt-cured, smoked, and nitrate-cured foods. In addition, regular guaiac testing for occult blood (hemoccult test) is recommended. Warning signals for this type of cancer include indigestion for 2 weeks or longer, blood in the stools, vomiting, and rapid weight loss.

Ovarian Cancer (women)

The ovaries are part of the female reproductive system that produces and releases the egg and the hormone estrogen. Ovarian cancer develops more frequently after menopause, and the highest incidence is seen between ages 55 and 64.

RISK FACTORS

1. *Age.* Risk increases with age and peaks in the eighth decade of life.
2. *History of ovarian problems.*
3. *Extensive history* of menstrual irregularities.
4. *Family history* of breast or ovarian cancer.
5. *Personal history* of breast, bowel, or endometrial cancer.
6. *Nulliparity* (no pregnancies).
7. *Hereditary non-polyposis colon cancer.*

PREVENTION AND WARNING SIGNALS

In most cases, ovarian cancer has no signs or symptoms. Therefore, regular pelvic examinations to detect signs of enlargement or other abnormalities are highly recommended. Some warning signals may be an enlarged abdomen, abnormal vaginal bleeding, unexplained digestive disturbances in women over age 40, and "normal"-size (pre-menopause size) ovaries after menopause.

Thyroid Cancer

The thyroid gland, located in the lower portion of the front of the neck, helps regulate growth and

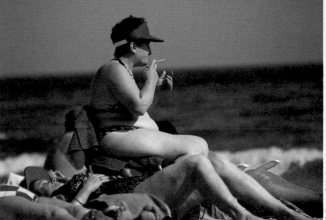

Cigarette smoking, obesity, and excessive sun exposure are major risk factors for cancer.

metabolism. Thyroid cancer occurs almost twice as often in women as in men. The incidence also is higher in whites than African Americans.

RISK FACTORS

1. *Aging.*
2. *Radiation therapy* of the head and neck region received in childhood or adolescence.
3. *Family history* of thyroid cancer.

PREVENTION AND WARNING SIGNALS

Regular inspection for thyroid tumors is done by palpating the gland and surrounding areas during a physical examination. Thyroid cancer is slow-growing; therefore, it is highly treatable. Nevertheless, any unusual lumps in front of the neck should be reported promptly to a physician. Although thyroid cancer does not have many warning signals (besides a lump), these may include difficulty swallowing, choking, labored breathing, and persistent hoarseness.

Liver Cancer

The incidence of liver cancer in the United States is low. Men are more prone then women to liver cancer, and the disease is more common after age 60.

RISK FACTORS

1. *History of cirrhosis* of the liver.
2. *History of hepatitis B virus.*
3. *Exposure to vinyl chloride* (industrial gas used in plastics manufacturing) and aflatoxin (natural food contaminant).

PREVENTION AND WARNING SIGNALS

Prevention consists primarily of avoiding the risk factors and being aware of warning signals. Possible signs and symptoms are a lump or pain in the upper right abdomen (which may radiate into the back and the shoulder), fever, nausea, rapidly deteriorating health, jaundice, and tenderness of the liver.

Leukemia

Leukemia is a type of cancer that interferes with blood-forming tissues (bone marrow, lymph nodes, and spleen) by producing too many immature white blood cells. People who have leukemia cannot fight infection very well. The causes of leukemia are mostly unknown, although suspected risk factors have been identified.

POSSIBLE RISK FACTORS

1. *Inherited susceptibility*, but not transmitted directly from parent to child.
2. *Greater incidence in children with Down syndrome* (mongolism) and a few other genetic abnormalities.
3. *Excessive exposure to ionizing radiation.*
4. *Environmental exposure* to chemicals such as benzene.

PREVENTION AND WARNING SIGNALS

Detection is not easy because early symptoms can be associated with other serious ailments. When leukemia is suspected, the diagnosis is made through blood tests and a bone marrow biopsy.

Early warning signals include fatigue, pallor, weight loss, easy bruising, nosebleeds, paleness, loss of appetite, repeated infections, hemorrhages, night sweats, bone and joint pain, and fever. At a more advanced stage, fatigue increases, hemorrhages become more severe, pain and high fever continue, the gums swell, and various skin disorders occur.

Lymphoma

Lymphomas are cancers of the lymphatic system. The lymphatic system consists of lymph nodes found throughout the body and a network of vessels that link these nodes. The lymphatic system participates in the body's immune reaction to foreign cells, substances, and infectious agents.

POSSIBLE RISK FACTORS

As with leukemia, the causes of lymphomas are unknown. People who have received organ transplants are at higher risk. Some researchers suspect that a form of herpes virus (called "Epstein–Barr virus") is active in the initial stages of lymphosarcomas. Risk of non-Hodgkin's lymphoma is higher in people who carry the human immunodeficiency virus (HIV) and human T-cell leukemia/lymphoma virus-I (HTLV-I) virus. Other researchers suggest that certain external factors may alter the immune system, making it more susceptible to the development and multiplication of cancer cells.

PREVENTION AND WARNING SIGNALS

Prevention of lymphoma is limited because little is known about its causes. Enlargement of a lymph node or a cluster of lymph nodes is the first sign of lymphoma. Other signs and symptoms are an enlarged spleen or liver, weakness, fever, back or abdominal pain, nausea/vomiting, unexplained weight loss, unexplained itching and sweating, and fever at night that lasts for a long time.

CRITICAL THINKING

You have learned about many of the risk factors major cancer sites. How will this information aff your health choices in t future? Will it be valuab to you, or will you quick forget all you have learn and remain in a Contem plation stage at the end this course?

What Can You Do?

If you are at high risk for any form of cancer, you are advised to discuss this with your physician. An ounce of prevention is worth a pound of cure. Although cardiovascular disease is the number-one killer in the country, cancer is the number-one fear. Of all cancers, 60 to 80 percent is preventable, and about 50 percent is curable. Most cancers are lifestyle-related, so being aware of the risk factors and following the screening guidelines (Table 12.2, page 372) and basic recommendations for preventing cancer will greatly decrease your risk for developing cancer.

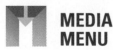

ASSESS YOUR KNOWLEDGE

1. Cancer can be defined as
   a. a process whereby some cells invade and destroy the immune system.
   b. an uncontrolled growth and spread of abnormal cells.
   c. the spread of benign tumors throughout the body.
   d. interference of normal body functions through blood-flow disruption caused by angiogenesis.
   e. All are correct choices.

2. Cancer treatment becomes more difficult when
   a. cancer cells metastasize.
   b. angiogenesis is disrupted.
   c. a tumor is encapsulated.
   d. cells are deficient in telomerase.
   e. cell division has stopped.

3. The leading cause of deaths from cancer in women is
   a. lung cancer.
   b. breast cancer.
   c. ovarian cancer.
   d. skin cancer.
   e. endometrial cancer.

4. Cancer
   a. is primarily a preventable disease.
   b. is often related to tobacco use.
   c. has been linked to dietary habits.
   d. risk increases with obesity.
   e. All are correct choices.

5. About 60 percent of cancers are related to
   a. genetics.
   b. environmental pollutants.
   c. viruses and other biological agents.
   d. ultraviolet radiation.
   e. diet, obesity, and tobacco use.

6. A cancer-prevention diet should include
   a. ample amounts of fruit and vegetables.
   b. cruciferous vegetables.
   c. phytochemicals.
   d. soy products.
   e. all of the above.

7. The biggest carcinogenic exposure in the workplace is
   a. asbestos fibers.
   b. cigarette smoke.
   c. biological agents.
   d. nitrosamines.
   e. pesticides.

8. Which of the following is *not* a warning signal for cancer?
   a. change in bowel or bladder habits
   b. nagging cough or hoarseness
   c. a sore that does not heal
   d. indigestion or difficulty in swallowing
   e. All of the above are warning signals for cancer.

9. The risk of breast cancer is higher in
   a. women under age 50.
   b. women with more than one family member with a history of breast cancer.
   c. minority groups than white women.
   d. women who had children prior to age 30.
   e. all of the above groups.

10. The risk for prostate cancer can be decreased by
    a. consuming selenium-rich foods.
    b. adding fatty fish to the diet.
    c. avoiding a high-fat diet.
    d. including tomato-rich foods in the diet.
    e. all of the above.

Correct answers can be found at the back of the book.

MEDIA MENU

PROFILE PLUS CD CONNECTIONS

▨ Assess your risk for cancer.

▨ Check how well you understand the chapter's concepts.

INTERNET CONNECTIONS

▨ American Cancer Society. This comprehensive site features fact sheets and information on a variety of cancer types. The site explores treatment options, including alternative or complementary therapies. It features the popular cancer profiler for personalized cancer treatment information, the cancer survivors' network, and a search engine for local resources.
   http://www.cancer.org

▨ National Cancer Institute. This government site, from the National Institutes of Health, provides statistics, frequently asked questions, as well as information on research and support resources. It includes links to Web pages with information about specific cancers.
   http://www.nci.nih.gov

▨ Cancer: Causes, Screening, and Prevention. This site, from the University of Pennsylvania Cancer Center, features information about cancer and diet, genetics, hormones, environment, drugs, smoking, and cancer epidemiology.
   http://www.oncolink.upenn.edu/causeprevent

▨ Susan G. Komen Breast Cancer Foundation. This site provides a wealth of breast cancer information including a video showing the correct way to perform a breast self exam, and the Komen NetQuiz which allows you to test your breast cancer knowledge.
   http://www.komen.org/bci/

Notes

1. American Cancer Society, *Cancer Facts & Figures—2004* (New York: ACS, 2004).

2. J. E. Enstrom, "Health Practices and Cancer Mortality among Active California Mormons," *Journal of the National Cancer Institute* 81 (1989): 1807–1814.

3. See note 1.

4. "Colorful Diet Helps Keep Cancer at Bay: Fruits and Vegetables Are Key," *Environmental Nutrition* 24, no. 6 (2001): 1, 6.

5. V. W. Setiawan et al., "Protective Effect of Green Tea on the Risks of Chronic Gastritis and Stomach Cancer," *International Journal of Cancer* 92 (2001): 600–604.

6. L. Mitscher and V. Dolby, *The Green Tea Book—China's Fountain of Youth* (New York: Avery Press, 1997).

7. J. H. Weisburger and G. M. Williams, "Causes of Cancer," *American Cancer Society Textbook of Clinical Oncology* (Atlanta: ACS, 1995): 10–39.

8. E. E. Calle, C. Rodriguez, K. Walker–Thurmond, and M. J. Thun, "Overweight, Obesity, and Mortality from Cancer in a Prospectively Studied Cohort of U.S. Adults," *New England Journal of Medicine* 348 (2003): 1625–1638.

9. American Cancer Society, *1995 Cancer Facts & Figures* (New York: ACS, 1995).

10. S. E. Whitmore, W. L. Morison, C. S. Potten, and C. Chadwick, "Tanning Salon Exposure and Molecular Alterations," *Journal of the American Academy of Dermatology* 44 (2001): 775–780.

11. See note 7.

Suggested Readings

American Cancer Society. *Cancer Facts & Figures—2005.* New York: ACS, 2005.

American Cancer Society. "Causes of Cancer," *Textbook of Clinical Oncology.* Atlanta: ACS, 1995.

American Heart Association and American Cancer Society. *Living Well, Staying Well.* New York: Random House, 1999.

American Institute for Cancer Research. *Stopping Cancer Before It Starts.* New York: Griffin, 2000.

Lab 12A

HEALTH QUESTIONNAIRES: CANCER PREVENTION AND EARLY WARNING SIGNS OF DISEASE

Name: _____   Date: _____   Grade: _____

Instructor: _____   Course: _____   Section: _____

Necessary Lab Equipment
None required.

Lab Preparation
None required.

Objective
To encourage healthy lifestyle practices that will help decrease the risk for cancer.

I. Cancer Prevention: Are You Taking Control?

Today, scientists think most cancers may be related to lifestyle and environment—what you eat and drink, whether you smoke, and where you work and play. The good news, then, is that you can help reduce your own cancer risk by taking control of things in your daily life.

12 Steps to a Healthier Life and Reduced Cancer Risk

	Yes	No
1. **Are you eating more cabbage-family vegetables?** They include broccoli, cauliflower, Brussels sprouts, all cabbages, and kale.	☐	☐
2. **Are high-fiber foods included in your diet?** Fiber is found in whole grains, fruits, and vegetables including peaches, strawberries, potatoes, spinach, tomatoes, wheat and bran cereals, rice, popcorn, and whole-wheat bread.	☐	☐
3. **Do you choose foods with vitamin A?** Fresh foods with beta-carotene, including carrots, peaches, apricots, squash, and broccoli are the best source—not vitamin pills.	☐	☐
4. **Is vitamin C included in your diet?** You'll find it naturally in lots of fresh fruits and vegetables including grapefruit, cantaloupe, oranges, strawberries, red and green peppers, broccoli, and tomatoes.	☐	☐
5. **Do you exercise and monitor calorie intake to avoid weight gain?** Walking is ideal exercise for many people.	☐	☐
6. **Are you cutting overall fat intake?** This is done by eating lean meat, fish, skinned poultry, and low-fat dairy products.	☐	☐
7. **Do you limit salt-cured, smoked, nitrite-cured foods?** Choose bacon, ham, hot dogs or salt-cured fish only occasionally if you like them a lot.	☐	☐
8. **If you smoke, have you tried quitting?**	☐	☐
9. **If you drink alcohol, are you moderate in your intake?**	☐	☐
10. **Do you respect the sun's rays?** Protect yourself with sunscreen (at least SPF 15) and wear long sleeves and a hat, especially during midday hours—10 A.M. to 2 P.M.	☐	☐
11. **Do you have a family history of any type of cancer? If so, have you brought this to the attention of your personal physician?**	☐	☐
12. **Are you familiar with the seven warning signals for cancer?**	☐	☐

If you answered "yes" to most of these questions, **congratulations**. You are taking control of simple lifestyle factors that will help you feel better and reduce your risk for cancer.

Adapted from the American Cancer Society, Texas Division.

II. Early Warning Signs of Possible Serious Illness

Many serious illnesses begin with apparently minor or localized symptoms that, if recognized early, can alert you to act in time for the disease to be cured or controlled. In most cases, nothing is seriously wrong. **If you experience any of the following symptoms, discuss the problem with your physician without delay.** Check only conditions that apply.

1. Rapid loss of weight—more than about 4 kg (10 lbs) in 10 weeks—without apparent cause.

2. A sore, scab, or ulcer, either in the mouth or on the body, that fails to heal within about 3 weeks.

3. A skin blemish or mole that begins to bleed or itch or that changes color, size, or shape.

4. Severe headaches that develop for no obvious reason.

5. Sudden attacks of vomiting, without preceding nausea.

6. Fainting spells for no apparent reason.

7. Visual problems such as seeing "haloes" around lights or intermittently blurred vision, especially in dim light.

8. Increasing difficulty with swallowing.

9. Hoarseness without apparent cause that lasts for a week or more.

10. A "smoker's cough" or any other nagging cough that has been getting worse.

11. Blood in coughed-up phlegm, or sputum.

12. Constantly swollen ankles.

13. A bluish tinge to the lips, the insides of the eyelids, or the nailbeds.

14. Extreme shortness of breath for no apparent reason.

15. Vomiting of blood or a substance that resembles coffee grounds.

16. Persistent indigestion or abdominal pain.

17. A marked change in normal bowel habits, such as alternating attacks of diarrhea and constipation.

18. Bowel movements that look black and tarry.

19. Rectal bleeding.

20. Unusually cloudy, pink, red, or smoky-looking urine.

21. In men, discomfort or difficulty when urinating.

22. In men, discharge from the tip of the penis.

23. In women, a lump or unusual thickening of a breast or any alteration in breast shape such as flattening, bulging, or puckering of skin.

24. In women, bleeding or unusual discharge from the nipple.

25. In women, vaginal bleeding or "spotting" that occurs between usual menstrual periods or after menopause.

From *American Medical Association Family Medical Guide* by The American Medical Association. Copyright © 1982 by The American Medical Association. Used by permission of Random House, Inc.

Lab 12B

CANCER RISK PROFILE

 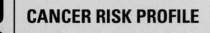

Name: _____ Date: _____ Grade: _____

Instructor: _____ Course: _____ Section: _____

Necessary Lab Equipment

None required.

Objective

To determine your risk for selected cancer sites.

I. Cancer Risk Profile

Instructions—Read the sections "Assessing Your Risks," "Common Sites of Cancer," and "Other Cancer Sites" (pages 371–382) and complete the Cancer Questionnaire: Assessing Your Risks in Figure 12.10 (pages 373–374). Copy your scores from Figure 12.10 into the blanks for those sites below. For all other sites, rate yourself on a scale from 1 to 3 (1 = low risk, 2 = moderate risk, 3 = high risk) according to the risk factors provided for each site under the *Other Cancer Sites* section.

Cancer Site	Total Points Men	Total Points Women	Risk Category
Lung			
Colon-Rectum			
Skin			
Breast			
Cervical			
Endometrial			
Prostate			
Testicular			
Pancreatic			
Kidney and Bladder			
Oral			
Esophageal and Stomach			
Ovarian			
Thyroid			
Liver			
Leukemia			
Lymphomas			

II. Stage of Change for Cancer Prevention

Using Figure 2.4 (page 41) and Table 2.3 (page 41), identify your current stage of change for participation in a cancer-prevention program:

III. Personal Interpretation

In the space provided below, discuss your results for the various cancer sites. State your feelings about cancer and comment on any experiences that you may have had with cancer patients.

IV. Cancer Prevention

Discuss lifestyle habits that you should eliminate and habits that you need to adopt to reduce your own risk of cancer. Also indicate how you can best implement and adhere to these changes.

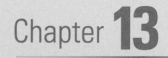

Chapter **13**

Addictive Behavior

Objectives

- Address the detrimental effects of addictive substances, including marijuana, cocaine, methamphetamine, Ecstasy, heroin, and alcohol.

- List the detrimental health effects of tobacco use in general.

- Recognize cigarette smoking as the largest preventable cause of premature illness and death in the United States.

- Enumerate the reasons people smoke.

- Explain the benefits and the significance of a smoking cessation program.

- Learn how to implement a smoking-cessation program, either for yourself (if you smoke), or to help others go through the quitting process.

Profile Plus CD Connections

- Find out if you're prone to addictive behavior.

- Plan for a smoke-free future.

- Check how well you understand the chapter's concepts.

389

© Rob Atkins/The Image Bank/Getty Images

At the beginning of the twenty-first century, chemical dependency remains one of the most serious health problems afflicting society. Substance abuse is an extremely destructive behavior that has ruined and ended millions of lives. Perhaps more than with any other unhealthy behavior, education is vital when addictive behaviors are at issue. Education concerning these subjects may assist in the search for answers, treatment, and a more productive and happier life. The information in this chapter will help you make informed decisions. The time to make healthy choices is *now*.

Addiction

When most people think of **addiction**, they probably think of dark and dirty alleys, an addict shooting drugs into a vein, or a wino passed out next to a garbage can after having spent an evening drinking alcohol. Psychotherapists have described addiction as a problem of imbalance or unease within the body and mind.

Almost anything can be addicting. Of the many types of addiction, some addictive behaviors are more detrimental than others. The most serious type is chemical dependency on drugs such as tobacco, alcohol, cocaine, methamphetamine, MDMA (Ecstasy), heroin, marijuana, or prescription drugs. Less serious are addictions to work, coffee, shopping, and even exercise.

People who are addicted to food eat to release stress or boredom or to reward themselves for every small personal achievement. Many people are addicted to television and the Internet. Others become so addicted to their jobs that all they think about is work. It may start out as enjoyable, but when it totally consumes a person's life, work can become an unhealthy behavior. If you find that you are readily irritated, moody, grouchy, constantly tired, not as alert as you used to be, or making more mistakes than usual, you may be becoming a workaholic and need to slow down or take time off work.

Even though exercise has enhanced the health and quality of life of millions of people, a relatively small number become obsessed with exercise, which has the potential for overuse and addiction. Compulsive exercisers feel guilty and uncomfortable when they miss a day's workout. Often, they continue to exercise even when they have injuries and sicknesses that require proper rest for adequate recovery. People who exceed the recommended guidelines for development and maintenance of fitness (see Chapters 6, 7, 8, and 9) are exercising for reasons other than health—including addictive behavior.

Addiction to caffeine can have undesirable side effects. In some individuals, caffeine doses in excess of 200 to 500 mg can produce an abnormally rapid heart rate, abnormal heart rhythms, higher blood pressure, and increased secretion of gastric acids, leading to stomach problems and possible birth defects in offspring. It also may induce symptoms of anxiety, depression, nervousness, and dizziness.

The caffeine content of drinks varies according to the product. In 6 ounces of coffee, for example, the content varies from 65 mg in instant coffee to as high as 180 mg in drip coffee. Soft drinks, mainly colas, range in caffeine content from about 30 to 70 mg per 12-ounce can.

These examples may be the first addictions you think of, but they are by no means the only kinds. Other addictions can be to gambling, pornography, sex, people, places, and on and on.

Risk Factors for Addiction

Although addictive behaviors cover a wide spectrum, they have factors in common that predispose people to addiction. Among these factors are the following:[1]

Profile Plus

Could you be prone to addictive behavior? Find out by completing the questionnaire on your CD-ROM.

- The behavior is reinforced.
- The addiction is an attempt to meet basic human needs, such as physical needs, the need to feel safe, the need to belong, the need to feel important, or the need to reach one's potential.
- The addiction seems to temporarily relieve stress.
- The addiction results from peer pressure.
- The addiction can be present within the person's value system (a person whose values wouldn't let him or her shoot heroin may be able to rationalize compulsive eating or obsessive television watching, for example).
- A serious physical illness is present, and the addiction may provide escape from pain or the fear of disfigurement.
- The addict feels pressured to perform or succeed.
- The addict hates himself or herself.
- A genetic link is present. Heredity might dictate susceptibility to some addictions.
- Society allows addiction. Advertising even encourages it (you can sleep better with a pill; snacking helps you enjoy life more fully; parties and sports are more fun with alcohol; shop 'til you drop; and so on).

The same general traits and behaviors are involved in all kinds of addictions, whether they involve food, sex, gambling, shopping, or drugs.

Most people with addictions deny their problem. Even when the addiction is clear to people around them, addicts continue to deny that they are addicted. Instead, they tend to get angry when someone tries to talk about the behavior and are likely to make excuses for their actions. Many addicts also blame others for their problem. In some cases, an addict admits the problem but fails to take any steps to change.

Recognizing that all forms of addiction are unhealthy, this chapter focuses on some of the most self-destructive addictive substances in our society: marijuana, cocaine, methamphetamine, MDMA, heroin, alcohol, and tobacco. About half a million Americans die each year from tobacco, alcohol, and illegal drug use.

Drugs and Dependence

A drug is any substance that alters the user's ability to function. Drugs encompass over-the-counter drugs, prescription medications, and illegal substances. Many drugs lead to physical and psychological dependence.

Any drug can be misused and abused. *Drug misuse* implies the intentional and inappropriate use of over-the-counter or prescribed medications.[2] Examples are taking more medication than prescribed, mixing drugs, not following prescription instructions, or discontinuing a drug prior to a physicians' approval.

Drug abuse is the intentional and inappropriate use of a drug resulting in physical, emotional, financial, intellectual, social, spiritual, or occupational consequences of the abuse.[3] Many substances, if used in the wrong manner, can be abused.

When drugs are used regularly, they integrate into the body's chemistry, increasing the user's tolerance to the drug and forcing the user to increase the dosage constantly to obtain similar results.

Drug abuse leads to serious health problems, and more than half of all adolescent suicides are drug-related. Often, drug abuse opens the gate to other illegal activities. According to the U.S. Department of Justice, the majority of convicted criminals —about 70 percent of federal inmates and 80 percent of state inmates—have abused drugs.

Approximately 60 percent of the world's production of illegal drugs is consumed in the United States. An estimated 15 million people in the United States use an illegal drug. Each year Americans spend more than $65 billion on illegal drugs.

According to the U.S. Department of Education, today's drugs are stronger and more addictive, and they pose a greater risk than ever before. If you are uncertain about addictive behavior(s) in your life, the Addictive Behavior Questionnaires in Lab 13A (page 413) can help you identify a potential problem. Some of the most commonly abused drugs in our society are discussed next.

Marijuana

Marijuana (pot or grass, as it is commonly called) is the most widely used illegal drug in the United States. Estimates by the Office of National Drug

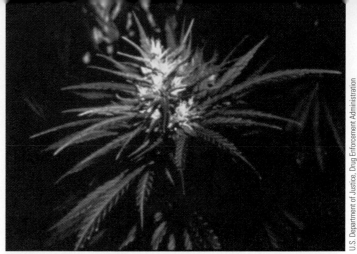

The flowering top of *Cannabis sativa*.

Control Policy indicate that 46 percent of Americans between ages 18 and 25 and 42 percent of those age 26 and older have smoked marijuana. Approximately 31 million people in the United States use marijuana regularly. Most users smoke loose marijuana that has been rolled into a joint or packed into a pipe. A few users bake it into foods such as brownies.

In small doses, marijuana has a sedative effect. Larger doses produce physical and psychological changes. Studies in the 1960s indicated that the potential effects of marijuana were exaggerated and that the drug was relatively harmless. The drug as it is used today, however, is as much as 10 times stronger than when the initial studies were conducted. Most of the research today shows marijuana to be dangerous and harmful.

The main, and most active, psychoactive and mind-altering ingredient in marijuana is thought to be delta-9-tetrahydrocannabinol (THC). In the 1960s, THC content in marijuana ranged from .02 to 2 percent. Users called the latter "real good grass." Today's THC content averages 4 to 6 percent, although it has been reported as high as 20 percent. The THC content in sinsemilla, a variety of high-potency marijuana grown from the seedless female cannabis plant, is approximately 6.7 percent.

THC reaches the brain within a few seconds after marijuana smoke is inhaled, and the psychic and physical changes reach their peak in about 2 or 3 minutes. THC then is metabolized in the liver to waste metabolites, but 30 percent of it remains in the body a week after the marijuana was smoked.

Addiction Compulsive and uncontrollable behavior(s) or use of substance(s).

Marijuana A psychoactive drug prepared from a mixture of crushed leaves, flowers, small branches, stems, and seeds from the hemp plant *cannabis sativa*.

THC is not completely eliminated until 30 days or longer after an initial dose of the drug. The drug always remains in the system of regular users.

Some of the short-term effects of marijuana are **tachycardia**, dryness of the mouth, reddened eyes, stronger appetite, decrease in coordination and tracking (the eyes' ability to follow a moving stimulus), difficulty in concentration, intermittent confusion, impairment of short-term memory and continuity of speech, interference with the physical and mental learning process during periods of intoxication, and increased risk of a heart attack for a full day after smoking the drug. Another common effect is the **amotivational syndrome**. This syndrome persists after periods of intoxication but usually disappears a few weeks after the individual stops using the drug.

Long-term harmful effects include atrophy of the brain (leading to irreversible brain damage), less resistance to infectious diseases, chronic bronchitis, lung cancer (marijuana smoke may contain as much as 50 percent more cancer-producing hydrocarbons than cigarette smoke), and possible sterility and impotence.

One of the most common myths about marijuana use is that it is not addictive. This myth has grown recently among young people as lobbyists work to convince the federal government to legalize marijuana for medicinal purposes. Ample scientific evidence clearly shows that regular users of marijuana do develop physical and psychological dependence. As with cigarette smokers, when regular users go without the drug, they crave the substance, go through mood changes, are irritable and nervous, and develop an obsession to get more.

CRITICAL THINKING

The legalization of marijuana for medical purposes is being heatedly debated across the United States. Do you think this decision should rest with the government, medical personnel, or the individuals themselves?

Cocaine

Similar to marijuana, **cocaine** was thought for many years to be relatively harmless. This misconception came to an abrupt halt in the mid-1980s when two well-known athletes—Len Bias (basketball) and Don Rogers (football)—died suddenly following cocaine overdoses. Currently, there are an estimated 2,707,000 chronic cocaine users and 3,035,000 occasional cocaine users in the United States. Between 5,000 and 7,000 people try the drug for the first time each year. Over the years, cocaine has been given several different names including, among others, coke, C, snow, blow, toot, flake, Peruvian lady, white girl, and happy dust. This drug can be sniffed or snorted, smoked, or injected.

When cocaine is snorted, it is absorbed quickly through the mucous membranes of the nose into the bloodstream. The drug is usually arranged in fine powder lines 1 to 2 inches long. Each line stimulates the autonomic nervous system for about 30 minutes. When cocaine is injected intravenously, larger amounts of cocaine can enter the body in a shorter time. The popularity of cocaine is based on the almost universal guarantee that users will find themselves in an immediate state of euphoria and well-being. It is an expensive drug—$400 to $1,800 per ounce for powdered cocaine. The addiction begins with a desire to get high, often at social gatherings, and usually with the assurance that "occasional use is harmless." At least 25 percent of these first-time users will become addicted in 4 years, and for many it is the beginning of a lifetime nightmare.

Animal research with cocaine has shown that all laboratory animals can become compulsive cocaine users. Animals work more persistently at pressing a bar for cocaine than bars for other drugs, including opiates. In one instance, an addicted monkey pressed the bar almost 13,000 times until it finally got a dose of cocaine. People respond similar to laboratory animals. Cocaine addicts prefer drug usage to any other activity and use the drug until the supply or the user is exhausted.

Cocaine users also exhibit unusual behaviors compared to their previous conduct, even to the point where a user has been known to sell a child to obtain more cocaine. Educated people are not immune to cocaine addiction. Some individuals (including lawyers, physicians, and athletes) have daily habits that cost them hundreds to thousands of dollars, with binges in the $20,000–$50,000 range. Cocaine addiction can lead to loss of a job and profession, loss of family, bankruptcy, and death.

Crack cocaine is a smokable form of cocaine that has become more popular over the past decade. It is many times more potent than cocaine and is highly addictive; two-thirds of users in the United States who are addicted to cocaine use crack. Because it is so potent, crack doses are smaller and, therefore, less expensive, at a price of $10 to $20 each, although users will still spend hundreds of dollars a day to support their addiction.

Crack typically is made by boiling cocaine hydrochloride in a solution of baking soda, then letting the solution dry. The residue is then broken up, to be smoked in a pipe. The high from crack comes within seconds, faster than the high from injected cocaine. The crack high lasts about 12 minutes, which is shorter than the high from snorted or injected cocaine. Choosing to use cocaine in this form heightens the risk for emphysema and heart attack.

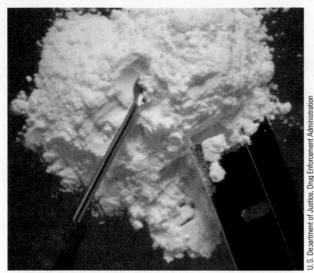

Powdered cocaine.

Cocaine seems to alleviate fatigue and raise energy levels, as well as lessen the need for food and sleep. Following the high comes a "crash," a state of physiological and psychological depression, often leaving the user with the desire to get more. This can produce a constant craving for the drug. Similar to alcoholics, cocaine users recover only by abstaining from the drug completely. A single "backslide" can result in renewed addiction.

Light-to-moderate cocaine use is commonly associated with feelings of pleasure and well-being. Sustained cocaine snorting can lead to a constant runny nose, nasal congestion and inflammation, and perforation of the nasal septum. Long-term consequences of cocaine use include loss of appetite, digestive disorders, weight loss, malnutrition, insomnia, confusion, anxiety, and cocaine psychosis, characterized by paranoia and hallucinations. In one type of hallucination, referred to as formication or "coke bugs," the chronic user perceives imaginary insects or snakes crawling on or underneath the skin.

High doses of cocaine can cause nervousness, dizziness, blurred vision, vomiting, tremors, seizures, strokes, angina, cardiac arrhythmias, and high blood pressure. As with smoking marijuana, the increased risk of having a heart attack following cocaine use is immediate. The user's risk may be 24 times higher than normal for up to 3 hours following cocaine use. Almost one-third of cocaine users who incurred a heart attack had no symptoms of heart disease prior to taking cocaine. In addition, intravenous users are at risk for hepatitis, HIV, and other infectious diseases.

Large overdoses of cocaine can precipitate sudden death from respiratory paralysis, cardiac arrhythmias, and severe convulsions. If individuals lack an enzyme used in metabolizing cocaine, as few as two to three lines of cocaine may be fatal.

Chronic users who constantly crave the drug often turn to crime, including murder, to sustain their habit. Some users view suicide as the only solution to this sad syndrome.

Methamphetamine

Methamphetamine, or "meth," is a more potent form of amphetamine and has become the fastest-growing drug threat in the United States. **Amphetamines** in general are part of a large group of synthetic agents used to stimulate the central nervous system. Amphetamines were widely given to soldiers during World War II to help them overcome fatigue, improve endurance, enhance battlefield ferocity, heighten mood, and keep them going. During the Vietnam War, U.S. soldiers used a greater amount of amphetamines than soldiers from all countries combined during World War II.

A powerfully addictive drug, methamphetamine falls under the same category of psychostimulant drugs as amphetamines and cocaine. It is also known as a "club drug," a group of illegal substances used at dance clubs, rock concerts, and raves (all-night dance parties). Other club drugs include MDMA (discussed on pages 394–396), LSD, GHB, Rohypnol, and ketamine.

Methamphetamine is typically a white, odorless, bitter-tasting powder that dissolves readily in water or alcohol. The drug is a potent central nervous system stimulant that produces a general feeling of well-being, decreases appetite, increases motor activity, and decreases fatigue and the need for sleep.

Based on the 2002 National Survey on Drug Use and Health (NSDUH) by the U.S. Department of Health and Human Services, more than 12 million Americans age 12 and older (5.3 percent of this population) have tried methamphetamines. Unlike most other drugs, methamphetamine use reaches rural and urban populations alike. Young people especially prefer methamphetamine because of its low cost and long-lasting effects—up to 12 hours following use.

Methamphetamine is easily manufactured with over-the-counter ingredients in clandestine "meth labs." These labs can be set up almost anywhere,

Tachycardia Faster-than-normal heart rate.

Amotivational syndrome A condition characterized by loss of motivation, dullness, apathy, and no interest in the future.

Cocaine 2-beta-carbomethoxy-3-betabenozoxytropane, the primary psychoactive ingredient derived from coca plant leaves.

Methamphetamine A potent form of amphetamine.

Amphetamines A class of powerful central nervous system stimulants.

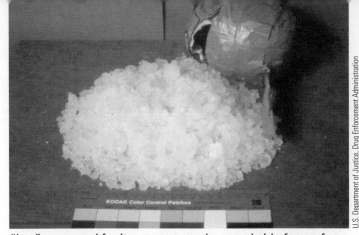

"Ice," so named for its appearance, is a smokable form of methamphetamine.

including garages, basements, or hotel rooms. The abundance of potential meth lab sites makes it difficult for drug enforcement agencies to locate many of these facilities. The risk of injury in a meth lab, however, is high, because potentially explosive environmental contaminants are discarded during production of the drug.

Methamphetamine can be snorted, swallowed, smoked, or injected. It is commonly referred to as "speed" or "crystal" when snorted or taken orally, "ice" or "glass" when smoked, and "crank" when injected. Depending on how it is taken, methamphetamine affects the body differently. Smoked or injected methamphetamines provide an immediate intense, pleasurable rush that lasts only a few minutes. Negative effects, nonetheless, can continue for several hours. When the drug is snorted or taken orally, the user does not experience a rush but develops a feeling of euphoria that lasts up to 16 hours.

Users of methamphetamines experience increases in body temperature, blood pressure, heart rate, and breathing rate; a decrease in appetite; hyperactivity; tremors; and violent behavior. High doses produce irritability, paranoia, irreversible damage to blood vessels in the brain (causing strokes), and risk of sudden death from hypothermia and convulsions if not treated at once.

Chronic abusers experience insomnia, confusion, hallucinations, inflammation to the heart lining, schizophrenia-like mental disorder, and brain-cell damage similar to that caused by a stroke. Physical changes to the brain may last months, or perhaps become permanent. Over time, methamphetamine use may reduce brain levels of **dopamine**, which can lead to symptoms similar to those of Parkinson's disease. In addition, users are frequently involved in violent crime, homicide, and suicide. Using methamphetamines during pregnancy may cause prenatal complications, premature delivery, and abnormal physical and emotional development of the child.

Similar to other stimulants, methamphetamines are often used in a binge cycle. Addiction takes hold quickly because tolerance to methamphetamines is developed within minutes of its initial use. The "high" disappears long before blood levels of the drug drop significantly. The user then attempts to maintain the pleasurable feelings by taking in more of the drug, and a binge cycle ensues.

The binge cycle, which can last for a couple of weeks, consists of several stages. The initial rush lasts 5 to 30 minutes. During this stage, heart rate, blood pressure, and metabolism increase and the user receives a great sense of pleasure. The high follows, lasting up to 16 hours. During this stage, users become arrogant and more argumentative. The binge stage sets in next and lasts between 2 and 14 days. Addicts continue to use the drug in an attempt to maintain the high for as long as possible.

When addicts can no longer achieve a satisfying high, they enter the "tweaking stage," the most dangerous stage in the cycle. At this point, users may have gone without food for several days and without sleep anywhere from 3 to 15 days. They become paranoid, irritable, and violent. Tweakers crave more of the drug, but no amount of amphetamines will restore the pleasurable, euphoric feelings achieved during the high. Thus, the addicts become increasingly frustrated, unpredictable, and dangerous to those around them (including police officers, medical personnel, and even to themselves). Once they finally crash, they are no longer dangerous. The users now become lethargic and sleep for 1 to 3 days.

Following the crash, addicts fall into a 1- to 3-month period of withdrawal. During this stage they can be paranoid, aggressive, fatigued, depressed, suicidal, and filled with an intense craving for another high. Re-use of the drug relieves these feelings. Therefore, the incidence of relapse in users who seek treatment is high.

MDMA (Ecstasy)

MDMA, also known as Ecstasy, became popular among teenagers and young adults in the United States in the mid-1980s, when it evolved into the most common "club drug." Although its use already constituted a serious drug problem in Europe, MDMA was not illegal in the United states until 1985. Prior to 1985, few Americans abused this drug. In the 1970s, some therapists used MDMA as a tool to help patients open up and feel at ease.

MDMA is named for its chemical structure: 3,4-methylenedioxymethamphetamine. Street names for the drug are X-TC, E, Adam, and love drug.

In 2002, more than 10 million persons aged 12 and older reported using Ecstasy at least once, up from 6.4 million in 2000. The number of users (used the drug within the last 30 days) in 2002 was estimated to be 676,000. Use of Ecstasy in the United States has been rising steadily since 1992, with 1.8 million new users in 2001. More than 1 in 23 eighth-graders have tried MDMA at least once, and more than 1 in 9 high school seniors have used the drug. Emergency-room mentions of MDMA in the United States also increased significantly—from 253 in 1994 to 4,026 in 2002.

Most users of MDMA are Hispanic American or white and are middle or high in socioeconomic rank. Typically, dealers are workers at nightclubs or raves. They push the drug as a way to increase energy, pleasure, and self-confidence. Some clubs have made an effort to protect their public image by hiring private ambulances to quickly treat and remove victims of overdose. As a result of increased awareness, communities are taking action to reduce the number of raves and to curb the use of club drugs at raves. Unfortunately, MDMA is now being pushed in new venues, including high schools, private homes, malls, and other popular gathering places for teenagers and young adults. The trafficking of MDMA is increasing at an alarming rate, and multiple agencies have reported large seizures of the drug.

Although MDMA is usually swallowed in the form of one or two pills in doses of up to 120 mg per pill, it can also be smoked, snorted, or, occasionally, injected. Because the drug is often prepared with other substances, users have no way of knowing the exact potency of the drug or additional substances found in each pill. Further, many users combine MDMA with alcohol, marijuana, or other drugs, which make its use even more dangerous.

MDMA shares characteristics with stimulants and hallucinogens. Its chemical structure closely parallels the hallucinogen **MDA** (methylenedioxyamphetamine) and methamphetamine, both man-made stimulants that damage the brain. MDMA's addictive properties and stimulation of hyperactivity have been compared to stimulants such as amphetamines and cocaine. The chemical structure of MDMA and its appeal, however, are similar to hallucinogens, but with milder psychedelic effects.

MDMA has a reputation among young people for being fun and harmless as long as it is used sensibly. But it is not a harmless drug. Current research is uncovering many negative side effects. The pleasurable effects peak about an hour after a pill is swallowed and last for 2 to 6 hours. Users claim to feel enlightened and introspective, accepting of themselves and trustful of others. Because they tend to act and feel closer to, or more intimate with, the people around them, some believe this drug to be an aphrodisiac, even though MDMA actually hampers sexual ability. MDMA also acts as a stimulant

by increasing brain activity and making users feel more energetic.

Like most addictive drugs, the effects of MDMA are said to diminish with each use. MDMA users may experience rapid eye movement, faintness, blurred vision, chills, sweating, nausea, muscle tension, and teeth-grinding. Users often bring infant pacifiers to raves to combat the latter side effect. Individuals with heart, liver, or kidney disease or high blood pressure are especially at risk because MDMA increases blood pressure, heart rate, and body temperature. Thus, its use may lead to seizures, kidney failure, a heart attack, or a stroke. The hot, crowded atmosphere at raves and dance clubs also heightens the user's risk. Deaths are more likely to occur when water is unavailable because the crowded atmosphere, combined with the stimulant effects of MDMA, causes dehydration (bottled water is often sold at inflated prices at raves). Other evidence suggests that a pregnant woman using MDMA may find long-term learning and memory difficulties in her child.

The damaging effects of the drug can be long-lasting and are possible after only a few uses. Long-term side effects, lasting for weeks after use, include confusion, depression, sleep disorders, anxiety, aggression, paranoia, and impulsive behavior. Questions still remain about other potential long-term effects. Verbal and visual memory may be significantly impaired for years after prolonged use. Researchers are now focusing on these lasting side effects, which may be the result of depleted serotonin, a neurotransmitter that is released with each dose of MDMA. The short-term effect of serotonin release is increased brain activity. Serotonin helps to regulate sleep cycles, pain, emotion, and appetite. Because MDMA may damage the neurons that release serotonin, long-term effects could be dangerous.

Advocates of MDMA are attempting to get approval to study medical uses of the drug. For example, MDMA could relieve suffering in terminally ill cancer patients. It also could help people in therapy for marital problems by encouraging introspection and conversation. Because MDMA is heralded as an instant antidepressant, it may help people who are in mourning. Opponents, meanwhile, question the value of MDMA as an effective

Dopamine A neurotransmitter that affects emotional, mental, and motor functions.

MDMA A synthetic hallucinogen drug with a chemical structure that closely resembles MDA and methamphetamine; also known as Ecstasy.

MDA A hallucinogenic drug that is structurally similar to amphetamines.

treatment modality because its effects diminish with continued use.

Heroin

For the first time in decades, **heroin** use is on the increase, and it is again being publicized by pop culture. Heroin started to make a comeback in 1991 and became increasingly stylish in 1995 following the arrests and deaths of prominent rock stars who abused the drug. According to the 2002 NSDUH, approximately 3.7 million Americans ages 12 and older (1.6 percent) reported trying heroin at least once. Approximately 404,000 reported past-year heroin use, and 166,000 reported past-month heroin use. Although the most common users are suburban, middle-class people and lower-income populations, its use is starting to appear in more affluent communities as well.

Common nicknames for heroin include diesel, dope, dynamite, white death, nasty boy, china white, H. Harry, gumball, junk, brown sugar, smack, tootsie roll, black tar, and chasing the dragon. Heroin is classified as a narcotic drug. It is synthesized from morphine, a natural substance found in the seedpod of several types of poppy plants. In its purest form, heroin is a white powder, but on the streets it is typically available in yellow or brown powders. The latter colors are attained when pure heroin is combined with other drugs or substances such as sugar, cornstarch, chalk, brick dust, or laundry soap. Heroin also is sold in a hardened or solid form (black tar), which is usually dissolved with other liquids for use in injectable form. Many users combine heroin with cocaine, a risky process commonly called "speedballing."

Today's heroin is more pure, powerful, and affordable than ever before. The average price has dropped by two-thirds over the last 10 years, which partially accounts for the increased popularity of the drug. For $100, drug users can get about 300 mg of heroin, an amount that will provide several "hits." Street-level heroin usually sells for $10 to $20 per dose, although prices vary throughout the country.

Highly dangerous, heroin is a significant health threat to users today in that they have no way of determining the strength of the drug purchased on the street, which places them at a constant risk for overdose and death. Based on a 2001 report from the Drug Abuse Warning Network, an estimated 15 percent of all drug-related cases seen in hospital emergency rooms that year involved heroin use.

Heroin can be injected intravenously or intramuscularly, sniffed/snorted, or smoked. Although injection is the predominant method of heroin use, users are turning away from intravenous injections because of the risk for HIV infection. The availability of relatively low-priced, high-purity heroin further contributes to the number of people who smoke or snort the drug. Some users have the misconception that heroin is less addictive when it is snorted or smoked. Whether injected, snorted, or smoked, heroin is an extremely addictive drug, and both physical and psychological dependence develop rapidly. Drug tolerance sets in quickly, and each time the drug is used, a higher dose is required to produce the same effects. Use of heroin induces a state of euphoria that comes within seconds of intravenous injection or within 5 to 15 minutes with other methods of administration. The drug is a sedative, so during the initial rush, the person has a sense of relaxation and does not feel any pain. In users who inhale the drug, however, the rush may be accompanied by nausea, vomiting, intense itching, and at times severe asthma attacks. As the rush wears off, users experience drowsiness, confusion, slowed cardiac function, and decreased breathing rate.

A heroin overdose can cause convulsions, coma, and death. During an overdose, heart rate, breathing, blood pressure, and body temperature drop dramatically. These physiological responses can induce vomiting and tight muscles and cause breathing to stop. Death is often the result of lack of oxygen or choking to death on vomit.

About 4 to 5 hours after the drug is taken, withdrawal sets in. Heroin withdrawal is painful and usually lasts up to 2 weeks—but could go on for several months. Symptoms of short-term use include red/raw nostrils, bone and muscle pains, muscle spasms and cramps, sweating, hot and cold flashes, runny nose and eyes, drowsiness, sluggishness, slurred speech, loss of appetite, nausea, diarrhea, restlessness and violent yawning. Heroin use can also kill a developing fetus or cause a spontaneous abortion.

Symptoms of long-term use of heroin include hallucinations, nightmares, constipation, sexual difficulties, impaired vision, reduced fertility, boils, collapsed veins, and a significantly elevated risk for lung, liver, and cardiovascular diseases, including bacterial infections in blood vessels and heart valves. The additives used in street heroin can clog vital blood vessels because these additives do not dissolve in the body, leading to infections and death of cells in vital organs. Sudden infant death syndrome (SIDS) is also seen more frequently in children born to addicted mothers.

Heroin addiction is treated with behavioral therapies and pharmaceutical agents. Medication helps suppress withdrawal symptoms, which makes it easier for patients to stop using heroin. The combination of these two treatment modalities helps the individual learn to lead a more stable, productive, and drug-free lifestyle.

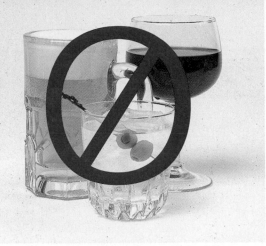

The sale of alcohol was illegal in the United States between 1920 and 1933.

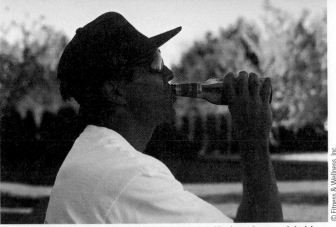

Approximately 14 million Americans will develop a drinking problem during their lifetime.

Alcohol

Drinking alcohol has been a socially acceptable behavior for centuries. **Alcohol** is an accepted accompaniment at parties, ceremonies, dinners, sport contests, the establishment of kingdoms or governments, and the signing of treaties between nations. Alcohol also has been used for medical reasons as a mild sedative or as a painkiller for surgery.

For a short period of 14 years, from 1920 to 1933, by constitutional amendment, the sale and use of alcohol were declared illegal in the United States. This amendment was repealed because drinkers and non-drinkers alike questioned the right of government to pass judgment on individual moral standards. In addition, organized crime activities to smuggle and sell alcohol illegally expanded enormously during this period.

Alcohol is the cause of one of the most significant health-related drug problems in the United States today. Based on the 2002 NSDUH, more than 120 million people 12 years and older (51.0 percent) use alcohol; 54 million (22.9 percent) participated in binge drinking at least once in the 30 days prior to the survey; 15.9 million (6.7 percent) were heavy drinkers; and 1 in 7 drove under the influence of alcohol at least once in the 12 months prior to the interview. The highest prevalence was among 21-year-olds, with almost 71 percent of this age group using alcohol. Furthermore, the number of adults who abuse alcohol or are alcohol dependent has risen from 13.8 million (7.41 percent) in 1991–1992 to 17.6 million (8.46 percent) in 2001–2002. Among younger people, about 7.2 million (19.3 percent) between the ages of 12 and 20 are binge drinkers.

Although modest health benefits are derived from moderate alcohol consumption, the media have extensively exaggerated these benefits. They like to discuss this topic because it seems to be "a vice that's good for you." The research data supports the assertion that consumption of no more than two alcoholic beverages a day for men and one for women provides modest benefits in decreasing the risk for cardiovascular disease. Not reported in the media, however, is that these modest health benefits do not always apply to African Americans.

The benefits of modest alcohol use can be equated to those obtained through a small daily dose of aspirin (about 81 mg per day, or the equivalent of a baby aspirin) or eating a small amount of nuts each day. And aspirin or a few nuts do not lead to impaired judgment or actions that you may later regret or have to live with for the rest of your life.

Effects of Alcohol Drinking

Alcohol is not for everyone. **Alcoholism** appears to have both a genetic and an environmental component. The reasons some people can drink for years without becoming addicted while others follow the downward spiral of alcoholism are not understood. The addiction to alcohol develops slowly. Most people think they are in control of their drinking habits and do not realize they have a problem until they become alcoholics, when they find themselves physically and emotionally dependent on the drug. This addiction is characterized by excessive use of, and constant preoccupation with, drinking. Alcohol abuse, in turn, leads to mental, emotional, physical, and social problems.

The effects of alcohol intake include impeded peripheral vision, decreased visual and hearing acuity,

Heroin A potent drug that is a derivative of opium.

Alcohol (ethyl alcohol) A depressant drug that affects the brain and slows down central nervous system activity; has strong addictive properties.

Alcoholism Disease in which an individual loses control over drinking alcoholic beverages.

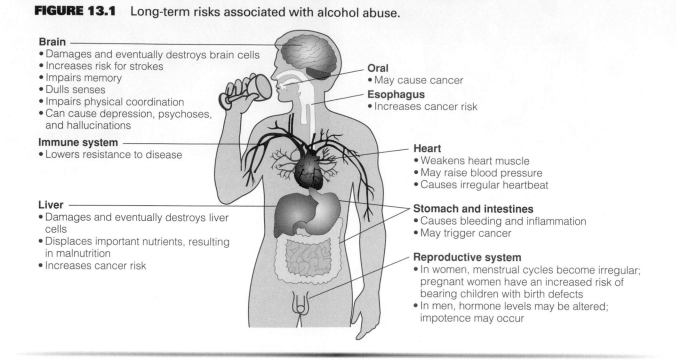

FIGURE 13.1 Long-term risks associated with alcohol abuse.

Brain
- Damages and eventually destroys brain cells
- Increases risk for strokes
- Impairs memory
- Dulls senses
- Impairs physical coordination
- Can cause depression, psychoses, and hallucinations

Immune system
- Lowers resistance to disease

Liver
- Damages and eventually destroys liver cells
- Displaces important nutrients, resulting in malnutrition
- Increases cancer risk

Oral
- May cause cancer

Esophagus
- Increases cancer risk

Heart
- Weakens heart muscle
- May raise blood pressure
- Causes irregular heartbeat

Stomach and intestines
- Causes bleeding and inflammation
- May trigger cancer

Reproductive system
- In women, menstrual cycles become irregular; pregnant women have an increased risk of bearing children with birth defects
- In men, hormone levels may be altered; impotence may occur

slower reaction time, impaired concentration and motor performance (including increased swaying), and impaired judgment of distance and speed of moving objects. Further, alcohol alleviates fear, increases risk-taking, stimulates urination, and induces sleep. A single large dose of alcohol also may decrease sexual function.

One of the most unpleasant, dangerous, and life-threatening effects of drinking is the **synergistic action** of alcohol when combined with other drugs, particularly central nervous system depressants. Each person reacts to a combination of alcohol and other drugs in a different way. The effects range from loss of consciousness to death.

Long-term effects of alcohol abuse are serious and often life-threatening (see Figure 13.1). Some of these detrimental effects are: lower resistance to disease; **cirrhosis** of the liver; higher risk for oral, esophageal, stomach, and liver cancer; **cardiomyopathy**; irregular heartbeat; elevated blood pressure; greater risk for strokes; inflammation of the esophagus, stomach, small intestine, and pancreas; stomach ulcers; sexual impotence; birth defects; malnutrition; damage to brain cells leading to loss of memory; depression; psychosis; and hallucinations.

Alcohol on Campuses

Alcohol is the number-one drug problem among college students. According to national surveys,

about 64 percent of full-time college students reported using alcohol within the past month, and 44 percent had engaged in binge drinking (5 or more drinks in a row). Alcohol is a factor in about 28 percent of all college dropouts. Today's student spends more on alcohol than on books.

A national survey involving about 94,000 college students from 197 colleges and universities conducted over 3 years showed that gradepoint average (GPA) is related to average number of drinks per week (see Figure 13.2).[4] Students with a "D" or "F" GPA reported a weekly consumption of almost 10 drinks. Students with "A" GPAs consumed about 4 drinks per week.

In another national survey of almost 55,000 undergraduate students from 131 colleges, close to 25 percent of students said that their academic problems resulted from alcohol misuse. Of greater concern, 29 percent of the surveyed students admitted driving while intoxicated. Of the 15 million college students in the United States, between 2 and 3 percent will eventually die from alcohol-related causes. This represents more students than those who will receive advanced degrees (master's and doctorate degrees combined).

Another major concern is that more than half of college students participate in games that involve heavy drinking (5 or more drinks in one sitting). Often, students take part because of peer pressure and fear of rejection. Almost 50 percent reported binge drinking at least once during the 2 weeks prior

FIGURE 13.2 Average number of drinks by college students per week by GPA.

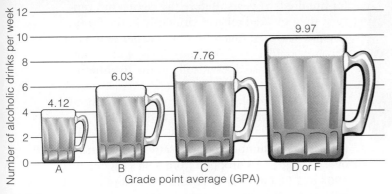

Source: C.A. Presley, J.S. Leichliter, and P. W. Meilman, *Alcohol and Drugs on American College Campuses: Findings from 1995, 1996, and 1997 (A Report to College Presidents)* (Carbondale, IL: Southern Illinois University, 1999).

BEHAVIOR MODIFICATION PLANNING

WHEN YOUR DATE DRINKS . . .

■ **Don't** make excuses for his/her behavior, no matter how embarrassing.

■ **Don't** allow embarrassment to put you in a situation with which you are uncomfortable.

■ **Do** be sure that body language and tone of voice match verbal messages you send.

■ **Do** leave as quickly as you can, without your date. **Don't** stop to argue. Intoxicated people can't listen to reason.

■ **Do** call a cab, a friend, or your parents. **Don't** ride home with your date.

For Women:

■ **Do** make your position clear. "No!" is much more effective than "Please stop!" or "Don't!"

■ **Do** make it clear that you will call the police if rape is attempted.

Source: "Sexuality Under the Influence of Alcohol." *Human Sexuality Supplement to Current Health* 2 (October 1990): p. 3.

to the survey. Excessive drinking can precipitate unplanned and unprotected sex (risking HIV infection) or date rape.

How to Cut Down on Drinking

To find out if drinking is a problem in your life, refer to the questionnaire in Lab 13A, page 414, developed by the American Medical Association. If you respond "yes" twice or more on this questionnaire, you may be jeopardizing your health.

If a person is determined to control the problem, it is not that difficult. The first and most important step is to want to cut down. If you want to do this but you cannot seem to do so, you had better accept the probability that alcohol is becoming a serious problem for you, and you should seek guidance from your physician or from an organization such as Alcoholics Anonymous. The next few suggestions also may help you cut down your alcohol intake.

1. *Set reasonable limits for yourself.* Decide not to exceed a certain number of drinks on a given occasion, and stick to your decision. No more than two beers or two cocktails a day is a reasonable limit. If you set a target such as this and consistently do not exceed it, you have proven to yourself that you can control your drinking.

2. *Learn to say no.* Many people have "just one more" drink because others in the group are doing this or because someone puts pressure on them, not because they really want a drink. When you reach the sensible limit you have set for yourself, politely but firmly refuse to exceed it. If you are being the generous host, pour yourself a glass of water or juice "on the rocks." Nobody will notice the difference.

3. *Drink slowly.* Don't gulp down a drink. Choose your drinks for their flavor, not their "kick," and savor the taste of each sip.

4. *Dilute your drinks.* If you prefer cocktails to beer, try tall drinks: Instead of downing gin or whiskey neat or nearly so, drink it diluted with a mixer such as tonic water or soda water in a tall glass. That way you can enjoy both the flavor and the act of drinking but you will take longer to finish each drink. Also, you can make your two-drink limit last all evening or switch to the mixer by itself.

5. *Do not drink on your own.* Confine your drinking to social gatherings. You may have a hard time resisting the urge to pour yourself a relaxing drink at the end of a hard day, but many formerly heavy drinkers have found that a soft drink satisfies the need as well as alcohol did. What may help you really unwind, even with no drink at all, is a comfortable chair, loosened

Synergistic action The effect of mixing two or more drugs, which can be much greater than the sum of two or more drugs acting by themselves.

Cirrhosis A disease characterized by scarring of the liver.

Cardiomyopathy A disease affecting the heart muscle.

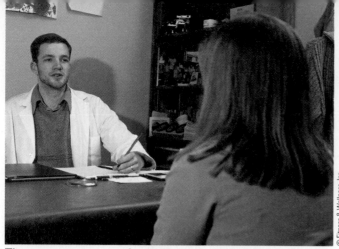

The sooner treatment for addiction is started, the longer the user stays in treatment, the better the chances for recovery and a more productive life.

clothing, and perhaps a soothing audiotape, television program, or good book to read.

Treatment of Addiction

Recovery from any addiction is more likely to be successful with professional guidance and support. The first step is to recognize the reality of the problem. The addictive behavior questionnaire in Lab 13A will help you recognize possible addictive behavior in yourself or someone you know. If the answers to more than half of these questions are positive, you may have a problem, in which case you should contact a physician, your institution's counseling center, or the local mental health clinic for a referral (see the Yellow Pages in your phone book).

You may also contact the Substance Abuse and Mental Health Services Administration (SAMHSA) at 1-800-662-HELP (1-800-662-4357) for referral to 24-hour substance abuse treatment centers in your local area. All information discussed during a phone call to this center is kept strictly confidential. Information is also available on the Internet at http://www.samhsa.gov. The national center provides printed information on drug abuse and addictive behavior.

About 5 million Americans have received treatment for addictive behavior.[5] An additional 7 million people are estimated to need treatment for substance abuse.[6] Among intervention and treatment programs for addiction are psychotherapy, medical care, and behavior modification. If addiction is a problem in your life, you need to act upon it without delay. Addicts do not have to resign themselves to a lifetime of addiction. The sooner you start, and the longer you stay in treatment, the better are your chances to recover and lead a healthier and more productive life.

Tobacco Use

People throughout the world have used tobacco for hundreds of years. Before the eighteenth century, they smoked tobacco primarily in the form of pipes or cigars. Cigarette smoking per se did not become popular until the mid-1800s, and its use started to increase dramatically in the twentieth century.

In 1900, people in the United States consumed 2.5 billion cigarettes, compared to 640 billion in 1981. This figure dropped to 487 billion in 1995. Per-capita consumption of cigarettes by Americans over the age of 18 dropped from 4,345 cigarettes in 1963 to 1,903 in 2003.[7] Nonetheless, more than 48 million Americans still smoke cigarettes.

When tobacco leaves are burned, hot air and gases containing **tar** (chemical compounds) and **nicotine** are released in the smoke. More than 1,200 toxic chemicals have been found in tobacco smoke. Tar contains about 60 chemical compounds that are proven carcinogens. The harmful effects of cigarette smoking and tobacco use in general were not exactly known until the early 1960s, when research began to show a link between tobacco use and disease. In 1964, the U.S. Surgeon General issued the first major report presenting scientific evidence that cigarettes were indeed a major health hazard in our society.

Morbidity and Mortality

Tobacco use in all its forms is considered a significant threat to life. World Health Organization estimates indicate that 10 percent of the 6 billion people presently living will die as a result of smoking-related illnesses, which kill approximately 5 million people each year. At the present rate of escalation, this figure is expected to climb to 10 million annual deaths by the year 2025. Tobacco will kill 150 million people in the first quarter of this century and another 300 million in the second quarter.

To gain some perspective on the seriousness of the tobacco problem, statistics indicate that overdoses of illegal drugs kill about 17,000 people per year in the United States and drug felonies and drug-related murders kill another 1,600 people each year. This brings drug-related deaths to a grand total of 18,600 annually. By comparison, tobacco, a legal drug, kills about 23 times as many people as all illegal drugs combined.

Cigarette smoking is the largest preventable cause of illness and premature death in the United States. Death rates from heart disease, cancer, stroke, aortic aneurysm, chronic bronchitis, emphysema, and peptic ulcers all increase with cigarette smoking.

FIGURE 13.3 Normal and diseased alveoli in lungs.

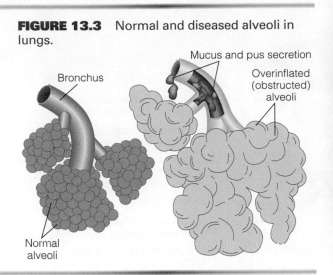

Bronchus

Mucus and pus secretion

Overinflated (obstructed) alveoli

Normal alveoli

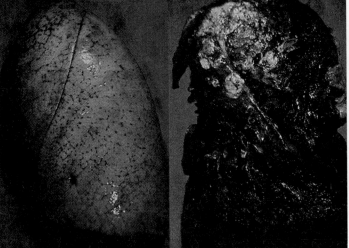

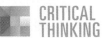
© "If You Smoke" slide show by Gordon Hewlett

Normal lung (left) is contrasted with diseased lung (right). The white growth near the top of the diseased lung is cancer; the dark appearance on the bottom half is emphysema.

In pregnant women, cigarette smoking has been linked to retarded fetal growth, higher risk for spontaneous abortion (miscarriage), and prenatal death. Smoking is also the most prevalent cause of injury and death from fire. The average life expectancy for a chronic smoker is as much as 15 years shorter than for a non-smoker, and the death rate among chronic smokers during their most productive years of life, between ages 25 and 65, is twice the national average. If we consider all related deaths, smoking is responsible for more than 435,000 unnecessary deaths each year—enough deaths to wipe out the entire population of Miami and Miami Beach in a single year.

Based on a report by U.S. government physicians, each cigarette shortens life by 7 minutes. This figure represents 5 million years of potential life that Americans lose to smoking each year. According to estimates by the American Heart Association, more than 30 percent of fatal heart attacks—or 120,000 in the United States annually—result from smoking. The risk for heart attack is 50 to 100 percent higher for smokers than for non-smokers. The mortality rate following heart attacks also is higher for smokers, because their attacks usually are more severe and their risk for deadly arrhythmias is much greater.

Cigarette smoking affects the cardiovascular system by increasing heart rate, blood pressure, and susceptibility to atherosclerosis, blood clots, coronary artery spasm, cardiac arrhythmia, and arteriosclerotic peripheral vascular disease. Evidence also indicates that smoking decreases high-density lipoprotein (HDL) cholesterol, the "good" cholesterol that lowers the risk for heart disease. Smoking further increases the amount of fatty acids, glucose, and various hormones in the blood. The carbon monoxide in smoke hinders the capacity of the blood to carry oxygen to body tissues. Both carbon monoxide and nicotine can damage the inner walls of the arteries and thus encourage the build-up of fat on them. Smoking also causes increased adhesiveness and clustering of platelets in the blood, decreases platelet survival and clotting time, and increases blood thickness. Any of these effects can precipitate a heart attack.

The American Cancer Society reports that 87 percent of lung cancer is attributable to smoking. Lung cancer is the leading cancer killer, accounting for approximately 173,770 deaths in the United States in the year 2004, or about 30 percent of all deaths from cancer.[8] Cigarette smoking also leads to chronic lower respiratory disease, the third leading cause of death in the United States (also see Chapter 1). Figure 13.3 illustrates normal and diseased **alveoli**.

The most common carcinogenic exposure in the workplace is cigarette smoke. Both fatal and non-fatal cardiac events are

CRITICAL THINKING

Cigarette smoking is the largest preventable cause of premature illness and death in the United States. Do you think the government should outlaw the use of tobacco in all forms? Or does the individual have the right to engage in self-destructive behavior?

Tar Chemical compound that forms during the burning of tobacco leaves.

Nicotine Addictive compound found in tobacco leaves.

Alveoli Air sacs in the lungs where gas exchange (oxygen and carbon dioxide) takes place.

FIGURE 13.4 The health effects of smoking.

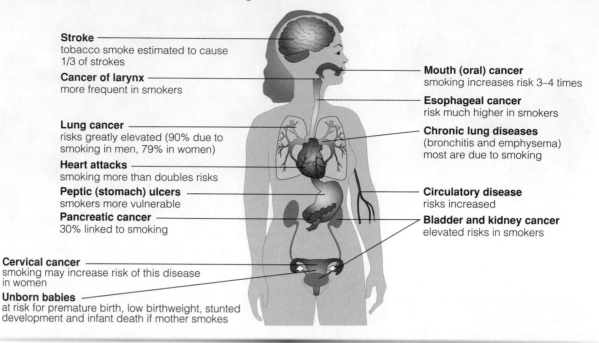

Stroke
tobacco smoke estimated to cause 1/3 of strokes

Cancer of larynx
more frequent in smokers

Lung cancer
risks greatly elevated (90% due to smoking in men, 79% in women)

Heart attacks
smoking more than doubles risks

Peptic (stomach) ulcers
smokers more vulnerable

Pancreatic cancer
30% linked to smoking

Cervical cancer
smoking may increase risk of this disease in women

Unborn babies
at risk for premature birth, low birthweight, stunted development and infant death if mother smokes

Mouth (oral) cancer
smoking increases risk 3–4 times

Esophageal cancer
risk much higher in smokers

Chronic lung diseases
(bronchitis and emphysema) most are due to smoking

Circulatory disease
risks increased

Bladder and kidney cancer
elevated risks in smokers

increased greatly in people who are exposed to passive smoke. Secondhand smoke is ranked behind active smoking and alcohol as the third leading preventable cause of death in the United States.[9] About 3,000 people die each year from lung cancer because of secondhand smoke, also known as environmental tobacco smoke (ETS). ETS is also a significant risk factor for heart disease in children and adults alike, causing an estimated 35,000 to 40,000 yearly deaths in non-smokers.[10]

Although half of all cancers are now curable, the 5-year survival rate for lung cancer is less than 13 percent. Furthermore, cigarette smoking is responsible for most cancers of the oral cavity, larynx, and esophagus (see Figure 13.4). Tobacco use also is related to the development of and deaths from bladder, pancreas, kidney, and cervical cancers.

Many tobacco users are aware of the health consequences of cigarette smoking but may fail to realize the risk of pipe smoking, cigar smoking, and tobacco chewing. As a group, pipe and cigar smokers have lower risks for heart disease and lung cancer than cigarette smokers. Nevertheless, blood nicotine levels in pipe and cigar smokers have been shown to approach those of cigarette smokers, because nicotine is still absorbed through the membranes of the mouth. Therefore, these tobacco users still have a higher risk for heart disease than non-smokers do.

Cigarette smokers who substitute pipe or cigar smoking for cigarettes usually continue to inhale the smoke, which actually results in more nicotine

and tar being brought into the lungs. Consequently, the risk for disease is even higher if pipe or cigar smoke is inhaled. The risk and mortality rates for lip, mouth, and larynx cancer for pipe smoking, cigar smoking, and tobacco chewing are actually higher than for cigarette smoking.

Heavy smokers use the health-care system, especially hospitals, twice as much as non-smokers do. The yearly cost to a given company has been estimated to be up to $5,000 per smoking employee. These costs include employee health care, absenteeism, additional health insurance, morbidity/disability and early mortality, on-the-job time lost, property damage/maintenance and depreciation, worker compensation, and the impact of secondhand smoke.

If every smoker were to give up cigarettes, in 1 year alone sick time would drop by approximately 90 million days, heart conditions would decrease by 280,000, chronic bronchitis and emphysema would number 1 million fewer cases, and total death rates from cardiovascular disease, cancer, and peptic ulcers would fall off drastically.

Every day more than 1,200 Americans die from smoking-related illnesses. That is the equivalent of three fully loaded jumbo jets crashing each day with no survivors.[11] Imagine what the coverage and concern would be if 435,000 people each year were to die in the United States alone because of airplane accidents! People would not even consider flying any more. Most individuals would think of it as a form of suicide.

Smoking kills more Americans in a single year than those who died in battle during World War II and the Vietnam War combined. Think of the public outrage if 435,000 Americans were to die annually in a meaningless war. What if a single non-prescription drug were to cause more than 138,000 deaths from cancer and 120,000 fatal heart attacks each year? The U.S. public would not tolerate these situations. We would mount an intense fight to prevent the deaths.

Yet, are we not committing slow suicide by smoking cigarettes? Isn't tobacco a non-prescription drug available to almost anyone who wishes to smoke, killing more than 435,000 people each year? If cigarettes were invented today, the tobacco industry would be put on trial for mass murder.

Trends

The fight against all forms of tobacco use has been gaining momentum in the last few years. This was not always the case. It has been difficult to fight an industry that has the enormous financial and political influence of the tobacco industry in the United States. Tobacco is the sixth largest cash crop in the United States, producing 2.5 percent of the gross national product. The tobacco industry has influenced elections cleverly by emphasizing the individual's right to smoke, avoiding the fact that so many people die because of it.

Philip Morris, one of the largest tobacco-producing companies in the world, receives nearly 70 percent of its profits from the sale of cigarettes. Philip Morris has donated millions of dollars to prominent organizations, so they no longer question the detrimental effects of tobacco use. Among the organizations that have received donations from Philip Morris are United Way, YMCA, Salvation Army, Pediatric AIDS Foundation, Red Cross, Cystic Fibrosis Foundation, March of Dimes, Easter Seals, Muscular Dystrophy Association, Multiple Sclerosis Society, Hemophilia Foundation, United Cerebral Palsy, American Civil Liberties Union, American Bar Association, Task Force for Battered Women, Boy Scouts, Boys and Girls Club, and Big Brothers and Big Sisters. We call Colombian drug-runners unprincipled scum (responsible for about 19,100 illegal drug-related deaths per year), yet we welcome Philip Morris with glee and we call it civic pride.[12]

Tobacco was socially accepted for many years. In the 1980s, however, cigarette smoking no longer was acceptable in many social circles. Some locales outlawed smoking in public places as non-smokers and ex-smokers alike fought for their rights to clean air and health.

Many smokers are unaware of, or simply do not care to realize, how much cigarette smoke bothers non-smokers. Smokers sometimes think that blowing the smoke off to the side is enough to get it out of the way. As a matter of fact, it is not enough. Smokers do not comprehend this until they quit and later find themselves in that situation. Suddenly they realize why cigarette smoke is so unpleasant and undesirable to most people.

In recent years, the Food and Drug Administration (FDA) Drug Abuse Advisory Committee has taken a strong stance against the use of all forms of tobacco products. Although the American Heart Association (AHA) commends the work initiated by the FDA, the AHA has further stated that the FDA and the federal government have an obligation to take regulatory action against the national problem of nicotine addiction and abuse of cigarettes and tobacco products in general. In a statement before the FDA Drug Abuse Advisory Committee, the AHA indicated that "it is a national health travesty that a product (tobacco), which accounts for over 435,000 deaths in the U.S. each year, has escaped regulation under every major health and safety law enacted by Congress to protect the public health.[13]

A U.S. Surgeon General's report for the year 2000 on reducing tobacco use stated that health education combined with social, economic, and regulatory approaches is imperative to offset the tobacco industry's marketing and promotion and to promote non-smoking environments.[14]

Smokeless Tobacco

Smokeless tobacco often is promoted as a safe alternative to cigarette smoking. According to the Advisory Committee to the U.S. Surgeon General, smokeless tobacco represents a significant health risk and is just as addictive as cigarette smoking.

Unlike smoking, the use of smokeless tobacco has increased during the last 15 years. Currently, some 15 million Americans use tobacco in this form. The greatest concern is the increase in use of "spit" tobacco, especially by young people. More than 2 million people under age 25 use spit tobacco, including nearly 20 percent of all males in grades 9 through 13. One-third of those who use spit tobacco started at age 5, and the average starting age was 9. One can of spit tobacco contains 2.5 times as much nicotine as a similarly priced pack of cigarettes.

Using smokeless tobacco can lead to gingivitis and periodontitis. It carries a fourfold increase in oral cancer, and in some cases even premature death. People who chew or dip also have a higher rate of cavities, sore gums, bad breath, and stained teeth. Their senses of smell and taste diminish; consequently, they tend to add more sugar and salt to food. These practices alone increase the risk for being overweight and having high blood pressure.

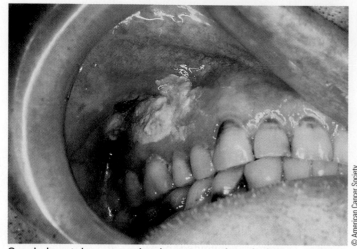

Smokeless tobacco can lead to gum and teeth damage as well as oral cancer (pictured).

Nicotine addiction and its related health risks also hold true for smokeless tobacco users. Nicotine blood levels approach those of cigarette smokers, increasing the risk for diseases of the cardiovascular system. Further, research has revealed changes in heart rate and blood pressure similar to those of cigarette smokers.

Using tobacco in any form can be addictive and poses a serious threat to health and well-being. Completely eliminating its use is the single most important lifestyle change a tobacco user can make to improve health, quality of life, and longevity.

Why People Smoke

People typically begin to smoke without realizing its detrimental effects on their health and life in general. Although people start to smoke for many different reasons, the three fundamental instigators are peer pressure, the desire to appear "grown up," and re-bellion against authority. Smoking only three packs of cigarettes can lead to physiological addiction, turning smoking into a nasty habit that has become the most widespread example of drug dependency in the United States.

Smoking Addiction and Dependency

The drug nicotine has strong addictive properties. Within seconds of inhalation, nicotine affects the central nervous system and can act simultaneously as a tranquilizer and a stimulant. The stimulating effect produces strong physiological and psychological dependency. The physical addiction to nicotine is 6 to 8 times more powerful than the addiction to alcohol, and most likely greater than that of some of the hard drugs currently used.

The psychological dependency develops over a longer time. People smoke to help themselves relax, and they also gain a certain amount of pleasure from the ritual of smoking. Smokers automatically associate many activities of daily life with cigarettes—typically, coffee drinking, alcohol drinking, being part of a social gathering, relaxing after a meal, talking on the telephone, driving, reading, and watching television. In many cases, the social rituals of smoking are the most difficult to eliminate. The dependency is so strong that years after people have stopped smoking, they may still crave cigarettes when they engage in certain social activities.

Most of the remaining information in this chapter is written directly to smokers. Non-smokers, however, will gain a better understanding of smokers by reading it. The following material also provides valuable information so you can help others implement a smoking cessation program.

"Why Do You Smoke?" Test

Most people smoke for a variety of reasons. To find out why people smoke, the National Clearinghouse for Smoking and Health developed the simple "Why Do You Smoke?" Test. This test, contained in Lab 13B, lists some statements by people, describing what they get out of smoking cigarettes. Smokers are asked to indicate how often they have the feelings described in each statement when they are smoking.

The scores obtained on this test assess smokers for each of six factors that describe people's feelings when they smoke. The first three highlight the positive feelings people derive from smoking. The fourth factor relates to reducing tension and relaxing. The fifth reveals the extent of dependence on cigarettes. The sixth factor differentiates habit smoking and purely automatic smoking. Each of the remaining factors fits one of the six reasons for smoking discussed next. A score of 11 or above on any factor indicates that smoking is an important source of satisfaction for you. The higher you score (15 is the highest), the more important a given factor is in your smoking and the more useful a discussion of that factor can be in your attempt to quit.

If you do not score high on any of the six factors, chances are that you do not smoke much or have not been smoking for very many years. If so, giving up smoking, and staying off, should be fairly easy.

1. *Stimulation.* If you score high or fairly high on the stimulation factor, you are one of those smokers who is stimulated by the cigarette. You think it helps wake you up, organize your energies, and keep you going. If you try to give up smoking, you may want a safe substitute—a

brisk walk or moderate exercise, for example—whenever you feel the urge to smoke.

2. *Handling.* Handling things can be satisfying, but you can keep your hands busy in many ways without lighting up or playing with a cigarette. Why not toy with a pen or pencil? Try doodling. Play with a coin, a piece of jewelry, or some other harmless object.

3. *Accentuation of pleasure/pleasurable relaxation.* Finding out whether you use the cigarette to feel good—get real, honest pleasure from smoking (Factor 3)—or to keep from feeling bad (Factor 4) is not always easy. About two-thirds of smokers score high or fairly high on accentuation of pleasure, and about half of those also score as high or higher on reduction of negative feelings. Those who do get real pleasure from smoking often find that honest consideration of the harmful effects of their habit is enough to help them quit. They substitute social and physical activities and find they do not seriously miss cigarettes.

4. *Reduction of negative feelings, or "a crutch."* Many smokers use cigarettes as a kind of crutch during moments of stress or discomfort. Ironically, the heavy smoker—the person who tries to handle severe personal problems by smoking many times a day—is apt to discover that cigarettes do not help deal with problems effectively. This kind of smoker may stop smoking readily when everything is going well but may be tempted to start again in a time of crisis. Again, physical exertion or social activity may be a useful substitute for cigarettes, especially in times of tension.

5. *Craving or dependence.* Quitting smoking is difficult for people who score high on this factor. The craving for a cigarette begins to build the moment the previous cigarette is put out, so tapering off is not likely to work. This smoker must go **cold turkey**. If you are dependent on cigarettes, you might try smoking more than usual for a day or two to spoil your taste for cigarettes, then isolating yourself completely from cigarettes until the craving is gone.

6. *Habit.* If you are smoking from habit, you no longer get much satisfaction from the cigarettes. You light them frequently without even realizing you are doing it. You may have an easy time quitting and staying off if you can break the habitual patterns you have built up. Cutting down gradually may be effective if you change the way you smoke cigarettes and the conditions under which you smoke them. The key to success is to become aware of each cigarette you smoke. You can do this by asking yourself, "Do I really want this cigarette?" You might be surprised at how many you do not want.

Smoking Cessation

If you are contemplating a smoking cessation program or are preparing to stop cigarette smoking, you need to know that quitting smoking is not easy. Annually, only about 20 percent of smokers who try to quit the first time succeed. The addictive properties of nicotine and smoke make quitting difficult.

The American Psychiatric Association and the National Institute on Drug Abuse have indicated that nicotine is perhaps the most addictive drug known to humans. The 1988 Surgeon General's Report on Nicotine Addiction concluded that[15]

■ Cigarettes and other forms of tobacco are addicting.
■ Nicotine is the drug responsible for the addictive behavior.
■ Pharmacologic and behavioral traits that determine addiction to tobacco are similar to those that determine addiction to drugs such as heroin and cocaine.

Smokers develop a tolerance to nicotine and tobacco smoke. They become dependent on both and get physical and psychological withdrawal symptoms when they stop smoking. Even though giving up smoking can be extremely difficult, it is by no means impossible, as attested by the many people who have quit.

During the last three decades, cigarette smoking in the United States has been declining gradually among smokers of all ages, with the exception of young women. Surveys have shown that between 75 and 90 percent of all smokers would like to quit. Forty percent of the adult population—53 percent of men and 32 percent of women—smoked in 1964 when the U.S. Surgeon General first reported the link between smoking and increased risk for disease and mortality. In 2003, only 25.8 percent of adult men and 21.6 percent of adult women smoked. More than 45 million Americans have given up cigarettes. More than 49 percent of all adults who have ever smoked have quit since 1964.

Further, more than 91 percent of successful ex-smokers have been able to do it on their own, either by quitting cold turkey or by using self-help kits available from

CRITICAL THINKING

You are in a designated non-smoking area and the person next to you lights up a cigarette. What can you say to this person to protect your right to clean air?

Cold turkey Eliminating a negative behavior all at once.

organizations such as the American Cancer Society, the American Heart Association, and the American Lung Association. Only 6.8 percent of ex-smokers have done so as a result of formal cessation programs. Smokers' information and treatment centers are listed in the Yellow Pages of the telephone book.

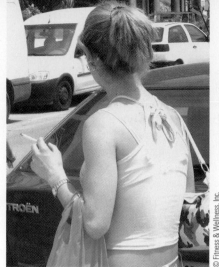

Cigarette smoking is the single largest preventable cause of illness and premature death in the United States.

"Do You Want To Quit?" Test

The most important factor in quitting cigarette smoking is the person's sincere desire to do so. Although a few smokers can simply quit, this is not usually the case. Those who can quit easily are primarily light or casual smokers. They realize that the pleasure of an occasional cigarette is not worth the added risk of disease and premature death. For heavy smokers, quitting most likely will be a difficult battle. Even though many do not succeed the first time around, the odds of quitting are much better for those who try to stop repeatedly.

If you are a smoker and want to find your readiness to quit, the "Do You Want To Quit?" test, developed by the National Clearinghouse for Smoking and Health and contained in Lab 13B, will measure your attitude toward the four primary reasons you want to quit smoking. The results give an indication of whether you are ready to start the program. On this test, the higher you score in any category, say, the Health category, the more important that reason is to you. A score of 9 or above in one of these categories indicates that this is one of the most important reasons you may want to quit.

1. *Health*. Knowing the harmful consequences of cigarettes, many people have stopped smoking and many others are considering doing so. If your score on the Health factor is 9 or above, the health hazards of smoking may be enough to make you want to quit now. If your score on this factor is low (6 or below), consider the hazards of smoking. You may be lacking important information or may even have incorrect information. If so, health considerations are not playing the role they should be in your decision to keep smoking or to quit.
2. *Example*. Some people stop smoking because they want to set a good example for others. Parents quit to make it easier for their children to resist starting to smoke. Doctors quit to be role models for their patients. Teachers quit to discourage their students from smoking. Sports stars want to set an example for their young fans. Husbands quit to influence their wives to quit, and vice versa. Examples have a significant influence on our behavior. Surveys show that almost twice as many high school students smoke if both parents are smokers, compared with those whose parents are non-smokers or former smokers.

If your score is low (6 or lower), you might not be interested in giving up smoking to set an example for others. Perhaps you do not realize how important your example could be.

3. *Aesthetics*. People who score high (9 or above) in this category recognize and are disturbed by some of the unpleasant aspects of smoking. The smell of stale smoke on their clothing, bad breath, and stains on their fingers and teeth might be reason enough to consider quitting.
4. *Mastery*. If you score 9 or above on this factor, you are bothered by knowing that you cannot control your desire to smoke. You are not your own master. Awareness of this challenge to your self-control may make you want to quit.

Breaking the Habit

The following seven-step plan has been developed as a guide to help you quit smoking. The total program should be completed in 4 weeks or less. Steps One through Four combined should take no longer than 2 weeks. A maximum of 2 additional weeks is allowed for the rest of the program.

STEP ONE

Decide positively that you want to quit. Avoid negative thoughts of how difficult this can be. Think positive. You can do it.

Now prepare a list of the reasons you smoke and why you want to quit (see Lab 13B, part IV). Make several copies of the list and keep them in places where you commonly smoke. Frequently review the reasons for quitting, because this will motivate and prepare you psychologically to quit.

When the reasons for quitting outweigh the reasons for smoking, you will have an easier time quitting. Read as much information as possible on the detrimental effects of tobacco and the benefits of quitting.

STEP TWO

Initiate a personal diet and exercise program. About one-third of the people who quit smoking gain weight. This could be caused by one or a combination of the following reasons:

1. Food becomes a substitute for cigarettes.
2. Appetite increases.
3. Basal metabolism may slow down.

If you start an exercise and weight-control program prior to quitting smoking, weight gain should not be a problem. If anything, exercise and lower body weight create more awareness of healthy living and strengthen the motivation for giving up cigarettes.

Even if you gain some weight, the harmful effects of cigarette smoking are much more detrimental to human health than a few extra pounds of body weight. Experts have indicated that, as far as the extra load on the heart is concerned, giving up one pack of cigarettes a day is the equivalent of losing between 50 and 75 pounds of excess body fat!

STEP THREE

Decide on the approach you will use to stop smoking. You may quit cold turkey or gradually cut down the number of cigarettes you smoke daily. Base your decision on your scores obtained on the "Why Do You Smoke?" Test. If you scored 11 points or higher in either the "Crutch: Tension Reduction" or the "Craving: Psychological Addiction" categories, your best chance for success is quitting cold turkey. If your highest scores occur in any of the other four categories, you may choose either approach.

People still argue about which approach is more effective. Quitting cold turkey may cause fewer withdrawal symptoms than tapering off gradually. When you are cutting down slowly, the fewer the cigarettes you smoke, the more important each one becomes. Therefore, you have a greater chance for relapse and returning to the original number of cigarettes smoked. But when the cutting-down approach is accompanied by a definite target date for quitting, the technique has been shown to be quite effective. Smokers who taper off without a target date for quitting are the most likely to relapse.

STEP FOUR

Keep a daily log of your smoking habit for a few days. This will help you understand the situations in which you smoke. To assist you in doing this, make copies of part V, Lab 13B, or develop your own form. Keep this form with you and, every time you smoke, record the required information. Keep track of the number of cigarettes you smoke, times of day you smoke them, events associated with smoking, amount of each cigarette smoked, and a

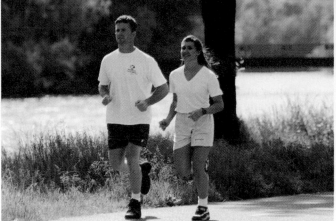

Starting an exercise program prior to giving up cigarettes encourages cessation and helps with weight control during the process.

rating of how badly you needed that cigarette. Rate each cigarette from 1 to 3:

1 means "desperately needed"
2 means "moderately needed"
3 means "no real need."

This daily log will assist you in three ways:

1. You will get to know your habit.
2. It will help you eliminate cigarettes you really do not crave.
3. It will help you find positive substitutes for situations that trigger your desire to smoke.

STEP FIVE

Set the target date for quitting. If you are going to taper off gradually, read the instructions under the "Cutting Down Gradually" discussion (see page 408) before you proceed to Step Six. When you set the target date, choose a special date to add a little extra incentive. An upcoming birthday, anniversary, vacation, graduation, family reunion—all are examples of good dates to free yourself from smoking. Dates when you are going to be away from events and environments that trigger your desire to smoke may be especially helpful. Once you have set the date, do not change it. Do not let anyone or anything interfere with this date.

Let your friends and relatives know of your intentions, and ask for their support. Consider asking someone else to quit with you. That way, you can support each other in your efforts to stop. Avoid anyone who will not support you in your effort to quit. When you are attempting to quit, other people can be a prime obstacle. Many smokers are intolerable when they first stop smoking, so some friends and relatives prefer that the person continue to smoke.

STEP SIX

Stock up on low-calorie foods—carrots, broccoli, cauliflower, celery, popcorn (butter- and salt-free), fruits, sunflower seeds (in the shell), sugarless gum—and drink plenty of water. Keep the food handy on the day you stop and the first few days following cessation. Substitute this food for a cigarette when you want one.

STEP SEVEN

On your quit day and the first few days thereafter, do not keep cigarettes handy. Stay away from friends and events that trigger your desire to smoke, and drink a lot of water and fruit juices. To replace the old behavior with new behavior, replace smoking time with new, positive substitutes that will make smoking difficult or impossible.

When you want a cigarette, take a few deep breaths and then occupy yourself by doing any of a number of things such as talking to someone else, washing your hands, brushing your teeth, eating a healthy snack, chewing on a straw, doing dishes, playing sports, going for a walk or a bike ride, going swimming, and so on. Engage in activities that require the use of your hands. Try gardening, sewing, writing letters, drawing, doing household chores, or washing the car. Visit non-smoking places such as libraries, museums, stores, and theaters. Plan an outing or a trip away from home. Any of these activities can keep your mind off cigarettes. Record your choice of activity or substitute under the Remarks/Substitutes column in part V of Lab 13B.

Quitting Cold Turkey

Many people have found that quitting all at once is the easiest way to do it. Most smokers have tried this approach at least once. Even though it might not work the first time, they do not allow themselves to get discouraged, and they eventually succeed. Many times after several attempts, all of a sudden they are able to overcome smoking without too much difficulty.

On the average, as few as three smokeless days are sufficient to break the physiological addiction to nicotine. The psychological addiction may linger for years but will get weaker as time goes by.

Cutting Down Gradually

Tapering off cigarettes can be done in several ways.

1. Eliminate cigarettes you do not strongly crave (those ranked numbers 3 and 2 on your daily log).
2. Switch to a brand lower in nicotine/tar every few days.
3. Smoke less of each cigarette.
4. Smoke fewer cigarettes each day.

Most people prefer a combination of these four suggestions.

Before you start cutting down, set a target date for quitting. Once the date is set, don't change it. The total time until your quit date should be no longer than 2 weeks. Reduce the total number of cigarettes you smoke each day by 10 to 25 percent. As you smoke less, be careful not to take more puffs or inhale more deeply as you smoke, because this would offset the principle of cutting down.

As an aid in tapering off, make several copies of Part V, Lab 13B. (By now you should have already completed the first daily log of your smoking habit—see Step Four under "Breaking the Habit" on page 407.) Start a new daily log, and every night review your data and set goals for the following day.

Decide and record which cigarettes will be easiest to give up, what brand you will smoke, the total number of cigarettes to be smoked, and how much of each you will smoke. Log any comments or situations you want to avoid, as well as any substitutes you could use to help you in the program. For example, if you always smoke while drinking coffee, substitute juice for coffee. If you smoke while driving, arrange for a ride or take a bus to work. If you smoke with a certain friend at lunch, avoid having lunch with that friend for a week or so. Continue using this log until you have stopped smoking completely.

Nicotine Substitution Products

Nicotine substitution drug products such as nicotine transdermal patches and nicotine gum have been developed to help people kick the tobacco habit. These products are most effective when they are used in a physician-supervised cessation program. As with tapering off, these products gradually decrease the amount of nicotine used until the person no longer craves the drug.

Nicotine patches supply a steady dose of nicotine through the skin. These patches are available in various dosages, delivering anywhere from about 5 to 21 mg of nicotine in a 24-hour period. A typical program lasts between 3 and 10 weeks, with an average weekly cost to the consumer of about $35. Sales of nicotine patches approximate $1 billion per year.

Public safety concerns regarding the use of nicotine patches, including indications, precautions, warnings, contraindications, potential abuse, and marketing and labeling issues are monitored and regulated by the FDA. People contemplating their use should pay careful attention to contraindications and potential side effects. Pregnant and lactating women and people with heart disease, high blood pressure, or who have had a recent heart attack should check with their physician prior to using nicotine substitution products. Skin redness, swelling, or rashes are sometimes associated with the use of nicotine patches. Other undesirable side effects are listed on the label and should be monitored closely.

Life After Cigarettes

When you first quit smoking, you can expect a series of withdrawal symptoms during the first few days; among them are lower heart rate and blood pressure, headaches, gastrointestinal discomfort, mood changes, irritability, aggressiveness, and difficulty sleeping.

The physiological addiction to nicotine is broken only 3 days following your last cigarette. Thereafter, you should not crave cigarettes as much. For the habitual smoker, the psychological dependency could be the most difficult to break. The first few days probably will not be as difficult as the first few months. Any of the activities of daily life that have been associated with smoking—either stress or relaxation, joy or unhappiness—may trigger a relapse even months, or at times years, after quitting.

Ex-smokers should realize that, even though some harm may have been done already, it is never too late to quit. The greatest early benefit is a lower risk for sudden death. Furthermore, the risk for illness starts to decrease the moment you stop smoking. You will have fewer sore throats and sores in the mouth, less hoarseness, no more cigarette cough, and lower risk for peptic ulcers.

Circulation to the hands and feet will improve, as will gastrointestinal and kidney and bladder functions. Everything will taste and smell better. You will have more energy, and you will gain a sense of freedom, pride, and well-being. You no longer will have to worry whether you have enough cigarettes to last through a day, a party, a meeting, a weekend, a trip.

When you first quit and you think how tough it is and how miserable you feel because you cannot have a cigarette, try the opposite: Think of the benefits and how great it is not to smoke! The ex-smoker's risk

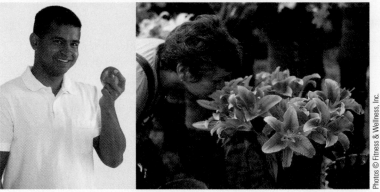

The simple pleasures of life, such as taste and smell, improve with smoking cessation.

for heart disease approaches that of a lifetime non-smoker 10 years following cessation, and for cancer, 15 years after cessation.

If you have been successful and stopped smoking, a lot of events can still trigger your urge to smoke. When confronted with these events, some people rationalize and think, "One cigarette won't hurt. I've been off for months (years in some cases)" or, "I can handle it. I'll smoke just today." It won't work! Before you know it, you will be back to the regular nasty habit. Be prepared to take action in those situations by finding substitutes such as those provided in the "Tips to Help Stop Smoking" (Figure 13.5).

Start thinking of yourself as a non-smoker—no "butts" about it. Remind yourself how difficult it has been and how long it has taken you to get to this point. If you have come this far, you certainly can resist brief moments of temptation. It will get easier rather than harder as time goes on.

CRITICAL THINKING

If you ever smoked or now smoke cigarettes, discuss your perceptions of how others accepted your behavior. If you smoked and have quit, how did you accomplish the task and has it changed the way you are viewed by others? If you never smoked, how do perceive smokers?

FIGURE 13.5 Tips to help stop smoking.

The following are different ways smokers retrained themselves to live without cigarettes. Any one or several of these methods in combination might be helpful to you. Check the ones you like and, from these, develop your own retraining program.

☐ Before you quit smoking, try wrapping your cigarettes with a sheet of paper like a Christmas present. Every time you want a cigarette, unwrap the pack and write down what you are doing, how you feel, and how important this cigarette is to you. Do this for 2 weeks and you'll have cut down as well as developed new insights into your smoking.

☐ If cigarettes give you an energy boost, try gum, modest exercise, a brisk walk, or a new hobby. Avoid eating new foods that are high in calories.

☐ If cigarettes help you relax, try eating, drinking new beverages, or joining social activities within reasonable bounds.

(continued)

FIGURE 13.5 (Continued)

- [ ] Try smoking an excess of cigarettes for a day or two before you quit so the taste of cigarettes is spoiled. Another opportune time to quit is when you are ill with a cold or flu and have lost your taste for cigarettes.

- [ ] On a 3" × 5" card, list what you like and dislike about smoking. Add to it and read it daily.

- [ ] Make up a short list of luxuries you have wanted or items you would like to purchase for a loved one. Next to each item, write down the cost. Now convert the cost to "packs of cigarettes." If you save the money each day from packs of cigarettes, you will be able to purchase these items. Use a special "piggy bank" for saving your money, or start a "Christmas Club" account at your bank.

- [ ] Don't smoke after you get a craving for a cigarette until 3 minutes have passed since you got the urge. During those 3 minutes, change your thinking or activity.

- [ ] Telephone an ex-smoker or somebody you can talk to until the craving subsides.

- [ ] Plan a memorable day for stopping. You might choose your vacation, New Year's Day, your birthday, a holiday, the birthday of your child, your anniversary. But don't make the date so distant that you lose momentum.

- [ ] If you smoke under stress at work, pick a date for stopping when you will be away from your work.

- [ ] Decide whether you are going to stop suddenly or gradually. If it is to be gradual, work out a tapering system so you have intermediate goals.

- [ ] Don't store cigarettes. Never buy a carton. Wait until one pack is finished before you buy another.

- [ ] Never carry cigarettes with you at home or at work. Keep your cigarettes as far from you as possible. Leave them with someone or lock them up.

- [ ] Until you quit, make yourself a "smoking corner" that is far from anything interesting. If you like to smoke with others, always smoke alone. If you like to smoke alone, always smoke with others, preferably if they are nonsmokers. Never smoke while watching television.

- [ ] Never carry matches or a lighter with you.

- [ ] Put away your ashtrays or fill them with objects so they cannot be used for ashes. Plant flowers in them or fill them with walnuts. The latter will give you something to do with your hands.

- [ ] Change your brand of cigarettes weekly so you always are smoking a brand of lower tar and nicotine content than the week before.

- [ ] Never say, "I quit smoking," because your resolution is broken if you have a cigarette. Better to say, "I don't want to smoke." This way you maintain your resolution even if you accidentally have a cigarette.

- [ ] Try to help someone else quit smoking, particularly your mate.

- [ ] Always ask yourself, "Do I need this cigarette or is this just a reflex?"

- [ ] Each day try to put off lighting your first cigarette.

- [ ] Decide arbitrarily that you will smoke only on even- or odd-numbered hours of the clock.

- [ ] Try going to bed early and rising a half hour earlier than usual to avoid hurrying through breakfast and rushing to work.

- [ ] Keep your hands occupied. Try playing a musical instrument, knitting, or fiddling with hand puzzles.

- [ ] Take a shower. You cannot smoke in the shower.

- [ ] Brush your teeth frequently to get rid of the tobacco taste and stains.

- [ ] If you have a sudden craving for a cigarette, take 10 deep breaths, holding the last breath while you strike a match. Exhale slowly, blowing out the match. Pretend the match was a cigarette by crushing it out in an ashtray. Now immediately get busy on some work or activity.

- [ ] Smoke only half a cigarette.

- [ ] After you quit, start using your lungs. Increase your activities and indulge in moderate exercise, such as short walks before or after a meal.

- [ ] Bet with someone that you can quit. Put the cigarette money in a jar each morning and forfeit it if you smoke. Keep the money if you don't smoke by the end of the week. Try to extend this period for a month.

- [ ] If you gain weight because you are not smoking, wait until you get over the craving before you diet. Dieting is easier then.

- [ ] If you are depressed or have physical symptoms that might be related to your smoking, relieve your mind by discussing this with your physician. It is easier to quit when you know your health status.

- [ ] After you quit, visit your dentist and have your teeth cleaned to get rid of the tobacco stains.

- [ ] If the cost of cigarettes is your motivation for quitting, purchase a money order equivalent to a year's supply of cigarettes. Give it to a friend. If you smoke in the next year, he or she cashes the money order and keeps the money. If you don't smoke, he or she gives back the money order at the end of the year.

- [ ] After you quit, redirect the temptation to smoke by calling or visiting someone.

- [ ] When you feel irritable or tense, shut your eyes and count backward from ten to zero as you imagine yourself descending a flight of stairs, or imagine that you are looking at the horizon as the sun sets in the west.

- [ ] Get out of your old habits. Seek new activities or perform old activities in a new way. Don't rely on the old ways of solving problems. Do things differently.

- [ ] If you are a "kitchen smoker" in the morning, volunteer your services to a school or nonprofit organization to get you out of the house.

- [ ] Stock up on light reading materials, crossword puzzles, and vacation brochures that you can read during your coffee breaks.

- [ ] Frequent places where you can't smoke, such as libraries, buses, theaters, swimming pools, department stores.

- [ ] Give yourself time to think and get fit by walking one-half hour each day. If you have a dog, take it for a walk with you.

Excerpted from *TIPS*, American Cancer Society, Texas Division.

rofile
lus

ing the
ssess Your
owledge"
d "Practice
izzes" op-
ns on your
)-ROM,
aluate how
ell you
derstand
e concepts
esented in
s chapter.

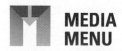

ASSESS YOUR KNOWLEDGE

1. The following is *not* a form of chemical dependency.
   a. Ecstasy
   b. alcohol
   c. cocaine
   d. heroin
   e. All are objects of chemical dependency.

2. The most widely used illegal drug in the United States is
   a. marijuana.
   b. alcohol.
   c. cocaine.
   d. heroine.
   e. Ecstasy.

3. Cocaine use
   a. causes lung cancer.
   b. leads to atrophy of the brain.
   c. can lead to sudden death.
   d. causes amotivational syndrome.
   e. All these things are possible.

4. Methamphetamine
   a. is less potent than amphetamine.
   b. increases fatigue.
   c. helps a person relax.
   d. is a central nervous system stimulant.
   e. increases the need for sleep.

5. Ecstasy
   a. is popular among middle-age people.
   b. is a relatively harmless drug.
   c. is used primarily by African American males.
   d. increases heart rate and blood pressure.
   e. All are correct choices.

6. Treatment of chemical dependency is
   a. accomplished primarily by the individual alone.
   b. most successful when there is peer pressure to stop.
   c. best achieved with the help of family members.
   d. seldom accomplished without professional guidance.
   e. usually done with the help of friends.

7. Cigarette smoking is responsible for about _____ unnecessary deaths in the United States each year.
   a. 10,000
   b. 80,000
   c. 250,000
   d. 435,000
   e. 1,000,000

8. Cigarette smoking increases death rates from
   a. heart disease.
   b. cancer.
   c. stroke.
   d. aortic aneurysm.
   e. all of the above.

9. The percentage of lung cancer attributed to cigarette smoking is
   a. 25 percent.
   b. 43 percent.
   c. 58 percent.
   d. 64 percent.
   e. 87 percent.

10. Following smoking cessation
    a. there is a decrease in sore throats.
    b. gastrointestinal function improves.
    c. there is a decrease in risk of sudden death.
    d. foods taste better.
    e. all of these changes occur.

Correct answers can be found at the back of the book.

MEDIA MENU

PROFILE PLUS CD CONNECTIONS

■ Find out if you're prone to addictive behavior.

■ Plan for a smoke-free future.

■ Check how well you understand the chapter's concepts.

INTERNET CONNECTIONS

■ National Institute on Alcohol Abuse and Alcoholism. This site, sponsored by the U.S. government, features information on research and education related to alcohol use and abuse.
   http://www.niaaa.nih.gov

■ CDC Page on Smoking and Health: Tobacco Information and Prevention Source. A comprehensive site featuring educational information, research, reports from the U.S. Surgeon General, tips on how to quit, and much more.
   http://www.cdc.gov/tobacco

■ NIDA Drug Pages. From the National Institute of Drug Abuse, this site features information about a comprehensive list of drugs, including alcohol, nicotine, marijuana, cocaine, ecstasy, amphetamines, steroids, prescription medications, and more. The site also features an excellent chart listing the common drugs of abuse according to category, examples of commercial and street names, as well as intoxication effects and potential health consequences.
   http://www.nida.nih.gov/Drugpages
   http://www.edc.org/hec/pubs/binge.htm

■ Facts On Tap: Alcohol and Your College Experience. This excellent site is geared to college students, featuring links to the following topics, and more: Risky Relationship: Alcohol and Sex, College Experience: Alcohol and Student Life, The Naked Truth: Alcohol and Your Body, and When Someone Else's Drinking Gives You a Hangover.
   http://www.factsontap.org

Notes

1. W. W. K. Hoeger, L. W. Turner, and B. Q. Hafen, *Wellness: Guidelines for a Healthy Lifestyle* (Belmont, CA: Wadsworth/Thomson Learning, 2002).

2. R. Goldberg, *Drugs Across the Spectrum* (Belmont, CA: Wadsworth/Thomson Learning, 2003).

3. See note 2.

4. C. A. Presley, J. S. Leichliter, and P. W. Meilman, *Alcohol and Drugs on American College Campuses: Findings from 1995, 1996, and 1997 (A Report to College Presidents)* (Carbondale, IL: Southern Illinois University, 1999).

5. *National Drug Control Strategy* (Washington, DC: U.S. Government Printing Office, 1998).

6. *Join Together: Results of the Fourth National Survey on Community Efforts to Reduce Substance Abuse and Gun Violence* (Boston: Join Together, 1999).

7. U.S. Department of Agriculture, *Tobacco Outlook Report.* (Washington DC: U.S. Department of Agriculture, Market and Trade Economics Division, Economic Research Service, 2004).

8. American Cancer Society, *Cancer Facts & Figures—2002* (New York: ACS, 2002).

9. S. A. Glantz and W. W. Parmley, "Passive Smoking and Heart Disease," *Journal of the American Medical Association* 273 (1995): 1047–1053.

10. See note 8.

11. "Wellness Facts," *University of California Berkeley Wellness Letter* 14 (1998): 1.

12. American Cancer Society, *World Smoking & Health* (Atlanta: ACS, 1993).

13. American Heart Association, *AHA Public Affairs/Coalition on Smoking: Health Position* (Dallas: AHA, 1996).

14. U.S. Department of Health and Human Services, *Reducing Tobacco Use: A Report of the Surgeon General* (Atlanta: U.S. Department of Health and Human Services; Centers for Disease Control and Prevention, National Center for Chronic Disease Prevention and Health Promotion, Office on Smoking and Health, 2000).

15. U.S. Department of Health and Human Services, *Nicotine Addiction, A Report of the Surgeon General* (Atlanta: U.S. Department of Health and Human Services, Centers for Disease Control and Prevention, National Center for Chronic Disease Prevention and Health Promotion, 1988).

Suggested Readings

American Cancer Society. *2002 Cancer Facts & Figures*. New York: ACS, 2002.

Doweiko, H. E. *Concepts of Chemical Dependence*. Pacific Grove, CA: Brooks/Cole, 2002.

Goldberg, R. *Drugs Across the Spectrum*. Belmont, CA: Wadsworth/Thomson Learning, 2002.

U.S. Public Health Service. *Why People Smoke Cigarettes*. Rockville, MD: U.S. Department of Health and Human Services, 1982.

U.S. Public Health Service. *A Self-Test for Smokers*. Rockville, MD: U.S. Department of Health and Human Services, 1983.

U.S. Public Health Service. *Chronic Obstructive Lung Disease: A Report of the Surgeon General*. Rockville, MD: U.S. Department of Health and Human Services, 1984.

U.S. Office on Smoking and Health. *Smoking and Health: A Report of the Surgeon General*. Washington, DC: U.S. Department of Health, Education and Welfare, 1979.

Lab 13A

ADDICTIVE BEHAVIOR QUESTIONNAIRES

Name: _____ Date: _____ Grade: _____

Instructor: _____ Course: _____ Section: _____

Necessary Lab Equipment

None required.

Objective

To determine possible addictive behavior.

Instruction

The following questionnaires are for your own personal information. Answer all questions on a separate sheet of paper and keep that sheet for yourself. Turn in only this page to your instructor as proof that you have read and completed the questionnaire. If you wish to do so, you may personally discuss the results of these questionnaires with your course instructor.

Stage of Change for Addictive Behavior

If chemical dependency is a problem in your life, use Figure 2.4 (page 41) and Table 2.3 (page 41) to identify your current stage of change for participation in a treatment program for addictive behavior.

I. Addictive Behavior: Could You Be An Addict?

The following test, designed by Dr. Lawrence J. Hatterer, is not a way to diagnose whether you are in the early, middle, or chronic stage of addictive disease. It is merely meant to help you understand addictive behavior better so you can recognize it in yourself or perhaps in people you know.

1. I am a person of excesses. I can't regulate what I do for pleasure and often use a substance or indulge in an activity heavily, in order to get high.

2. I am an extremely self-involved person. People tell me that I am into myself too much.

3. I am compulsive. I must have what I want when I want it, regardless of the consequences.

4. I am excessively dependent on or independent of others.

5. I am preoccupied. I spend a lot of time thinking or fantasizing about a particular activity or substance. Also, I will work my day around doing it or go to pains to make sure it's available.

6. I deny that I do this and lie about it when others ask me.

7. I have been involved in this behavior for at least 1 year.

8. I've told myself I could easily stop, even though I've shown no signs of slowing down.

9. Once I start indulging in this behavior or substance, I find I have trouble stopping.

10. One or more members of my family are also involved in some kind of excessive behavior or substance abuse.

11. I find I gravitate mostly toward people who have the same behavior or take the same substance as I.

12. I seem to be developing a tolerance of the behavior or substance. I have had a need to steadily increase the amounts I take or the time I spend doing it.

13. I have found that my excessive use of highs has, in fact, only made my problems worse.

14. If someone tries to keep me from obtaining the substance or practicing the activity, I get angry and reject or abuse them.

15. I experience withdrawal symptoms if I cannot indulge in the substance or activity.

16. This has gotten in the way of my functioning. I have missed something important—days at work or time with my friends, family, or children—because of it.

17. The substance/activity is destroying my home life. I know I am hurting those closest to me.

18. I have failed in many goals in life, lost money, given up many social and occupational contacts, all because of my excessive behavior.

19. I have tried to stop or cut down on my excesses but have been unsuccessful.

20. I have physically endangered myself or others in accidents that were a direct result of my excessive behavior.

How To Score

If you answer "yes" to half or more of the questions, you may have a problem with addictive disease and should seek immediate professional help. For a referral, contact your local mental health clinic (look in the Yellow Pages) or speak to your doctor.

From *McCall's Magazine*, November 1986.

II. Alcohol Abuse: Are You Drinking Too Much?

Using a separate sheet of paper, specifically indicate the steps that you are going to take to correct addictive behavior(s) and identify people or organizations that you will contact to help you get started.

1. When you are holding an empty glass at a party, do you always actively look for a refill instead of waiting to be offered one?
2. If given the chance, do you frequently pour out a more generous drink for yourself than seems to be the "going" amount for others?
3. Do you often have a drink or two when you are alone, either at home or in a bar?
4. Is your drinking ever the direct cause of a family quarrel, or do quarrels often seem to occur, if only by coincidence, after you have had a drink or two?
5. Do you feel that you must have a drink at a specific time every day—right after work, for instance?
6. When worried or under unusual stress, do you almost automatically take a stiff drink to "settle your nerves"?
7. Are you untruthful about how much you have had to drink when questioned on the subject?
8. Does drinking ever cause you to take time off work or to miss scheduled meetings or appointments?
9. Do you feel physically deprived if you cannot have at least one drink every day?
10. Do you sometimes crave a drink in the morning?
11. Do you sometimes have "mornings after" when you cannot remember what happened the night before?

How to Score

You should regard a "yes" answer to any one of the above questions as a warning sign. Do not increase your consumption of alcohol. Two "yes" answers suggest that you already may be becoming dependent on alcohol. Three or more "yes" answers indicate that you may have a serious problem and you should get professional help. Also refer to pages 399–400 for general guidelines to cut down your drinking.

From *American Medical Association Family Medical Guide* by The American Medical Association. Copyright © 1982 by The American Medical Association. Used by permission of Random House, Inc.

III. Changing Addictive Behavior

Using a separate sheet of paper, specifically indicate the steps that you are going to take to correct addictive behavior(s) and identify people or organizations that you will contact to help you get started.

Lab 13B

SMOKING CESSATION QUESTIONNAIRES

Name: _____ Date: _____ Grade: _____

Instructor: _____ Course: _____ Section: _____

Necessary Lab Equipment
None required.

Objective
To develop a smoking cessation program either for yourself or for friends and relatives.

I. Introduction

The forms provided in this lab have been designed to help smokers identify reasons why they smoke and their readiness to initiate a smoking cessation program. These forms should be filled out prior to initiating a smoking cessation program. Interpretation of the results are given in this chapter (pages 404–406). The daily cigarette smoking log, Part V of this lab, has been developed to help smokers get to know their habit, cut down on cigarettes not really needed, and find positive substitutes when confronted with situations that trigger their desire to smoke.

II. "Why Do You Smoke?" Test

	Always	Fre-quently	Occa-sionally	Seldom	Never
A. I smoke cigarettes to keep myself from slowing down.	5	4	3	2	1
B. Handling a cigarette is part of the enjoyment of smoking it.	5	4	3	2	1
C. Smoking cigarettes is pleasant and relaxing.	5	4	3	2	1
D. I light up a cigarette when I feel angry about something.	5	4	3	2	1
E. When I have run out of cigarettes, I find it almost unbearable until I can get them.	5	4	3	2	1
F. I smoke cigarettes automatically without even being aware of it.	5	4	3	2	1
G. I smoke cigarettes for stimulation, to perk myself up.	5	4	3	2	1
H. Part of the enjoyment of smoking a cigarette comes from the steps I take to light up.	5	4	3	2	1
I. I find cigarettes pleasurable.	5	4	3	2	1
J. When I feel uncomfortable or upset about something, I light up a cigarette.	5	4	3	2	1
K. I am very much aware of the fact when I am not smoking a cigarette.	5	4	3	2	1
L. I light up a cigarette without realizing I still have one burning in the ashtray.	5	4	3	2	1
M. I smoke cigarettes to give me a "lift."	5	4	3	2	1
N. When I smoke a cigarette, part of the enjoyment is watching the smoke as I exhale it.	5	4	3	2	1
O. I want a cigarette most when I am comfortable and relaxed.	5	4	3	2	1
P. When I feel "blue" or want to take my mind off cares and worries, I smoke cigarettes.	5	4	3	2	1
Q. I get a real gnawing hunger for a cigarette when I haven't smoked for a while.	5	4	3	2	1
R. I've found a cigarette in my mouth and didn't remember putting it there.	5	4	3	2	1

How to Score: (See pages 404–405 to interpret your test results.)

Enter the numbers you have circled on the test questions in the spaces provided below, putting the number you have circled to question A on line A, to question B on line B, and so on. Add the three scores on each line to get a total for each factor. For example, the sum of your scores over lines A, G, and M gives you your score on "Stimulation"; lines B, H, and N give the score on "Handling." Scores can vary from 3 to 15. Any score 11 and above is high; any score 7 and below is low.

A ____	+ G ____	+ M ____	= ____	Stimulation
B ____	+ H ____	+ N ____	= ____	Handling
C ____	+ I ____	+ O ____	= ____	Pleasure/Relaxation
D ____	+ J ____	+ P ____	= ____	Crutch: Tension Reduction
E ____	+ K ____	+ Q ____	= ____	Craving: Psychological Addiction
F ____	+ L ____	+ R ____	= ____	Habit

From *A Self-Test for Smokers*, U.S. Department of Health and Human Services, 1983.

III. "Do You Want to Quit?" Test

	Strongly Agree	Mildly Agree	Mildly Disagree	Strongly Disagree
A. Cigarette smoking might give me a serious illness.	4	3	2	1
B. My cigarette smoking sets a bad example for others.	4	3	2	1
C. I find cigarette smoking to be a messy kind of habit.	4	3	2	1
D. Controlling my cigarette smoking is a challenge to me.	4	3	2	1
E. Smoking causes shortness of breath.	4	3	2	1
F. If I quit smoking cigarettes, it might influence others to stop.	4	3	2	1
G. Cigarettes cause damage to clothing and other personal property.	4	3	2	1
H. Quitting smoking would show that I have willpower.	4	3	2	1
I. My cigarette smoking will have a harmful effect on my health.	4	3	2	1
J. My cigarette smoking influences others close to me to take up or continue smoking.	4	3	2	1
K. If I quit smoking, my sense of taste or smell will improve.	4	3	2	1
L. I do not like the idea of feeling dependent on smoking.	4	3	2	1

How to Score (See page 406 to interpret your test results.)

Write the number you have circled after each statement on the test in the corresponding space to the right. Add the scores on each line to get your totals. For example, the sum of your scores A, E, and I gives you your score for the Health factor. Scores can vary from 3 to 12. Any score of 9 or over is high; any score 6 or under is low.

A		+ E		+ I		=		Health
B		+ F		+ J		=		Example
C		+ G		+ K		=		Aesthetics
D		+ H		+ L		=		Mastery

From *A Self-Test for Smokers*, U.S. Department of Health and Human Services, 1983.

IV. Reasons to Smoke, Reasons to Quit

Reasons to Smoke Cigarettes

1. _____
2. _____
3. _____
4. _____
5. _____

Reasons to Quit Cigarette Smoking

1. _____
2. _____
3. _____
4. _____
5. _____

V. Daily Cigarette Smoking Log

Today's Date: _____   Quit Date: _____   Decision Date: _____

Cigarettes to be smoked today: _____   Brand: _____

No.	Time	Activity	Rating[a]	Amount Smoked[b]	Remarks/Substitutes
1.					
2.					
3.					
4.					
5.					
6.					
7.					
8.					
9.					
10.					
11.					
12.					
13.					
14.					
15.					
16.					
17.					
18.					
19.					
20.					

[a]Rating: 1 = desperately needed, 2 = moderately needed, 3 = no real need
[b]Amount Smoked: entire cigarette, two-thirds, half, etc.

Additional comments, list of friends and/or activities to avoid.

_____

_____

_____

_____

_____

VI. Conclusion

In a few sentences, indicate your feelings about cigarette smoking and what you have learned from the previous questionnaires.

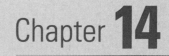

Chapter **14**

Preventing Sexually Transmitted Diseases

Objectives

- Name and describe the most common sexually transmitted diseases.
- Outline the health consequences of sexually transmitted diseases.
- Define the difference between HIV and AIDS.
- Explain the seriousness of the AIDS epidemic in the United States and worldwide.
- Describe ways to prevent acquiring sexually transmitted diseases.

Profile Plus CD Connections

- Evaluate your risk of HIV/AIDS.
- Check how well you understand the chapter's concepts.

Sexually transmitted diseases (STDs) have reached epidemic proportions in the United States. Of the more than 25 known STDs, some are still incurable. The American Social Health Association stated that 25 percent of all Americans will acquire at least one STD in their lifetime. Each year, more than 19 million people in the United States are newly infected with STDs, and almost half of them are seen in young people between the ages of 15 and 24.[1]

Based on estimates by the World Health Organization, 1 million people worldwide are infected daily with STDs not including HIV. These infections include more than 4 million cases of chlamydia, 800,000 cases of gonorrhea, between one-half and 1 million cases of genital warts, half a million cases of herpes, and nearly 15,000 cases of syphilis. Attracting most of the attention because of its life-threatening potential is HIV infection, which leads to AIDS.

Following are brief descriptions of the leading STDs, their symptoms, and their treatment (if any).

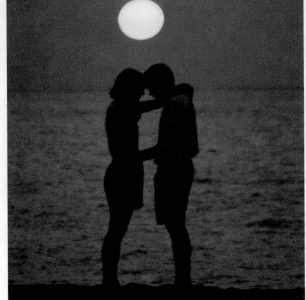

More than 25 diseases are spread through sexual contact. About 1 in 4 adults in the United States has a sexually transmitted disease.

Chlamydia

Chlamydia is a bacterial infection that spreads during vaginal, anal, or oral sex, or from the vagina to a newborn baby during childbirth. Chlamydia can damage the reproductive system seriously. This disease is considered to be a major factor in male and female infertility. Because it may have no symptoms, three of four people with the disease don't know they're ill until the infection has become quite serious. Each year there are 2.8 million new cases of chlamydia in the United States.[2] Furthermore, according to the U.S. Centers for Disease Control and Prevention (CDC), 15- to 19-year-old girls represent 46 percent of infections and 20- to 24-year-old women represent another 33 percent.[3]

When symptoms are present, they tend to mimic other STDs, so the disease can be mistreated. Symptoms of serious infection include abdominal pain, fever, nausea, vaginal bleeding, and arthritis. Although chlamydia can be treated successfully with oral antibiotics, its damage to the reproductive system is irreversible. Regular testing for chlamydia is recommended for all sexually active women under the age of 25, for older women with multiple sexual partners and/or previous STDs, and for those who do not regularly use condoms.[4]

Gonorrhea

One of the oldest STDs, **gonorrhea** is caused by a bacterial infection. Gonorrhea is transmitted through vaginal, anal, and oral sex. Approximately 650,000 new cases are seen each year in the United States.

Typical symptoms in men include a pus-like secretion from the penis and painful urination. Infected women also may have discharge and painful urination. Up to 80 percent of infected women, however, don't experience any symptoms until the infection has become fairly serious. At this stage, women develop fever, severe abdominal pain, and pelvic inflammatory disease (discussed next).

If untreated, gonorrhea can produce widespread bacterial infection, infertility, heart damage, and arthritis in men and women, and blindness in children born to infected women. Gonorrhea is treated successfully with penicillin and other antibiotics.

Pelvic Inflammatory Disease

Each year about 1 million women in the United States develop a condition known by the umbrella term **pelvic inflammatory disease (PID).**[5] PID is not truly an STD but, rather, refers to complications resulting from chlamydia or gonorrhea infection. PID often develops when the STD spreads to the fallopian tubes, uterus, and ovaries.

Complications associated with PID typically include scarring and obstruction of the fallopian tubes (which may lead to infertility), ectopic pregnancies, and chronic pelvic pain. If a woman with PID becomes pregnant, she could have an ectopic (tubal) pregnancy, which destroys the embryo and can kill the woman.

Typical symptoms of PID are fever, nausea, vomiting, chills, spotting between menstrual periods, heavy bleeding during periods, and pain in the lower abdomen during sexual intercourse, between menstrual periods, or during urination. Many times, however, women do not know they have PID because these symptoms are not always present.

PID is treated with antibiotics, bed rest, and sexual abstinence. Further, surgery may be required to remove infected or scarred tissue or to repair or remove the fallopian tubes or uterus.

Human Papillomavirus and Genital Warts

Human papillomavirus (HPV) is one of the most common causes of sexually transmitted infection.

There are more than 100 types of HPV, and though most of them are harmless, some cause **genital warts**. Approximately 5.5 million new cases of HPV are reported each year, and at least 20 million Americans are infected with the virus.

Genital warts show up anywhere from 1 to 8 months after exposure. These warts may be flat or raised and usually are found on the penis or around the vulva and the vagina. They also can appear in the mouth, throat, rectum, on the cervix, or around the anus.

Based on data from the CDC, as many as one million new cases of genital warts are diagnosed in the United States each year. In some cities, nearly half of all sexually active teenagers have genital warts. Similar to chlamydia, the virus is spread through vaginal, anal, or oral sex, or from the vagina to a newborn baby.

Health problems associated with genital warts include increased risk for cancers of the cervix, vulva, and penis, and enlargement and spread of the warts, leading to obstruction of the urethra, vagina, and anus. Because babies born to infected mothers commonly develop warts over their bodies, Cesarean section is recommended for childbirth.

Treatment requires completely removing all warts. This can be done by freezing them with liquid nitrogen, dissolving them with chemicals, or removing them through electrosurgery or laser surgery. Infected patients may have to be treated more than once, because genital warts can recur.

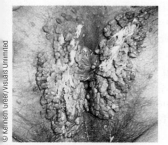

An advanced case of genital warts on the female.

Genital Herpes

One of the most common STDs, **genital herpes** is caused by the herpes simplex virus (HSV). The several types of HSV produce different ailments, including genital herpes, oral (lip) herpes, shingles, and chicken pox. The two most common forms of HSV are Types I and II. In Type I—the HSV most often known to cause oral herpes—cold sores or fever blisters appear on the lips and mouth.

Approximately 135 million Americans over the age of 12 carry HSV Type I.[6] HSV Type II is better known as the virus that causes genital herpes. About 20 percent of the population over the age of 12, or 45 million people, are infected with HSV Type II, and more than 1 million new cases are diagnosed each year.

HSV is a highly contagious virus. Victims are most contagious during an outbreak, and HSV spreads by contact with an active sore. The disease can also be spread through virus-containing secretions from the vagina or penis. A few days following infection, sores appear on the infected areas, most notably the mouth, genitals, and rectum, but can also surface on other parts of the body.

In conjunction with the sores, victims usually have mild fever, swollen glands, and headaches. The symptoms usually disappear within a few weeks, causing some people to believe they are cured. Presently, though, herpes is incurable, and its victims remain infected. The virus can remain dormant for extended periods, but repeated outbreaks are common. Excessive stress and illness can precipitate new outbreaks.

HSV Types I and II both can cause oral and genital sores. People who have an outbreak of oral herpes should not touch their genitals or someone else's after touching the oral cold sores, as doing so can lead to herpes infection of the genitals. Oral sex can result in transmission of HSV from the lips to the genitals, and vice versa. People with cold sores on the lips or mouth should take care not to touch these sores. Following contact with cold or herpes

Sexually transmitted diseases (STDs) Communicable diseases spread through sexual contact.

Chlamydia A sexually transmitted disease, caused by a bacterial infection, that can cause significant damage to the reproductive system.

Gonorrhea A sexually transmitted disease caused by a bacterial infection.

Pelvic inflammatory disease (PID) An overall designation referring to the effects of other STDs, primarily chlamydia and gonorrhea.

Human papillomavirus (HPV) A group of viruses that can cause sexually transmitted diseases.

Genital warts A sexually transmitted disease caused by a viral infection.

Genital herpes A sexually transmitted disease caused by a viral infection of the herpes simplex virus Types I and II. The virus can attack different areas of the body, but commonly causes blisters on the genitals.

sores, individuals should carefully wash themselves with soap.

Syphilis

Another common type of STD, also caused by bacterial infection, is **syphilis**. Approximately 3 weeks after infection, a painless sore appears where the bacteria entered the body. This sore disappears on its own in a few weeks. If untreated, more sores may appear within 6 months of the initial outbreak but again will disappear by themselves.

A latent stage, during which the victim is not contagious, may last up to 30 years, lulling victims into thinking they are healed. During the last stage of the disease, some people develop paralysis, crippling, blindness, heart disease, brain damage, and insanity, and they even can die as a direct result of the disease. One of the oldest known STDs, syphilis once killed its victims, but now penicillin and other antibiotics are used to treat it.

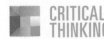

CRITICAL THINKING

Many individuals who have sexually transmitted diseases withhold this information from potential sexual partners. Do you think it should be considered a criminal action if an individual knowingly transmits a STD to someone else?

HIV and AIDS

Of all sexually transmitted diseases, AIDS is the most frightening because in most cases it is fatal and it has no known cure. **AIDS**—which stands for **acquired immunodeficiency syndrome**—is the end stage of infection by the **human immunodeficiency virus (HIV).** In Lab 14A you will have the opportunity to evaluate your basic understanding of HIV and AIDS.

HIV is a chronic infectious disease that is passed from one person to another through blood-to-blood and sexual contact. The virus spreads most commonly among individuals who engage in risky behavior such as having unprotected sex or sharing hypodermic needles. When a person becomes infected with HIV, the virus multiplies and attacks and destroys white blood cells. These cells are part of the immune system, and their function is to fight off infections and diseases in the body.

As the number of white blood cells that are killed increases, the body's immune system gradually breaks down or may be destroyed completely. Without an immune system, a person becomes susceptible to various **opportunistic diseases** and to cancers.

HIV is a progressive disease. At first, people who become infected with HIV might not know they are

Profile Plus

How much do you know about HIV/AIDS? Find answers and evaluate your risks using the activity on your CD-ROM.

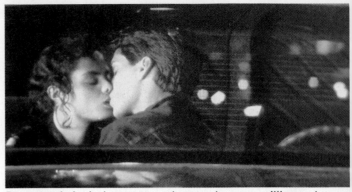

VANESSA WAS IN A FATAL CAR ACCIDENT LAST NIGHT. ONLY SHE DOESN'T KNOW IT YET.

Drugs and alcohol use can make people more willing to have unplanned and unprotected sex, thereby risking HIV infection.

infected. An incubation period of weeks, months, or years may pass during which no symptoms appear. The virus may live in the body 10 years or longer before symptoms emerge.

When the infection progresses to a point at which certain diseases develop, the person is said to have AIDS. HIV itself doesn't kill. Nor do people die from AIDS. "AIDS" is the term designating the final stage of HIV infection. Death is caused by a weakened immune system that is unable to fight off these opportunistic diseases.

Earliest symptoms of AIDS include unexplained weight loss, constant fatigue, mild fever, swollen lymph glands, diarrhea, and sore throat. Advanced symptoms include loss of appetite, skin diseases, night sweats, and deterioration of mucous membranes.

Most of the illnesses that AIDS patients develop are harmless and rare in the general population but are fatal to AIDS victims. The two most common fatal conditions in AIDS patients are pneumocystis carinii pneumonia (a parasitic infection of the lungs) and Kaposi's sarcoma (a type of skin cancer). The AIDS virus also may attack the nervous system, causing damage to the brain and spinal cord.

On the average, the individual develops the symptoms that fit the case definition of AIDS about 10 years following infection. From that point on, the person might live another 3 years or so. In essence, from the point of infection, the individual might endure a chronic disease for about 12 years.

The only means to determine whether someone has HIV is through an HIV antibody test. Being HIV-positive does not necessarily mean the person has AIDS. Several years can go by before the person develops the diseases that fit the case definition of AIDS.

Upon becoming infected, the immune system forms antibodies that bind to the virus. HIV antibodies can be detected in the blood as soon as 25 days following infection. According to the CDC, all except 5 percent of infected individuals will show these antibodies within 12 to 14 weeks of infection. In some cases, they are not detectable until after 6 months or longer.

If HIV infection is suspected, a person should wait 6 months to be tested, when the test is believed to be almost 100 percent accurate. During this time, and from then on, individuals should refrain from further endangering themselves and others through risky behaviors. Some people are tested to reassure themselves that their risky behaviors are acceptable. Even if the test turns up negative for HIV, this does not represent a "license" to continue risky behaviors.

No one has to become infected with HIV. At present, once infected, a person cannot become uninfected. There is no second chance. Everyone must protect himself or herself against this chronic disease. If they do not, and are so ignorant as to believe it can never happen to them, they are putting themselves and their partners at risk.

New therapies are preventing AIDS from developing in a growing number of HIV-infected persons. Professionals, however, disagree as to how many HIV carriers actually will develop AIDS. Even if individuals have not developed AIDS, they can pass on the virus to others, who could then easily develop AIDS.

Transmission of HIV

HIV is transmitted by the exchange of cellular body fluids including blood, semen, vaginal secretions, and maternal milk, and other body fluids containing blood. These fluids can be exchanged during sexual intercourse, by using hypodermic needles that infected individuals have used previously, between a pregnant woman and her developing fetus, by infection of a baby from the mother during childbirth, less frequently during breast feeding, and, rarely, from a blood transfusion or organ transplant.

The primary modes of HIV transmission in reported AIDS cases in the United States are presented in Figures 14.1 and 14.2. Approximately 42,000 new infections are reported each year. Of these new infections, 45 percent are reported in men who have sex with men, 30 percent in men and women through heterosexual sex, and 24 percent by injection drug use.

The proportion of AIDS cases by race/ethnicity is given in Figures 14.3 and 14.4. More than 50 percent of the new infections occur in African Americans, followed by Caucasians (26 percent), and Hispanics (19 percent).

Today, the risk of being infected with HIV from a blood transfusion is slight. Prior to 1985, several cases of HIV infection came from blood transfusions

FIGURE 14.1 Primary modes of HIV transmission by exposure category and year of transmission.*

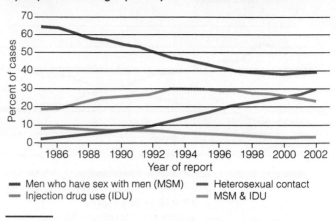

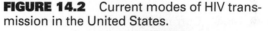

*Data adjusted for reporting delays and proportional redistribution of cases reported without a risk.

Source: http://www.cdc.gov/hiv/graphics/surveill.htm. Downloaded Nov. 27, 2004.

FIGURE 14.2 Current modes of HIV transmission in the United States.

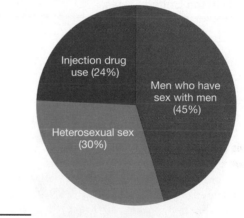

Source: Centers for Disease Control, Atlanta, GA.

because the blood was donated by HIV-infected individuals. Now, all individuals who donate blood are first tested for HIV. To be absolutely safe, people who are planning to have surgery might consider

Syphilis A sexually transmitted disease caused by a bacterial infection.

Acquired immunodeficiency syndrome (AIDS) Any of a number of diseases that arise when the body's immune system is compromised by HIV; the final stage of HIV infection.

Human immunodeficiency virus (HIV) Virus that leads to acquired immunodeficiency syndrome (AIDS).

Opportunistic diseases Diseases that arise in the absence of a healthy immune system, which would fight them off in healthy people.

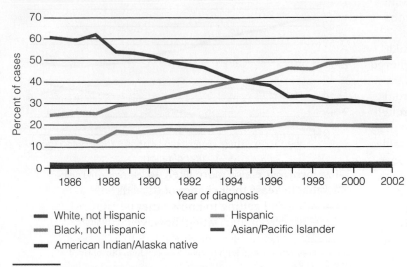

FIGURE 14.3 Proportion of AIDS cases by race/ethnicity in the United States, 1985–2002.

Legend:
- White, not Hispanic
- Black, not Hispanic
- American Indian/Alaska native
- Hispanic
- Asian/Pacific Islander

Source: http://www.cdc.gov/hiv/graphics/surveill.htm. Downloaded Nov 27, 2004.

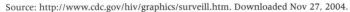

FIGURE 14.4 Current proportion of new HIV infections in the United States.

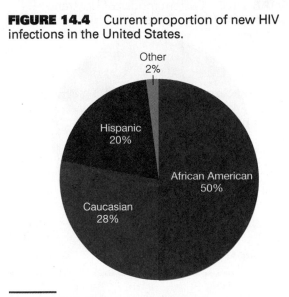

Other 2%
Hispanic 20%
African American 50%
Caucasian 28%

Source: Centers for Disease Control, Atlanta, GA.

storing their own blood in advance so safe blood will be available if a transfusion becomes necessary.

A myth regarding HIV is that it can be transmitted by donating blood. People cannot get HIV from giving blood. Health professionals use a brand-new needle every time they withdraw blood from a person. They use these needles only once and destroy them immediately after each person has donated blood.

People do not get HIV because of who they are but, rather, because of what they *do*. HIV and AIDS can threaten anyone, anywhere: men, women, children, teenagers, young people, older adults, Caucasians, African Americans, Hispanic Americans, Asian Americans, Native Americans, Africans, Europeans, homosexuals, heterosexuals, bisexuals, drug users. Nobody is immune to HIV.

HIV can be transmitted between males, between females, from male to female, or from female to male. Although HIV and AIDS are preventable, almost all of the people who get HIV do so because they engage in risky behaviors.

Risky Behaviors

You cannot tell if people are infected with HIV or have AIDS by simply looking at them or taking their word. Not you, not a nurse, not even a doctor can tell without an HIV antibody test. Therefore, every time you engage in risky behavior, you run the risk of contracting HIV. The two most basic risky behaviors are the following.

1. *Having unprotected vaginal, anal, or oral sex with an HIV-infected person.* Unprotected sex means having sex without using a condom properly. A person should select only latex (rubber or prophylactic) condoms that state "disease prevention" on the package. Although you might have unprotected sex with an infected person and not get the virus, you can get it by having unprotected sex only once with an infected individual.

Rubbing during sexual intercourse often damages mucous membranes and causes unseen bleeding (even in the mouth). During vaginal, anal, or oral sexual contact, infected blood, semen, or vaginal fluids can penetrate the mucous membranes that line the vagina, the penis, the rectum, the mouth, or the throat. From the membrane, HIV then travels into the previously uninfected person's blood.

Health experts believe that unprotected anal sex is the riskiest type of sex. Even though bleeding is not visible in most cases, anal sex almost always causes tiny tears and bleeding in the rectum. This happens because the rectum does not stretch easily, the mucous membrane is quite thin, and small blood vessels lie directly beneath the membrane. Condoms also are more likely to break during anal intercourse because more friction is produced in a smaller cavity. All of these factors greatly enhance the risk of transmitting HIV.

Although latex condoms, if used correctly, provide for "safer" sex, they are not 100 percent foolproof. Abstaining from sex is the only 100 percent sure way to protect yourself from HIV infection and other STDs.

2. *Sharing hypodermic needles or other drug paraphernalia with someone who is infected.* Following an injection, a small amount of blood remains in the needle, and sometimes in the syringe itself. If the person who used the syringe is infected with HIV and someone else uses that same syringe to shoot up, regardless of the drug used (legal or illegal), that small amount of blood is sufficient to spread the virus. All used syringes should be destroyed and disposed of immediately.

In addition, a person must be cautious when getting acupuncture, getting a tattoo, or having the ears or other body parts pierced. If the needle used was used previously on someone who is HIV-infected and the needle was not disinfected properly, the person risks getting HIV.

Otherwise prudent people often act irrationally and engage in risky behaviors when they are under the influence of drugs. Getting high can make you willing to have sex when you really didn't plan to—thereby running the risk of contracting HIV.

Small concentrations of the virus have been found in saliva and teardrops. In principle, if both people have open cuts on the lips or in the mouth or gums, HIV could be transmitted through open-mouthed kissing. Prolonged open-mouth kissing can damage the mouth or lips and allow HIV to be transmitted from an infected person to a partner through cuts or sores in the mouth. These cases, however, are rare.

Myths about HIV Transmission

The virus cannot be transmitted through perspiration. Sporting activities with no physical contact pose no risk to uninfected individuals unless they both have open wounds through which blood from an infected person can come in direct contact with the open wound of the uninfected person. The skin is an excellent line of defense against HIV. Blood from an infected person cannot penetrate the skin except through an opening in the skin. As an extra precaution, a person should use vinyl or latex gloves when performing work that requires direct contact with someone else's blood or open wound.

HIV is not transmitted through casual contact. HIV cannot be caught by spending time with, shaking hands with, or hugging an infected person; from a toilet seat, dishes, or silverware used by an HIV patient; or by sharing a drink, food, a towel, or clothes with a person who has HIV.

Some people fear getting HIV from health-care professionals. The chances of getting infected during physical or medical procedures are practically nil.

Health-care workers take extra care to protect themselves and their patients from HIV.

Another myth regarding HIV transmission is that you can get it from insects or animals. The H in HIV stands for "human." You cannot catch HIV from insects or animals. Animals do not get infected with HIV.

Wise Dating

With the advent of the Internet, people now search for sex partners online. Use of the Internet to find sexual partners may further increase the risk of contracting an STD. A recent study showed that those who seek sex partners over the Internet are at a greater risk. These people are also more likely to have characteristics that increase their chance of transmitting STDs.[7]

Dating and getting to know other people are normal aspects of life. Dating, however, does not mean the same thing as having sex. Sexual intercourse as a part of dating can be risky, and one of the risks is AIDS. You can't tell if someone you are dating or would like to date has been exposed to HIV. The good news is that as long as you avoid sexual activity and don't share drug needles, you are not at risk for contracting HIV.

Trends in HIV and AIDS Infection

Estimates indicate that more than 40 million people worldwide are infected with HIV, and more than 20 million have died from AIDS since the epidemic began. Women are becoming increasingly affected by HIV. Almost 50 percent, or 18.5 million of all HIV cases worldwide, have been reported in women.

According to the CDC, between 800,000 and 900,000 people in the United States are infected with HIV. One in every 300 Americans is presently infected, and about 26 percent of the newly reported cases are women. Through the end of 2002, a cumulative total of 859,000 AIDS cases had been diagnosed in the United States (see Figure 14.5), and 487,725 people had died from the diseases caused by HIV. About 70 percent of the people who died are in the 25- to 44-year-old age group. Of the reported AIDS cases, 666,026 were in males.

Although initially more than half of all AIDS cases in the United States occurred in homosexual or bisexual men, HIV infection is now spreading at a faster rate in heterosexuals. Many heterosexuals practice unprotected sex because they don't believe it can happen to their segment of the population. HIV is an epidemic that does not discriminate by sexual orientation. Worldwide, up to 80 percent of the AIDS cases have been reported in heterosexuals.[8]

AIDS experts are turning their attention to the population of sub-Saharan Africa, where 70 percent of the world's HIV victims live. Within 10 years, life

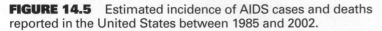

FIGURE 14.5 Estimated incidence of AIDS cases and deaths reported in the United States between 1985 and 2002.

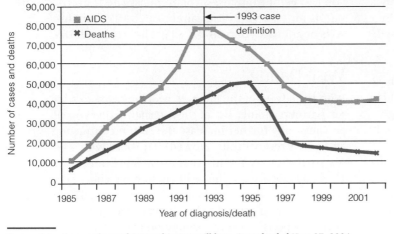

Source: http://www.cdc.gov/hiv/graphics/surveill.htm. Downloaded Nov. 27, 2004.

expectancy is predicted to hit its lowest point in a century in that part of the world, and the number of AIDS orphans will accelerate dramatically. The AIDS epidemic could also ruin the economies of these already impoverished countries. The medications used to treat victims in Western countries are unaffordable in sub-Saharan Africa. Public-awareness programs may be the only answer to the HIV epidemic there.

As with any other serious illness, HIV infected people and AIDS patients deserve respect, understanding, and support. Rejection and discrimination are traits of immature, hateful, and ignorant people. Education, knowledge, and responsible behaviors are the best ways to minimize fear and discrimination.

HIV Testing

A person can be tested for HIV in several ways. You may look up your local Public Health Department or AIDS Information Service (or related names) in the phone book. Testing is usually free of charge, and the results are kept confidential.

Many states also conduct anonymous testing. Your name is never recorded. You can call several toll-free hotlines for more information on anonymous testing, treatment programs, support services, and information about HIV, AIDS, and STDs in general. All information discussed during a phone call to these hotlines is kept strictly confidential. The numbers to call are:

> National AIDS Hotline: 1-800-342-AIDS
>   (1-800-342-2437)
> or La Linea Nacional de SIDA: 1-800-344-SIDA
>   (1-800-344-7432) for Spanish-speaking people
> STD Hotline: 1-800-227-8922.

HIV Treatment

Even though several drugs are being tested to treat and slow the disease process, AIDS has no known cure. Approximately 40 different approaches to an AIDS vaccine are being explored. The best advice at this point is to take a preventive approach.

Although HIV has no cure, medications are available that delay the progress of infection, allow HIV-infected patients to live longer, and even keep some people from developing AIDS. The sooner the treatment is initiated, the better is the prognosis for a longer life.

Developing a vaccine to prevent HIV infection or AIDS seems highly unlikely within the decade. People should not expect a medical breakthrough. Treatment modalities, however, should continue to improve and allow HIV-infected persons and AIDS patients to live longer and more productive lives.

Presently, several AIDS clinical trials are available in the United States. These projects are co-sponsored by the CDC, the Food and Drug Administration, the National Institute of Allergy and Infectious Diseases, the National Library of Medicine, and the National Institutes of Health. The purpose of AIDS clinical trials is to evaluate experimental drugs and various therapies for people at all stages of HIV infection. Interested individuals can call 1-800-TRIALS-A. As with all HIV testing, calls are completely confidential. Eligibility to participate in an AIDS clinical trial varies, and all applicants are evaluated individually. By calling the telephone number given, an interested person will receive information on the purpose and location of the trials (studies) that are open, eligibility requirements and exclusion criteria, and names and telephone numbers of persons to contact.

Guidelines for Preventing Sexually Transmitted Diseases

The good news is that you can do things to prevent the spread of STDs and take precautions to keep yourself from becoming a victim. The facts are in: The best prevention technique is a mutually **monogamous** sexual relationship. This one behavior will remove you almost completely from any risk for developing an STD.

Unfortunately, in today's society, trust is elusive. You may be led to believe you are in a safe, monogamous relationship when your partner actually (a) may cheat on you and get infected, (b) has a one-night stand with someone who is infected, (c) got

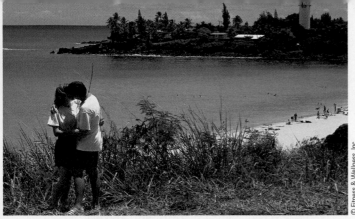

A monogamous sexual relationship almost completely removes people from risking HIV infection and the danger of developing other sexually transmitted diseases.

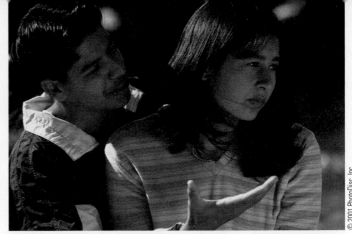

If someone does not respect your choice to wait, he or she certainly does not deserve your friendship or, for that matter, anything else.

the virus several years ago before the current relationship and still doesn't know about the infection, (d) may choose not to tell you about the infection, or (e) shoots up drugs and becomes infected. In any of these cases, HIV can be passed on to you.

Because your future and your life are at stake, and because you may never know if your partner is infected, you should give serious and careful consideration to postponing sex until you believe you have found an uninfected person with whom you can have a lifetime monogamous relationship. In doing so, you will not have to live with the fear of catching HIV or other STDs or deal with an unplanned pregnancy.

As strange as this may seem to some, many people postpone sexual activity until they are married. This is the best guarantee against HIV. Young people should understand that married life will provide plenty of time for fulfilling and rewarding sex.

If you choose to delay sex, do not let peers pressure you into having sex. Some people would have you believe that you are not a "real" man or woman if you don't have sex. Manhood and womanhood are not proven during sexual intercourse but, instead, through mature, responsible, and healthy choices.

Other people lead you to believe that love doesn't exist without sex. Sex in the early stages of a relationship is not the product of love. It is simply the fulfillment of a physical, and often selfish, drive. A loving relationship develops over a long time with mutual respect for each other.

Then there are those who enjoy bragging about their sexual conquests and mock people who choose to wait. Many of these conquests are only fantasies expounded in an attempt to gain popularity with peers.

Teenagers are especially susceptible to peer pressure leading to premature sexual intercourse. The result: more than 860,000 teen pregnancies per year and a 33 percent pregnancy rate for all girls at least once as a teenager. Presently, the U.S. teen pregnancy rate is one of the highest among industrialized nations. Too many young people wish they had postponed sex and silently admire those who do. Sex lasts only a few minutes. The consequences of irresponsible sex may last a lifetime. And in some cases, they are fatal!

Sexual promiscuity never leads to a trusting, loving, and lasting relationship. Mature people respect others' choices. If someone does not respect your choice to wait, he or she certainly does not deserve your friendship or, for that matter, anything else.

There is no greater sex than that between two loving and responsible individuals who mutually trust, admire, and love each other. Contrary to many beliefs, these relationships are possible. They are built upon unselfish attitudes and behaviors.

As you look around, you will find that many people hold these values. Seek them out and build your friendships and future around people who respect you for who you are and what you believe. You don't have to compromise your choices or values. In the end, you will reap the greater rewards of a lasting relationship free of AIDS and other STDs.

Also, be prepared so you will know your course of action before you get into an intimate situation. Look for common interests and work together toward them. Express your feelings openly: "I'm not ready for sex; I just want to have fun, and kissing is fine with me." If your friend does not accept your answer and is not willing to stop the advances, be prepared with a strong response. Statements like, "Please stop" or "Don't!" are for the most part ineffective. Use a firm statement such as, "No, I'm not willing to have sex" or "I've already thought about this and I'm not going to have sex." If this still doesn't work, label the behavior as rape and say, "This is rape, and I'm going to call the police."

Monogamous A sexual relationship in which two people have sexual relations only with each other.

Reducing the Risk for STDs

What about those who do not have—or do not desire—a monogamous relationship? Some other things can be done to lower, but not completely eliminate, the risk for developing STDs in general:

1. *Plan before you get into a sexual situation.* Determine the conditions under which you will allow sex to take place. Ask yourself: "Am I willing to have sex with this person?" If you decide to have sex, practice safer sex. There is no reason to accept anything else. You will feel better about yourself.

2. *Know your partner.* The days are gone when safe sex resulted from anonymous encounters at a bathhouse or a singles bar. Limit your sexual relationships, and always practice safer sex.

3. *Discuss STDs with the person you are contemplating having sex with before you do so.* Even though talking about STDs might be awkward, the short-lived embarrassment of addressing intimate questions can keep you from contracting or spreading disease. If you do not know the person well enough to address this issue or you are uncertain about the answers, do not have sex with this individual.

4. *Limit the number of sexual partners you have.* Having one partner lowers your chances of becoming infected. The more partners you have, the greater are your chances for infection.

5. *If you are sexually promiscuous*, have periodic physical check-ups. You can easily get exposed to an STD from a person who does not have any symptoms and who is unaware of the infection. Sexually promiscuous men and women between ages 15 and 35 are considered to be a particularly high-risk group for developing STDs.

6. *Use "barrier" methods of contraception to help prevent the disease from spreading.* Condoms, diaphragms, and spermicidal suppositories, foams, and jellies can all deter the spread of certain STDs. Spermicidal agents may act as a disinfectant as well. Many physicians are encouraging promiscuous teenagers, especially, to use condoms. Traditionally, teenagers do not use birth-control methods at all and therefore remain at high risk for STDs. Take a few minutes at this time and list at least three ways you might bring up the subject of condom use with your partner. Also, think of ways you might convince a person to use one. If your partner refuses to use a condom, your answer should be quite simple: "No condom, no sex."

7. *Negotiate safer sex.* Focus on the problem and not the person. Describe your feelings about the problem, using "I" instead of "you." For example, you might say, "I'm feeling awkward and uncomfortable. The only way I can feel comfortable is by using a condom." You also can offer options and provide alternative solutions. You might indicate to your partner, "We can work this out together. Let's go for a drive and get a condom with a spermicide agent. We'll feel better about what we're doing."

8. *If you know you have an infection, be responsible enough to abstain from sexual activity.* Go to a physician or a clinic for treatment, and ask your doctor when you can safely resume sexual activity. Abstain until it is safe. Just as you want to be protected in a sexual relationship, you should want to protect your partner as well.

   If you are diagnosed with an STD and you believe you know the person who gave it to you, think of ways you might bring up the subject of STDs with this person. You need to take responsibility and discuss this matter with your partner. As a result of your conversation, medical treatment can be initiated and other people can be protected from infection as well.

9. *Urinate immediately following sexual intercourse.* Although this is not an entirely reliable method, it may help flush bacteria and viruses from the urinary tract.

10. *Thoroughly wash immediately after sexual activity.* Although washing with hot, soapy water will not guarantee safety against STDs, it can prevent you from spreading certain germs on your fingers and might wash away bacteria and viruses that have not entered the body yet.

11. *If you suspect that your partner is infected with an STD, ask.* He or she may not even be aware of the infection, so look for signs of infection, such as sores, redness, inflammation, a rash, growths, warts, or a discharge. If you are unsure, abstain.

12. *Consider abstaining from sexual relations if you have any kind of an illness or disease*, even a common cold. Any kind of illness makes you more susceptible to other illnesses, and lower immunity can make you more vulnerable to STDs. The same holds true for times when you are under extreme stress, when you are fatigued, and when you are overworked. Drugs and alcohol also can lower your resistance to disease.

13. *Wear loose-fitting clothes made from natural fibers.* Tight-fitting clothing made from synthetic fibers (especially underwear and nylon pantyhose) can create conditions that encourage the growth of bacteria and can actually aggravate STDs.

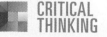 **CRITICAL THINKING**

Discuss how the information presented in this chapter has affected your feelings and perceptions about sex. What impact will this information have on your wellness lifestyle?

Reducing the Risks for HIV

Based upon recommendations from health experts, observing the following precautions can reduce your risk for getting HIV and, subsequently, AIDS:

1. Postpone sex until you and your uninfected partner are prepared to enter into a lifetime monogamous relationship.

2. Unless you are in a monogamous relationship and you know your partner is not infected (which you may never know for sure), practice safer sex every time you have sex. This means you should use a latex condom from start to finish for each sexual act. If you think your partner should use a condom but refuses to do so, say no to sex with that person.

3. Don't have multiple and anonymous sexual partners. Keep in mind that anyone you have sex with could be infected with HIV.

4. Don't have sexual contact with anyone who doesn't practice safer sex.

5. Avoid sexual contact with anyone who has had sex with people at risk for getting HIV, even if they are now practicing safer sex.

6. Don't have sex with prostitutes.

7. If you do have sex with someone who might be infected with HIV or whose history is unknown to you, avoid exchange of body fluids.

8. Don't share toothbrushes, razors, or other implements that could become contaminated with blood, with anyone who is, or who might be, infected with HIV.

9. Be cautious regarding procedures (such as acupuncture, tattooing, and ear piercing) in which needles or other non-sterile instruments may be used again and again to pierce the skin or mucous membranes. These procedures are safe if proper sterilization methods are followed or disposable needles are used. Before undergoing the procedure, ask what precautions are being taken.

10. If you are planning to undergo artificial insemination, insist that frozen sperm be obtained from a laboratory that tests all donors for infection with HIV. Donors should be tested twice before the lab accepts the sperm—once at the time of donation and again a few months later.

11. If you know you will be having surgery in the near future, and if you are able, consider donating blood for your own use. This will eliminate completely the already small risk of contracting HIV through a blood transfusion. It also will eliminate the more substantial risk for contracting other bloodborne diseases, such as hepatitis, from a transfusion.

Avoiding risky behaviors that destroy quality of life and life itself is crucial to a healthy lifestyle. Learning the facts, and acting upon your personal values so you can make responsible choices, can protect you and those around you from painful, embarrassing, startling, unexpected, or fatal conditions.

---

ofile
us

aluate how
ell you
derstand
e concepts
esented in
s chapter
ing the
ssess Your
owledge"
d "Practice
izzes"
tions
your
-ROM.

ASSESS YOUR KNOWLEDGE

1. What percentage of Americans will develop at least one STD in their lifetime?
   a. 30 percent
   b. 17 percent
   c. 25 percent
   d. 15 percent
   e. 20 percent

2. Which of the following sexually transmitted diseases is not caused by a bacterial infection?
   a. chlamydia
   b. genital warts
   c. syphilis
   d. gonorrhea
   e. All of the above are caused by bacterial infections.

3. Chlamydia
   a. treatment, even if successful, will not reverse any damage that has occurred to the reproductive system.
   b. can cause infertility.
   c. may occur without symptoms.
   d. may cause arthritis.
   e. All choices are correct.

4. Gonorrhea can cause
   a. widespread bacterial infection.
   b. infertility.
   c. heart damage.
   d. arthritis.
   e. all of the above.

5. Treatment of genital warts is done by
   a. dissolving the warts with chemicals.
   b. electrosurgery.
   c. freezing the warts with liquid nitrogen.
   d. All of the above choices apply.
   e. None of the above choices is correct.

6. Herpes
   a. is incurable.
   b. sores are treated with electrosurgery.
   c. requires antibiotics for successful treatment and cure.
   d. is caused by a bacterial infection.
   e. is not a serious STD because the person becomes uninfected once the sores heal.

7. Cold sores
   a. can cause genital herpes.
   b. are not highly contagious.
   c. that are caused by bacterial infection are treatable.
   d. All of the above choices are correct.
   e. None of the above choices is correct.

8. The only way to determine whether someone is infected with HIV is through
   a. an AIDS outbreak.
   b. a physical exam by a physician.
   c. a bacterial culture test.
   d. an HIV antibody test.
   e. All choices are correct.

9. HIV
   a. attacks and destroys white blood cells.
   b. readily multiplies in the human body.

   c. breaks down the immune system.
   d. increases the likelihood of developing opportunistic diseases and cancers.
   e. All of the above are correct.

10. The best way to protect yourself against sexually transmitted diseases is
    a. through the use of condoms with a spermicide.
    b. by knowing about the people who have previously had sex with your partner.
    c. through a mutually monogamous sexual relationship.
    d. by having sex only with an individual who has no symptoms of STDs.
    e. All of the above choices provide equal protection against STDs.

Correct answers can be found at the back of the book.

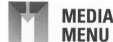

MEDIA MENU

PROFILE PLUS CD CONNECTIONS

▪ Evaluate your risk of HIV/AIDS.

▪ Check how well you understand the chapter's concepts.

INTERNET CONNECTIONS

▪ Sexuality Information from Columbia University Health Education Department "Go Ask Alice". This site presents a series of questions and answers about sex, organized into several categories, including sexual intercourse, abstinence, kissing, and genital wonderings.

   http://www.goaskalice.columbia.edu/

▪ The Body: Safer Sex and Prevention. This site features information for consumers, gay men, and health care professionals on a variety of prevention issues, including safer

sex and general prevention measures, condoms, sexual communication skills, sexual and non-sexual prevention, effective educational programs, treatment, and research.

   http://www.thebody.com/safesex.html

▪ American Social Health Association. This site features information on a variety of sexually transmitted diseases, a comprehensive frequently asked questions section, as well as information about STD hotlines. It also features a link to iwannaknow.org, the ASHA STD prevention Web site for teens.

   http://www.ashastd.org

▪ CDC National Center for HIV, STD, and TB Prevention. This comprehensive site features a variety of links to information regarding HIV/AIDS prevention, including the latest statistics.

   http://www.cdc.gov/hiv/dhap.htm

Notes

1. H. Weinstock, S. Berman, and W. Cates, "Sexually Transmitted Diseases Among American Youth: Incidence and Prevalence Estimates, 2000," *Perspectives on Sexual and Reproductive Health* 36 (2004): 6–10.

2. See note 1.

3. Unless otherwise indicated, all the statistics regarding STDs are from the U.S. Centers for Disease Control and Prevention, Atlanta.

4. "Chlamydia Screening for Young Women," *American Journal of Preventive Medicine* 20 (2001): 90.

5. V. Igra, "Pelvic Inflammatory Disease in Adolescents," *AIDS Patient Care & STDs* (February 1998): 109–124.

6. "Taming Herpes," *Mayo Clinic Women's HealthSource*, September 2001.

7. M. McFarlane, S. S. Bull, and C. A. Rietmeijer, "The Internet as a Newly Emerging Risk Environment for Sexually Transmitted Diseases," *Journal of the American Medical Association* 284 (2000): 443–446.

8. P. Philpott, "Heterosexual Transmission Studies," *Reappraising AIDS* 6, no. 1 (1998): 1.

Suggested Readings

Blona, R., and J. Levitan. *Healthy Sexuality*. Belmont, CA: Wadsworth/Thomson Learning, 2005.

Hoeger, W. W. K., L. W. Turner, and B. Q. Hafen. *Wellness: Guidelines for a Healthy Lifestyle*. Belmont, CA: Wadsworth/Thomson Learning, 2002.

Institute of Medicine. *The Hidden Epidemic: Confronting Sexually Transmitted Diseases*. Washington, DC: National Academy Press, 1997.

Lab 14A

SELF-QUIZ ON HIV AND AIDS

Name: _____   Date: _____   Grade: _____

Instructor: _____   Course: _____   Section: _____

Necessary Lab Equipment
None required.

Instruction
Please answer all of the following questions.

Objective
To evaluate basic understanding of HIV and AIDS.

	Yes	No
1. AIDS—acquired immunodeficiency syndrome—is the end stage of infection caused by the human immunodeficiency virus, HIV.	☐	☐
2. HIV is a chronic infectious disease that spreads among individuals who choose to engage in risky behavior such as unprotected sex or the sharing of hypodermic needles.	☐	☐
3. There is a cure for AIDS.	☐	☐
4. Abstaining from sex is the only 100 percent sure way to protect yourself from sexually-transmitted HIV infection.	☐	☐
5. Using drugs and alcohol can make you willing to have sex when you really don't plan to.	☐	☐
6. Condoms are 100 percent effective in protecting you against HIV infection.	☐	☐
7. Using drugs and alcohol makes a person less likely to use a condom and use it correctly.	☐	☐
8. If you're sexually active, latex condoms provide the best protection against HIV infection.	☐	☐
9. Using drugs and alcohol can make you more likely to have unplanned and unprotected sex.	☐	☐
10. Each year more and more teens are infected with HIV.	☐	☐
11. You can become HIV-infected by donating blood.	☐	☐
12. You can tell by looking at someone if he/she is HIV-infected.	☐	☐
13. The only means to determine whether someone has HIV is through an HIV antibody test.	☐	☐
14. HIV can completely destroy the immune system.	☐	☐
15. The HIV virus may live in the body 10 years or longer before AIDS symptoms develop.	☐	☐
16. People infected with HIV have AIDS.	☐	☐
17. Once infected with HIV, a person never becomes uninfected.	☐	☐
18. HIV infection is preventable.	☐	☐

Selected items on this questionnaire are adapted from *Test Your Survival Smarts: Self-Quiz on Drugs and AIDS*, National Institute on Drug Abuse, U. S. Department of Health & Human Services.

Answers:

1. Yes. AIDS is the term used to define the manifestation of opportunistic diseases and cancers that occur as a result of HIV infection (also referred to as "HIV disease").

2. Yes. People do not get HIV because of who they are, but because of what they do. Almost all of the people who get HIV do so because they choose to engage in risky behaviors.

3. No. There is no cure for AIDS, and there doesn't appear to be one in the foreseeable future.

4. Yes. Abstinence will protect you from HIV infection. But you may still get the disease by sharing hypodermic needles.

5. Yes. When you use alcohol or drugs, you can forget what you know about safer sex and do things you normally wouldn't do. If you're drunk or high, you might have sex even though you really don't plan to.

6. No. Only abstaining from sex gives you 100 percent protection, but condoms are effective in protecting against HIV infection if they're used correctly.

7. Yes. Individuals who are drunk or high are less likely to use condoms because, under the influence, they forget or feel that nothing "bad" can happen.

8. Yes. Proper use, however, is necessary to minimize the risk of infection.

9. Yes. Otherwise-prudent people often act irrationally and engage in risky behaviors when they are under the influence of drugs and alcohol.

10. Yes. In the early 1990s, the number of infected teens increased by 96 percent over a short span of 2 years. One reason for the increase may be that teens who are under the influence of drugs or alcohol often engage in risky sex. It is believed that about 20 percent of the AIDS patients today were infected as teenagers.

11. No. A myth regarding HIV is that it can be transmitted by donating blood. People cannot get HIV from giving blood. A brand-new needle is used by health professionals every time blood is taken. These needles are only used once and are destroyed and thrown away immediately after each individual has donated blood.

12. No. The symptoms of AIDS are often not noticeable until several years after a person has been infected with HIV. That's why, no matter who your partner is, it's important to always protect yourself against HIV and the risk of developing AIDS—either by abstaining from sex or by using condoms if you decide to have sex.

13. Yes. Not you, not a nurse, not even a doctor can tell, unless an HIV antibody test is done. Upon HIV infection, the immune system's line of defense against the virus is the formation of antibodies that bind to the virus. On the average it takes 3 months for the body to manufacture enough antibodies to show positive in an HIV antibody test. Sometimes it takes 6 months or longer.

14. Yes. The virus multiplies, attacks, and destroys white blood cells. These cells are part of the immune system, and their function is to fight off infections and diseases in the body. As the number of white blood cells killed increases, the body's immune system gradually breaks down or may be completely destroyed.

15. Yes. Ten years or longer may go by before the person develops AIDS.

16. No. Being HIV-positive does not necessarily mean that the person has AIDS. It may be 10 years or longer following infection before the individual develops the symptoms that fit the case definition of AIDS. From that point on, the person may live another 2 to 3 years. In essence, from the point of infection, the individual may endure a chronic disease for about 12 or more years.

17. Yes. There is no second chance. Everyone must protect him- or herself against HIV infection.

18. Yes. The best prevention technique is abstaining from sex until the time comes for a mutually monogamous sexual relationship (two people having a sexual relationship only with each other). That one behavior will almost completely remove you from any risk of HIV infection or developing any other sexually transmitted disease.

Lifetime Fitness and Wellness

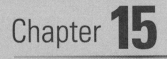

Objectives

- Describe the effects of a healthy lifestyle on longevity.
- Differentiate between physiological age and chronological age.
- Estimate your life expectancy and determine your real physiological age.
- Describe complementary and alternative medicine practices.
- Outline some guidelines for preventing consumer fraud.
- List factors to consider when selecting a health/fitness club.
- Know how to select appropriate exercise equipment.
- Review health/fitness accomplishments and chart a personal wellness program for the future.

Profile Plus CD Connections

- Discover how you've changed and plan for a healthy future.
- Check how well you understand the chapter's concepts.

433

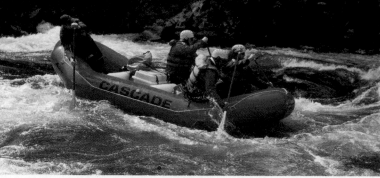

Good physical fitness provides freedom to enjoy many of life's recreational and leisure activities without limitations.

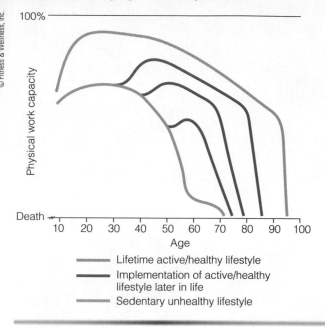

© Fitness & Wellness, Inc.

FIGURE 15.1 Relationships between physical work capacity, aging, and lifestyle habits.

Legend:
- Lifetime active/healthy lifestyle
- Implementation of active/healthy lifestyle later in life
- Sedentary unhealthy lifestyle

The three most important benefits to be derived from a lifetime fitness and wellness program are better health, a higher quality of life, and longevity. You have learned that physical fitness in itself does not always lower the risk for chronic diseases and ensure better health. Thus, implementation of healthy behaviors is the only way to attain your highest potential for well-being. The real challenge will come now that you are about to finish this course: maintaining your own lifetime commitment to fitness and wellness. Adhering to a program in a structured setting is a lot easier, but from now on, you will be on your own.

This chapter will help you evaluate how well you are adhering to health-promoting behaviors and the impact these behaviors may have on your **physiological age** and length of life. You will also learn how to chart a personal wellness program for the future.

Research data indicate that healthy (and un-healthy) lifestyle actions you take today will have an impact on your health and quality of life in middle and advanced age. In that most young people don't seem to worry much about health and longevity, you may want to take a closer look at the quality of life of your parents or other middle-aged and older friends and relatives you know. Though you may have a difficult time envisioning yourself at that age, their health status and **functional capacity** may help you determine how you would like to live when you reach your fourth, fifth, and subsequent decades of life.

Although previous research has documented declines in physiologic function and motor capacity as a result of aging, no hard evidence at present proves that large declines in physical work capacity are related primarily to aging alone. Lack of physical activity—a common phenomenon in our society as people age—is accompanied by decreases in physical work capacity that are greater by far than the effects of aging itself.

Data on individuals who have taken part in systematic physical activity throughout life indicate that these people maintain a higher level of functional capacity and do not experience the typical declines in later years. From a functional point of view, typical sedentary people in the United States are about 25 years older than their **chronological age** indicates. Thus, an active 60-year-old person can have a physical work capacity similar to that of a sedentary 35-year-old person.

Unhealthy behaviors precipitate premature aging. For sedentary people, any type of physical activity is seriously impaired by age 40 and produc-tive life ends before age 60. Most of these people hope to live to be age 65 or 70 but often must cope with serious physical ailments. These people "stop living at age 60 but are buried at age 70" (see the theoretical model in Figure 15.1).

Scientists believe that a healthy lifestyle allows people to live a vibrant life—a physically, intellectu-ally, emotionally, socially active, and functionally independent existence—to age 95. Such are the re-wards of a wellness way of life. When death comes to active people, it usually is rather quick and not as a result of prolonged illness. In Figure 15.1, note the low, longer slope of the "unhealthy lifestyle" before death.

Life Expectancy and Physiological Age

Aging is a natural process, but some people seem to age better than others. Most likely, you know someone who looks much younger than his or her

A healthy lifestyle enhances functional capacity, health, quality of life, and longevity.

chronological age indicates and, vice versa, someone who appears much older than their chronological age indicates. For example, you may have an instructor whom you would have guessed to be about 40, but in reality is 52 years old. Conversely, you may have a relative who looks 60 but who is actually 50 years old. Why the differences?

During the aging process, natural biological changes occur within the body. Although no one measurement can predict how long you will live, the rate at which the changes associated with aging take place depends on a combination of genetic and lifestyle factors. Your lifestyle habits will determine to a great extent how your genes will affect your aging process. Hundreds of research studies now point to critical lifestyle behaviors that will determine your statistical chances of dying at a younger age or living a longer life. Research also shows that lifestyle behaviors have a far greater impact on health and longevity than your genes alone.

Throughout this book, you have studied many of these factors. The question that you now need to ask yourself is: Are your lifestyle habits accelerating or decelerating the rate at which your body is aging? To help you determine how long and how well you may live the rest of your life, the Life Expectancy and Physiological Age Prediction Questionnaire, provided in Lab 15A, can help answer this question. By looking at 46 critical genetic and lifestyle factors, you will be able to estimate your **life expectancy** and your real physiological age. Of greater importance, most of these factors are under your own control and you can do something to make them work for you instead of against you.

CRITICAL THINKING

How long would you like to live, and are you concerned about how you will live the rest of your life?

As you fill out the questionnaire, you must be completely honest with yourself. Your life expectancy and physiological age prediction is based on your present lifestyle habits, should you continue those habits for life. Using the questionnaire, you will review factors that you can modify or implement in daily living and that may add years and health to your life. Please note that the questionnaire is not a precise scientific instrument but, rather, an estimated life expectancy analysis according to the impact of lifestyle factors on health and longevity. Also, the questionnaire is not intended as a substitute for advice and tests conducted by medical and health care practitioners.

Complementary and Alternative Medicine (CAM)

Conventional Western medicine, also known as **allopathic medicine**, has seen major advances in

Physiological age The biological and functional capacity of the body as it should be in relation to the person's maximal potential at any given age in the lifespan.

Functional capacity The ability to perform ordinary and unusual demands of daily living without limitations and excessive fatigue or injury.

Chronological age Calendar age.

Life expectancy How many years a person is expected to live.

Conventional Western medicine Traditional medical practice based on methods that are tested through rigorous scientific trials; also called **allopathic medicine**.

care and treatment modalities during the last few decades. Conventional medicine is based on scientifically proven methods, wherein medical treatments are tested through rigorous scientific trials. In addition to a **primary care physician** (medical doctor), people seek advice from other practitioners of conventional medicine, including **osteopaths, dentists, oral surgeons, orthodontists, ophthalmologists, optometrists, physician assistants**, and **nurses**.

Notwithstanding modern technological and scientific advancements, many medical treatments either do not improve the patient's condition or create other ailments caused by the treatment itself. Only about 20 percent of conventional treatments have been proven to be clinically effective in scientific trials.[1] Thus, millions of consumers are turning to **complementary and alternative medicine** or **CAM** (also called "unconventional," or "nonallopathic," or "integrative" medicine) in search of answers to their health problems.

The reasons for seeking complementary and alternative treatments are diverse. Among the reasons commonly given by patients who seek unconventional treatments are lack of progress in curing illnesses and disease, frustration and dissatisfaction with physicians, lack of personal attention, testimonials about the effectiveness of alternative treatments, and rising health care costs.

Unconventional medicine is referred to as CAM because patients use it to either augment their regular medical care (complementary medicine) or to replace conventional practices (alternative medicine).

According to the Centers for Disease Control and Prevention, 36 percent of American adults aged 18 and over used some form of CAM services in 2002. This figure increased to 62 percent when prayer was specifically included for health reasons.[2] People who use CAM tend to be more educated and believe that body, mind, and spirit all contribute to good health.

The National Center for Complementary and Alternative Medicine (NCCAM) was established under the National Institutes of Health to examine methods of healing that previously were unexplored by science. CAM includes treatments and health care practices not widely taught in medical schools, not generally used in hospitals, and not usually reimbursed by medical insurance companies. The five domains of CAM are given in Figure 15.2. Many physicians now endorse complementary and alternative treatments, and an ever-increasing number of medical schools are offering courses in this area.

Alternative medicine practices have not gone through the same standard scrutiny as conventional medicine. Nonallopathic treatments are often based on theories that have not been scientifically proven.

FIGURE 15.2 The five domains of complementary and alternative medicine.

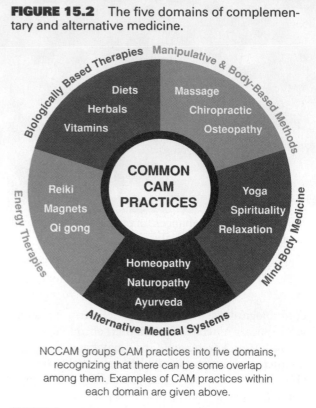

NCCAM groups CAM practices into five domains, recognizing that there can be some overlap among them. Examples of CAM practices within each domain are given above.

Source: Downloaded August 9, 2004 from http://nccam.nih.gov/news/camssurvey_fs1.htm

This does not imply that unconventional medicine practices are unhelpful. Many people have found relief from ailments or have been cured through unconventional treatments. In due time, however, these theories will have to be investigated using scientific trials similar to those in conventional medicine.

CAM includes a wide range of healing philosophies, approaches, and therapies. The practices most often associated with nonallopathic medicine are **acupuncture, chiropractics, herbal medicine, homeopathy, naturopathic medicine, ayurveda, magnetic therapy**, and **massage therapy**. Each of these practices offers a different approach to treatments, based on its beliefs about the body, some of which are hundreds or thousands of years old.

Many practitioners of these unconventional treatments believe that their modality aids the body in performing its own natural healing process. Inherent in these approaches, alternative treatments usually take longer than conventional allopathic medical care. Nonallopathic treatments are usually less harsh on the patient, and practitioners tend to avoid surgery and extensive use of medications.

Unconventional therapies are frequently called "holistic," implying that the practitioner looks at all the dimensions of wellness when evaluating a person's condition. Practitioners often persuade patients to adopt healthier lifestyle habits that will help them improve current conditions and also prevent other ailments from occurring. CAM further allows patients to better understand the treatments, and patients often are allowed to administer self-treatment.

Costs for CAM practices are typically lower than costs associated with conventional medicine. With the exception of acupuncture and chiropractic care, most nonallopathic treatments are not covered by health insurance. Typically, patients pay directly for these services. Conservative estimates indicate that $21.2 billion a year is spent on alternative medical treatments, with at least $12.2 billion paid out-of-pocket.[3] These costs exceeded the out-of-pocket expenses for all hospitalizations in the United States. If you are considering alternative medical therapies, consult your health-care insurance provider to determine which therapies are reimbursable.

CAM does have shortcomings, among them:

1. Many of the practitioners do not have the years of education given to conventional medical personnel and often know less about physiological responses that occur in the body.

2. Some practices are completely void of science; hence, the practitioner can rarely explain the specific physiologic benefits of the treatment used. Much of the knowledge is based on experiences with previous patients.

3. The practice of CAM is not regulated like that of conventional medicine. The training and certification of practitioners, malpractice liability, and evaluation of tests and methods used in treatments are not routinely standardized. Many states do license practitioners in the areas of chiropractic services, acupuncture, naturopathy, homeopathy, herbal therapy, and massage therapy, but other therapies are unmonitored.

4. Unconventional medicine lacks regulation of natural and herbal products. The word "natural" does not imply that the product is safe. Many products, including some herbs, can be toxic in large doses.

5. An estimated 15 million Americans (about one-fifth of all prescription users) combine high-dose vitamins and/or herbal supplements with prescription drugs.[4] Such combinations can yield undesirable side effects. Therefore, individuals should always let their health care practitioners know which medications and alternative (including vitamin and mineral) supplements are being taken in combination.

Herbal medicine has been around for centuries. Through trial and error, by design, or by accident, people have found that certain plant substances have medicinal properties. Today, many of these plant substances have been replaced by products that are safer, more effective, and have fewer negative side effects. Although science has found the mechanisms whereby some herbs work, much research remains to be done.

Many herbs and herbal remedies are not safe for human use and continue to meet resistance from the scientific community. One of the main concerns is that active ingredients in drug therapy

Primary care physician A medical practitioner who provides routine treatment of ailments; typically, the patient's first contact for health care.

Osteopath A medical practitioner with specialized training in musculoskeletal problems who uses diagnostic and therapeutic methods of conventional medicine in addition to manipulative measures.

Dentist Practitioner who specializes in diseases of the teeth, gums, and oral cavity.

Oral surgeon A dentist who specializes in surgical procedures of the oral–facial complex.

Orthodontist A dentist who specializes in the correction and prevention of teeth irregularities.

Ophthalmologist Medical specialist concerned with diseases of the eye and prescription of corrective lenses.

Optometrist Health care practitioner who specializes in the prescription and adaptation of lenses.

Physician assistant Health care practitioner trained to treat most standard cases of care.

Nurse Health care practitioner who assists in the diagnosis and treatment of health problems and provides many services to patients in a variety of settings.

Complementary and alternative medicine (CAM) A group of diverse medical and health care systems, practices, and products that are not presently considered to be part of conventional medicine; also called unconventional, nonallopathic, or integrative medicine.

Acupuncture Chinese medical system that requires body piercing with fine needles during therapy to relieve pain and treat ailments and diseases.

Chiropractics Health care system that believes that many diseases and ailments are related to misalignments of the vertebrae and emphasizes the manipulation of the spinal column.

Herbal medicine Unconventional system that uses herbs to treat ailments and disease.

Homeopathy System of treatment based on the use of minute quantities of remedies that in large amounts produce effects similar to the disease being treated.

Naturopathic medicine Unconventional system of medicine that relies exclusively on natural remedies to treat disease and ailments.

Ayurveda Hindu system of medicine based on herbs, diet, massage, meditation, and yoga to help the body boost its own natural healing.

Magnetic therapy Unconventional treatment that relies on magnetic energy to promote healing.

Massage therapy The rubbing or kneading of body parts to treat ailments.

must be administered in accurate dosages. With herbal medicine, the potency cannot always be adequately controlled.

Also, some herbs produce undesirable side effects. For example, ephedra (ma huang), a previously popular weight loss and energy supplement, caused high blood pressure, rapid heart rate, tremors, seizures, headaches, insomnia, stroke, and even death. About 1,400 reports of adverse effects linked to herbal products containing ephedra, including 81 ephedra-related deaths, prompted its removal from the marketplace. St. John's wort, commonly taken as an antidepressant, can produce serious interactions with drugs used to treat heart disease. Ginkgo biloba impairs blood clotting; thus, it can cause bleeding in people who are already on regular blood-thinning medication or aspirin therapy. Other herbs, such as yohimbe, chaparral, comfrey, and jin bu juan have been linked to adverse events.

Increasingly, conventional health-care providers will refer you to someone who is familiar with alternative treatments, but you have to be an informed consumer. Ask your primary care physician to obtain valid information regarding the safety and effectiveness of a given treatment. At times, the medical community will resist and reject unconventional therapies. If your physician is unable or unwilling to provide you with this information, other sources to search for this information include medical, college, or public libraries and popular bookstores. In any case, you need to educate yourself about the advantages and disadvantages of alternative treatments, risks, side effects, expected results, and length of therapy.

Information on a wide range of medical conditions or specific diseases also can be obtained by calling the National Institutes of Health (NIH) at 301-496-4000. Ask the operator to direct you to the appropriate NIH office. The NCCAM office provides a Web site (nccam.nih.gov) with access to more than 180,000 bibliographic records of research published on CAM during the last 35 years.

When you select a primary care physician or a nonallopathic practitioner, consult local and state medical boards, other health regulatory boards and agencies, and consumer affairs departments for information about a given practitioner's education, accreditation, and license and about complaints that may have been filed against this health care provider. Many of the unconventional medical fields also have a national organization that provides guidelines for practitioners and health consumers. These organizations can guide you to the appropriate regulatory agencies within your state where you can obtain information regarding a specific practitioner.

You may also talk to other individuals who have undergone similar therapies and learn about the

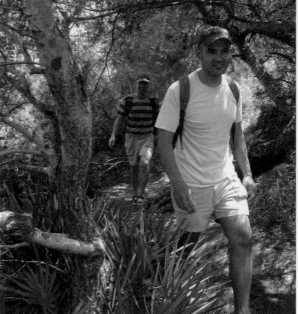

Frequent participation in recreational activities is important for health and wellness.

competence of the practitioner in question. Keep in mind, however, that patient testimonials do not adequately assess the safety and effectiveness of alternative treatments. Whenever possible, search for results of controlled scientific trials of the therapy in question and use this information in making your decision.

When undergoing any type of treatment or therapy, always disclose this information with all of your health care providers, whether conventional or unconventional. Adequate health care management requires that health care providers be informed of all concurrent therapies, so they will have a complete picture of the treatment plan. Lack of knowledge by one health care provider regarding treatments by another provider can interfere with the healing process or even worsen a given condition.

Millions of Americans have benefited from CAM practices. You may also benefit from such services, but you need to make careful and educated decisions about the available options. By finding well-trained (and preferably licensed) practitioners, you increase your chances for recovery from ailments and disease.

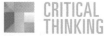

CRITICAL THINKING

Have you or someone you know ever used complementary or alternative medicine treatments? What experiences did you have with such treatment modalities, and would you use them in the future?

Quackery and Fraud

The rapid growth of the fitness and wellness industry during the last three decades has spurred the promotion of fraudulent products that deceive consumers into "miraculous," quick, and easy ways to achieve total well-being. **Quackery** and **fraud** are conscious promotions of unproven claims for profit.

Today's market is saturated with "special" foods, diets, supplements, pills, cures, equipment, books, and videos that promise quick, dramatic results. Advertisements for these products often are based on testimonials, unproven claims, secret research, half-truths, and quick-fix statements that the uneducated consumer wants to hear. In the meantime, the organization or enterprise making the claims stands to make a large profit from consumers' willingness to pay for astonishing and spectacular solutions to problems related to their unhealthy lifestyle.

Television, magazine, and newspaper advertisements arc not necessarily reliable. For instance, one piece of equipment sold through television and newspaper advertisements promised to "bust the gut" through 5 minutes of daily exercise that appeared to target the abdominal muscle group. This piece of equipment consisted of a metal spring attached to the feet on one end and held in the hands on the other end. According to handling and shipping distributors, the equipment was "selling like hotcakes" and companies could barely keep up with consumer demands.

Three problems became apparent to the educated consumer: First, there is no such thing as spot reducing; therefore, the claims could not be true. Second, exercising 5 minutes daily burns hardly any calories and, therefore, has no effect on weight loss. Third, the intended abdominal (gut) muscles were not really involved; the exercise engaged mostly the gluteal and lower back muscles. This piece of equipment now can be found at garage sales for about a tenth of its original cost!

Although people in the United States tend to be firm believers in the benefits of physical activity and positive lifestyle habits as a means to promote better health, most do not reap these benefits because they simply do not know how to put into practice a sound fitness and wellness program that will give them the results they want. Unfortunately, many uneducated wellness consumers are targets of deception by organizations making fraudulent claims for their products.

Deception is not limited to advertisements. Deceit is all around us—in newspaper and magazine articles, trade books, radio, and television. To make a profit, popular magazines occasionally exaggerate health claims or leave out pertinent information to avoid offending advertisers. Some publishers print books on diets or self-treatment approaches that have no scientific foundation. Consumers should even be cautious about news reports of the latest medical breakthroughs. Reporters have been known to overlook important information or give certain findings more credence than they deserve.

Precautions must also be taken when seeking health advice on the Internet. The Internet is full of both credible and dubious information. The following tips can help as you conduct a search on the Internet:

- Look for credentials of the person or organization sponsoring the site.
- Check when the site was last updated. Credible sites are updated often.
- Check the appearance of the information on the site. It should be presented in a professional manner. For instance, if every sentence ends with an exclamation mark, you have a good cause for suspicion.
- Be cautious if the site's sponsor is trying to sell a product. Be leery of opinions posted on the site. They could be biased, given that the company's main objective is to sell a product. Credible companies trying to sell a product on the Internet usually reference their sources of health information and provide additional links that support their product.
- Compare the content of a site to other credible sources. The content should be generally similar to that of other reputable sites or publications.
- Note the address and contact information for the company. A reliable company will list more than a post office box, an 800 number, and the company's email address. When only this information is provided, consumers may never be able to locate the company for questions, concerns, or refunds.
- Be on the alert for companies that claim to be innovators while criticizing competitors or the government for being close-minded or trying to keep them from doing business.
- Watch for advertisers that use valid medical terminology in an irrelevant context or use vague pseudomedical jargon to sell their product.

Not all people who promote fraudulent products, however, know they are doing so. Some may be convinced that the product they are promoting is effective. If you have questions or concerns about a health product, you may write to the National Council Against Health Fraud (NCAHF), 119 Foster Street, Peabody, MA 01960. The purpose of this organization is to provide the consumer with responsible, reliable, evidence-driven health information. The organization also monitors deceitful advertising, investigates complaints, and offers public information regarding fraudulent health claims. You may also report any type of quackery to NCAHF on its Web site at http://www.ncahf.org/. The site contains

Quackery/fraud The conscious promotion of unproven claims for profit.

an updated list of reliable and unreliable health Web sites for the consumer.

Other consumer-protection organizations offer to follow up on complaints about quackery and fraud. The assurance of these organizations, however, should not give the consumer a false sense of security. The overwhelming number of complaints they receive each year makes it impossible for them to follow up on each case individually. The FDA's Center for Drug Evaluation Research, for example, has developed a priority system to determine which health fraud product it should regulate first. Products are rated on how great a risk they pose to the consumer. With this in mind, you can use the following list of organizations to make an educated decision before you spend your money. You can also report consumer fraud to these organizations:

■ Food and Drug Administration (FDA). The FDA regulates safety and labeling of health products and cosmetics. You can search for the office closest to you in the federal government listings (blue pages) of the phone book.

■ Better Business Bureau (BBB). The BBB can tell you whether other customers have lodged complaints about a product, a company, or a salesperson. You can find a listing for the local office in the business section of the phone book, or you can check the BBB Web site at http://www.betterbusinessbureau.com/.

■ Consumer Product Safety Commission (CPS). This independent federal regulatory agency targets products that threaten the safety of American families. Unsafe products can be researched and reported on its Web site at http://www.cpsc.gov/.

Another way to get informed before making your purchase is to seek the advice of a reputable professional. Ask someone who understands the product but does not stand to profit from the transaction. As examples, a physical educator or an exercise physiologist can advise you regarding exercise equipment; a registered dietician can provide information on nutrition and weight-control programs; a physician can offer advice on nutritive supplements. Also, be alert to those who bill themselves as "experts." Look for qualifications, degrees, professional experience, certifications, and reputation.

Keep in mind that if it sounds too good to be true, it probably is. Fraudulent promotions often rely on testimonials or scare tactics and promise that their products will cure a long list of unrelated ailments; they use words like quick-fix, time-tested, new-found, miraculous, special, secret, all-natural, mail-order only, and money-back guarantee. Deceptive companies move often so customers have no way of contacting the company to request a reimbursement.

RELIABLE SOURCES OF HEALTH, FITNESS, NUTRITION, AND WELLNESS INFORMATION

Newsletter	Approx. Yearly Issues	Annual Cost
Bottom Line / Health BottomLineSecrets.com 800-289-0409	12	$29.95
Consumer Reports on Health www.ConsumerReports.org/health 800-234-2188	12	$24
Environmental Nutrition www.environmentalnutrition.com 800-829-5384	12	$30
Tufts University Health & Nutrition Letter www.healthletter.tufts.edu 800-274-7581	12	$28
University of California Berkeley Wellness Letter www.WellnessLetter.com 386-447-6328	12	$28

When claims are made, ask where the claims are published. Refereed scientific journals are the most reliable sources of information. When a researcher submits information for publication in a refereed journal, at least two qualified and reputable professionals in the field conduct blind reviews of the manuscript. A blind review means that the author does not know who will review the manuscript and the reviewers do not know who submitted the manuscript. Acceptance for publication is based on this input and relevant changes.

Deciding Your Fitness Future

Once you've decided to pursue a lifetime wellness program, you'll face several more decisions about exactly how to accomplish it. Following are some issues you'll encounter.

Health/Fitness Club Memberships

You may want to consider joining a health/fitness facility. Or, if you have mastered the contents of this book and your choice of fitness activity is one you can pursue on your own (walking, jogging, cycling), you may not need to join a health club. Barring injuries, you may continue your exercise program

FIGURE 15.3 American College of Sports Medicine standards for health and fitness facilities.

1. A facility must have an appropriate emergency plan.
2. A facility must offer each adult member a preactivity screening that is relevant to the activities that will be performed by the member.
3. Each person who has supervisory responsibility must be professionally competent.
4. A facility must post appropriate signs in those areas of a facility that present potential increased risk.
5. A facility that offers services or programs to the youth must provide appropriate supervision.
6. A facility must conform to all relevant laws, regulations, and published standards.

Adapted from ACSM's *Health/Fitness Facility Standards and Guidelines.* (Champaign, IL: Human Kinetics, 1997).

RELIABLE HEALTH WEB SITES

- American Cancer Society
  http://www.cancer.org/
- American Heart Association
  http://americanheart.org
- American College of Sports Medicine
  http://acsm.org
- Clinical Trials Listing Service
  http://www.centerwatch.com
- Healthfinder—Your Guide to Reliable Health Information
  http://www.healthfinder.gov
- HospitalWeb
  http://neuro-www.mgh.harvard.edu/hospitalweb.shtml
- National Cancer Institute
  http://www.cancer.gov
- National Center for Complementary and Alternative Medicine
  http://nccam.nih.gov/
- The National Library of Medicine
  http://www.nlm.nih.gov/
- The National Institutes of Health
  http://www.nih.gov/
- The Centers for Disease Control and Prevention
  http://www.cdc.gov/
- The Medical Matrix
  http://www.medmatrix.org/
- The National Council Against Health Fraud
  http://www.ncahf.org/
- The Food and Drug Administration
  http://www.fda.gov/
- WebMD
  http://webmd.com/
- World Health Organization
  http://www.who.int/en/

outside the walls of a health club for the rest of your life. You also can conduct strength training and stretching programs (see Chapters 7 and 8) in your own home.

To stay up-to-date on fitness and wellness developments, you probably should buy a reputable and updated fitness/wellness book every 4 to 5 years. You may subscribe to a credible health, fitness, nutrition, or wellness newsletter to stay current. You also can surf the World Wide Web, but be sure that the sites you are searching are from credible and reliable organizations.

If you are contemplating membership in a fitness facility, do all of the following:

- Make sure that the facility complies with the standards established by the American College of Sports Medicine (ACSM) for health and fitness facilities. These standards are given in Figure 15.3.
- Examine all exercise options in your community: health clubs/spas, YMCAs, gyms, colleges, schools, community centers, senior centers, and the like.
- Check to see if the facility's atmosphere is pleasurable and nonthreatening to you. Will you feel comfortable with the instructors and other people who go there? Is it clean and well kept up? If the answer is no, this may not be the right place for you.
- Analyze costs versus facilities, equipment, and programs. Take a look at your personal budget. Will you really use the facility? Will you exercise there regularly? Many people obtain memberships and permit dues to be withdrawn automatically from a local bank account, yet seldom attend the fitness center.
- Find out what types of facilities are available: walking/running track, basketball/tennis/racquetball courts, aerobic exercise room, strength training room, pool, locker rooms, saunas, hot tubs, handicapped access, and so on.
- Check the aerobic and strength-training equipment available. Does the facility have treadmills, bicycle ergometers, stair climbers, cross-country skiing simulators, free weights, strength-training machines? Make sure the facilities and equipment meet your activity interests.
- Consider the location. Is the facility close, or do you have to travel several miles to get there? Distance often discourages participation.
- Check on times the facility is accessible. Is it open during your preferred exercise time (for example, early morning or late evening)?

- Work out at the facility several times before becoming a member. Are people standing in line to use the equipment, or is it readily available during your exercise time?
- Inquire about the instructors' qualifications. Do the fitness instructors have college degrees or professional certifications from organizations such as the American College of Sports Medicine or the International Dance Exercise Association (IDEA)? These organizations have rigorous standards to ensure professional preparation and quality of instruction.
- Consider the approach to fitness (including all health-related components of fitness). Is it well-rounded? Do the instructors spend time with members, or do members have to seek them out constantly for help and instruction?
- Ask about supplementary services. Does the facility provide or contract out for regular health and fitness assessments (cardiovascular endurance, body composition, blood pressure, blood chemistry analysis)? Does it offer wellness seminars (nutrition, weight control, stress management)? Do these have hidden costs?

Personal Trainers

In recent years, personal trainers have been in high demand by health and fitness participants. A **personal trainer** is a health/fitness professional who evaluates, motivates, educates, and trains clients to help them meet individualized healthy lifestyle goals. Rates typically start at $40 an hour and go up from there. Exercise sessions are usually conducted at a health/fitness facility or at the client's own home. Experience and the ability to design safe and effective programs based on the client's current fitness level, health status, and fitness goals are important. Personal trainers also recognize their limitations and refer clients to other health care professionals as necessary.

Currently, anyone who prescribes exercise can call himself or herself a personal trainer without proof of education, experience, or certification. Although good trainers should strive to maximize their own health and fitness, a good physique and previous athletic experience do not certify a person as a personal trainer.

Because of the high demand for personal trainers, more than 200 organizations now provide some type of certification to fitness specialists. This has led to great confusion by clients on how to evaluate the credentials of personal trainers. There is also a clear distinction between "certification" and a "certificate." Certification implies that the individual has met educational and professional standards of performance and competence. A certificate is typically awarded to individuals who attend a conference or workshop but are not required to meet any professional standards.

Presently, there is no licensing body that oversees personal trainers. Thus, it is easy to become a personal trainer. At a minimum, personal trainers should have an undergraduate degree and certification from a reputable organization such as ACSM or IDEA. Undergraduate (and graduate) degrees should be conferred in a fitness-related area such as exercise science, exercise physiology, kinesiology, sports medicine, or physical education.

ACSM offers three certification levels: group exercise leader, health/fitness instructor, and health/fitness director. IDEA offers four levels: professional, advanced, elite, and master. For both ACSM and IDEA, each level of certification is progressively more difficult to obtain. A third organization, the National Strength and Conditioning Association (NSCA), also offers a personal trainer's certification program. When looking for a personal trainer, always inquire about the trainer's education and certification credentials.

As a final word of caution when seeking fitness advice from a health/fitness trainer via the Internet: Be aware that certain services cannot be provided over the Internet. An Internet trainer is not able to directly administer fitness tests, motivate, observe exercise limitations, or respond effectively in an emergency situation (spotting, administering first-aid or CPR), and thus, is not able to design the most safe and effective exercise program for you.

Purchasing Exercise Equipment

A final consideration addressed in this book is that of purchasing your own exercise equipment. The first question to ask yourself is: Do I really need this piece of equipment? Most people buy on impulse because of television advertisements or because a salesperson has convinced them it is a great piece of equipment that will do wonders for their health and fitness. Ignore claims that an exercise device or machine can provide "easy/no-sweat" results in only a few minutes. Keep in mind that the benefits of exercise are obtained only if you do exercise. With some creativity, you can implement an excellent and comprehensive exercise program with little, if any, equipment (see Chapters 6, 7, 8, and 9).

Many people buy expensive equipment only to find that they really do not enjoy that mode of activity. They do not remain regular users. A few years ago, stationary bicycles (lower body only) and rowing ergometers were among the most popular pieces of equipment. Most of them now are seldom used and have become "fitness furniture" somewhere in the basement. Furthermore, be skeptical of testimonials and before-and-after pictures from "satisfied" customers. These results may not be typical, and they don't mean that you will like the equipment as well.

Exercise equipment does have its value for people who prefer to exercise indoors, especially during the winter months. It supports some people's motivation and adherence to exercise. The convenience of having equipment at home also allows for flexible scheduling. You can exercise before or after work or while you watch your favorite television show.

If you are going to purchase equipment, the best recommendation is to actually try it out several times before buying it. Ask yourself several questions: Did you enjoy the workout? Is the unit comfortable? Are you too short, tall, or heavy for it? Is it stable, sturdy, and strong? Do you have to assemble the machine? If so, how difficult is it to put together? How durable is it? Ask for references—people or clubs that have used the equipment extensively. Are they satisfied? Have they enjoyed using the equipment? Talk with professionals at colleges, sports medicine clinics, or health clubs.

Another consideration is to look at used units for signs of wear and tear. Quality is important. Cheaper brands may not be durable, so your investment would be wasted.

Finally, watch out for expensive gadgets. Monitors that provide exercise heart rate, work output, caloric expenditure, speed, grade, and distance may help motivate you, but they are expensive, need frequent repairs, and do not enhance the actual fitness benefits of the workout. Look at maintenance costs, and check for service personnel in your community.

CRITICAL THINKING

Are there people around you whom you admire and would like to emulate for their wellness lifestyle? What behaviors do these people exhibit that would help you adopt a healthier lifestyle? What keeps you from emulating these behaviors, and how can you overcome these barriers?

Self-Evaluation and Behavioral Goals for the Future

The main objective of this book is to provide the information and experiences necessary to implement your personal fitness and wellness program. If you have implemented the programs in this book, including exercise, you should be convinced that a wellness lifestyle is the only way to attain a higher quality of life.

Most people who engage in a personal fitness and wellness program experience this new quality of life after only a few weeks of training and practicing healthy lifestyle patterns. In some instances, however—especially for individuals who have led a poor lifestyle for a long time—a few months may be required to establish positive habits and feelings of well-being. In the end, though, everyone who applies the principles of fitness and wellness will reap the desired benefits.

Self-Evaluation

Throughout this course you have had an opportunity to assess various fitness and wellness components and write goals to improve your quality of life. You now should take the time to evaluate how well you have achieved your own goals. Ideally, if time allows and facilities and technicians are available, reassess the health-related components of physical fitness. If you are unable to reassess these components, determine subjectively how well you accomplished your objectives. You will find a self-evaluation form in part I of Lab 15B.

Profile Plus

Has this course brought you closer to a healthier lifestyle? Discover how you've changed, and plan for a healthy future with the activity on your CD-ROM.

Behavioral Goals for the Future

If you have not yet achieved all of your goals during this course, or if you need to reach beyond your current achievements, a final assignment should be conducted to help you chart the future. To complete this assignment, fill out the Wellness Compass in part II of Lab 15b. This compass provides a list of various wellness components, each illustrating a scale from 5 to 1; "5" indicates a low or poor rating and "1" indicates an excellent or "wellness" rating for that component. Using the Wellness Compass, rate yourself for each component according to the following instructions:

1. Color in red a number from 5 to 1 to indicate where you stood on each component at the beginning of the semester. For example, if at the start of this course, you rated poor in cardiorespiratory endurance, color the number 5 in red.
2. Color in blue a second number from 5 to 1 to indicate where you stand on each component at the present time. If your level of cardiorespiratory endurance improved to average by the end of the semester, color the number 3 in blue. If you were not able to work on a given component, simply color in blue on top of the previous red.
3. Select one or two components you intend to work on during the next 2 months. Developing

Personal trainer A health/fitness professional who evaluates, motivates, educates, and trains clients to help them meet individualized, healthy, lifestyle goals.

new behavioral patterns takes time, and trying to work on too many components at once most likely will lower your chances for success.

Start with components in which you think you will have a high chance for success. Next, color in yellow the intended goal (number) to accomplish by the end of the 2 months. If your goal is to achieve a "good" level of cardiorespiratory endurance, color the number 2 in yellow. When you achieve this level, you may later color the number 1, also in yellow, to indicate your next goal.

After you have completed the previous exercise, write goals and objectives for the two components you intend to work on during the next 2 months (use the form in part III of Lab 15B). As you write and work on these goals, review the SMART Goals section provided in Chapter 2, pages 42–43.

As a final assignment, to summarize your feelings about your past and present lifestyle, what you have learned in this course, and changes you were able to implement successfully, use part IV of Lab 15B for this evaluation. Keep this summary handy so you can review it in months and years to come.

The Fitness/Wellness Experience and a Challenge for the Future

Patty Neavill is a typical example of someone who often tried to change her life but was unable to do so because she did not know how to implement a sound exercise and weight control program. At age 24 and at 240 pounds, she was discouraged with her weight, level of fitness, self-image, and quality of life in general. She had struggled with her weight most of her life. Like thousands of other people, she had made many unsuccessful attempts to lose weight.

Patty put her fears aside and decided to enroll in a fitness course. As part of the course requirement, a battery of fitness tests was administered at the beginning of the semester. Patty's cardiovascular fitness and strength ratings were poor, her flexibility classification was average, and her percent body fat was 41.

Following the initial fitness assessment, Patty met with her course instructor, who prescribed an exercise and nutrition program like the one in this book. Patty fully committed herself to carry out the prescription. She walked/jogged five times a week. She enrolled in a weight-training course that met twice a week. Her daily caloric intake was set in the range of 1,500 to 1,700 calories.

Determined to increase her level of activity further, Patty signed up for recreational volleyball and basketball courses. Besides being fun, these classes provided 4 additional hours of activity per week.

She took care to meet the minimum required servings from the basic food groups each day, which contributed about 1,200 calories to her diet. The remainder of the calories came primarily from complex carbohydrates.

At the end of the 16-week semester, Patty's cardiovascular fitness, strength, and flexibility ratings had all improved to the "good" category, she had lost 50 pounds, and her percent body fat had decreased to 22.5!

Patty was tall. At 190 pounds, most people would have thought she was too heavy. Her percent body fat, however, was lower than the average for college female physical education major students (about 23 percent body fat).

A thank-you note from Patty to the course instructor at the end of the semester read:

Thank you for making me a new person. I truly appreciate the time you spent with me. Without your kindness and motivation, I would have never made it. It is great to be fit and trim. I've never had this feeling before, and I wish everyone could feel like this once in their life.

Thank you,
Your trim Patty!

Patty had never been taught the principles governing a sound weight-loss program. In Patty's case, not only did she need this knowledge, but, like most Americans who have not experienced the process of becoming physically fit, she needed to be in a structured exercise setting to truly feel the joy of fitness.

Even more significant, Patty maintained her aerobic and strength-training programs. A year after ending her calorie-restricted diet, her weight increased by 10 pounds, but her body fat decreased from 22.5 to 21.2 percent. As you may recall from Chapter 5, this weight increase is related mostly to gains in lean tissue that she had lost during the weight-reduction phase.

In spite of only a slight drop in weight during the second year following the calorie-restricted diet, the 2-year follow-up revealed a further decrease in body fat, to 19.5 percent. Patty understood the new quality of life reaped through a sound fitness program, and, at the same time, she finally learned how to apply the principles that regulate weight maintenance.

If you have read and successfully completed all of the assignments set out in this book, including a regular exercise program, you should be convinced of the value of exercise and healthy lifestyle habits in achieving a new quality of life.

Perhaps this new quality of life was explained best by the late Dr. George Sheehan, when he wrote:[5]

For every runner who tours the world running marathons, there are thousands who run to hear

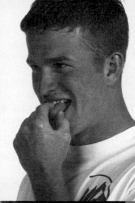
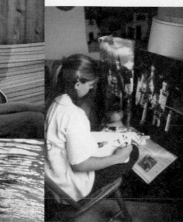
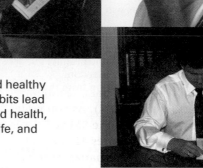

Fitness and healthy lifestyle habits lead to improved health, quality of life, and wellness.

the leaves and listen to the rain, and look to the day when it is all suddenly as easy as a bird in flight. For them, sport is not a test but a therapy, not a trial but a reward, not a question but an answer.

The real challenge will come now: a lifetime commitment to fitness and wellness. To make the commitment easier, enjoy yourself and have fun along the way. If you implement your program based on your interests and what you enjoy doing most, adhering to your new lifestyle will not be difficult.

Your activities over the last few weeks or months may have helped you develop "positive addictions" that will carry on throughout life. If you truly experience the feelings Dr. Sheehan expressed, there will be no looking back. If you don't get there, you won't know what it's like. Fitness and wellness is a process, and you need to put forth a constant and deliberate effort to achieve and maintain a higher quality of life. Improving the quality of your life, and most likely your longevity, is in your hands. Only you can take control of your lifestyle and thereby reap the benefits of wellness.

ASSESS YOUR KNOWLEDGE

1. From a functional point of view, typical sedentary people in the United States are about _____ years older than their chronological age indicates.
   a. 2
   b. 8
   c. 15
   d. 20
   e. 25

2. Which one of the following factors has the greatest impact on health and longevity?
   a. genetics
   b. the environment
   c. lifestyle behaviors
   d. chronic diseases
   e. gender

3. Your real physiological age is determined by
   a. your birthdate.
   b. lifestyle habits.
   c. the amount of physical activity.
   d. your family's health history.
   e. your ability to obtain proper medical care.

4. Complementary and alternative medicine is
   a. also known as allopathic medicine.
   b. referred to as Western medicine.
   c. based on scientifically proven methods.
   d. a method of unconventional medicine.
   e. All are correct choices.

5. Complementary and alternative medicine health-care practices and treatments are
   a. not widely taught in medical schools.
   b. endorsed by many physicians.
   c. not generally used in hospitals.
   d. not usually reimbursed by medical insurance companies.
   e. All of the above choices are correct.

6. In complementary and alternative medicine
   a. practitioners believe that their treatment modality aids the body as it performs its own natural healing process.
   b. treatments are usually shorter than with typical medical practices.
   c. practitioners rely extensively on the use of medications.
   d. patients are often discouraged from administering self-treatment.
   e. All of the above choices are correct.

ofile
ıs

luate how
I you
erstand
concepts
sented in
chapter
ıg the
sess Your
wledge"
"Practice
izes"
ons
our
ROM.

7. When the word "natural" is used with a product
   a. it implies that the product is safe.
   b. it cannot be toxic, even when taken in large doses.
   c. it cannot yield undesirable side effects when combined with prescription drugs.
   d. there will be no negative side effects with its use.
   e. All of the above choices are incorrect.

8. To protect yourself from consumer fraud when buying a new product,
   a. get as much information as you can from the salesperson.
   b. obtain details about the product from another salesperson.
   c. ask someone who understands the product but does not stand to profit from the transaction.
   d. obtain all the research information from the manufacturer.
   e. All of these choices are correct.

9. Which of the following should you consider when looking to join a health/fitness center?
   a. location
   b. instructor's certifications
   c. type and amount of equipment available
   d. verify that the facility complies with ACSM standards
   e. All choices are correct.

10. When purchasing exercise equipment, the most important factor is
   a. to try it out several times before buying it.
   b. a recommendation from an exercise specialist.
   c. cost-effectiveness.
   d. that it provides accurate exercise information.
   e. to find out how others like this piece of equipment.

Correct answers can be found at the back of the book.

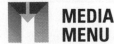

MEDIA MENU

PROFILE PLUS CD CONNECTIONS

■ Discover how you've changed and plan for a healthy future.

■ Check how well you understand the chapter's concepts.

INTERNET CONNECTIONS

■ American College of Sports Medicine (ACSM). This site provides information on sport safety and research projects. This organization is committed to the practical application of sports medicine and exercise science to maintain and enhance physical fitness, health, and quality of life.

   http://www.acsm.org

■ Getting Started with an Exercise Program. This comprehensive site, from the Department of Kinesiology and Health of Georgia State University, features information on the benefits of exercise, how to choose a personal trainer, exercise safety and precautions, and lots more.

   http://www.gsu.edu/~wwwfit/getstart.html

■ RealAge. This site features diet and exercise assessment tools, such as BMI calculator and exercise estimator, as well as RealAge assessment quizzes on a variety of health topics to help determine your risk of disease and what you can do to reduce this risk. The main feature is an interactive online personal assessment of a variety of lifestyle behaviors that also gives you options for growing younger.

   http://www.realage.com

■ National Center for Complementary and Alternative Medicine. This comprehensive site features information about a variety of complementary therapies geared for consumers, clinical practitioners, and investigators. The site also features a complementary medicine database, clinical trials information, and a list of resources.

   http://nccam.nih.gov/

Notes

1. R. J. Donatelle and L. G. Davis, *Access to Health* (Boston: Allyn and Bacon, 2000).

2. U.S. Department of Health and Human Services, Centers for Disease Control and Prevention, National Center for Health Statistics, *Complementary and Alternative Medicine Use among Adults: United States, 2002* 343 (May 27, 2004).

3. D. M. Eisenberg et al., "Trends in Alternative Medicine Use in the United States, 1990–1997," *Journal of the American Medical Association* 280, no. 18 (1998): 1569–1575.

4. See note 3.

5. Human Relations Media, *Dynamics of Fitness: The Body in Action* (Pleasantville, NY, 1980).

Suggested Readings

Bloomer, R. "Successful Attributes of a Professional Fitness Trainer." *Fitness Management* 19 (1999): 40–45.

Janowiak, J. *Alternative Medicines: The Mindbody Prescription.* Belmont, CA: Wadsworth/Thomson, 2001.

Roizen, M. F. *Real Age: Are You As Young As You Can Be?* New York: Cliff Street Books, 1999.

Lab 15A

LIFE EXPECTANCY AND PHYSIOLOGICAL AGE PREDICTION QUESTIONNAIRE*

Name: _____ Date: _____ Grade: _____

Instructor: _____ Course: _____ Section: _____

Necessary Lab Equipment
None required.

Objective
To estimate the total number of years that you will live and your real physiological age based on your present lifestyle habits.

Instructions
Circle the points to the correct answer to each question. At the end of each page, obtain a net score for that page. Be completely honest with yourself. Your age prediction is based on your lifestyle habits, should you continue those habits for life. Using this questionnaire, you will learn about factors that you can modify or implement that can add years and health to your life. The scoring system is provided at the end of the questionnaire. Please note that the questionnaire is not a precise scientific instrument, but rather an estimated life expectancy analysis according to the impact of lifestyle factors on health and longevity. This questionnaire is not intended to substitute for advice and tests conducted by medical and health care practitioners.

I. Questionnaire

1. What is your current health status?
   - A. Excellent   + 2
   - B. Good   + 1
   - C. Average   0
   - D. Fair   − 1
   - E. Poor   − 2
   - F. Bad   − 3

2. How many days per week do you accumulate 30 minutes of moderate-intensity physical activity (50 to 60% of heart rate reserve—see Chapter 6)?
   - A. 6 to 7   + 3
   - B. 3 to 5   + 1
   - C. 1 to 2   0
   - D. Less than once per week   − 3

3. How often do you participate in a high-intensity cardio-respiratory exercise (over 60% of heart rate reserve) for at least 20 minutes?
   - A. 3 or more times per week   + 2
   - B. 2 times per week   + 1
   - C. Once a week   − 1
   - D. Less than once per week   − 2

4. How often do you perform strength-training exercises per week (a minimum of 8 exercises using 8 to 12 repetitions to near-fatigue on each exercise)?
   - A. 1–2 times   + 2
   - B. Less than once or less than 8 exercises with 8 to 12 reps per session   0
   - C. Do not strength train   − 1

5. How many times per week do you perform flexibility exercises (at least 15 minutes per stretching session)?
   - A. 3 or more   + 1
   - B. 1 to 3 times   + .5
   - C. Less than 1   0
   - D. Do not perform flexibility exercises   − .5

6. How many servings of fruits and vegetables do you eat on a daily basis?
   - A. 9 or more   + 3
   - B. 6 to 8   + 2
   - C. 5   + 1
   - D. 3 to 4   0
   - E. 2 or less   − 2

7. How many grams of fiber do you consume on an average day?
   - A. 25 or over   + 1
   - B. Between 13 and 24   0
   - C. 10 to 12 or don't know   − 1
   - D. Less than 10   − 2

8. As a percentage of total calories, what is your average fat intake on a daily basis?
   - A. 20% to 30%   + 1
   - B. 30%   0
   - C. 30% to 35% or don't know   − 1
   - D. Over 35%   − 2

9. As a percentage of total calories, what is your average saturated fat intake on a daily basis?
   - A. 5% or less   + 1
   - B. More than 5% but less than 10%   0
   - C. Don't know   − 1
   - D. Over 10%   − 2

10. How many servings of red meat (3 to 6 ounces) do you consume on a weekly basis?
    - A. 1 or less   + 1
    - B. 2 to 3   0
    - C. 4 to 7   − 1
    - D. More than 7   − 2

Page score: _____

*Source: Fitness & Wellness, Inc., Boise, Idaho, ©2000. Reproduced with permission.

11. How many servings of fish (3 to 6 ounces) do you consume on a weekly basis?
    A. 2 or more — + 1
    B. 1 — 0
    C. None — − 1

12. How many alcoholic drinks (a 12-ounce bottle of beer, a 4-ounce glass of wine, or a 1.5-ounce shot of 80 proof liquor) do you consume per day?
    A. Men 2 or less, women 1 or less — + 1
    B. None — 0
    C. Men 3–4, women 2–4 — − 1
    D. 5 or more — − 3

13. How many international units of vitamin E do you get from supplements on a daily basis?
    A. 400 — + 2
    B. Over 200 but less than 400 — + 1
    C. Between 50 and 200 — 0
    D. None — − 1

14. How many milligrams of vitamin C do you get from food on a daily basis?
    A. Between 250 and 500 — + 1
    B. Over 90 but less than 250 — +.5
    C. Less than 90 — − 1

15. How many micrograms of selenium do you get on a daily basis (preferably from food)?
    A. Between 100 and 200 — + 1
    B. Between 50 and 99 — +.5
    C. Less than 50 — − 1

16. How many milligrams of calcium and how many international units of vitamin D do you get from food and supplements on an average day?
    A. Calcium = 1,200, Vitamin D = 400 or more — + 1
    B. Calcium = 1,200, Vitamin D = unknown — +.5
    C. Calcium = 800 to 1,200, Vitamin D = less than 400 — 0
    D. Calcium = less than 800, Vitamin D = less than 400 — − 1

17. How many times per week do you eat breakfast?
    A. 7 — + 1
    B. 5 to 6 — +.5
    C. 3 to 5 — 0
    D. Less than 3 — −.5

18. How many cigarettes do you smoke each day?
    A. Never smoked cigarettes or more than 15 years since giving up cigarettes — + 2
    B. None for 5 to 15 years — + 1
    C. None for 1 to 5 years — 0
    D. None for 0 to 1 year — − 1
    E. Smoker, less than 1 pack per day — − 3
    F. Smoker, 1 pack per day — − 5
    G. Smoker, up to 2 packs per day — − 7
    H. Smoker, more than 2 packs per day — − 10

19. Do you use tobacco products other than cigarettes?
    A. Never have — 0
    B. Less than once per week — − 1
    C. Once per week — − 2
    D. 2 to 6 times per week — − 3
    E. More than 6 times per week — − 5

20. How often are you exposed to secondhand smoke or other environmental pollutants?
    A. Less than 1 hour per month — 0
    B. Between 1 and 5 hours per month — − 1
    C. Between 5 and 29 hours per month — − 2
    D. Daily — − 3

21. Do you use addictive drugs, other than tobacco or alcohol?
    A. None — 0
    B. 1 — − 3
    C. 2 or more — − 5

22. What is the age of your parents (or how long did they live)?
    A. Both over 76 — + 3
    B. Only one over 76 — + 1
    C. Both are still alive and under 76 — 0
    D. Only one under 76 — − 1
    E. Neither one lived past 76 — − 3

23. What is your body composition category (see Table 4.9 in Chapter 4)?
    A. Excellent — + 2
    B. Good — + 1
    C. Average — 0
    D. Overweight — − 1
    E. Significantly overweight — − 2

24. What is your blood pressure?
    A. 120/80 or less (both numbers) — + 2
    B. 120–140 or 80–90 (either number) — − 1
    C. Greater than 140/90 (either number) — − 3

25. What is your HDL cholesterol?
    A. Men greater than 45, women over 55 — + 2
    B. Men 35 to 44, women 45 to 54 — 0
    C. Don't know — − 1
    D. Men less than 35, women below 45 — − 2

26. What is your LDL cholesterol?
    A. Less than 130 — + 2
    B. Don't know — − 1
    C. 130 to 159 — − 1
    D. 160 or higher — − 2

27. Do you floss and brush your teeth regularly?
    A. Every day — +.5
    B. 3 to 6 days per week — 0
    C. Less than 3 days per week — −.5

28. Are you a diabetic?
    A. No — 0
    B. Yes, well-controlled — − 1
    C. Yes, poorly or not controlled — − 3

29. How often do you sunbathe (tan)?
    A. Not at all — + 1
    B. Between 1 and 3 times per year — −.5
    C. More than 3 times per year — − 1

30. How often do you wear a seat belt?
    A. All the time — + 1
    B. Most of the time — −.5
    C. Less than half the time — − 1

31. How fast do you drive?
    A. Always at or below the speed limit — 0
    B. Up to 5 mph over the speed limit — −.5
    C. Between 5 and 10 mph over the speed limit — − 1
    D. More than 10 mph over the speed limit — − 2

Page score:

32. Do you drink and drive?
    A. Never   0
    B. Yes (even if only once)   − 5

33. In terms of your sexual activity:
    A. I am not sexually active
       or I am in a monogamous
       sexual relationship   + 1
    B. I have more than one
       sexual partner but I always
       practice safer sex   − 1
    C. I have multiple sexual
       partners and I do not
       practice safer sex
       techniques   − 3

34. What is your marital status?
    A. Happily married   + 1
    B. Single and happy   0
    C. Single and unhappy   −.5
    D. Divorced   − 1
    E. Widowed with a belief
       in life hereafter   − 1
    F. Widowed   − 2
    G. Married and unhappy   − 2

35. On the average, how many
    hours of sleep do you get
    each night?
    A. 7 to 8   + 1
    B. 7   0
    C. 6 to 7   − 1
    D. Less than 6   − 2

36. Your stress rating according
    to the Life Experiences Survey
    (see Lab 10A) is:
    A. Excellent   + 1
    B. Good   0
    C. Average   −.5
    D. Fair   − 1
    E. Poor   − 2

37. Your Type A behavior rating
    (see Lab 10A) is:
    A. Low   0
    B. Medium   − 1
    C. High   − 2

38. When under stress (distress),
    how often do you practice stress
    management techniques?
    A. Always   + 1
    B. Most of the time   +.5
    C. Not applicable (don't
       suffer from stress)   0
    D. Sometimes   − 1
    E. Never   − 2

39. Do you suffer from depression?
    A. Not at all   0
    B. Mild depression   − 1
    C. Severe depression   − 2

40. How often do you associate
    with people who have a
    positive attitude about life?
    A. Always   +.5
    B. Most of the time   0
    C. About half of the time   −.5
    D. Less than half the time   − 1

41. Do you have close family or
    personal relationships whom
    you can trust and rely on for
    help in times of need?
    A. Yes   + 1
    B. No   − 1

42. Do you feel loved and can
    you routinely give affection
    and love?
    A. Yes   + 1
    B. No   − 1

43. Do you have a good sense
    of humor?
    A. Yes   + 1
    B. No   − 1

44. How satisfied are you with
    your school work?
    A. Satisfied   +.5
    B. It's okay   0
    C. Not satisfied   −.5

45. How do you rate your
    present job satisfaction?
    A. Love it   + 1
    B. Like it   0
    C. It's okay   −.5
    D. Don't like it   − 1
    E. Hate it   − 2
    F. Not applicable   0

46. How do you rate yourself
    spiritually?
    A. Very spiritual   + 1
    B. Spiritual   0
    C. Somewhat spiritual   −.5
    D. Not spiritual at all   − 1

Page score:

Net score for all questions:

II. How To Score

To estimate the total number of years that you will live, (a) determine a net score by totaling the results from all 46 questions, (b) obtain an age change score by multiplying the net score by the age correction factor given below, and (c) add or subtract this number from your base life expectancy age (73 for men and 80 for women—the current life expectancies in the United States). For example, if you are a 20-year-old male and the net score from the answers to all questions was −16, your estimated life expectancy would be 68.2 years (age change score = −16 × .3 = −4.8, life expectancy = 73 − 4.8 = 68.2).

You can also determine your real physiological age by subtracting a positive age-change score or adding a negative age-change score to your current chronological (calendar) age. For instance, in the previous example, the real physiological age would be 24.8 years (20 + 4.8). If the age change score had been +4.8, the real physiological age would have been 16.2 years. Thus, a healthy lifestyle will always make your physiological age younger than your chronological age. Your real physiological age will have much greater significance in middle and older age, when it is not uncommon to see real-age reductions of 10 to 25 years in people who lead healthy lifestyles. Thus a 50-year-old person could easily have a real physiological age of 30.

Age Correction Factor (ACF)*

Age	ACF
≤30	.3
31–40	.4
41–50	.5
51–60	.6
61–70	.6
71–80	.5
81–90	.4
≥91	.3

*Adapted from: M. F. Roizen, *RealAge*, New York: Cliff Street Books, 1999.

Age Change Score (ACS) = _____ (net score) × _____ (ACF) = _____

Life expectancy

Men   = 73 ± _____ (ACS) = _____ years

Women = 80 ± _____ (ACS) = _____ years

Real physiological age**

Men   = _____ (your age) ± _____ (ACS) = _____ years

Women = _____ (your age) ± _____ (ACS) = _____ years

**Subtract a positive ACS from, or add a negative ACS to, your current age.

State your feelings about the experience of taking this questionnaire, analyze your results, and list lifestyle factors that you can work on that will positively affect your health and longevity.

Lab 15B

SELF-EVALUATION AND BEHAVIORAL GOALS FOR THE FUTURE

Name: _____   Date: _____ Grade: _____

Instructor: _____   Course: _____ Section: _____

Necessary Lab Equipment
None required unless fitness tests are repeated.

Objective
To conduct a self-evaluation of the goals achieved in this course and to write behavioral goals for the future.

Lab Preparation
Review the section on SMART Goals in Chapter 2 (pages 42–43) prior to completing this lab. If time allows and technicians are available, repeat the assessments for the health-related components of fitness.

I. Fitness Evaluation

Conduct a self-evaluation of the fitness goals you accomplished in this course. Fill in the required information on the health-related fitness components below. If you were unable to repeat your fitness assessments, subjectively determine how well you reached your goals.

1. Did you accomplish your objective for:

Cardiorespiratory Endurance (see Lab 6A)   ☐ Yes ☐ No

Pre-assessment VO_{2max}: _____ ml/kg/min   Fitness Classification: _____

Post-assessment VO_{2max}: _____ ml/kg/min   Fitness Classification: _____

Body Composition (see Labs 4A and 4B)   ☐ Yes ☐ No

Pre-assessment Percent Body Fat: _____   Body Composition Classification: _____

Post-assessment Percent Body Fat: _____   Body Composition Classification: _____

Muscular Strength and Endurance (see Lab 7A)   ☐ Yes ☐ No

Pre-assessment Percentile Total Points: _____   Fitness Classification: _____

Post-assessment Percentile Total Points: _____   Fitness Classification: _____

Muscular Flexibility (see Lab 8A)   ☐ Yes ☐ No

Pre-assessment Percentile Total Points: _____   Fitness Classification: _____

Post-assessment Percentile Total Points: _____   Fitness Classification: _____

II. Wellness Evaluation

Using the Wellness Compass, rate yourself for each component and plan goals and objectives for the future according to the following instructions:

1. Color in red a number from 5 to 1 to indicate where you stood on each component at the beginning of the semester (5 = poor rating, 1 = excellent or ideal rating).
2. Color in blue a second number from 5 to 1 to indicate where you stand on each component at the present time.
3. Select one or two components that you intend to work on in the next 2 months. Start with components in which you think you will have a high chance for success. Color in yellow the intended goal (number) to accomplish by the end of the 2 months. Once you achieve your objective, you later may color another number, also in yellow, to indicate your next objective.

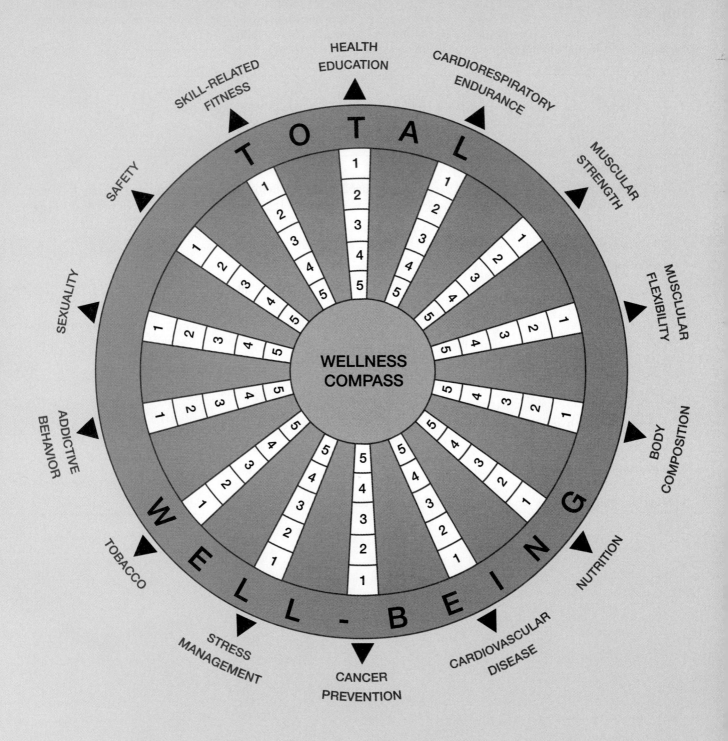

III. Wellness Lifestyle Self-Assessment

1. Explain the exercise program that you implemented in this course, indicate your feelings about the outcomes of this program, and evaluate how well you accomplished your fitness goals.

2. List nutritional or dietary changes that you were able to implement this term and the effects of these changes on your body composition and personal wellness.

3. List other lifestyle changes that you were able to make this term that may decrease your risk for disease. In a few sentences, explain how you feel about these changes and their impact on your overall well-being.

IV. Behavioral Goals for the Future

Identify one or two goals you will work on during the next couple of months and write specific objectives that you will use to accomplish each goal (you may not need six objectives; write only as many as needed).

Goal:

Objectives:

1. _____
2. _____
3. _____
4. _____
5. _____
6. _____

Goal:

Objectives:

1. _____
2. _____
3. _____
4. _____
5. _____
6. _____

V. This Course and Your Future Lifestyle

Briefly evaluate this course and its impact on your quality of life. Indicate what you feel will be needed for you to continue to adhere to an active and healthy lifestyle.

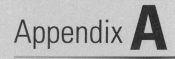

Nutritive Value
of Selected Foods

Food	Amount	Weight (g)	Calories	Protein (g)	Fat (g)	Sat. Fat (g)	Choles-terol (g)	Carbo-hydrate (g)	Fiber (g)	Cal-cium (mg)	Iron (mg)	Sodi-um (mg)	Vit A (IU)	Thia-min (Vit B₁) (mg)	Ribo-flavin (Vit B₂) (mg)	Niacin (mg)	Vit C (mg)	Folate (mcg)
Apples, fresh, w/peel, lrg	1 ea	150	88	0.3	1	0.1	0	23	4.1	10	0.3	0	80	0.03	0.02	0.1	9	4.2
Applesauce, swtnd, w/o salt, cnd	1 cup	255	194	0.5	0	0.1	0	51	3.1	10	0.9	8	28	0.03	0.07	0.5	4	1.53
Apricots, pitted, fresh, whole	3 ea	114	55	1.6	0	0	0	13	2.7	16	0.6	1	2978	0.03	0.05	0.7	11	9.8
Apricots, w/skin, in heavy syrup, cnd, whole	½ cup	120	100	0.6	0	0	0	26	1.9	11	0.4	5	1476	0.02	0.03	0.5	4	2.04
Asparagus, spears, ckd w/o salt	4 ea	60	14	1.6	0	0	0	3	1	12	0.4	7	323	0.07	0.08	0.6	6	87.6
Avocado, Calif, fresh	½ ea	120	212	2.5	21	3.1	0	8	5.9	13	1.4	14	734	0.13	0.15	2.3	9	78.6
Bagel, plain, 3½" diameter	1 ea	68	187	7.1	1	0.1	0	36	1.6	50	2.4	363	0	0.37	0.21	3.1	0	59.84
Banana, fresh, med	1 ea	140	129	1.4	1	0.3	0	33	3.4	8	0.4	1	113	0.06	0.14	0.8	13	26.74
Bar, granola, hard	1 ea	24	113	2.4	5	0.6	0	15	1.3	15	0.7	71	36	0.06	0.03	0.4	0	5.52
Beans, black, mature, ckd w/o salt	1 cup	172	227	15.2	1	0.2	0	41	15	46	3.6	2	10	0.42	0.1	0.9	0	255.9
Beans, chickpea/garbanzo, mature, ckd	1 cup	164	269	14.5	4	0.4	0	45	12.5	80	4.7	11	44	0.19	0.1	0.9	2	282.0
Beans, frijoles/refried, cnd	½ cup	145	136	8	2	0.7	12	23	7.7	51	2.4	434	0	0.04	0.02	0.5	9	15.95
Beans, green, snap/string, ckd	½ cup	65	23	1.2	0	0	0	5	2.1	30	0.8	2	433	0.05	0.06	0.4	6	21.64
Beans, kidney, red, mature, cnd	1 cup	185	157	9.7	1	0.1	0	29	11.8	44	2.3	631	0	0.19	0.16	0.8	2	93.61
Beans, lima, fordhook, immature, ckd f/fzn w/o salt, drained	½ cup	85	85	5.2	0	0.1	0	16	4.9	19	1.2	45	162	0.06	0.05	0.9	11	18.02
Beans, mung, mature, sprouted, raw	½ cup	52	16	1.6	0	0	0	3	0.9	7	0.5	3	11	0.04	0.06	0.4	7	31.62
Beans, pinto, mature, ckd w/o salt	1 cup	171	234	14	1	0.2	0	44	14.7	82	4.5	3	3	0.32	0.16	0.7	4	294.1
Beef, chuck arm pot roast, brsd, choice, ¼" trim	3 oz	85	296	22.9	22	8.6	84	0	0	8	2.6	50	0	0.06	0.2	2.7	0	7.65
Beef, corned, cnd	3 oz	85	212	23	13	5.3	73	0	0	10	1.8	855	0	0.02	0.12	2.1	0	7.65
Beef, ground, hamburger patty, brld, well done, 16% fat	3 oz	85	225	24.3	13	5.3	84	0	0	8	2.4	70	0	0.06	0.27	5	0	9.35
Beef, ground, hamburger patty, brld, well done, 18% fat	3 oz	85	238	24	15	5.9	86	0	0	10	2.1	76	0	0.05	0.2	5.1	0	9.35
Beef, liver, fried	3 oz	85	184	22.7	7	2.3	410	7	0	9	5.3	90	30689	0.18	3.52	12.3	20	187
Beef, T-bone steak, brld, choice, ¼" trim	3 oz	85	263	19.7	20	7.7	57	0	0	7	2.3	54	0	0.08	0.18	3.4	0	5.95
Beef, top sirloin steak, lean, brld, choice, ¼" trim	3 oz.	85	172	25.8	7	2.6	76	0	0	9	2.9	56	0	0.11	0.25	3.6	0	8.5
Beer	12 fl-oz	360	148	1.1	0	0	0	13	0.7	18	0.1	18	0	0.02	0.09	1.6	0	21.6
Beer, light	12 fl-oz	354	99	0.7	0	0	0	5	0	18	0.1	11	0	0.03	0.11	1.4	0	14.51
Beets, cnd, drained, diced	½ cup	80	25	0.7	0	0	0	6	1.4	12	1.5	155	9	0.01	0.03	0.1	3	24.16
Biscuits, homemade	1 ea	35	124	2.5	6	1.5	1	16	0.5	82	1	203	29	0.12	0.11	1	0	21.35
Blueberries, fresh, bilberries	½ cup	73	41	0.5	0	0	0	10	2	4	0.1	4	73	0.04	0.04	0.3	9	4.67
Brandy, 86 proof	1 oz	28	70	0	0	0	0	0	0	7	0.1	0	0	0	0	0	0	0
Bread, banana, prep f/recipe w/veg shortening	1 pce	50	169	2.2	6	1.5	22	28	0.7	9	0.7	99	46	0.09	0.1	0.7	1	5.5
Bread, cracked wheat	1 pce	25	65	2.2	1	0.2	0	12	1.4	11	0.7	134	0	0.09	0.06	0.9	0	15.25
Bread, French	1 pce	35	96	3.1	1	0.2	0	18	1	26	0.9	213	0	0.18	0.12	1.7	0	33.25
Bread, mixed grain	1 pce	26	65	2.6	1	0.2	0	12	1.7	24	0.9	127	0	0.11	0.09	1.1	0	20.8
Bread, pita pocket, white	1 ea	60	165	5.5	1	0.1	0	33	1.3	52	1.6	322	0	0.36	0.2	2.8	0	57
Bread, pumpernickel	1 pce	32	80	2.8	1	0.1	0	15	2.1	22	0.9	215	0	0.1	0.1	1	0	25.6
Bread, rye	1 pce	25	65	2.1	1	0.2	0	12	1.5	18	0.7	165	2	0.11	0.08	1	0	21.5
Bread, white, f/recipe w/2% milk	1 pce	25	71	2	1	0.3	1	12	0.5	14	0.7	90	20	0.1	0.1	0.9	0	22.75
Bread, whole wheat	1 pce	25	62	2.4	1	0.2	0	12	1.7	18	0.8	132	0	0.09	0.05	1	0	12.5
Broccoli, med stalk, 8" long, ckd w/o add salt	1 ea	140	39	4.2	0	0.1	0	7	4.1	64	1.2	36	1943	0.08	0.16	0.8	104	70
Broccoli, spear, raw, 5" long	1 ea	114	32	3.4	0	0.1	0	6	3.4	55	1	31	1758	0.07	0.14	0.7	106	80.94
Brownie, chocolate, w/walnuts, prep f/rec	1 ea	20	93	1.2	6	1.5	15	10	0.4	11	0.4	69	153	0.03	0.04	0.2	0	5.8
Brussels Sprouts, ckd, drained	½ cup	78	30	2	0	0.1	0	7	2	28	0.9	16	561	0.08	0.06	0.5	48	46.8
Buns, hamburger	1 ea	40	114	3.4	2	0.5	0	20	1.1	56	1.3	224	0	0.19	0.12	1.6	0	38

APPENDIX A NUTRITIVE VALUE OF SELECTED FOODS

Food	Amount	Weight (g)	Calories	Protein (g)	Fat (g)	Sat. Fat (g)	Choles-terol (g)	Carbo-hydrate (g)	Fiber (g)	Cal-cium (mg)	Iron (mg)	Sodi-um (mg)	Vit A (IU)	Thia-min (Vit B1) (mg)	Ribo-flavin (Vit B2) (mg)	Niacin (mg)	Vit C (mg)	Folate (mcg)
Buns, hot dog/frankfurter	1 ea	40	114	3.4	2	0.5	0	20	1.1	56	1.3	224	0	0.19	0.12	1.6	0	38
Burger/Patty, vegetarian, Gardenburger, original	1 ea	71	130	8	3	1	11	18	5	84	0	290	50	0.11	0.15	1.1	0	10.08
Burger/Patty, vegetarian, soy	1 ea	71	142	14.9	6	1	11	6	3.3	21	1.5	390	0	0.64	0.43	7.1	0	55.38
Butter, salted	1 Tbs	5	36	0	4	2.5	11	0	0	1	0	41	153	0	0	0	0	0.15
Buttermilk, skim, cultured	1 cup	245	99	8.1	2	1.3	9	12	0	285	0.1	257	81	0.08	0.38	0.1	2	12.25
Cabbage, ckd w/o add salt, drained, shredded	½ cup	85	19	0.9	0	0	0	4	2	26	0.1	7	112	0.05	0.05	0.2	17	17
Cabbage, raw, shredded	½ cup	45	11	0.6	0	0	0	2	1	21	0.3	8	60	0.02	0.02	0.1	14	19.35
Cake, angel food, cmrcl prep	1 pce	60	155	3.5	0	0.1	0	35	0.9	84	0.3	449	0	0.06	0.29	0.5	0	21
Cake, carrot, w/cream cheese icing	1 pce	96	419	4.4	25	4.7	52	45	1.2	24	1.2	236	3310	0.13	0.15	1	1	11.52
Cake, chocolate, w/chocolate icing, 1/8th	1 pce	69	253	2.8	11	3.3	29	38	1.9	30	1.5	230	59	0.02	0.09	0.4	0	11.73
Cake, devils food, marshmallow iced	1 pce	99	408	3.5	21	5.8	52	52	1.2	47	1.3	338	0	0.04	0.07	0.4	0	12.3
Cake, pound, w/butter	1 pce	30	116	1.7	6	3.5	66	15	0.1	10	0.4	119	182	0.05	0.07	0.3	0	2.11
Cake, white, w/chocolate icing	1 pce	71	259	1.8	8	3.7	13	46	0.8	55	0.5	219	166	0.08	0.69		0	21
Calamari/Squid, fried, mixed species	1 cup	150	262	26.9	11	2.8	390	12	2	58	1.5	459	52	0.01	0.06	3.9	6	9.5
Candy Bar, Almond Joy, fun size	1½ oz	42	196	1.8	11	7.3	8	24	2	26	0.6	61	5	0.02	0.16	0.2	0	6
Candy Bar, Mars almond	1 ea	50	234	4.1	12	3.6	8	31	1	84	0.6	85	94	0.02	0.13	0.5	1	0.82
Candy Bar, Milky Way, 2.1 oz bar	1 ea	60	254	2.7	10	4.7	8	43	1	78	0.5	144	65	0.01	0.03	0.2	0	1.4
Candy Bar, Special Dark sweet chocolate	1 ea	41	226	2	13	8.3	0	25	2	11	1	3	14	0	0.05	0.2	0	0
Candy, caramels, plain/chocolate	1 oz	28	107	1.3	2	1.8	2	22	0.3	39	0.1	69	9	0.02	0	0.1	0	2.24
Candy, hard, all flvrs	1 oz	28	110	0	0	0	0	27	0	1	0.1	11	0	0	0	0	0	9.8
Candy, Kisses, milk chocolate	1 oz	28	144	1.9	9	5.2	6	17	1	53	0.4	23	52	0.02	0.08	0	0	1.68
Candy, M & M's peanut chocolate	1 oz	28	144	2.7	7	2.9	3	17	1	28	0.3	13	26	0.03	0.05	1	0	3.36
Candy, M & M's plain chocolate	1 oz	28	138	1.2	6	3.7	4	20	0.7	29	0.3	17	57	0.02	0.06	0.1	0	10.15
Candy, milk chocolate, w/almonds	1 oz	28	147	2.5	10	4.8	5	15	1.7	63	0.5	21	21	0.02	0.12	0.2	0	11.34
Carrots, ckd w/o add salt, drained, slices	½ cup	73	33	0.8	0	0	0	8	2.4	23	0.5	48	17924	0.02	0.04	0.4	2	
Carrots, raw, whole, 7½" long	1 ea	81	35	0.8	0	0	0	8	2.4	22	0.4	28	22784	0.08	0.05	0.8	8	
Catsup/Ketchup	1 Tbs	15	16	0.2	0	0	0	4	0.2	3	0.1	178	152	0.01	0.01	0.2	2	2.25
Cauliflower, ckd, drained	½ cup	63	14	1.2	0	0	0	3	1.7	10	0.2	9	11	0.03	0.03	0.3	28	27.72
Celery, raw, med stalk, 8" long	1 ea	40	6	0.3	0	0	0	1	0.7	16	0.2	35	54	0.02	0.02	0.1	3	11.2
Cereal, 100% Bran, rte, dry	½ cup	33	89	4.1	2	0.3	0	24	9.8	23	4.1	229	0	0.79	0.89	10.5	31	23.43
Cereal, All-Bran, rte, dry	¼ cup	21	55	2.6	1	0.1	0	16	6.8	74	3.1	43	525	0.27	0.29	3.5	10	63
Cereal, Alpha-Bits, rte, dry	1 cup	28	110	2.2	1	0.1	0	24	1.2	8	2.7	178	1235	0.36	0.42	4.9	0	98.84
Cereal, bran flakes, rte, dry	¾ cup	30	96	2.8	1	0.1	0	24	5.3	17	8.1	220	750	0.38	0.43	5	0	99.9
Cereal, Cheerios	1 cup	23	84	2.4	1	0.3	0	18		42	6.2	218	958	0.29	0.33	3.8	12	76.59
Cereal, Chex, corn, rte, dry	1 cup	28	105	2	0	0.1	0	24	0.5	94	8.4	270	0	0.35	0	4.7	6	93.24
Cereal, Chex, wheat, rte, dry	1 cup	46	159	4.8	1	0.2	0	37	5.1	92	13.8	412	0	0.34	0.06	4.6	6	92
Cereal, corn flakes, rte, dry	1 cup	25	91	1.6	0	0.1	0	22	0.7	1	7.8	266	625	0.32	0.35	4.2	12	88.25
Cereal, Corn Pops, rte, dry	1 cup	28	107	1	0	0.1	0	26	0.4	2	1.7	111	700	0.36	0.39	4.7	14	98.84
Cereal, Cream of Wheat, quick, ckd w/water	1 cup	244	132	3.7	0	0.1	0	27	1.2	51	10.5	142	0	0.24	0	1.5	0	109.8
Cereal, Crispy Rice, rte, dry	¾ cup	22	87	1.4	0	0	0	19	0.3	4	0.6	161	971	0.41	0.46	5.4	12	108.6
Cereal, Frosted Flakes, rte, dry	1 cup	35	135	1.4	0	0.1	0	32	0.7	1	5.1	226	847	0.42	0.49	5.6	17	105
Cereal, Frosted Mini Wheats, rte, dry	1 cup	55	186	5.2	1	0.2	0	45	5.9	20	15.4	2	0	0.38	0.44	5.4	0	110
Cereal, granola, rte, dry	½ cup	57	257	6	10	1.3	0	38	3.6	43	1.8	92	0	0.18	0.06	0.6	0	8.55
Cereal, Grape Nuts, rte, dry	½ cup	57	205	6.2	1	0.2	0	46	5	19	15.9	348	737	0.37	0.42	4.9	0	98.04
Cereal, Honey Bran, rte, dry	½ cup	30	102	2.6	1	0.2	0	25	3.3	14	4.8	173	1323	0.39	0.45	5.3	16	20.1
Cereal, Life, plain, rte, dry	1 cup	44	167	4.3	2	0.3	0	35	2.8	134	12.3	240	16	0.55	0.62	7.3	0	146.9
Cereal, Mueslix, five grain muesli, rte, dry	1 cup	82	289	6.2	5	0.7	0	63	5.6	67	8.9	107	2488	0.75	0.84	9.8	1	196.8
Cereal, Nutri-Grain, wheat, rte, dry	1 oz	28	101	2.4	0	0.1	0	24	1.8	8	0.8	190	0	0.36	0.42	4.9	15	98.84
Cereal, oatmeal, unsalted, ckd w/water	½ cup	120	74	3.1	1	0.2	0	13	2	10	0.8	1	19	0.13	0.02	0.2	0	4.8

Food	Amount	Weight (g)	Calories	Protein (g)	Fat (g)	Sat. Fat (g)	Choles-terol (g)	Carbo-hydrate (g)	Fiber (g)	Cal-cium (mg)	Iron (mg)	Sodium (mg)	Vit A (IU)	Thia-min (Vit B_1) (mg)	Ribo-flavin (Vit B_2) (mg)	Niacin (mg)	Vit C (mg)	Folate (mcg)
Cereal, raisin bran, rte, dry	1 cup	49	155	3.9	1	0.1	0	38	6.4	22	9	299	623	0.31	0.35	4.2	0	82.81
Cereal, Shredded Wheat, sml biscuits, rte, dry	1 cup	19	68	2.1	0	0.1	0	15	1.9	7	0.8	2	0	0.05	0.05	1	0	9.5
Cereal, Smacks, rte, dry	1 cup	37	141	2.4	1	0.4	0	32	1.3	4	2.5	70	1028	0.52	0.59	6.8	21	136.9
Cereal, Special K, rte, dry	1 cup	21	78	4.3	0	0	0	15	0.7	3	5.9	169	508	0.36	0.4	4.7	10	63
Cereal, Total, wheat, rte, dry	1 cup	33	116	3.3	1	0.2	0	26	2.9	284	19.8	218	1375	1.65	1.87	22.1	66	439.8
Cereal, Wheaties, rte, dry	1 cup	29	106	3.1	1	0.2	0	23	2	53	7.8	215	725	0.36	0.41	4.8	14	96.57
Cheese Puffs/Cheetos	1 oz	28	155	2.1	10	1.8	1	15	0.3	16	0.7	294	74	0.07	0.1	0.9	0	33.6
Cheese Spread, low fat, low sod	1 pce	34	61	8.4	2	1.5	12	1	0	233	0.1	2	92	0.01	0.13	0	0	3.06
Cheese, American, proc, shredded	1 oz	28	105	6.2	9	5.5	26	0	0	172	0.1	401	339	0.01	0.1	0	0	2.18
Cheese, blue	1 oz	28	99	6	8	5.2	21	1	0	148	0.1	391	202	0.01	0.11	0.3	0	10.19
Cheese, cheddar, diced	1 oz	28	113	7	9	5.9	29	0	0	202	0.2	174	297	0.01	0.11	0	0	5.1
Cheese, feta	1 oz	28	74	4	6	4.2	25	1	0	138	0.2	313	125	0.04	0.24	0.3	0	8.96
Cheese, monterey jack, shredded	1 oz	28	105	6.9	8	5.3	25	0	0	209	0.2	150	266	0	0.11	0	0	5.1
Cheese, mozzarella, part skm milk, low moist, shredded	1 oz	28	78	7.7	5	3	15	1	0	205	0.1	148	197	0.01	0.1	0	0	2.77
Cheese, parmesan, grated	1 Tbs	5	23	2.1	2	1	4	0	0	69	0	93	35	0	0.02	0	0	0.4
Cheese, ricotta, part skm	1 oz	28	39	3.2	2	1.4	9	1	0	76	0.1	35	121	0.01	0.05	0	0	3.67
Cheese, Swiss, shredded	1 oz	28	105	8	8	5	26	1	0	269	0	73	237	0.01	0.1	0	0	1.79
Cheesecake	1 pce	85	273	4.7	19	8.4	47	22	0.4	43	0.5	176	465	0.02	0.16	0.2	0	15.3
Cherries, sweet, fresh	10 ea	75	54	0.9	1	0.2	0	12	1.7	11	0.3	0	160	0.04	0.04	0.3	5	3.15
Chicken, broiler/fryer, breast, rstd	1 ea	98	193	29.2	8	2.1	82	0	0	14	1	70	91	0.06	0.12	12.5	0	3.92
Chicken, broiler/fryer, dark meat, w/o skin, rstd	3 oz	85	174	23.3	8	2.3	79	0	0	13	1.1	79	61	0.06	0.19	5.6	0	6.8
Chicken, broiler/fryer, drumstick, rstd	1 ea	52	112	14.1	6	1.6	47	0	0	6	0.7	47	52	0.04	0.11	3.1	0	4.16
Chicken, broiler/fryer, meat only, w/o skin, rstd	3 oz	85	162	24.6	6	1.7	76	0	0	13	1	73	45	0.06	0.15	7.8	0	5.1
Chips, corn	1 oz	28	151	1.8	9	1.3	0	16	1.4	36	0.4	176	26	0.01	0.04	0.3	0	5.6
Chips, tortilla, chili & lime	18 pce	28	110	2	2		0	22	2	60	3.6	200	0	0.02	0.05	0.4	0	2.8
Chips, tortilla, plain	1 oz	28	140	2	7	1.4	0	18	1.8	43	0.4	148	55	0.07	0.1	2.3	0	8.71
Cod, batter fried	3½ oz	100	173	17.4	7	1.6	50	7	0.2	29	0.7	91	30	0.02	0.05	2.2	2	6.6
Cod, stmd/poached	3½ oz	100	102	22.4	1	0.1	46	0	0	9	0.3	80	28	0	0	0.4	3	0.18
Coffee, brewed	¾ cup	180	4	0.2	0	0	0	1	0	4	0.1	4	0			0.5	0	
Collards, ckd w/o add salt	½ cup	95	25	2	0	0	0	5	2.7	113	0.4	9	2973	0.04	0.1	0.5	17	88.35
Cone, ice cream, wafer/cake type	1 ea	115	480	9.3	8	1.4	0	91	3.4	29	4.1	164	0	0.29	0.41	5.1	0	117.3
Cookie, chocolate chip, prep w/marg f/rec	2 ea	20	98	1.1	8	1.6	6	12	0.6	8	0.5	72	127	0.04	0.04	0.3	0	6.6
Cookie, chocolate sandwich, creme filled	4 ea	40	189	1.9	8	1.5	0	28	1.3	10	1.6	242	1	0.03	0.07	0.8	0	17.2
Cookie, fig bar	4 ea	56	195	2.1	4	0.6	0	40	2.6	36	1.6	196	18	0.09	0.12	1	0	15.12
Cookie, oatmeal raisin, prep f/rec	2 ea	26	113	1.7	4	0.8	9	18	0.8	26	0.7	140	167	0.06	0.04	0.3	0	7.8
Cookie, peanut butter, prep f/rec	2 ea	24	114	2.2	6	1.1	7	14	0.5	9	0.5	124	144	0.05	0.05	0.8	0	13.2
Cookie, shortbread, cmrcl, plain	4 ea	32	161	2	8	2	6	21	0.6	11	0.9	146	28	0.11	0.11	1.1	0	18.88
Cookie, vanilla wafer type, 12–17% fat	10 ea	40	176	2	6	1.5	20	29	0.8	19	1	125	11	0.11	0.13	1.2	0	20
Coriander, raw	¼ cup	4	1	0.1	0.1	0.1	0	0.1	0.1	4	0.1	4	111		0	0	7	0.41
Corn, yellow, vac pack, cnd	½ cup	83	66	2	2	0.1	0	16	1.7	4	0.3	226	200	0.03	0.06	1	7	40.92
Cornbread, prep f/dry mix	1 ea	60	188	4.3	6	1.6	37	29	1.4	44	1.1	467	123	0.15	0.16	1.2	0	33
Cornmeal, yellow, degermed, enrich, dry	½ cup	120	439	10.2	2	0.3	0	93	8.9	6	5	4	496	0.86	0.49	6	0	224.4
Cottage Cheese, 2% fat	½ cup	113	101	15.5	2	1.4	9	4	0	77	0.2	459	79	0.03	0.21	0.2	0	14.8
Cottage Cheese, creamed, sml curd	½ cup	105	109	13.1	5	3	16	3	0	63	0.1	425	171	0.02	0.17	0.1	0	12.81
Crab, blue, cnd, drained	1 cup	135	134	27.7	2	0.3	120	0	0	136	1.1	450	7	0.11	0.11	1.8	4	57.38

Profile Plus

More information on thousands of additional foods can be found on your Profile Plus CD-ROM.

Food	Amount	Weight (g)	Calories	Protein (g)	Fat (g)	Sat. Fat (g)	Cholesterol (g)	Carbohydrate (g)	Fiber (g)	Calcium (mg)	Iron (mg)	Sodium (mg)	Vit A (IU)	Thiamin (Vit B$_1$) (mg)	Riboflavin (Vit B$_2$) (mg)	Niacin (mg)	Vit C (mg)	Folate (mcg)
Crackers, cheese	1 ea	10	50	1	3	0.9	1	6	0.2	15	0.5	100	16	0.06	0.04	0.5	0	8
Crackers, graham, plain/honey, 2½ square	2 ea	14	59	1	1	0.2	0	11	0.4	3	0.5	85	0	0.03	0.04	0.6	0	8.4
Crackers, matzoh, plain, svg	1 ea	28	111	2.8	0	0.1	0	23	0.8	4	0.9	1	0	0.11	0.08	1.1	0	32.76
Crackers, rye, wafers	2 ea	14	47	1.3	0	0	0	11	3.2	6	0.8	111	1	0.06	0.04	0.2	0	6.3
Crackers, saltine	1 ea	11	48	1	1	0.3	0	8	0.3	13	0.6	143	0	0.06	0.05	0.6	0	13.64
Crackers, standard, reg. snack type, round	1 ea	3	15	0.2	1	0.1	0	2	0	4	0.1	25	0	0.01	0.01	0.1	0	2.31
Crackers, triscuit	1 ea	5	24	0.5	1	0.2	0	3	0.5	1	0.2	26	0	0.01	0.01	0.1	0	0.36
Crackers, wheat	1 ea	2	9	0.2	0	0.1	0	1	0.1	1	0.1	16	0	0	0.06	0	0	3.7
Cream Cheese	1 oz	28	98	2.1	10	6.2	31	1	0	22	0.3	83	400	0.01	0.06	0	0	0.34
Cream, light	1 Tbs	15	29	0.4	3	1.8	10	1	0	14	0	6	95	0	0.02	0	0	0.56
Cream, whipping, heavy	1 Tbs	15	52	0.3	6	3.5	21	0	0	10	0	6	221	0	0.02	0	0	
Croissant, butter	1 ea	57	231	4.7	12	6.6	38	26	1.5	21	1.2	424	424	0.22	0.14	1.2	0	35.34
Cucumber, w/o skin, raw, sliced	½ cup	60	7	0.3	0	0	0	2	0.4	8	0.1	1	44	0.01	0.01	0.1	2	8.4
Dates, fresh, whole	10 ea	83	228	1.6	0	0.2	0	61	6.2	27	1	2	42	0.07	0.08	1.8	0	10.46
Dinner, chicken, cacciatore, w/noodles, low cal, fzn	1 ea	308	311	22.5	10	2.4	59	33	3.4	29	3.2	934	732	0.28	0.4	8	26	32.22
Doughnut, cake	1 ea	47	198	2.3	11	1.7	17	23	0.7	21	0.9	257	27	0.1	0.11	0.9	0	22.09
Doughnut, raised, glazed	1 ea	60	242	3.8	14	3.5	4	27	0.7	26	1.2	205	8	0.22	0.13	1.7	0	25.8
Egg Substitute, Egg Beaters, new	¼ cup	61	30	6	0	0	0	1	0	20	1.1	125	300	0	0.85	0	0	32.0
Egg Whites, raw	1 ea	33	16	3.5	0	0	0	0	0	2	0	54	0	0	0.15	0	0	0.99
Egg Yolks, raw, lrg	1 ea	17	61	2.8	5	1.6	218	0	0	23	0.6	7	331	0.03	0.11	0	0	24.82
Eggs, hard ckd/bld, lrg	1 ea	50	78	6.3	5	1.6	212	1	0	25	0.6	62	280	0.03	0.26	0	0	22
Eggs, scrambled, plain, lrg	1 ea	64	106	7.1	8	2.4	225	1	0	45	0.8	179	436	0.03	0.28	0.1	0	19.2
Eggs, whole, fried	1 ea	46	92	6.2	7	1.9	211	1	0	25	0.7	162	394	0.03	0.24	0	0	17.48
Entree, lasagna, w/meat, prep f/rec	1 pce	220	352	20.7	14	7.2	52	36	2.5	243	2.8	351	902	0.21	0.3	3.8	13	17.82
Entree, macaroni & cheese, prep f/rec w/margarine	½ cup	100	215	8.4	11	4.4	21	20	0.6	181	0.9	543	430	0.1	0.2	0.9	0	5.15
Entree, meatloaf, beef	1 pce	111	232	20.2	14	5.6	107	5	0.2	37	2.1	185	148	0.06	0.28	3.3	0	14.28
Entree, quiche, lorraine	1 pce	242	724	20.5	56	25.9	304	34	1	318	2.6	303	1323	0.36	0.67	2.8	1	26.48
Entree, spaghetti, w/meatballs, prep f/rec	1 cup	248	332	18.6	12	3.3	74	39	7.7	124	3.7	1009	1587	0.25	0.3	4	22	9.99
Entree, spaghetti, w/tomato sauce & cheese, prep f/rec	1 cup	250	260	8.8	9	2	8	37	2.5	80	2.2	955	1075	0.25	0.17	2.2	12	8
Figs, dried, unckd	1 ea	21	54	0.6	0	0	0	14	2.5	30	0.5	2	28	0.01	0.02	0.1	0	1.57
Fish Sticks/Portions, heated f/fzn, 4x1x.5	2 ea	56	152	8.8	7	1.8	63	13	0	11	0.4	326	59	0.07	0.1	1.2	0	10.19
Flour, all purpose, white, bleached, enrich	1 cup	125	455	12.9	1	0.2	0	95	3.4	19	5.8	2	0	0.98	0.62	7.4	0	192.5
Flour, whole wheat	1 cup	120	407	16.4	2	0.4	0	87	14.6	41	4.7	6	0	0.54	0.26	7.6	0	52.8
Frankfurter/Hot Dog, beef & pork, 10 pack	1 ea	57	182	6.4	17	6.1	28	1	0	6	0.7	638	0	0.11	0.07	1.5	0	2.28
Frankfurter/Hot Dog, beef, 8 pack	1 ea	57	180	6.8	16	6.9	35	1	0	11	0.8	585	0	0.03	0.06	1.4	0	2.28
Frankfurter/Hot Dog, turkey	1 ea	45	102	6.4	8	2.7	48	1	0	48	0.8	642	0	0.02	0.08	1.9	0	3.6
Frozen Yogurt, vanilla/strawberry, nonfat, sml scoop	4 oz	113	112	5.6	0	0.1	2	22	0	196	0.1	75	7	0.05	0.23	0.1	1	11.99
Fruit Cocktail, in heavy syrup, cnd	1 cup	245	179	1	0	0	0	46	2.5	15	0.7	15	502	0.04	0.05	0.9	5	6.37
Fruit Cocktail, in juice	1 cup	248	114	1.1	0	0	0	29	2.5	20	0.5	10	756	0.03	0.04	1	7	6.2
Fruit Punch, prep f/pwd	1 cup	240	89	0	0	0	0	23	0	38	0.1	34	0	0	0	0	28	0.24
Fudge, chocolate, prep f/rec	1 oz	28	107	0.5	2	1.4	4	22	0.2	12	0.1	17	53	0	0.02	0	0	0.56
Grapefruit, pink, fresh, 3¾" diameter	½ ea	123	37	0.7	0	0	0	9	1.7	14	0.1	0	319	0.04	0.02	0.2	47	15.01
Grapes, tokay/empress/red flame, fresh	10 ea	50	36	0.3	0	0.1	0	9	0.5	6	0.1	1	36	0.05	0.03	0.2	5	1.95
Haddock, fillet, brd, fried	3 oz	85	184	17.1	9	1.9	65	7	0.2	53	1.5	145	69	0.08	0.09	3.7	0	11.6
Halibut, Greenland, fillet, bkd/brld	3 oz	85	203	15.7	15	2.6	50	0	0	3	0.7	88	51	0.06	0.09	1.6	0	0.85
Honey, strained, extracted	1 Tbs	21	64	0.1	0	0	0	17	0	1	0.1	1	0	0	0.01	0	0	0.42
Hot Cocoa/Choc, prep f/rec w/whole milk	1 cup	250	192	9.8	6	3.6	20	29	2	315	1.1	128	515	0.1	0.44	0.4	2	15
Hummus/Hummos, raw	1 cup	246	421	12.1	21	3.1	0	50	12.5	123	3.9	600	62	0.23	0.13	1	19	146.1

Food	Amount	Weight (g)	Calories	Protein (g)	Fat (g)	Sat. Fat (g)	Choles- terol (mg)	Carbo- hydrate (g)	Fiber (g)	Cal- cium (mg)	Iron (mg)	Sodi- um (mg)	Vit A (IU)	Thia- min (Vit B₁) (mg)	Ribo- flavin (Vit B₂) (mg)	Niacin (mg)	Vit C (mg)	Folate (mcg)
Instant Breakfast, prep f/dry mix w/nonfat milk	1 cup	282	216	15.7	1	0.7	9	36	0.2	407	4.8	268	2343	0.4	0.42	5.5	31	118.2
Instant Breakfast, prep f/dry mix w/whole milk	1 cup	281	280	15.4	9	5.4	38	36	0.2	396	4.9	262	2151	0.41	0.47	5.5	31	117.7
Jam/Preserves, pkt	1 ea	14	39	0.1	0	0	0	10	0.2	3	0.1	4	2	0	0	0	2	4.62
Jelly	1 Tbs	18	51	0	0	0	0	13	0.2	1	0	5	3	0	0	0	0	0.18
Juice, apple, unswtnd, cnd/btld	½ cup	124	58	0.1	0	0	0	14	0.1	9	0.5	4	1	0.03	0.02	0.1	1	0.12
Juice, cranberry cocktail	1 cup	253	144	0	0	0	0	36	0.3	8	0.4	5	10	0.02	0.02	0.1	90	0.51
Juice, grape, unswtnd, btld/cnd	½ cup	127	77	0.7	0	0	0	19	0.1	11	0.3	4	10	0.03	0.05	0.3	0	3.3
Juice, grapefruit, unswtnd, cnd	½ cup	124	47	0.6	0	0	0	11	0.1	9	0.2	1	9	0.05	0.02	0.3	36	12.9
Juice, grapefruit, unswtnd, prep f/fzn conc	1 cup	247	101	1.4	0	0	0	24	0.2	20	0.3	2	22	0.1	0.05	0.5	83	8.89
Juice, lemon, fresh	1 Tbs	15	4	0.1	0	0	0	1	0.1	1	0	0	3	0	0	0	7	1.94
Juice, orange, prep f/fzn	½ cup	125	56	0.9	0	0	0	13	0.2	11	0.1	1	98	0.1	0.02	0.3	49	54.75
Juice, prune, w/o pulp	½ cup	88	60	0.7	0	0	0	14	0.5	2	0.9	4	54	0.03			3	
Juice, tomato, w/salt, cnd	1 cup	244	41	1.9	0	0	0	10	1	22	1.4	881	1357	0.11	0.08	1.6	45	48.56
Kale, ckd w/o add salt, drained	½ cup	55	15	1	0	0	0	3	1.1	40	0.5	13	4070	0.03	0.04	0.3	23	7.32
Kiwifruit/Chinese Gooseberries, fresh, med	1 ea	76	46	0.8	0	0	0	11	2.6	20	0.3	4	133	0.02	0.04	0.4	74	28.88
Lamb, leg, whole, lean, rstd, choice, ¼" trim	3 oz	85	162	24.1	7	2.3	76	0	0	7	1.8	58	0	0.09	0.25	5.4	0	19.55
Lamb, loin chop, lean, brld, choice, ¼" trim	3 oz	84	181	25.2	8	2.9	80	0	0	16	1.7	71	0	0.09	0.24	5.8	0	20.16
Lemonade, white, fzn conc	12 oz	340	615	1	1	0.1	0	160	1.4	24	2.4	14	0	0.05	0.33	0.3	60	34
Lentils, sprouts, stir fried	1 cup	124	125	10.9	1	0.1	0	26	4.8	17	3.8	12	51	0.27	0.11	1.5	16	83.08
Lentils, unsalted, ckd	1 cup	200	232	18	1	0.1	0	40	15.8	38	6.7	4	16	0.34	0.15	2.1	3	361.6
Lettuce, butterhead, Boston/bibb, leaf, raw	2 pce	15	2	0.2	0	0	0	0	0.2	5	0.2	1	146	0.01	0.01	0	1	11
Lettuce, romaine, raw, chpd	1 cup	55	8	0.9	0	0	1	1	0.9	20	0.6	4	1430	0.06	0.06	0.3	13	74.64
Lobster, northern, stmd	1 cup	145	142	29.7	1	0.2	104	2	0	88	0.6	551	126	0.01	0.1	1.6	0	16.1
Lunchmeat Spread, liverwurst, cnd	1 oz	28	87	3.6	7	2.5	33	2	0.5	3	2.3	193	3818	0.05	0.04		1	
Lunchmeat, bologna, beef & pork	1 pce	28	88	3.3	8	3	15	1	0	3	0.4	285	0	0.05	0.04	0.7	0	1.4
Lunchmeat, bologna, turkey	2 pce	57	113	7.8	9	2.9	56	1	0	48	0.9	500	0	0.03	0.09	2	0	3.99
Lunchmeat, roast beef, deli style, pouch	3 oz	85	96	17.2	3	1.1	41	1	0	5	1.6	860	0				0	
Lunchmeat, turkey breast, rstd, fat free	1 pce	28	24	4.2	0	0.1	9	1	0	3	0.3	334	0				0	
Mayonnaise, imit, low cal	1 Tbs	15	35	0	3	0.5	4	2	0	0	0	75	14	0	0	0	0	
Mayonnaise, soybean oil, w/salt	1 tsp	5	36	0.1	4	0.6	3	0	0	1	0	28	0	0	0	0	0	0.38
Melon, cantaloupe/musk, med 5" diameter	¼ ea	239	84	2.1	1	0.2	0	20	1.9	26	0.5	22	7705	0.09	0.05	1.4	101	40.63
Melon, honeydew, fresh, wedge, 1/8 melon	1 pce	129	45	0.6	0	0	0	12	0.8	8	0.1	13	52	0.1	0.02	0.8	32	7.74
Milk Shake, chocolate, fast food	10 fl-oz	340	432	11.6	13	7.9	44	70	2.7	384	1.1	330	316	0.2	0.83	0.5	1	11.9
Milk, evaporated, whole, w/add vit A, cnd	½ cup	126	169	8.6	10	5.8	37	13	0	329	0.2	133	500	0.06	0.4	0.2	2	9.95
Milk, low fat, 1%, w/add vit A	1 cup	244	102	8	3	1.6	10	12	0	300	0.1	123	500	0.1	0.41	0.2	2	12.44
Milk, low fat, 2%, chocolate	1 cup	250	179	8	5	3.1	17	26	1.2	284	0.6	150	500	0.09	0.41	0.3	2	12
Milk, low fat, 2%, w/add vit A	1 cup	244	121	8.1	5	2.9	18	12	0	297	0.1	122	500	0.1	0.4	0.2	2	12.44
Milk, nonfat/skim, w/add vit A	1 cup	245	86	8.4	0	0.3	4	12	0	302	0.1	126	500	0.09	0.34	0.2	2	12.74
Milk, whole, 3.3%	1 cup	244	150	8	8	5.1	33	11	0	291	0.1	120	307	0.09	0.4	0.2	2	12.2
Milkshake, strawberry, fast food	10 fl-oz	340	384	11.6	10	5.9	37	64	1.4	384	0.4	282	408	0.15	0.66	0.6	3	10.2
Mixed Vegetables, cnd, drained	1 cup	182	86	4.7	1	0.1	0	17	5.5	49	1.9	271	21198	0.08	0.09	1.1	9	42.95
Muffin, English, plain	1 ea	57	134	4.4	1	0.1	0	26	1.5	99	1.4	264	0	0.25	0.16	2.2	0	46.17
Muffin, English, plain, tstd	1 ea	52	133	4.4	1	0.1	0	26	1.5	98	1.4	262	0	0.2	0.14	2	0	38.48
Muffin, wheat bran, prep f/rec w/whole milk	1 ea	45	130	3.2	6	1.2	16	19	3.2	84	1.9	265	363	0.2	0.2	1.8	4	23.4
Mushrooms, raw, pces/slices	1 cup	35	9	1	0	0	0	1	0.4	2	0.4	1	0	0.03	0.15	1.4	1	4.2
Mustard Greens, ckd w/o add salt, drained	½ cup	70	10	1.6	0	0	0	1	1.4	52	0.5	11	2122	0.03	0.04	0.3	18	51.38
Nuts, almonds, dried, unblanched, whole	¼ cup	36	208	7.7	18	1.4	0	7	4.2	89	1.5	0	4	0.09	0.29	1.4	0	10.44
Nuts, Brazil, dried, shelled, 32 kernels	1 oz	28	184	4	19	4.5	0	4	1.5	49	1	1	0	0.28	0.03	0.5	0	1.12

Food	Amount	Weight (g)	Calories	Protein (g)	Fat (g)	Sat. Fat (g)	Cholesterol (g)	Carbohydrate (g)	Fiber (g)	Calcium (mg)	Iron (mg)	Sodium (mg)	Vit A (IU)	Thiamin (Vit B_1) (mg)	Riboflavin (Vit B_2) (mg)	Niacin (mg)	Vit C (mg)	Folate (mcg)
Nuts, cashews, dry rstd, salted	1 cup	137	786	21	63	12.5	0	45	4.1	62	8.2	877	0	0.27	0.27	1.9	0	94.8
Nuts, coconut, unswtnd, dried	½ cup	65	429	4.5	42	37.2	0	16	10.6	17	2.2	24	0	0.04	0.06	0.4	1	5.85
Nuts, peanuts, oil rstd, unsalted, chpd	1 oz	28	163	7.4	14	1.9	0	5	1.9	25	0.5	2	0	0.07	0.03	4	0	35.2
Nuts, pecans, dried, halves	1 oz	28	193	2.6	20	1.7	0	4	2.7	20	0.7	0	22	0.18	0.04	0.3	0	6.16
Nuts, walnuts, black, dried, chpd	1 oz	28	170	6.8	16	1	0	3	1.4	16	0.9	0	83	0.06	0.03	0.2	1	18.34
Oil, canola	1 cup	218	1927	0	218	15.5	0	0	0	0	0	0	0	0	0	0	0	0
Oil, corn	1 Tbs	15	133	0	15	1.9	0	0	0	0	0	0	0	0	0	0	0	0
Oil, olive	1 Tbs	15	133	0	15	2	0	0	0	0	0.1	0	0	0	0	0	0	0
Oil, peanut	1 cup	216	1909	0	216	36.5	0	0	0	0	0.1	0	0	0	0	0	0	0
Oil, safflower, greater than 70% linoleic	1 Tbs	15	133	0	15	0.9	0	0	0	0	0	0	0	0	0	0	0	0
Oil, soybean	1 tsp	5	44	0	5	0.7	0	0	0	0	0	0	0	0	0	0	0	0
Okra, bindi, ckd w/o add salt f/raw, drained, pods	8 ea	85	27	1.6	0	0	0	6	2.1	54	0.4	4	489	0.11	0.05	0.7	14	38.85
Olives, w/o pits, ripe, lrg, cnd	10 ea	44	51	0.4	5	0.6	0	3	1.4	39	1.5	384	177	0	0	0	0	0
Olives, w/o pits, ripe, sml, cnd	10 ea	32	37	0.3	3	0.5	0	2	1	28	1.1	279	129	0	0	0	0	0
Onions, yellow, ckd w/o add salt, drained, chpd	½ cup	105	46	1.4	0	0	0	11	1.5	23	0.3	3	0	0.04	0.02	0.2	5	15.75
Oranges, fresh, med	1 ea	180	85	1.7	0	0	0	21	4.3	72	0.2	0	369	0.16	0.07	0.5	96	54.54
Oysters, eastern, brd, fried, med	1 ea	45	89	3.9	6	1.4	36	5	0.1	28	3.1	188	136	0.07	0.09	0.7	2	13.95
Oysters, eastern, raw, wild	½ cup	120	82	8.5	3	0.9	64	5	0	54	8	253	120	0.12	0.11	1.7	4	12
Pancake, buckwheat, prep f/incomplete dry mix, 4"	1 ea	27	56	2.1	2	0.5	18	8	0.6	69	0.5	144	63	0.05	0.07	0.4	0	4.59
Pancake, plain, homemade, 4"	1 ea	73	166	4.7	7	1.5	43	21	1.1	160	1.3	320	143	0.15	0.21	1.1	0	27.74
Papaya, fresh, med	½ ea	227	89	1.4	0	0.1	0	22	4.1	54	0.2	7	645	0.06	0.07	0.8	140	86.26
Pasta, egg noodles, enrich, ckd	½ cup	80	106	3.8	1	0.2	26	20	0.9	10	1.3	6	16	0.15	0.07	1.2	0	51.2
Pasta, macaroni noodles, enrich, ckd	½ cup	70	99	3.3	0	0.1	0	20	0.9	5	1	1	0	0.14	0.07	1.2	0	49
Pasta, spaghetti noodles, enrich, salted, ckd	1 cup	140	197	6.7	1	0.1	0	40	2.4	10	2	140	0	0.29	0.14	2.3	0	98
Pasta, spaghetti noodles, whole wheat, ckd	1 cup	125	155	6.7	1	0.1	0	33	5.6	19	1.3	4	0	0.14	0.06	0.9	0	6.25
Pastry, cinnamon danish	1 ea	110	443	7.7	25	6.2	23	49	1.4	78	2.2	408	13	0.33	0.29	3.2	0	68.2
Peaches, fresh, sliced	½ cup	85	37	0.6	0	0	0	9	1.7	4	0.1	0	455	0.01	0.03	0.8	6	2.89
Peaches, in heavy syrup, cnd	½ tsp	96	71	0.4	0	0	0	19	1.2	3	0.3	6	319	0.01	0.02	0.6	3	3.07
Peaches, in juice, cnd, whole	½ tsp	77	34	0.5	0	0	0	9	1	5	0.2	3	293	0.01	0.01	0.4	3	2.62
Peanut Butter, smooth, salted	1 Tbs	32	190	8.1	16	3.3	0	6	1.9	12	0.6	149	0	0.03	0.03	4.3	0	23.68
Pears, bartlett, fresh, med	1 ea	180	106	0.7	1	0	0	27	4.3	20	0.4	0	36	0.04	0.07	0.2	7	13.14
Pears, in heavy syrup, cnd, halves	½ ea	103	76	0.2	0	0	0	20	1.6	5	0.2	5	0	0.01	0.02	0.2	1	1.24
Pears, in juice, cnd, halves	½ ea	77	38	0.3	0	0	0	10	1.2	7	0.2	3	5	0.01	0.01	0.2	1	0.92
Peas, cnd, drained	½ cup	85	59	3.8	0	0.1	0	11	3.5	17	0.8	214	653	0.1	0.07	0.6	8	37.65
Peas, green, ckd f/fzn w/o add salt, drained	½ cup	80	62	4.1	0	0	0	11	4.4	19	1.3	70	534	0.23	0.08	1.2	8	46.88
Peppers, bell, green, sweet, raw, med	1 ea	200	54	1.8	0	0.1	0	13	3.6	18	0.9	4	1264	0.13	0.06	1	179	44
Peppers, bell, red, sweet, raw, sml	1 ea	74	20	0.7	0	0	0	5	1.5	7	0.3	1	4218	0.05	0.02	0.4	141	16.28
Peppers, bell, yellow, sweet, raw, lrg	1 ea	186	50	1.9	0	0.1	0	12	1.7	20	0.9	4	443	0.05	0.05	1.7	341	48.36
Pickles, dill	1 ea	135	24	0.8	0	0.1	0	6	1.6	12	0.7	1731	444	0.02	0.04	0.1	3	1.35
Pickles, sweet, med	1 ea	35	41	0.1	0	0	0	11	0.4	1	0.2	329	44	0	0.01	0.1	0	0.35
Pie, apple, bkd f/fzn, 1/6th of 8"	1 pce	118	280	2.2	13	4.5	0	40	1.9	13	0.5	314	146	0.03	0.03	0.3	4	25.96
Pie, bluberry, prep f/rec, 1/8th of 9"	1 pce	158	387	4.3	19	4.6	0	53	2.2	11	1.9	292	66	0.24	0.21	1.9	1	36.34
Pie, cherry, prep f/rec, 1/8th of 9"	1 pce	118	319	3.3	14	3.5	0	45	1.8	12	2.2	225	483	0.17	0.15	1.5	1	31.86
Pie, chocolate cream, rts, 1/6th of 8"	1 pce	175	532	4.5	34	8.7	9	59	3.5	63	1.9	238	0	0.06	0.19	1.2	0	22.75
Pie, lemon meringue, rts, 1/6th of 8"	1 pce	140	375	2.1	12	2.5	63	66	1.7	78	0.9	204	245	0.09	0.29	0.9	4	18.2
Pie, pecan, rts, 1/6th of 8"	1 pce	138	552	5.5	26	4.9	44	79	4.8	23	1.4	585	242	0.13	0.17	0.3	2	37.26
Pie, pumpkin, rts, 1/6th of 8"	1 pce	114	239	4.4	11	2	23	31	3.1	68	0.9	321	3915	0.06	0.17	0.2	1	22.8
Pineapple, chunks, fresh	½ cup	78	38	0.3	0	0	0	10	0.9	5	0.3	1	18	0.07	0.03	0.3	12	8.27
Pineapple, in heavy syrup, cnd, tidbits	½ cup	128	100	0.4	0	0	0	26	1	18	0.5	1	18	0.12	0.03	0.4	9	5.89
Pineapple, in juice, cnd	½ cup	125	75	0.5	0	0	0	20	1	18	0.3	1	48	0.12	0.02	0.4	12	6

Food	Amount	Weight (g)	Calories	Protein (g)	Fat (g)	Sat. Fat (g)	Cholesterol (g)	Carbohydrate (g)	Fiber (g)	Calcium (mg)	Iron (mg)	Sodium (mg)	Vit A (IU)	Thiamin (Vit B₁) (mg)	Riboflavin (Vit B₂) (mg)	Niacin (mg)	Vit C (mg)	Folate (mcg)
Popcorn, air popped, plain	1 cup	6	23	0.7	0	0	0	5	0.9	1	0.2	0	12	0.01	0.02	0.1	0	1.38
Popcorn, ckd in oil, salted	1 cup	11	55	1	3	0.5	0	6	1.1	1	0.3	97	17	0.01	0.01	0.2	0	1.87
Pork, bacon/cracklings, brld/pan fried/rstd	2 pce	15	86	4.6	7	2.6	13	0	0	2	0.2	239	0	0.1	0.04	1.1	0	0.75
Pork, cured, ham, reg, 11% fat, rstd	3 oz	85	151	19.2	8	2.7	50	0	0	7	1.1	1275	8	0.62	0.28	5.2	0	2.55
Pork, ham, whole, rstd	3 oz	85	232	22.8	15	5.5	80	0	0	12	0.9	51	8	0.54	0.27	3.9	0	8.5
Pork, ribs, spareribs, brsd	3 oz	85	337	24.7	26	9.5	103	0	0	40	1.6	79	8	0.35	0.32	4.7	0	3.4
Potato Chips, plain, salted	10 pce	20	107	1.4	7	2.2	0	11	0.9	5	0.3	119	0	0.03	0.04	0.8	6	9
Potatoes, au gratin, prep w/milk & butter f/dry mix	1 cup	245	228	5.6	10	6.3	37	31	2.2	203	0.8	1076	522	0.05	0.2	2.3	8	16.17
Potatoes, baked, w/flesh & skin, long	1 ea	202	220	4.6	0	0.1	0	51	4.8	20	2.7	16	0	0.22	0.07	3.3	26	22.22
Potatoes, hash browns, prep f/fzn	½ cup	78	170	2.5	9	3.5	0	22	1.6	12	1.2	27	0	0.09	0.02	1.9	5	5.07
Potatoes, mashed, w/whole milk	½ cup	105	81	2	1	0.3	2	18	2.1	27	0.3	318	20	0.09	0.04	1.2	7	8.61
Potatoes, sweet, flesh, bkd in skin, med, peeled	1 ea	146	150	2.5	0	0	0	35	4.4	41	0.7	15	31860	0.11	0.19	0.9	36	33
Pretzels, hard, salted, twisted	1 oz	28	107	2.5	1	0.2	0	22	0.9	10	1.2	480	0	0.13	0.17	1.5	0	47.88
Prunes, dried	5 ea	61	146	1.6	0	0	0	38	4.3	31	1.5	2	1212	0.05	0.1	1.2	2	2.26
Pudding, choc, rte, 5oz can	5 oz	142	189	3.8	6	1	4	32	1.4	128	0.7	183	51	0.04	0.22	0.5	3	4.26
Pudding, tapioca, 5oz can	5 oz	142	169	2.8	5	0.9	1	28	0.1	119	0.3	226	0	0.03	0.14	0.4	1	4.26
Pudding, vanilla, 5oz can	5 oz	142	185	3.3	5	0.8	10	31	0.1	125	0.2	192	30	0.03	0.2	0.4	0	0
Raisins, seedless, unpacked	1 oz	28	84	0.9	0	0	0	22	1.1	14	0.6	3	2	0.04	0.02	0.2	1	0.92
Raspberries, fresh	1 cup	123	60	1.1	1	0	0	14	8.3	27	0.7	0	160	0.04	0.11	1.1	31	31.98
Raspberries, swtnd, fzn	1 cup	250	400	10	15	9.1	12	62	5.5	368	3.1	245	400	0.09	0.53	0.8	1	27.5
Rice, brown, ckd	½ cup	96	107	2.5	1	0.2	0	22	1.7	10	0.4	5	0	0.09	0.02	1.5	0	3.84
Rice, white, reg, ckd	½ cup	103	134	2.8	0	0.1	0	29	0.4	10	1.2	1	0	0.17	0.01	1.5	0	59.74
Rice, wild, ckd	½ cup	100	101	4	0	0	0	21	1.8	3	0.6	3	0	0.05	0.09	1.3	0	26
Rolls, hard, white	1 ea	50	146	4.9	2	0.3	0	26	1.1	48	1.6	272	0	0.24	0.17	2.1	0	47.5
Salad Dressing, blue cheese/roquefort	1 Tbs	15	76	0.7	8	1.5	3	1	0	12	0.1	164	32	0	0.02	0	0	1.21
Salad Dressing, french	1 Tbs	16	69	0.1	7	1.5	0	3	0	2	0.1	219	208	0	0	0	0	0.67
Salad Dressing, French, low cal	1 Tbs	15	20	0	1	0.1	0	3	0	2	0.1	118	195	0	0	0	0	
Salad Dressing, Italian	1 Tbs	15	70	0.1	7	1.1	0	2	0	2	0	118	12	0	0	0	0	0.73
Salad Dressing, Italian, diet, 2cal/tsp, cmrcl	1 Tbs	15	16	0	1	0.2	1	1	0	0	0	118	0	0	0	0	0	0
Salad Dressing, ranch	1 Tbs	15	80	0	8	1.2	5	0	0	0	0	105	0	0	0	0	0	
Salad Dressing, thousand island	1 Tbs	15	57	0.1	5	0.9	4	2	0	2	0.1	105	48	0	0	0	0	0.94
Salad Dressing, thousand island, low cal	1 Tbs	15	24	0.1	1	0.2	2	2	0.2	2	0.1	150	48	0	0	0	0	0.84
Salad, chicken, w/celery	½ cup	78	268	10.6	25	3.1	48	1	0.2	16	0.6	201	155	0.03	0.07	3.3	1	8.46
Salad, pasta, garden primavera, prep f/dry	¾ cup	142	280	8	12	2.5	2	34	2	80	1.8	730	200	0.15	0.17	2	1	
Salad, potato	½ cup	125	179	3.4	10	1.8	85	14	1.6	24	0.8	661	261	0.1	0.07	1.1	12	8.38
Salad, tuna	1 cup	205	383	32.9	19	3.2	27	19	0	35	2	824	199	0.06	0.14	13.7	5	16.4
Salami, beef & pork, dry	1 oz	28	117	6.4	10	3.4	22	1	0	2	0.4	521	0	0.17	0.08	1.4	0	0.56
Salmon, pink, w/bone, cnd, not drained	3 oz	85	118	16.8	5	1.3	47	0	0	181	0.7	471	47	0.02	0.16	5.6	0	13.09
Salmon, sockeye, fillet, bkd/brld	3 oz	85	184	23.2	9	1.6	74	0	0	6	0.5	56	178	0.18	0.15	5.7	0	4.25
Salsa, homemade, Mexican sauce	1 Tbs	15	3	0.1	0	0	0	1	0.2	1	0.3	1	57	0.01		0.1	2	1.74
Sandwich, bacon, lettuce & tomato, on soft white	1 ea	130	323	10.8	18	4.7	22	30	1.7	54	2.1	619	271	0.36	0.2	3.4	12	35.5
Sandwich, egg salad, on soft white	1 ea	111	361	9.1	24	4.2	149	29	1.2	67	2.1	499	239	0.25	0.3	1.9	0	35.39
Sandwich, peanut butter & jam, on soft white, unsalted	1 ea	100	348	11.5	15	3.1	2	46	3	60	2.2	290	2	0.27	0.17	5.3	0	40.04
Sandwich, reuben, grilled	1 ea	237	458	27.6	29	9.8	80	25	2.2	286	4.2	1933	453	0.21	0.34	2.8	13	37.79
Sardines, Atlantic, w/bones, cnd in oil, drained	1 oz	28	58	6.9	3	0.4	40	0	0	107	0.8	141	63	0.02	0.06	1.5	0	3.3
Sauce, soy, made f/soy & wheat	1 Tbs	16	9	1.3	0	0	0	1	0.1	3	0.3	871	0	0.01	0.03	0.4	0	2.56
Sauce, teriyaki, rts	1 Tbs	18	15	1.1	0	0	0	3	0	4	0.3	690	0	0.01	0.01	0.2	0	3.6

Food	Amount	Weight (g)	Calories	Protein (g)	Fat (g)	Sat. Fat (g)	Cholesterol (g)	Carbohydrate (g)	Fiber (g)	Calcium (mg)	Iron (mg)	Sodium (mg)	Vit A (IU)	Thiamin (Vit B_1) (mg)	Riboflavin (Vit B_2) (mg)	Niacin (mg)	Vit C (mg)	Folate (mcg)
Sauerkraut, w/liquid, cnd	½ cup	118	22	1.1	0	0	0	5	2.9	35	1.7	780	21	0.02	0.03	0.2	17	27.97
Sausage, pork, smkd, link	1 ea	68	265	15.1	22	7.7	46	1	0	20	0.8	1020	0	0.48	0.17	3.1	1	3.4
Scallops, brd, fried, mixed species, lrg	2 ea	31	67	5.6	3	0.8	19	3	0	13	0.3	144	23	0.01	0.03	0.5	1	11.47
Seaweed, spirulina, dried	1 cup	119	345	68.4	9	3.2	0	28	4.3	143	33.9	1247	678	2.83	4.37	15.3	12	111.8
Shrimp/Prawns, brd, fried, lrg	7 ea	85	206	18.2	10	1.8	150	10	0.3	57	1.1	292	161	0.11	0.12	2.6	1	6.89
Shrimp/Prawns, ckd, lrg	3 oz	85	84	17.8	1	0.2	166	0	0	33	2.6	190	186	0.03	0.03	2.2	2	2.98
Soda, cola	12 fl-oz	369	151	0	0	0	0	38	0	11	0.1	15	0	0	0	0	0	0
Soda, cola/Coke, diet, w/sacc, low sod	12 fl-oz	340	0	0	0	0	0	0	0	14	0.1	54	0	0	0	0	0	0
Soda, ginger ale	12 fl-oz	366	124	0	0	0	0	32	0	11	0.7	26	0	0	0	0	0	0
Soda, lemon lime	12 fl-oz	340	136	0	0	0	0	35	0	7	0.2	37	0	0	0	0.1	0	0
Soda, root beer	12 fl-oz	340	139	0	0	0	0	36	0	17	0.2	44	0	0	0	0	0	0
Sole/Flounder, fillet, bkd/brld	3 oz	85	99	20.5	1	0.3	58	0	0	15	0.3	89	32	0.07	0.1	1.9	0	7.82
Soup, beef bouillon/broth, cnd, prep w/water	1 cup	240	17	2.7	1	0.3	0	0	0	14	0.4	782	0	0	0.05	1.9	0	4.8
Soup, chicken noodle, prep w/water	1 cup	241	75	4	2	0.7	7	9	0.7	17	0.8	1106	711	0.05	0.06	1.4	0	21.69
Soup, clam chowder, Manhattan, prep f/cnc	1 cup	244	112	12.3	2	0	10	11	3.1	41	1.8	725	2297				4	
Soup, clam chowder, New England, prep w/milk	1 cup	248	164	9.5	7	3	22	17	1.5	186	1.5	992	164	0.07	0.24	1	3	9.67
Soup, cream of chicken, prep w/milk	1 cup	248	191	7.5	11	4.6	27	15	0.2	181	0.7	1047	714	0.07	0.26	0.9	1	7.69
Soup, cream of mushroom, prep w/milk	1 cup	245	201	6	13	5.1	20	15	0.5	176	0.6	906	152	0.08	0.28	0.9	2	9.8
Soup, minestrone, prep w/water	1 cup	241	82	4.3	3	0.6	2	11	1	34	0.9	911	2338	0.05	0.04	0.9	1	36.15
Soup, pea, split, w/ham, prep w/water	1 cup	245	184	10	4	1.7	7	27	2.2	22	2.2	975	431	0.14	0.07	1.4	1	2.45
Soup, tomato, prep w/milk	1 cup	248	161	6.1	6	2.9	17	22	2.7	159	1.8	744	848	0.13	0.25	1.5	68	20.83
Soup, tomato, prep w/water	1 cup	245	86	2.1	2	0.4	0	17	0.5	12	1.8	698	691	0.09	0.05	1.4	67	14.7
Soup, vegetable beef, prep w/water	1 cup	245	78	5.6	2	0.9	5	10	0.5	17	1.1	794	1899	0.04	0.05	1	2	10.54
Soup, vegetable, vegetarian, prep w/water	1 cup	250	75	2.2	2	0.3	0	12	0.5	22	1.1	852	3118	0.05	0.05	0.9	2	11
Sour Cream, cultured	1 Tbs	14	30	0.4	3	1.8	6	1	0	16	0	7	111	0	0.02	0	0	1.51
Spinach, ckd w/o add salt, drained	½ cup	103	24	3.1	0	0	0	4	2.5	140	3.7	72	8436	0.1	0.24	0.5	10	150.1
Spinach, raw, chpd	1 cup	55	12	1.6	0	0	0	2	1.5	54	1.5	43	3693	0.04	0.1	0.4	15	106.9
Spinach, w/o add salt, cnd, drained	½ cup	103	24	2.9	1	0.1	0	4	2.5	131	2.4	28	9039	0.02	0.14	0.4	15	100.7
Squash, acorn, ckd	1 cup	245	83	1.6	0	0	0	22	6.4	64	1.4	7	632	0.25	0.02	1.3	16	27.69
Squash, summer, ckd w/o add salt, drained	½ cup	90	18	0.8	0	0.1	0	4	1.3	24	0.3	1	258	0.04	0.04	0.5	5	18.09
Squash, winter, avg, bkd, mashed	½ cup	103	40	0.9	1	0.1	0	9	2.9	14	0.3	1	3664	0.09	0.02	0.7	10	28.84
Strawberries, fresh, whole	1 cup	149	45	0.9	1	0	0	10	3.4	21	0.6	1	40	0.03	0.1	0.3	84	26.37
Strawberries, slices, swtnd, fzn	1 cup	250	240	1.3	0	0	0	65	4.8	28	1.5	8	60	0.04	0.13	1	104	37.25
Stuffing, bread, prep f/dry mix	½ cup	70	125	2.2	6	1.2	0	15	2	22	0.8	380	219	0.1	0.07	1	0	70.7
Sugar, beet/cane, brown, packed	1 tsp	5	19	0	0	0	0	5	0	4	0.1	2	0	0	0	0	0	0.05
Sugar, white, granulated	1 tsp	4	15	0	0	0	0	4	0	0	0	0	0	0	0	0	0	0
Syrup, maple	1 Tbs	20	52	0	0	0	0	13	0	13	0.2	2	0	0	0	0	0	0
Taco Shells	1 ea	10	47	0.7	2	0.3	0	7	0.7	20	0.2	67	33					
Tangerines/Mandarin oranges, fresh, med	1 ea	116	51	0.7	0	0	0	13	2.7	16	0.1	1	1067	0.12	0.03	0.2	36	23.66
Tea, brewed	¼ cup	180	2	0	0	0	0	1	0	0	0	5	0	0	0.03	0	0	9.36
Tempeh	1 cup	166	320	30.8	18	3.7	0	16	9	184	4.5	15	0	0.13	0.59	4.4	0	39.67
Tofu, firm, silken	½ cup	126	78	8.7	3	0.5	0	3	0.1	40	1.3	45	0	0.13	0.05	0.3	0	
Tomatoes, red, ripe, raw, med, whole	1 ea	100	21	0.9	0	0	0	5	1.1	5	0.4	9	623	0.06	0.05	0.6	19	15
Tomatoes, red, ripe, w/o add salt, cnd, in liquid	½ cup	121	23	1.1	0	0	0	5	1.2	36	0.7	179	720	0.05	0.04	0.9	17	9.44
Tortilla/Taco/Tostada Shell, corn	1 ea	148	693	10.7	33	5	0	92	11.1	237	3.7	543	518	0.34	0.08	2	0	8.88
Trout, rainbow, fillet, bkd/brld, wild	3 oz	85	128	19.5	5	1.4	59	0	0	73	0.3	48	42	0.13	0.08	4.9	2	16.15
Tuna, light, cnd in oil, drained	3 oz	85	168	24.8	7	1.3	15	0	0	11	1.2	301	66	0.03	0.1	10.5	0	4.51
Tuna, light, cnd in water, drained	3½ oz	99	115	25.3	1	0.2	30	0	0	11	1.5	335	55	0.03	0.07	13.1	0	3.96
Turkey, average, w/o skin, rstd	3 oz	85	144	24.9	4	1.4	65	0	0	21	1.5	60	0	0.05	0.15	4.6	0	5.95

Food	Amount	Weight (g)	Calories	Protein (g)	Fat (g)	Sat. Fat (g)	Cholesterol (g)	Carbohydrate (g)	Fiber (g)	Calcium (mg)	Iron (mg)	Sodium (mg)	Vit A (IU)	Thiamin (Vit B₁) (mg)	Riboflavin (Vit B₂) (mg)	Niacin (mg)	Vit C (mg)	Folate (mcg)
Turnip Greens, ckd f/fzn, drained	½ cup	73	22	2.4	0	0.1	0	4	2.5	111	1.4	11	5822	0.04	0.05	0.3	16	28.76
Turnips, ckd w/add salt, raw, cubes	½ cup	78	16	0.6	0	0	0	4	1.6	17	0.2	39	0	0.02	0.02	0.2	9	7.18
Veal, loin, brsd	3 oz	85	241	25.7	15	5.7	100	0	0	24	0.9	68	0	0.03	0.26	7.7	0	11.9
Veal, loin, lean, brsd	3 oz	85	192	28.5	8	2.2	106	0	0	27	0.9	71	0	0.04	0.29	8.5	0	12.75
Vinegar, balsamic, 60 grain	1 Tbs	15	21	0	0	0	0	5	0		0.1	3	0	0.08	0.08	0.1	0	
Watermelon, fresh, diced	1 cup	160	51	1	1	0.1	0	11	0.8	13	0.3	3	586	0.13	0.03	0.3	15	3.52
Wheat, bulgur, ckd	1 cup	135	112	4.2	0	0.1	0	25	6.1	14	1.3	7	0	0.08	0.04	1.4	0	24.3
Wheat, flakes, rolled, dry	1 cup	30	97	3.5	0	0	0	21	4.4	18	1	7	0	0.13	0.03	1.4	0	
Wheat, germ, tstd	1 Tbs	6	23	1.7	1	0.1	0	3	0.8	3	0.5	0	0	0.1	0.05	0.3	0	21.12
Whiskey, 90 proof	2 fl-oz	42	110	0	0	0	0	0	0			0	0			0	0	0
Wine, cooler	4 oz	113	56	0.1	0	0	0	7	0	6	0.3	9	1	0.01	0.01	0.1	2	1.34
Wine, red	⅙ cup	30	22	0.1	0	0	0	1	0	2	0.1	2	0	0	0.01	0	0	0.6
Wine, Rose	2 fl-oz	59	42	0.1	0	0	0	1	0	5	0.2	3	0	0	0.01	0	0	0.65
Wine, white, med	2 fl-oz	59	40	0.1	0	0	0	0	0	5	0.2	3	0	0	0	0	0	0.12
Yogurt, fruit, low fat, 10g prot/8 oz	1 cup	227	231	9.9	2	1.6	10	43	0	345	0.2	133	104	0.08	0.4	0.2	1	21.11
Yogurt, plain, low fat, 12g prot/8 oz	8 oz	226	143	11.9	4	2.3	14	16	0	413	0.2	159	149	0.1	0.48	0.3	2	25.31
FAST FOOD RESTAURANTS																		
General																		
Burrito, bean	1 ea	166	342	10.8	10	5.3	3	55	6.3	86	3.5	754	254	0.48	0.46	3.1	1	66.4
Chili, con carne	1 cup	255	258	24.8	8	3.5	135	22	4	69	5.2	1015	1675	0.13	1.15	2.5	2	45.9
Cole Slaw, fast food	1 cup	120	178	1.8	13	1.9	6	15	2	41	0.9	324	409	0.05	0.04	0.1	10	46.8
English Muffin, w/butter	1 ea	63	189	4.9	6	2.4	13	30	1.9	103	1.6	386	136	0.25	0.31	2.6	1	56.7
Entree, enchilada, cheese	1 ea	230	451	13.6	27	14.9	62	40		458	1.9	1106	1638	0.12	0.6	2.7	1	92
Hot Dog, plain	1 ea	98	242	10.4	15	5.1	44	18		24	2.3	670	0	0.24	0.27	3.6	0	48.02
Pancake, w/butter & syrup	2 ea	232	520	8.3	14	5.9	58	91	1.2	128	2.6	1104	281	0.39	0.56	3.4	3	51.04
Sandwich, chicken, fillet, plain	1 ea	157	444	20.8	25	7.4	52	33	1.1	52	4	826	86	0.28	0.2	5.9	8	86.35
Sundae, hot fudge, fast food	1 ea	164	295	5.9	9	5.2	21	49	0	215	0.6	189	230	0.07	0.31	1.1	2	9.84
Arby's																		
Salad, chef	1 ea	273	136	12.3	6	2.6	84	9	0.9	113	3.3	529	3321	0.26	0.25	4.6	35	
Sandwich, beef, Arby Q	1 ea	190	389	17.6	15	5.4	29	48		70	9.2	1268		0.27	0.39	9.2		
Sandwich, beef, French dip & swiss cheese	1 ea	154	369	24.7	16	7.5	58	31	0.9	232	3.6	1237	0	0.18	0.47	7.4	0	16.35
Sandwich, beef 'n cheddar	1 ea	194	508	24.6	26	7.7	52	43		150	6.1	1166	339	0.42	0.63	9.8	1	
Sandwich, chicken, grilled, deluxe	1 ea	195	365	20	17	3	37	35	1.1	59	2.1	764		0.27	0.25	11.5	7	
Sandwich, roast beef, regular	1 ea	155	383	22	18	6.9	43	35		60	4.9	936	0	0.28	0.48	11	1	14
Sauce, Arby's	½ oz	14	15	0.1	0	0	0	3			0.4	113						
Sauce, horsey	½ oz	14	110	0.1	5	1.2	0	3		20		105						
Burger King Corporation																		
Cheeseburger, Whopper	1 ea	294	730	33	46	16	115	46	3	250	4.5	1350	750	0.34	0.48	7	9	
Croissant, w/egg, sausage & cheese	1 ea	110	375	13.8	29	10	162	16	0.6	94	2.2	712	250				0	
Hamburger, Whopper	1 ea	270	640	27	39	11	90	45	3	80	4.5	870	500	0.33	0.41	7	9	
Onion Rings, reg svg	3 ea	30	75	1	3	0.5	0	10	1.5	24	0.3	196	0					
Potatoes, french fries, salted, med svg	1 ea	116	370	5	20	5	0	43	3	0	1.1	240	0				4	
Sandwich, chicken, broiler	1 ea	168	373	20.3	20	4.1	54	28	1.4	41	3.7	325	203				4	
Sandwich, fish, big	1 ea	255	700	26	41	6	90	56	3	60	2.7	980	100				1	
Dunkin Donuts, Inc.																		
Croissant, plain	1 ea	18	81	1.2	5	1.2	2	8	0	6	0.5	78	0				0	
Hidden Valley																		
Salad Dressing, ranch, reduced fat & cal	2 Tbs	28	58	0.5	5	0.9	10	2	0	11	0.1	237	15				0	
International Dairy Queen Inc.																		
Frozen Yogurt Cone, med	4 oz	113	148	5.1	1	0.3	3	32	0	143	1	91	0	0.05	0.2		1	

Food	Amount	Weight (g)	Calories	Protein (g)	Fat (g)	Sat. Fat (g)	Cholesterol (mg)	Carbohydrate (g)	Fiber (g)	Calcium (mg)	Iron (mg)	Sodium (mg)	Vit A (IU)	Thiamin (Vit B_1) (mg)	Riboflavin (Vit B_2) (mg)	Niacin (mg)	Vit C (mg)	Folate (mcg)
Frozen Yogurt, nonfat	4 oz	113	133	4	0	0		28	0	133	1	93	0	0.29	0.25	3.9	0	
Hamburger, homestyle	1 ea	138	290	17	12	5	45	29	2	60	2.7	630	200	0.06	0.26	0.1	4	
Ice Cream Cone, vanilla, med	1 ea	142	237	5.7	6	4.3	22	38	0	179	1.3	115	538	0.12	0.6	0.8	2	
Milk Shake, vanilla, med	1 ea	397	520	12	14	8	45	88	0.3	400	1.4	230	400	0.09	0.05	0.4	0	
Onion Rings, svg	3 oz	85	241	3.8	12	3	0	29	2.3	15	1.1	135	0					
Sandwich, fish, fillet	1 ea	182	396	17.1	17	3.7	48	42	2.1	43	1.9	674	0	0.32	0.24	3.2	0	
Sundae, chocolate, med	1 ea	184	315	6.3	8	4.7	24	56	0	197	1.1	165	590	0.06	0.27	0.3	0	
Jack In the Box																		
Bowl, chicken teriyaki	1 ea	502	670	26	4	1	15	128	3	100	4.5	1730	6500				24	
Cheeseburger, Jumbo Jack	1 ea	296	640	31	38	15	105	44	2	250	4.5	1340	750	0.44	0.54	2	9	
Hamburger	1 ea	104	250	12	9	3.5	30	30	2	100	3.6	610	0	0.16	0.28	2.1	0	
Hamburger, sourdough, jack	1 ea	233	690	34	45	15	105	37	2	200	4.5	1180	750	0.68	0.5	8.4	9	
Sandwich, chicken, supreme	1 ea	305	830	33	49	7	65	66	3	200	3.6	2140	500	0.49	0.4	13.7	9	
Kentucky Fried Chicken Corporation																		
Chicken, leg, original recipe	1 ea	54	124	11.5	8	1.8	66	4	0	18	0.6	374	89				1	27.73
Chicken, wing, hot & spicy	1 ea	55	210	10	15	4	55	9	1	20	0.7	350	100				1	22.37
Chicken, wing, original recipe	1 ea	45	134	8.6	10	2.4	53	5	0	19	0.3	396	96				1	31.06
Long John Silver's																		
Dinner, fish & fries, batter fried, 2pce	1 ea	261	610	27	37	7.9	60	52		40	1.8	1480		0.38	0.34	8	9	
McDonald's Nutrition Information Center																		
Biscuit, sausage & egg	1 ea	175	541	17.7	36	9.8	241	34	1	98	2.7	1140	295	0.53	0.57	4.1	0	46.53
Cheeseburger	1 ea	115	304	14.3	12	5.7	38	33	1.9	190	2.6	779	285	0.31	0.29	3.6	2	25.63
Cheeseburger, Quarter Pounder	1 ea	186	493	26	28	12.1	88	35	1.9	279	4.2	1200	465	0.37	0.4	6.3	2	33.47
Chicken, nuggets, McNuggets, 4 pce, svg	1 ea	71	190	12	11	2.5	40	10			0.7	340		0.08	0.11	5	0	18.95
Danish, apple	1 ea	115	394	5.5	18	5.5	44	56	1.1	88	1.2	318	548	0.33	0.19	2.2	1	
Frozen Yogurt Cone, vanilla, low fat	3 oz	85	142	3.8	4	2.8	19	22	0	94	0.3	71	283				1	
Hamburger, Big Mac	1 ea	204	529	24.6	29	9.4	80	42	2.8	236	4.2	1011	283	0.46	0.42	5.7	3	5.03
Hamburger, Quarter Pounder	1 ea	160	391	21.4	20	7.4	65	34	1.9	140	4.2	763	93	0.37	0.3	6.3	2	33.16
McMuffin, egg	1 ea	138	294	17.2	12	4.6	238	27	1	203	2.7	802	507	0.5	0.45	3.3	1	25.57
McMuffin, sausage	1 ea	135	434	15.7	28	9.6	54	31	1.2	241	2.2	892	241	0.68	0.33	4.5	1	8.64
Milk Shake, vanilla, sml	1 ea	289	355	10.8	9	5.9	39	58		345	0.4	246	296	0.12	0.5	0.3	1	
Muffin, apple bran, fat free	1 ea	75	197	3.9	2	0.3	0	40	2	66	0.9	250	0	0.14	0.14	1.3	1	
Pie, apple	3 oz	307	1037	12	52	14	0	136	4	80	4.3	797		0.71	0.43	5.6	96	
Potatoes, french fries, sml svg	1 ea	68	210	3	10	1.5	0	26	2	9	0.4	135	0	0.05	0	1.9	9	
Potatoes, hash browns	1 ea	55	135	1	8	1.6	0	15	1	7	0.4	342		0.08	0.02	0.9	2	
Salad, garden, shaker	1 ea	149	100	7	6		75	4	2	150	1.1	120	1500				15	26.73
Sandwich, Filet O Fish	1 ea	131	378	13.4	21	3.8	42	35	1.7	126	1.5	731	168	0.29	0.21	2.3	0	
Sauce, sweet & sour, pkt 1	1⅙ oz	32	57	0	0	0	0	13	0	2	0.2	160	343	0	0.01	0.1	0	
Pizza Hut, Inc.																		
Pizza, cheese, pan, med, 12"	2 pce	205	495	22.8	21	9.5	47	53	3.8	273	2.8	951	1000	0.57	0.61	5.2	7	
Pizza, cheese, thin n' crispy, med, 12"	2 pce	148	350	18.8	14	6.8	43	36	3.4	247	1.8	911	922	0.39	0.39	4.8	5	
Pizza, pepperoni, pan, med, 12"	2 pce	211	539	22.4	24	8.1	49	57	4.1	209	3.3	1157	966	0.63	0.49	5.4	8	0
Pizza, pepperoni, personal pan	1 ea	255	637	27	28	10	55	69	5	250	5	1339	1164	0.56	0.66	8.2	10	
Pizza, supreme, pan, med, 12"	2 pce	255	581	28	28	11.2	56	52	5.6	219	4.3	1428	912	0.8	0.79	6	10	
Subway International																		
Sandwich, chicken breast, rstd, on white, 6"	1 ea	246	332	26	6	1	48	41	3	35	3	967	617				15	
Sandwich, Italian bmt, on white, 6"	1 ea	246	445	21	21	8	56	39	3	44	4	1652	753				15	
Sandwich, meatball, on white, 6"	1 ea	260	404	18	16	6	33	44	3	32	4	1035	712				16	
Sandwich, roast beef, deli style	1 ea	180	245	13	4	1	13	38	2	23	3	638	565				14	
Sandwich, tuna, w/lt mayonnaise, on wheat, 6"	1 ea	253	391	19	15	2	32	46	3	38	3	940	729				15	
Sandwich, turkey, on white, 6"	1 ea	232	273	17	4	1	19	40	3	30	4	1391	601				15	

Food	Amount	Weight (g)	Calories	Protein (g)	Fat (g)	Sat. Fat (g)	Choles-terol (g)	Carbo-hydrate (g)	Fiber (g)	Cal-cium (mg)	Iron (mg)	Sodi-um (mg)	Vit A (IU)	Thia-min (Vit B$_1$) (mg)	Ribo-flavin (Vit B$_2$) (mg)	Niacin (mg)	Vit C (mg)	Folate (mcg)
Taco Bell Inc.																		
Burrito, beef, big supreme	1 ea	298	520	24	23	10	55	54	11	150	2.7	1520	3000				5	
Burrito, seven layer	1 ea	234	438	13.2	19	5.8	21	55	10.7	165	3	1058	1240				5	
Burrito, supreme	1 ea	255	440	17	19	8	35	51	10	150	9	1230	2500	0.4	2.1	2.9	5	
Taco	1 ea	83	192	9.6	11	4.3	27	13	3.2	85	1.1	351	532	0.05	0.15	1.3	0	
Taco, soft	1 ea	92	225	9.2	10	4.1	26	12	3.1	82	1.1	337	511	0.39	0.22	2.7	0	
Wendy's Foods International																		
Cheeseburger, w/bacon, jr	1 ea	170	393	20.5	19	7.5	58	35	1.9	171	3.6	895	390	0.31	0.32	6.6	9	28.85
Chicken, nuggets	6 pce	94	292	13.9	20	3.6	37	14	0	24	0.5	589	0	0.15	0.14	9	1	
Frosty, dairy dessert, med	1 ea	298	440	11	11	7	50	73	0	410	1.4	260	1000	0.14	0.62	0.4	0	22.9
Hamburger, bacon classic, big	1 ea	251	517	30.1	26	10.7	88	41	2.4	206	4.5	1298	622	0.4	1.36	5.3	13	
Salad, caesar, w/o dressing, side	1 ea	130	151	12.4	8	3.4	25	9	2	190	1.6	538	2501				22	
Salad, chicken, grilled, w/o dressing	1 ea	338	195	22.1	8	1.7	46	10	4	188	2.1	676	5872				35	
Salad, garden, deluxe, w/o dressing	1 ea	271	110	6.7	6	1	1	10	3.9	189	1.5	319	5883				35	
Salad, taco, w/o chips	1 ea	510	411	28.7	20	10.5	69	31	8.7	403	4.5	1132	2582	0.29	0.5	3.2	28	88.27
Sandwich, chicken, brd	1 ea	208	433	27.4	16	3.1	54	47	1.8	93	2.7	754	217	0.43	0.32	13.3	13	
Sandwich, chicken, club	1 ea	220	483	30.6	20	4.4	64	48	1.9	95	2.9	957	222				14	
Sandwich, chicken, grilled	1 ea	177	283	22.6	7	1.5	61	34	1.8	84	2.7	698	201				9	
CONVENIENCE FOODS & MEALS																		
El Charrito																		
Entree, enchilada, beef, family size, 6 pack	1 ea	200	353	11.8	17	6.5	33	39	5.2	196	2.4	837	1961				3	
Healthy Choice																		
Dinner, fish, herb baked, fzn	1 ea	273	300	14.1	6	1.3	31	48	4.4	35	0.6	424	2650				0	
Dinner, meatloaf, traditional, fzn	1 ea	340	316	15.3	5	2.5	37	52	6.1	48	2.2	459	745				55	
Entree, burrito, chicken, con queso, fzn	1 ea	216	253	10.1	4	1.8	25	43	4.3	29	1.3	426	1084				4	
Entree, lasagna, roma, fzn	1 ea	284	311	19.3	7	2.2	26	44	4.4	111	2.7	430	371	0.22	0.19	1.5	4	
Entree, spaghetti, bolognese, fzn	1 ea	284	280	14	6	2	30	43	5	40	3.6	470	500				15	
Lean Cuisine																		
Entree, chow mein, chicken, w/rice	1 ea	241	198	12.3	5	0.9	33	26	1.9	19	0.3	482	95	0.14	0.16	4.7	6	
Entree, lasagna, w/meat sauce	1 ea	291	270	19	6	2.5	25	34	5	150	1.8	560	500	0.15	0.25	3	12	
Entree, ravioli, cheese	1 ea	241	250	12	8	3	55	32	4	200	1.1	500	750	0.06	0.25	1.2	6	
Entree, spaghetti, w/meatballs, fzn	1 ea	290	322	19.4	8	2.2	6	43	4.9	102	2.6	502	0					48
The Budget Gourmet																		
Dinner, chicken, teriyaki, 3 dish	1 ea	340	360	20	12		55	44		80	1.4	610	1500	0.15	0.34	6	12	
Dinner, veal, parmigiana, 3 dish	1 ea	340	440	26	20		165	39		30	4.5	1160	5000	0.45	0.6	6	6	
Entree, beef, sirloin tips, w/country gravy	1 ea	334	365	18.8	21		47	25		71	0.4	670	882	0.18	0.2	4.7	3	
Entree, linguini, w/shrimp	1 ea	284	330	15	15		75	33		10	3.6	1250	5000	0.3	0.17	3	2	
The Budget Gourmet-Slim Select																		
Entree, stroganoff, beef	1 ea	238	269	17.3	10		58	28		58	2.6	537	288	0.25	0.33	3.8	9	
Weight Watchers																		
Entree, chow mein, chicken	1 ea	255	200	12	2	0.5	25	34	3	40	0.7	430	1499				36	

This food composition table has been prepared for West-Wadsworth Publishing Company and is copyrighted by ESHA Research in Salem, Oregon—the developer and publisher of the Food Processor®, Genesis® R&D, and the Computer Chef® nutrition software systems. The major sources for the data are from the USDA, supplemented by more than 1200 additional sources of information. Because the list of references is so extensive, it is not provided here, but is available from the publisher.

Computer Data Form

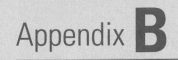
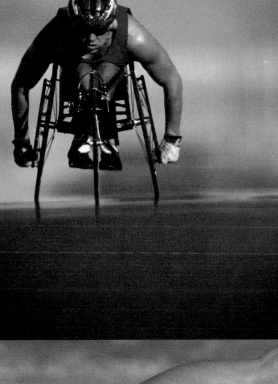
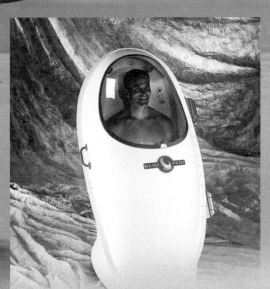

Preliminary Information

Data Disk Drive   A   B   C   (circle drive)

Pre-test _____   Post-test _____

Date (mm-dd-year)   _____-_____-_____

Course name _____

Section number _____

Instructor _____

General Information

Name _____

I.D. (9 digits or less) _____

Age   _____

Male or female (circle one)   M   F

Body weight (pounds)   _____

Resting heart rate   _____

Systolic blood pressure   _____

Diastolic blood pressure   _____

Cardiorespiratory Endurance (circle one)

1. 1.5-mile run   Time _____:_____
2. 1.0-mile walk   Time _____:_____   HR _____
3. Step test   Recov. HR _____
4. Astrand test   WLoad _____
      5th min HR _____   6th min HR _____   Avg. HR _____
5. 12-min swim test   Distance _____

Muscular Strength (circle 1 or 2)

1. Muscular strength and endurance

Exercise	BW	$\times$	%BW	= Resist.	Reps
			MEN WOMEN		
Lat pull down	_____:_____	$\times$	.70 .45	= _____	_____
Leg extension	_____:_____	$\times$	.65 .50	= _____	_____
Bench press	_____:_____	$\times$	.75 .45	= _____	_____
Abd curl/crunch	_____:_____		NA		_____
Leg curl	_____:_____	$\times$	.32 .25	= _____	_____
Arm curl	_____:_____	$\times$	.35 .18	= _____	_____

2. Muscular endurance

MEN		WOMEN	
Bench jumps	_____	Bench jumps	_____
Chair dips	_____	Mod. push-ups	_____
Abd curl/crunch	_____	Abd curl/crunch	_____

Muscular Flexibility

Sit and reach   _____:_____

Right or left body rotation (circle one)   R   L

Right body rotation   _____:_____

Left body rotation   _____:_____

Shoulder width   _____:_____

Shoulder rotation   _____:_____

Body Composition (circle 1   2   or   3)

1. Skinfolds

MEN		WOMEN	
Chest	_____	Triceps	_____
Abdomen	_____	Suprailium	_____
Thigh	_____	Thigh	_____

2. Girth measurements

MEN (use inches)		WOMEN (use cm)	
Waist	_____	Upper arm	_____
Wrist	_____	Hip	_____
		Wrist	_____

3. Other technique

   Indicate percent body fat   _____

Skill Fitness

Agility	_____	Power _____ ft. _____ in.
Balance	_____	Reaction time _____
Coordination	_____	Speed _____

Cardiovascular Disease (see pp. 357–360)

   CHD risk score: _____

Cancer Risk (see pp. 371–382)

Rate each site from 1 to 3.

   Low risk = 1   Moderate risk = 2   High risk = 3

	MEN	WOMEN
Lung	_____	_____
Colon-Rectum	_____	_____
Skin	_____	_____
Breast		_____
Cervical		_____
Endometrial		_____
Prostate	_____	
Testicular	_____	
Pancreatic	_____	_____
Kidney and bladder	_____	_____
Oral	_____	
Esophageal and stomach	_____	_____
Ovarian		_____
Thyroid	_____	_____
Liver	_____	_____
Leukemia	_____	_____
Lymphomas	_____	_____

Stress

Life Experiences Survey (p. 371)   _____

Type A personality assessment (p. 320) _____

Stress vulnerability (p. 323)   _____

Smoking (circle one)

Never smoked	= 1
Quit smoking	= 2
Cigarette smoker	= 3
Pipe smoker	= 4
Cigar smoker	= 5
Chew or dip tobacco	= 6

NUTRIENT ANALYSIS DATA

Use the computer form provided on page 92 and follow the instructions on page 62 of the book.

CARDIORESPIRATORY EXERCISE PRESCRIPTION DATA

Date (mm-dd-year)   _____-_____-_____

Name _____

Age   _____

Resting heart rate   _____

Male or female (circle one)   M   F

Current cardiorespiratory fitness (circle one)

   Excellent = 1   Average = 3   Poor = 5

   Good   = 2   Fair   = 4

EXERCISE LOG DATA

Use the activity list provided on page 141. Keep track of the exercise date, body weight, mode of exercise (activity), duration of exercise and exercise heart rate. Then simply follow the computer instructions.

Preliminary Information

Data Disk Drive   A B C   (circle drive)

Pre-test _____   Post-test _____

Date (mm-dd-year)   _____-_____-_____

Course name _____

Section number _____

Instructor _____

General Information

Name _____

I.D. (9 digits or less) _____

Age   _____

Male or female (circle one)   M   F

Body weight (pounds)   _____

Resting heart rate   _____

Systolic blood pressure   _____

Diastolic blood pressure   _____

Cardiorespiratory Endurance (circle one)

1. 1.5-mile run   Time _____:_____
2. 1.0-mile walk   Time _____:_____   HR _____
3. Step test   Recov. HR _____

4. Astrand test   WLoad _____
   5th min HR _____ 6th min HR _____ Avg. HR _____
5. 12-min swim test   Distance _____

Muscular Strength (circle 1 or 2)

1. Muscular strength and endurance

   Exercise   BW   ×   %BW = Resist. Reps
                   MEN WOMEN

   Lat pull down _____:_____ × .70 .45 = _____ _____
   Leg extension _____:_____ × .65 .50 = _____ _____
   Bench press   _____:_____ × .75 .45 = _____ _____
   Abd curl/crunch_____:_____   NA   _____
   Leg curl   _____:_____ × .32 .25 = _____ _____
   Arm curl   _____:_____ × .35 .18 = _____ _____

2. Muscular endurance

   MEN   **WOMEN**
   Bench jumps _____   Bench jumps _____
   Chair dips   _____   Mod. push-ups _____
   Abd curl/crunch_____   Abd curl/crunch _____

Muscular Flexibility

Sit and reach   _____:_____

Right or left body rotation (circle one)   R   L

Right body rotation   _____:_____

Left body rotation   _____:_____

Shoulder width   _____:_____

Shoulder rotation   _____:_____

Body Composition (circle 1 2 or 3)

1. Skinfolds

   MEN   **WOMEN**
   Chest   _____   Triceps   _____
   Abdomen   _____   Suprailium _____
   Thigh   _____   Thigh   _____

2. Girth measurements

   MEN (use inches)   **WOMEN** (use cm)
   Waist   _____   Upper arm   _____
   Wrist   _____   Hip   _____
                                Wrist   _____

3. Other technique
   Indicate percent body fat   _____

Skill Fitness

Agility   _____   Power _____ ft. _____ in.
Balance   _____   Reaction time   _____
Coordination   _____   Speed   _____

Cardiovascular Disease (see pp. 357–360)

CHD risk score: _____

Cancer Risk (see pp. 371–382)

Rate each site from 1 to 3.

   Low risk = 1   Moderate risk = 2   High risk = 3

	MEN	WOMEN
Lung	_____	_____
Colon-Rectum	_____	_____
Skin	_____	_____
Breast		_____
Cervical		_____
Endometrial		_____
Prostate	_____	
Testicular	_____	
Pancreatic	_____	_____
Kidney and bladder	_____	_____
Oral	_____	_____
Esophageal and stomach	_____	_____
Ovarian		_____
Thyroid	_____	_____
Liver	_____	_____
Leukemia	_____	_____
Lymphomas	_____	_____

Stress

Life Experiences Survey (p. 317)   _____

Type A personality assessment (p. 320)_____

Stress vulnerability (p. 323)   _____

Smoking (circle one)

Never smoked   = 1
Quit smoking   = 2
Cigarette smoker   = 3
Pipe smoker   = 4
Cigar smoker   = 5
Chew or dip tobacco   = 6

NUTRIENT ANALYSIS DATA

Use the computer form provided on page 92 and follow the instructions on page 62 of the book.

CARDIORESPIRATORY EXERCISE PRESCRIPTION DATA

Date (mm-dd-year)   _____-_____-_____

Name _____

Age   _____

Resting heart rate   _____

Male or female (circle one)   M   F

Current cardiorespiratory fitness (circle one)
   Excellent = 1   Average = 3   Poor = 5
   Good   = 2   Fair   = 4

EXERCISE LOG DATA

Use the activity list provided on page 141. Keep track of the exercise date, body weight, mode of exercise (activity), duration of exercise and exercise heart rate. Then simply follow the computer instructions.

glossary

A

Acquired immunodeficiency syndrome (AIDS) Any of a number of diseases that arise when the body's immune system is compromised by HIV; the final stage of HIV infection.

Action stage Stage of change in the transtheoretical model in which people are actively changing a negative behavior or adopting a new, healthy behavior.

Activities of daily living Everyday behaviors that people normally do to function in life (cross the street, carry groceries, lift objects, do laundry, sweep floors).

Acupuncture Chinese medical system that requires body piercing with fine needles during therapy to relieve pain and treat ailments and diseases.

Addiction Compulsive and uncontrollable behavior(s) or use of substance(s).

Adenosine triphosphate (ATP) A high-energy chemical compound that the body uses for immediate energy.

Adequate Intakes (AI) The recommended amount of a nutrient intake when sufficient evidence is not available to calculate the EAR and subsequent RDA.

Addiction Compulsive and uncontrollable behavior(s) or use of substance(s).

Adipose tissue Fat cells in the body.

Aerobic Exercise that requires oxygen to produce the necessary energy (ATP) to carry out the activity.

Agility Ability to change body position and direction quickly and efficiently.

Air displacement Technique to assess body composition by calculating the body volume from the air displaced by an individual sitting inside a small chamber.

Alcohol (ethyl alcohol) A depressant drug that affects the brain and slows down central nervous system activity; has strong addictive properties.

Alcoholism Disease in which an individual loses control over drinking alcoholic beverages.

Allopathic medicine See Conventional Western medicine.

Altruism True concern for the welfare of others.

Alveoli Air sacs in the lungs where oxygen is taken up and carbon dioxide (produced by the body) is released from the blood.

Amenorrhea Cessation of regular menstrual flow.

Amino acids Chemical compounds that contain nitrogen, carbon, hydrogen, and oxygen; the basic building blocks the body uses to build different types of protein.

Amotivational syndrome A condition characterized by loss of motivation, dullness, apathy, and no interest in the future.

Amphetamines A class of powerful central nervous system stimulants.

Anabolic steroids Synthetic versions of the male sex hormone testosterone, which promotes muscle development and hypertrophy.

Anaerobic Exercise that does not require oxygen to produce the necessary energy (ATP) to carry out the activity.

Angina pectoris Chest pain associated with coronary heart disease.

Angiogenesis Formation of blood vessels (capillaries).

Angioplasty A procedure in which a balloon-tipped catheter is inserted, then inflated, to widen the inner lumen of one or more arteries.

Anorexia nervosa An eating disorder characterized by self-imposed starvation to lose and maintain very low body weight.

Anthropometric measurement techniques Measurement of body girths at different sites.

Anticoagulant Any substance that inhibits blood clotting.

Antioxidants Compounds such as vitamins C and E, beta-carotene, and selenium that prevent oxygen from combining with other substances in the body to form harmful compounds.

Aquaphobic Having a fear of water.

Arrhythmias Irregular heart rhythms.

Arterial-venous oxygen difference (a-$\overline{v}O_2$diff) The amount of oxygen removed from the blood as determined by the difference in oxygen content between arterial and venous blood.

Atherosclerosis Fatty/cholesterol deposits in the walls of the arteries leading to formation of plaque.

Atrophy Decrease in the size of a cell.

Autogenic training A stress management technique using a form of self-suggestion, wherein an individual is able to place himself or herself in an autohypnotic state by repeating and concentrating on feelings of heaviness and warmth in the extremities.

Ayurveda Hindu system of medicine based on herbs, diet, massage, meditation, and yoga to help the body boost its own natural healing.

B

Balance Ability to maintain the body in proper equilibrium.

Ballistic (dynamic) stretching Exercises done with jerky, rapid, bouncy movements, or slow, short, and sustained movements.

Basal metabolic rate (BMR) The lowest level of oxygen consumption necessary to sustain life.

Behavior modification The process of permanently changing negative behaviors to positive behaviors that will lead to better health and well-being.

Benign Noncancerous.

Binge-eating disorder An eating disorder characterized by uncontrollable episodes of eating excessive amounts of food within a relatively short time.

Bioelectrical impedance Technique to assess body composition by running a weak electrical current through the body.

Biofeedback A stress-management technique in which a person learns to influence physiological responses that are not typically under voluntary control or responses that typically are regulated but for which regulation has broken down as a result of injury, trauma, or illness.

Blood lipids (fat) Cholesterol and triglycerides.

Blood pressure A measure of the force exerted against the walls of the vessels by the blood flowing through them.

Bod Pod Commercial name of the equipment used for the assessment of body composition through the air displacement technique.

Body composition The fat and nonfat components of the human body; important in assessing recommended body weight.

Body mass index (BMI) A technique to determine thinness and excessive fatness that incorporates height and weight to estimate critical fat values at which the risk for disease increases.

Bradycardia Slower heart rate than normal.

Breathing exercise A stress management technique wherein the individual concentrates on "breathing away" the tension and inhaling fresh air to the entire body.

Bulimia nervosa An eating disorder characterized by a pattern of binge eating and purging in an attempt to lose weight and maintain low body weight.

C

Calorie The amount of heat necessary to raise the temperature of 1 gram of water 1 degree Centigrade; used to measure the energy value of food and cost (energy expenditure) of physical activity.

Cancer Group of diseases characterized by uncontrolled growth and spread of abnormal cells.

Capillaries Smallest blood vessels carrying oxygenated blood to the tissues in the body.

Carbohydrate loading Increasing intake of carbohydrates during heavy aerobic training or prior to aerobic endurance events that last longer than 90 minutes.

Carbohydrates A classification of dietary nutrient containing carbon, hydrogen, and oxygen; the major source of energy for the human body.

Carcinogens Substances that contribute to the formation of cancers.

Carcinoma in situ Encapsulated malignant tumor that has not spread.

Cardiac output Amount of blood pumped by the heart in one minute.

Cardiomyopathy A disease affecting the heart muscle.

Cardiorespiratory endurance The ability of the lungs, heart, and blood vessels to deliver adequate amounts of oxygen to the cells to meet the demands of prolonged physical activity.

Cardiorespiratory training zone The recommended training intensity range, in terms of exercise heart rate, to obtain adequate cardiorespiratory endurance development.

Cardiovascular diseases The array of conditions that affect the heart and the blood vessels.

Carotenoids Pigment substances in plants that are often precursors to vitamin A. More than 600 carotenoids are found in nature, about 50 of which are precursors to vitamin A, the most potent one being beta-carotene.

Catecholamines "Fight-or-flight" hormones, including epinephrine and norepinephrine.

Cellulite Term frequently used in reference to fat deposits that "bulge out"; these deposits are nothing but enlarged fat cells from excessive accumulation of body fat.

Chiropractics Health care system that believes that many diseases and ailments are related to misalignments of the vertebrae and emphasizes the manipulation of the spinal column.

Chlamydia A sexually transmitted disease, caused by a bacterial infection, that can cause significant damage to the reproductive system.

Cholesterol A waxy substance, technically a steroid alcohol, found only in animal fats and oil; used in making cell membranes, as a building block for some hormones, in the fatty sheath around nerve fibers, and in other necessary substances.

Chronic diseases Illnesses that develop and last a long time.

Chronic Lower Respiratory Disease (CLRD) A general term that includes chronic obstructive pulmonary disease, emphysema, and chronic bronchitis (all diseases of the respiratory system).

Chronological age Calendar age.

Chylomicron Triglyceride-transporting molecules.

Circuit training Alternating exercises by performing them in a sequence of three to six or more.

Cirrhosis A disease characterized by scarring of the liver.

Cocaine 2-beta-carbomethoxy-3-betabenozoxytropane, the primary psychoactive ingredient derived from coca plant leaves; crack cocaine is the most popular form.

Cold turkey Eliminating a negative behavior all at once.

Complementary and alternative medicine (CAM) A group of diverse medical and health care systems, practices, and products that are not presently considered to be part of conventional medicine; also called unconventional, nonallopathic, or integrative medicine.

Complex carbohydrates Carbohydrates formed by three or more simple sugar molecules linked together; also referred to as polysaccharides.

Concentric Shortening of a muscle during muscle contraction.

Contemplation stage Stage of change in the transtheoretical model in which people are considering changing behavior within the next 6 months.

Contraindicated exercises Exercises that are not recommended because that may cause injury to a person.

Controlled ballistic stretching Exercises done with slow, short, and sustained movements.

Conventional Western medicine Traditional medical practice based on methods that are tested through rigorous scientific trials; also called allopathic medicine.

Cool-down Tapering off an exercise session slowly.

Coordination The integration of the nervous and the muscular systems to produce correct, graceful, and harmonious body movements.

Core strength training A training program designed to strengthen the abdominal, hip, and spinal muscles (the core of the body).

Coronary heart disease (CHD) Condition in which the arteries that supply the heart muscle with oxygen and nutrients are narrowed by fatty deposits, such as cholesterol and triglycerides.

C-reactive protein (CRP) A protein whose blood levels increase with inflammation, at times hidden deep in the body; elevation of this protein is an indicator of potential cardiovascular events.

Creatine An organic compound derived from meat, fish, and amino acids that combines with inorganic phosphate to form creatine phosphate.

Creatine phosphate (CP) A high-energy compound that the cells use to resynthesize ATP during all-out activities of very short duration.

Cruciferous vegetables Plants that produce cross-shaped leaves (cauliflower, broccoli, cabbage, Brussels sprouts, and kohlrabi); they seem to have a protective effect against cancer.

D

Daily Values (DVs) Reference values for nutrients and food components used in food labels.

Dentist Practitioner who specializes in diseases of the teeth, gums, and oral cavity.

Deoxyribonucleic acid (DNA) Genetic substance of which genes are made; molecule that contains cell's genetic code.

Diabetes mellitus A disease in which the body doesn't produce or utilize insulin properly.

Diastolic blood pressure Pressure exerted by the blood against the walls of the arteries during the relaxation phase (diastole) of the heart; lower of the two numbers in blood pressure readings.

Dietary fiber A complex carbohydrate in plant foods that is not digested but is essential to the digestion process.

Dietary Reference Intakes (DRIs) A general term that describes four types of nutrient standards that establish adequate amounts and maximum safe nutrient intakes in the diet. These standards are Estimated Average Requirements (EAR), Recommended Dietary Allowances (RDA), Adequate Intakes (AI), and Tolerable Upper Intake Levels (UL).

Disaccharides Simple carbohydrates formed by two monosaccharide units linked together, one of which is glucose. The major disaccharides are sucrose, lactose, and maltose.

Distress Negative stress: Unpleasant or harmful stress under which health and performance begin to deteriorate.

Dopamine A neurotransmitter that affects emotional, mental, and motor functions.

Dual energy X-ray absorptiometry (DEXA) Method to assess body composition that uses very low-dose beams of X-ray energy to measure total body fat mass, fat distribution pattern, and bone density.

Dynamic training Strength-training method referring to a muscle contraction with movement.

Dysmenorrhea Painful menstruation.

E

Eccentric Lengthening of a muscle during muscle contraction.

Ecosystem A community of organisms interacting with each other in an environment.

Ecstacy See MDMA.

Elastic elongation Temporary lengthening of soft tissue.

Electrocardiogram (ECG or EKG) A recording of the electrical activity of the heart.

Emotional wellness The ability to understand one's own feelings, accept limitations, and achieve emotional stability.

Endorphins Morphine-like substances released from the pituitary gland (in the brain) during prolonged aerobic exercise; thought to induce feelings of euphoria and natural well-being.

Energy-balancing equation A principle holding that as long as caloric input equals caloric output, the person will not gain or lose weight. If caloric intake exceeds output, the person gains weight; when output exceeds input, the person loses weight.

Environmental wellness The capability to live in a clean and safe environment that is not detrimental to health.

Enzymes Catalysts that facilitate chemical reactions in the body.

Essential fat Minimal amount of body fat needed for normal physiological functions; constitutes about 3 percent of total weight in men and 12 percent in women.

Estimated Average Requirements (EAR) The amount of a nutrient that meets the dietary needs in half the people.

Estimated Energy Requirement (EER) The average dietary energy (caloric) intake that is predicted to maintain energy balance in a healthy adult of defined age, gender, weight, height, and level of physical activity, consistent with good health.

Estrogen Female sex hormone essential for bone formation and conservation of bone density.

Eustress Positive stress: Health and performance continue to improve, even as stress increases.

Exercise A type of physical activity that requires planned, structured, and repetitive bodily movement with the intent of improving or maintaining one or more components of physical fitness.

Exercise intolerance Inability to function during exercise because of excessive fatigue or extreme feelings of discomfort.

F

Fast-twitch fibers Muscle fibers with greater anaerobic potential and fast speed of contraction.

Fats A classification of nutrients containing carbon, hydrogen, some oxygen, and sometimes other chemical elements.

Ferritin Iron stored in the body.

Fight or flight Physiological response of the body to stress that prepares the individual to take action by stimulating the body's vital defense systems.

Fixed resistance Type of exercise in which a constant resistance is moved through a joint's full range of motion.

Flexibility Refers to the achievable range of motion at a joint or group of joints without causing injury.

Folate One of the B vitamins.

Fortified foods Foods that have added nutrients that either were not present or were present in insignificant amounts with the intent of preventing nutrient deficiencies.

Fraud/quackery The conscious promotion of unproven claims for profit.

Free weights Barbells and dumbbells.

Frequency How many times per week a person engages in an exercise session.

Functional capacity The ability to perform ordinary and unusual demands of daily living without limitations and excessive fatigue or injury.

Functional foods Foods or food ingredients containing physiologically active substances that provide specific health benefits beyond those supplied by basic nutrition.

Functional independence Ability to carry out activities of daily living without assistance from other individuals.

G

General adaptation syndrome (GAS) A theoretical model that explains the body's adaptation to sustained stress which includes three stages: Alarm reaction, resistance, and exhaustion/recovery.

Genetically modified foods (GM foods) Foods whose basic genetic material (DNA) is manipulated by inserting genes with desirable traits from one plant, animal, or microorganism into another one either to introduce new traits or to enhance existing ones.

Genital herpes A sexually transmitted disease caused by a viral infection of the herpes simplex virus Types I and II. The virus can attack different areas of the body, but commonly causes blisters on the genitals.

Genital warts A sexually transmitted disease caused by a viral infection.

Girth measurements Technique to assess body composition by measuring circumferences at specific body sites.

Glucose intolerance A condition characterized by slightly elevated blood glucose levels.

Glycemic index An index that is used to rate the plasma glucose response of carbohydrate-containing foods with the response produced by the same amount of carbohydrate from a standard source, usually glucose or white bread.

Glycogen Form in which glucose is stored in the body.

Goals The ultimate aims toward which effort is directed.

Gonorrhea A sexually transmitted disease caused by a bacterial infection.

H

Hatha yoga A form of yoga that incorporates specific sequences of static-stretching postures to help induce the relaxation response.

Health A state of complete well-being, and not just the absence of disease or infirmity.

Health fitness standards The lowest fitness requirements for maintaining good health, decreasing the risk for chronic diseases, and lowering the incidence of muscular-skeletal injuries; also referred to as criterion-referenced standards.

Health-related fitness Fitness programs that are prescribed to improve the individual's overall health; components are cardiorespiratory endurance, muscular strength and endurance, muscular flexibility, and body composition.

Healthy Life Expectancy (HLE) Number of years a person is expected to live in good health; this number is obtained by subtracting ill-health years from overall life expectancy.

Heart rate reserve (HRR) The difference between the maximal heart rate and the resting heart rate.

Heat cramps Muscle spasms caused by heat-induced changes in electrolyte balance in muscle cells.

Heat exhaustion Heat-related fatigue.

Heat stroke Emergency situation resulting from the body being subjected to high atmospheric temperatures.

Hemoglobin Protein–iron compound in red blood cells that transports oxygen in the blood.

Herbal medicine Unconventional system that uses herbs to treat ailments and disease.

Heroin A potent drug that is a derivative of opium.

High-density lipoproteins (HDLs) Cholesterol-transporting molecules in the blood ("good" cholesterol) that help clear cholesterol from the blood.

Homeopathy System of treatment based on the use of minute quantities of remedies that in large amounts produce effects similar to the disease being treated.

Homeostasis A natural state of equilibrium; the body attempts to maintain this equilibrium by constantly reacting to external forces that attempt to disrupt this fine balance.

Homocysteine An amino acid that, when allowed to accumulate in the blood, may lead to plaque formation and blockage of arteries.

Human immunodeficiency virus (HIV) Virus that leads to acquired immunodeficiency syndrome (AIDS).

Human papillomavirus (HPV) A group of viruses that can cause sexually transmitted diseases.

Hydrostatic weighing Underwater technique to assess body composition; considered the most accurate of the body composition assessment techniques.

Hypertension Chronically elevated blood pressure.

Hypertrophy An increase in the size of the cell, as in muscle hypertrophy.

Hypokinetic diseases "Hypo" denotes "lack of"; therefore, lack of physical activity.

Hypotension Low blood pressure.

Hypothermia A breakdown in the body's ability to generate heat; a drop in body temperature below 95° F.

I

Imagery Mental visualization of relaxing images and scenes to induce body relaxation in times of stress or as an aid in the treatment of certain medical conditions such as cancer, hypertension, asthma, chronic pain, and obesity.

Insulin A hormone secreted by the pancreas; essential for proper metabolism of blood glucose (sugar) and maintenance of blood glucose level.

Insulin resistance Inability of the cells to respond appropriately to insulin.

Intensity In cardiorespiratory exercise, how hard a person has to exercise to improve or maintain fitness.

Intensity (for flexibility exercises) Degree of stretch when doing flexibility exercises.

International unit (IU) Measure of nutrients in foods.

Interval training A training program where high intensity speed intervals are followed by short recovery intervals.

Isokinetic training Strength-training method in which the speed of the muscle contraction is kept constant because the equipment (machine) provides an accommodating resistance to match the user's force (maximal) through the range of motion.

Isometric training Strength-training method referring to a muscle contraction that produces little or no movement, such as pushing or pulling against an immovable object.

L

Lactic acid End product of anaerobic glycolysis (metabolism).

Lactovegetarians Vegetarians who eat foods from the milk group.

Lean body mass Body weight without body fat.

Life expectancy Number of years a person is expected to live based on the person's birth year.

Life Experiences Survey A questionnaire used to assess sources of stress in life.

Lipoproteins Lipids covered by proteins, they transport fats in the blood; types are LDL, HDL, and VLDL.

Locus of control A concept examining the extent to which a person believes he or she can influence the external environment.

Low-density lipoproteins (LDLs) Cholesterol-transporting molecules in the blood ("bad" cholesterol) that tend to increase blood cholesterol.

M

Magnetic therapy Unconventional (CAM) treatment that relies on magnetic energy to promote healing.

Maintenance stage Stage of change in the transtheoretical model in which people maintain behavioral change for up to 5 years.

Malignant Cancerous.

Mammogram Low-dose X-rays of the breasts used as a screening technique for the early detection of breast cancer.

Marijuana A psychoactive drug prepared from a mixture of crushed leaves, flowers, small branches, stems, and seeds from the hemp plant *cannabis sativa*.

Massage therapy The rubbing or kneading of body parts to treat ailments.

Maximal heart rate (MHR) Highest heart rate for a person, related primarily to age.

Maximal oxygen uptake (VO$_{2max}$) Maximum amount of oxygen the body is able to utilize per minute of physical activity, commonly expressed in ml/kg/min; the best indicator of cardiorespiratory or aerobic fitness.

MDA A hallucinogenic drug that is structurally similar to amphetamines.

MDMA A synthetic hallucinogen drug with a chemical structure that closely resembles

MDA and methamphetamine; also known as Ecstacy.

Meditation A stress management technique used to gain control over one's attention by clearing the mind and blocking out the stressor(s) responsible for the increased tension.

Mediterranean diet Typical diet of people around the Mediterranean region that focuses on olive oil, red wine, grains, legumes, vegetables, and fruits, with limited amounts of meat, fish, milk, and cheese.

Megadoses For most vitamins, 10 times the RDA or more; for vitamins A and D, 5 and 2 times the RDA, respectively.

Melanoma The most virulent, rapidly spreading form of skin cancer.

Mental wellness A state in which one's mind is engaged in lively interaction with the surrounding world; also called intellectual wellness.

MET Represents the rate of resting energy expenditure at rest; MET is the equivalent of 3.5 ml/kg/min.

Metabolic fitness Denotes improvements in the metabolic profile through a moderate-intensity exercise program in spite of little or no improvement in physical fitness standards.

Metabolic profile A measurement to assess risk for diabetes and cardiovascular disease through plasma insulin, glucose, lipid, and lipoprotein levels.

Metabolic syndrome *See* Syndrome X.

Metabolism All energy and material transformations that occur within living cells; necessary to sustain life.

Metastasis The movement of cells from one part of the body to another.

Methamphetamine A potent form of amphetamine.

METs Short for metabolic equivalents, an alternative method of prescribing exercise intensity in multiples of the resting metabolic rate.

Minerals Inorganic nutrients essential for normal body functions; found in the body and in food.

Mitochondria Structures within the cells where energy transformations take place.

Mode Form or type of exercise.

Moderate physical activity Activity that uses 150 calories of energy per day, or 1,000 calories per week.

Monogamous A sexual relationship in which two people have sexual relations only with each other.

Monosaccharides The simplest carbohydrates (sugars), formed by five- or six-carbon skeletons. The three most common monosaccharides are glucose, fructose, and galactose.

Morbidity A condition related to, or caused by, illness or disease.

Motivation The desire and will to do something.

Motor neurons Nerves connecting the central nervous system to the muscle.

Motor unit The combination of a motor neuron and the muscle fibers that neuron innervates.

Muscular endurance The ability of a muscle to exert submaximal force repeatedly over time.

Muscular strength The ability of a muscle to exert maximum force against resistance (for example, 1 repetition maximum [or 1 RM] of the bench press exercise).

Myocardial infarction Heart attack; damage to or death of an area of the heart muscle as a result of an obstructed artery to that area.

Myocardium Heart muscle.

N

Naturopathic medicine Unconventional system of medicine that relies exclusively on natural remedies to treat disease and ailments.

Negative resistance The lowering or eccentric phase of a repetition during a strength training exercise.

Neustress Neutral stress; stress that is neither harmful nor helpful.

Nicotine Addictive compound found in tobacco leaves.

Nitrosamines Potentially cancer-causing compounds formed when nitrites and nitrates, which are used to prevent the growth of harmful bacteria in processed meats, combine with other chemicals in the stomach.

Nonallopathic medicine See complementary and alternative medicine.

Nonmelanoma skin cancer Cancer that spreads or grows at the original site but does not metastasize to other regions of the body.

Nonresponders Individuals who exhibit small or no improvements in fitness as compared to others who undergo the same training program.

Nurse Health care practitioner who assists in the diagnosis and treatment of health problems and provides many services to patients in a variety of settings.

Nutrient density A measure of the amount of nutrients and calories in various foods.

Nutrients Substances found in food that provide energy, regulate metabolism, and help with growth and repair of body tissues.

Nutrition Science that studies the relationship of foods to optimal health and performance.

O

Obesity An excessive accumulation of body fat, usually at least 30 percent above recommended body weight; body mass index (BMI) 30 or higher.

Objectives Steps required to reach a goal.

Occupational wellness The ability to perform one's job skillfully and effectively under conditions that provide personal and team satisfaction and adequately reward each individual.

Oligomenorrhea Irregular menstrual cycles.

Omega-3 fatty acids Polyunsaturated fatty acids found primarily in cold-water seafood, flaxseed, and flaxseed oil; thought to lower blood cholesterol and triglycerides.

Omega-6 fatty acids Polyunsaturated fatty acids found primarily in corn and sunflower oils and most oils in processed foods.

Oncogenes Genes that initiate cell division.

One repetition maximum (1 RM) The maximum amount of resistance an individual is able to lift in a single effort.

Ophthalmologist Medical specialist concerned with diseases of the eye and prescription of corrective lenses.

Opportunistic diseases Diseases that arise in the absence of a healthy immune system, which would fight them off in healthy people.

Optometrist Health care practitioner who specializes in the prescription and adaptation of lenses.

Oral surgeon A dentist who specializes in surgical procedures of the oral–facial complex.

Orthodontist A dentist who specializes in the correction and prevention of teeth irregularities.

Osteopath A medical practitioner with specialized training in musculoskeletal problems who uses diagnostic and therapeutic methods of conventional medicine in addition to manipulative measures.

Osteoporosis Softening, deterioration, or loss of bone mineral density that leads to disability, bone fractures, and even death from medical complications.

Overload principle Training concept that the demands placed on a system (cardiorespiratory or muscular) must be increased systematically and progressively over time to cause physiological adaptation (development or improvement).

Overtraining An emotional, behavioral, and physical condition marked by increased fatigue, decreased performance, persistent muscle soreness, mood disturbances, and feelings of "staleness" or "burnout" as a result of excessive physical training.

Overweight An excess amount of weight against a given standard, such as height or recommended percent body fat; body mass index (BMI) greater than 25 but less than 30.

Ovolactovegetarians Vegetarians who include eggs and milk products in their diet.

Ovovegetarians Vegetarians who allow eggs in their diet.

Oxygen free radicals Substances formed during metabolism that attack and damage proteins and lipids, in particular the cell membrane and DNA, leading to diseases such as heart disease, cancer, and emphysema.

Oxygen uptake (VO₂) The amount of oxygen used by the human body.

P

Pelvic inflammatory disease (PID) An overall designation referring to the effects of other STDs, primarily chlamydia and gonorrhea.

Percent body fat Proportional amount of fat in the body based on the person's total weight; includes both essential fat and storage fat; also termed fat mass.

Periodization A training approach that divides the season into three cycles (macrocycles, mesocycles, and microcycles) using a systematic variation in intensity and volume of training to enhance fitness and performance.

Peripheral vascular disease Narrowing of the peripheral blood vessels, excluding the cerebral and coronary arteries.

Peristalsis Involuntary muscle contractions of intestinal walls that facilitate excretion of wastes.

Personal trainer A health/fitness professional who evaluates, motivates, educates, and trains clients to help them meet individualized, healthy, lifestyle goals.

Physical activity Bodily movement produced by skeletal muscles; requires expenditure of energy and produces progressive health benefits.

Physical fitness The ability to meet the ordinary as well as the unusual demands of daily life safely and effectively without being overly fatigued and still have energy left for leisure and recreational activities.

Physical fitness standards A fitness level that allows a person to sustain moderate-to-vigorous physical activity without undue fatigue and the ability to closely maintain this level throughout life.

Physical wellness Good physical fitness and confidence in one's personal ability to take care of health problems.

Physician assistant Health care practitioner trained to treat most standard cases of care.

Physiological age The biological and functional capacity of the body as it should be in relation to the person's maximal potential at any given age in the lifespan.

Phytochemicals Chemical compounds thought to prevent and fight cancer; found in large quantities in fruits and vegetables.

Pilates A training program that uses exercises designed to help strengthen the body's core by developing pelvic stability and abdominal control; exercises are coupled with focused breathing patterns.

Plastic elongation Permanent lengthening of soft tissue.

Plyometric exercise Explosive jump training, incorporating speed and strength training to enhance explosiveness.

Positive resistance The lifting, pushing, or concentric phase of a repetition during a strength-training exercise.

Power The ability to produce maximum force in the shortest time.

Prayer Sincere and humble communication with a higher power.

Precontemplation stage Stage of change in the transtheoretical model in which people are unwilling to change behavior.

Preparation stage Stage of change in the transtheoretical model in which people are getting ready to make a change within the next month.

Primary care physician A medical practitioner who provides routine treatment of ailments; typically, the patient's first contact for health care.

Principle of individuality Training concept that states that genetics plays a major role in individual responses to exercise training and these differences must be considered when designing exercise programs for different people.

Processes of change Actions that help you achieve change in behavior.

Progressive muscle relaxation A stress management technique that involves progressive contraction and relaxation of muscle groups throughout the body.

Progressive resistance training A gradual increase of resistance over a period of time.

Proprioceptive neuromuscular facilitation (PNF) Mode of stretching that uses reflexes and neuromuscular principles to relax the muscles that are being stretched.

Proteins A classification of nutrients consisting of complex organic compounds containing nitrogen and formed by combinations of amino acids; the main substances used in the body to build and repair tissues.

Pro-vitamin A compound that can be converted into a vitamin.

Q

Quackery/fraud The conscious promotion of unproven claims for profit.

R

Range of motion Entire arc of movement of a given joint.

Rate of perceived exertion (RPE) A perception scale to monitor or interpret the intensity of aerobic exercise.

Reaction time The time required to initiate a response to a given stimulus.

Recommended body weight Body weight at which there seems to be no harm to human health; healthy weight.

Recommended Dietary Allowances (RDA) The daily amount of a nutrient (statistically determined from the EARs) considered adequate to meet the known nutrient needs of almost 98 percent of all healthy people in the United States.

Recovery time Amount of time the body takes to return to resting levels after exercise.

Registered dietician (RD) A person with a college degree in dietetics who meets all certification and continuing education requirements of the American Dietetic Association or Dietitians of Canada.

Relapse (v.) To slip or fall back into unhealthy behavior(s); or (n.) failure to maintain healthy behaviors.

Repetitions Number of times a given resistance is performed.

Resistance Amount of weight that is lifted.

Responders Individuals who exhibit improvements in fitness as a result of exercise training.

Resting heart rate (RHR) Heart rate after a person has been sitting quietly for 15–20 minutes.

Resting metabolic rate (RMR) The energy requirement to maintain the body's vital processes in the resting state.

Resting metabolism Amount of energy (expressed in milliliters of oxygen per minute or total calories per day) an individual requires during resting conditions to sustain proper body function.

Reverse cholesterol transport A process in which HDL molecules attract cholesterol and carry it to the liver, where it is changed to bile and eventually excreted in the stool.

Ribonucleic acid (RNA) Genetic material that guides the formation of cell proteins.

RICE An acronym used to describe the standard treatment procedure for acute sports injuries: Rest, Ice (cold application), Compression, and Elevation.

Risk factors Lifestyle and genetic variables that may lead to disease.

S

Sarcopenia Age-related loss of lean body mass, strength, and function.

Sedentary A lifestyle characterized by relative inactivity and a lot of sitting.

Sedentary Death Syndrome (SeDS) A term used to describe deaths that are attributed to a lack of regular physical activity.

Semivegetarians Vegetarians who include milk products, eggs, and fish and poultry in the diet.

Set A fixed number of repetitions; one set of bench presses might be 10 repetitions.

Setpoint Weight control theory that the body has an established weight and strongly attempts to maintain that weight.

Sexually transmitted diseases (STDs) Communicable diseases spread through sexual contact.

Shin splints Injury to the lower leg characterized by pain and irritation in the shin region of the leg.

Side stitch A sharp pain in the side of the abdomen.

Simple carbohydrates Formed by simple or double sugar units with little nutritive value; divided into monosaccharides and disaccharides.

Skill-related fitness Fitness components important for success in activities and athletic events requiring high skill levels; encompasses agility, balance, coordination, power, reaction time, and speed.

Skinfold thickness Technique to assess body composition by measuring a double thickness of skin at specific body sites.

Slow-sustained stretching Exercises in which the muscles are lengthened gradually through a joint's complete range of motion.

Slow-twitch fibers Muscle fibers with greater aerobic potential and slow speed of contraction.

SMART An acronym used in reference to Specific, Measurable, Attainable, Realistic, and Time-specific goals.

Social wellness The ability to relate well to others, both within and outside the family unit.

Specific adaptation to imposed demand (SAID) training Training principle stating that, for improvements to occur in a specific activity, the exercises performed during a strength-training program should resemble as closely as possible the movement patterns encountered in that particular activity.

Specificity of training Principle that training must be done with the specific muscle the person is attempting to improve.

Speed The ability to propel the body or a part of the body rapidly from one point to another.

Sphygmomanometer Inflatable bladder contained within a cuff and a mercury gravity manometer (or aneroid manometer) from which the pressure is read.

Spiritual wellness The sense that life is meaningful, that life has purpose, and that some power brings all humanity together; the ethics, values, and morals that guide one and give meaning and direction to life.

Spot reducing Fallacious theory that exercising a specific body part will result in significant fat reduction in that area.

Sterols Derived fats, of which cholesterol is the best-known example.

Storage fat Body fat in excess of essential fat; stored in adipose tissue.

Strength training A program designed to improve muscular strength and/or endurance through a series of resistance (weight) training exercises that overload the muscular system and cause physiological development.

Stress The mental, emotional, and physiological response of the body to any situation that is new, threatening, frightening, or exciting.

Stress electrocardiogram An exercise test during which the workload is gradually increased until the individual reaches maximal fatigue, with blood pressure and 12-lead electrocardiographic monitoring throughout the test.

Stressor Stress-causing event.

Stretching Moving the joints beyond the accustomed range of motion.

Stroke volume Amount of blood pumped by the heart in one beat.

Structured interview Assessment tool used to determine behavioral patterns that define Type A and B personalities.

Subluxation Partial dislocation of a joint.

Substrates Substances acted upon by an enzyme (examples: carbohydrates, fats).

Sun protection factor (SPF) Degree of protection offered by ingredients in sunscreen lotion; at least SPF 15 is recommended.

Supplements Tablets, pills, capsules, liquids, or powders that contain vitamins, minerals, amino acids, herbs, or fiber that are taken to increase the intake of these nutrients.

Suppressor genes Genes that deactivate the process of cell division.

Syndrome X (metabolic syndrome) An array of metabolic abnormalities that contribute to the development of atherosclerosis triggered by insulin resistance. These conditions include low HDL-cholesterol, high triglycerides, high blood pressure, and an increased blood clotting mechanism.

Synergistic action The effect of mixing two or more drugs, which can be much greater than the sum of two or more drugs acting by themselves.

Synergy A reaction in which the result is greater than the sum of its two parts.

Syphilis A sexually transmitted disease caused by a bacterial infection.

Systolic blood pressure Pressure exerted by blood against walls of arteries during forceful contraction (systole) of the heart; higher of the two numbers in blood pressure readings.

T

Tachycardia Faster-than-normal heart rate.

Tar Chemical compound that forms during the burning of tobacco leaves.

Techniques of change Methods or procedures used during each process of change.

Telomerase An enzyme that allows cells to reproduce indefinitely.

Telomeres A strand of molecules at both ends of a chromosome.

Termination/adoption stage Stage of change in the transtheoretical model in which people have eliminated an undesirable behavior or maintained a positive behavior for more than 5 years.

Thermogenic response Amount of energy required to digest food.

Transfatty acid Solidified fat formed by adding hydrogen to monounsaturated and polyunsaturated fats to increase shelf life.

Triglycerides Fats formed by glycerol and three fatty acids; also called free fatty acids.

Type 1 diabetes Insulin-dependent diabetes mellitus (IDDM), a condition in which the pancreas produces little or no insulin; also known as juvenile diabetes.

Type 2 diabetes Non-insulin-dependent diabetes mellitus (NIDDM), a condition in which insulin is not processed properly; also known as adult-onset diabetes.

Type A Behavior pattern characteristic of a hard-driving, overambitious, aggressive, at times hostile, and overly competitive person.

Type B Behavior pattern characteristic of a calm, casual, relaxed, and easy-going individual.

Type C Behavior pattern of individuals who are just as highly stressed as the Type A but do not seem to be at higher risk for disease than the Type B.

U

Ultraviolet B (UVB) rays Portion of sunlight that causes sunburn and encourages skin cancers.

Unconventional medicine See complementary and alternative medicine.

Underweight Extremely low body weight.

Upper Intake Level (UL) The highest level of nutrient intake that appears safe for most healthy people, beyond which exists an increased risk of adverse effects.

V

Variable resistance Training using special machines equipped with mechanical devices that provide differing amounts of resistance through the range of motion.

Vegans Vegetarians who eat no animal products at all.

Vegetarians Individuals whose diet is of vegetable or plant origin.

Very low-calorie diet A diet that only allows an energy intake (consumption) of 800 or less calories per day.

Very low-density lipoproteins (VLDLs) Triglyceride, cholesterol, and phospholipid-transporting molecules in the blood that tend to increase blood cholesterol.

Vigorous activity Any exercise that requires a MET level equal to or greater than 6 METs (21 ml/kg/min); 1 MET is the energy expenditure at rest, 3.5 ml/kg/min, whereas METs are defined as multiples of the resting metabolic rate (examples of activities that require a 6-MET level are aerobics, walking uphill at 3.5 mph, cycling at 10 to 12 mph, playing doubles in tennis, and vigorous strength training).

Vigorous exercise Cardiorespiratory exercise that requires an intensity level above 60 percent of maximal capacity.

Vitamins Organic nutrients essential for normal metabolism, growth, and development of the body.

Volume (in strength training) The sum of all the repetitions performed multiplied by the resistances used during a strength-training session.

Volume (of training) The total amount of training performed in a given work period (day, week, month, or season).

W

Waist-to-hip ratio (WHR) A measurement to assess potential risk for disease based on distribution of body fat.

Warm-up Starting a workout slowly.

Water The most important classification of essential body nutrients, involved in almost every vital body process.

Weight-regulating mechanism (WRM) A feature of the hypothalamus of the brain that controls how much the body should weigh.

Wellness The constant and deliberate effort to stay healthy and achieve the highest potential for well-being. It encompasses seven dimensions—physical, emotional, mental, social, environmental, occupational, and spiritual—and integrates them all into a quality life.

Workload Load (or intensity) placed on the body during physical activity.

Y

Yoga A school of thought in the Hindu religion that seeks to help the individual attain a higher level of spirituality and peace of mind.

Yo-yo dieting Constantly losing and gaining weight.

answer key

	1	2	3	4	5	6	7	8	9	10	11	12	13	14	15
1.	a	a	b	e	b	a	c	b	d	a	e	b	e	c	e
2.	e	a	e	b	c	d	d	e	a	c	b	a	a	b	c
3.	c	e	c	d	e	c	a	a	b	c	a	a	c	c	b
4.	e	d	d	a	a	c	b	a	e	e	e	e	d	e	d
5.	b	c	d	b	b	c	d	b	d	e	e	e	d	d	e
6.	c	d	a	e	e	e	a	e	b	e	e	e	d	a	a
7.	a	a	a	b	a	c	c	c	a	a	e	b	d	a	e
8.	d	b	c	b	c	d	c	b	e	a	e	e	e	d	c
9.	c	e	a	e	d	c	e	e	a	b	e	b	e	e	e
10.	b	e	e	e	e	c	e	d	e	c	a	e	e	c	a

index